‘A smorgasbord of insights into the world of healthcare, this volume begins with an informative explanation of political economy with its focus on class power and class struggle, and proceeds to offer a wealth of studies from veterans in the field as well as a sprinkle of contributions from early, and very promising, career academics. The chapters offer a plurality of theoretical approaches, demonstrating the diversity and versatility of the interdisciplinary basis of political economy, and cover issues from many different regions and countries of the world. The *Handbook* is, indeed, a convincing portrayal of health and healthcare under the exorbitant and inexorable demands of capitalism, particularly as experienced with the historically recent shift to neoliberal governance. It is a celebration of the very best of political economy with its capacity to make sense of economic and social issues with immediate relevance for the health and well-being of humans.’

Fran Collyer, *Professor of Sociology, University of Wollongong, and President RC08 International Sociological Association*

‘Coming fifteen years after the report of the 2008 World Health Organization (WHO) Commission on the Social Determinants of Health, and the all-too-predictable soft-pedaling and depoliticization of this widely-adopted framework, this volume constitutes a timely return to – and expansion of – critical political economy critiques of health and healthcare. Mainly concerned with the harmful impacts of neoliberal/market fundamentalist capitalism, its rich chapters usefully build a case for systemic political-economic change, mindful of the interdependent material and ecological world that provides the basis for life and death on this planet.’

Nancy Krieger, *Professor of Social Epidemiology and American Cancer Society Clinical Research Professor, Harvard University*

‘Challenged by capitalism and chipped away by neoliberalism, the global COVID-19 pandemic brought into sharp focus longstanding concerns with the political economy of health and healthcare. This *Handbook* rises to the occasion by providing readers with theory- and problem-driven coverage that does not sacrifice depth for breadth, offering a comprehensive analysis befitting its pressing subject matter. The book will surely move studies in political economy, and be of interest to anyone seeking to better understand the contours of health and healthcare today.’

Heather Whiteside, *Associate Professor of Political Science, University of Waterloo*

The Routledge Handbook of the Political Economy of Health and Healthcare

This handbook provides a comprehensive and critical overview of the gamut of contemporary issues around health and healthcare from a political economy perspective. Its contributions present a unique challenge to prevailing economic accounts of health and healthcare, which narrowly focus on individual behaviour and market processes. Instead, the capacity of the human body to reach its full potential and the ability of society to prevent disease and cure illness are demonstrated to be shaped by a broader array of political-economic processes. The material conditions in which societies produce, distribute, exchange, consume, and reproduce – and the operation of power relations therein – influence all elements of human health: from food consumption and workplace safety, to inequality, healthcare and housing, and even the biophysical conditions in which humans live.

This volume explores these concerns across five sections. First, it introduces and critically engages with a variety of established and cutting-edge theoretical perspectives in political economy to conceptualise health and healthcare – from neoclassical and behavioural economics, to Marxist and feminist approaches. The next two sections extend these insights to evaluate the neoliberalisation of health and healthcare over the past 40 years, highlighting their individualisation and commodification by the capitalist state and powerful corporations. The fourth section examines the diverse manifestation of these dynamics across a range of geographical contexts. The volume concludes with a section devoted to outlining more progressive health and healthcare arrangements, which transcend the limitations of both neoliberalism and capitalism.

This volume will be an indispensable reference work for students and scholars of political economy, health policy and politics, health economics, health geography, the sociology of health, and other health-related disciplines.

David Primrose is in the Menzies Centre for Health Policy and Economics, University of Sydney, Australia.

Rodney Loeppky is in the Department of Political Science, York University, Canada.

Robin Chang is in the Department of Political Science, York University, Canada.

THE ROUTLEDGE HANDBOOK OF THE POLITICAL ECONOMY OF HEALTH AND HEALTHCARE

Edited by David Primrose, Rodney Loeppky and Robin Chang

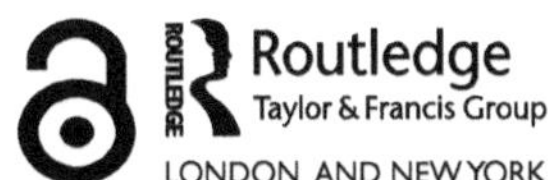

Designed cover image: © Getty Images

First published 2024
by Routledge
4 Park Square, Milton Park, Abingdon, Oxon OX14 4RN

and by Routledge
605 Third Avenue, New York, NY 10158

Routledge is an imprint of the Taylor & Francis Group, an informa business

British Library Cataloguing-in-Publication Data
A catalogue record for this book is available from the British Library

ISBN: 9780367861360 (hbk)
ISBN: 9781032650678 (pbk)
ISBN: 9781003017110 (ebk)

DOI: 10.4324/9781003017110

Typeset in Times New Roman
by codeMantra

The Open Access version of chapters 1 and 8 were funded by University of Sydney Library.

CONTENTS

ILLUSTRATIONS

Figures

Tables

Box

CONTRIBUTORS

Jean-Louis Aillon is a medical doctor and psychotherapist, PhD in Social Science at Università degli Studi di Genova, Genoa, and researcher at the Interdisciplinary Research Institute on Sustainability, Torino.

Clare Bambra is Professor of Public Health in the Faculty of Medical Sciences, Newcastle University.

Olivia Banner is Associate Professor of Critical Media Studies at the University of Texas at Dallas.

Rama V. Baru is Professor at the Centre of Social Medicine and Community Health, Jawaharlal Nehru University, and Honorary Fellow at the Institute of Chinese Studies, Delhi.

Philippe Batifoulier is Professor of Economics and Deputy Director of the CEPN Society, Pluralism and Institutions Team, Université Sorbonne Paris Nord.

Fran Baum is Professor of Health Equity at Stretton Institute, University of Adelaide.

Anne-Emanuelle Birn is Professor of Global Development Studies, and Social and Behavioural Health Sciences at the University of Toronto.

Mauro Bonaiuti is Professor of Economics and Statistics at the University of Turin, and a co-founder of the Italian Degrowth Association.

Arnel M. Borras is Assistant Professor in the School of Nursing, St. Francis Xavier University.

Jackie Brown is an independent researcher who received her MES in Environmental Studies from York University.

Robin Chang is a PhD candidate in the Department of Political Science at York University.

Isaac Christiansen is Associate Professor of Sociology at Midwestern State University.

Tamara Daly is Professor in the School of Health Policy and Management, York University.

Raju Das is Professor in the Faculty of Environmental and Urban Change, York University.

Nicolas Da Silva is Lecturer in Economics at Université Sorbonne Paris Nord.

John B. Davis is Professor Emeritus of Economics at Marquette University, and Professor and Chair of History and Philosophy of Economics at the University of Amsterdam.

Kevin Deane is Senior Lecturer in Economics at Open University, UK.

Jana Fey is Lecturer in Public Health at the Brighton and Sussex Medical School, University of Sussex.

Jonathan Filippon is Senior Lecturer in Health Systems at the Wolfson Institute of Population Health, Queen Mary University of London.

Timon Forster is Postdoctoral Research Fellow in the School of Economics and Political Science, University of St. Gallen.

Nick J. Fox is Professor of Sociology at the University of Huddersfield.

Toby Freeman is Senior Research Fellow of Health Equity at Stretton Institute, University of Adelaide.

Marc-André Gagnon is Associate Professor in the School of Public Policy and Administration, Carleton University.

Deborah Gleeson is Associate Professor in the School of Psychology and Public Health, La Trobe University.

Scott L. Greer is Professor of Health Management and Policy, Global Public Health, and Political Science at the University of Michigan, and Senior Expert Advisor on Health Governance for the European Observatory on Health Systems and Policies.

Jean-Germain Gros is Professor of Political Science and Public Policy Administration at the University of Missouri-St. Louis.

Geoffrey M. Hodgson is Professor Emeritus in Management at Loughborough University, and Editor-in-Chief of the *Journal of Institutional Economics.*

Shailender Kumar Hooda is Associate Professor at the Institute for Studies in Industrial Development, New Delhi.

Alexandros E. Kentikelenis is Associate Professor of Political Economy and Sociology at Bocconi University.

Lawrence King is Professor in the Department of Economics, University of Massachusetts Amherst, and former Professor of Sociology and Political Economy at the University of Cambridge.

John M. Kirk is Professor Emeritus of Latin American Studies at Dalhousie University.

Jennifer Lacy-Nichols is Research Fellow in the Melbourne School of Population and Global Health, Faculty of Medicine, Dentistry and Health Sciences, University of Melbourne.

David G. Legge is Scholar Emeritus in Public Health at La Trobe University.

Rodney Loeppky is Associate Professor in the Department of Politics, York University.

Margitta Mätzke is Professor of Politics and Social Policy, and Chair of the Institute of Politics and Social Policy, Johannes Kepler University of Linz.

Gerry McCartney is Professor of Wellbeing Economy in Sociology at the University of Glasgow.

Robert McMaster is Professor of Political Economy in the Adam Smith Business School, University of Glasgow.

Lindsay Naylor is Associate Professor in the Department of Geography and Spatial Sciences at the University Delaware.

Laura Nervi is Associate Professor in the College of Population Health at the University of New Mexico, United States.

Patrick Neveling is Senior Lecturer in the Department of Social Sciences, Bournemouth University.

Madhurima Nundy is Fellow at the Centre for Social and Economic Progress, New Delhi, and Visiting Fellow at the Institute of Chinese Studies, Delhi.

Steven Pressman is Professor Emeritus of Economics and Finance at Monmouth University, and Part-Time Professor of Economics at the New School for Social Research.

David Primrose recently completed his PhD in the Department of Political Economy, and is an Academic Fellow in the Menzies Centre for Health Policy and Economics, at the University of Sydney.

Sarah Redikopp is a PhD candidate in Gender, Feminist, and Women's Studies at York University.

Gabor Scheiring is an Assistant Professor at Georgetown University Qatar, and a former member of the Hungarian Parliament.

Gyorgy Scrinis is Associate Professor of Food Politics and Policy at the University of Melbourne.

Thomas H. Stubbs is Reader in Global Political Economy at Royal Holloway, University of London, and Research Associate in Political Economy at the Centre for Business Research, University of Cambridge.

Ben Spies-Butcher is Associate Professor of Economy and Society at Macquarie University.

Chris Thomas is Head of the Commission of Health and Prosperity at the Institute for Public Policy Research, and Editor of *Progressive Review*.

Belinda Townsend is Fellow in the School of Regulation and Global Governance, Australian National University.

Georgia van Toorn is a Lecturer in the School of Social Sciences, University of New South Wales.

Howard Waitzkin is Distinguished Professor Emeritus in the Department of Sociology, University of New Mexico, and Adjunct Professor in the Department of Internal Medicine, University of Illinois.

Young Soon Wong is an independent researcher and community development worker who received his PhD at the School of Medicine and Health Sciences, Monash University Malaysia.

Volkan Yilmaz is Lecturer (Assistant Professor) in Social Policy at the School of Applied Social and Policy Sciences, Ulster University.

1

REVITALIZING THE POLITICAL ECONOMY OF HEALTH AND HEALTHCARE IN A CONTEXT OF CRISIS

David Primrose and Rodney Loeppky

Exasperated by the teleological assumption of neoclassical economics that, free from government 'intervention', markets will *eventually* return to equilibrium, John Maynard Keynes (2013 [1923]: 65) sardonically quipped: 'in the long run we are all dead'. The ongoing Global Coronavirus Crisis (GCC) – the most pervasive and lethal epidemiological calamity since the 1918–19 Spanish Influenza pandemic – has recently reinforced a parallel, if more morbid, precept. As recurrently demonstrated throughout the history of capitalism (Szreter 2005; Leys 2009; Chernomas and Hudson 2013), the GCC grimly confirmed that restructuring socio-ecological life around market processes increases the likelihood of illness and death in the *short run*, too. Put differently, contrary to the assumption of both mainstream political discourse and media outlets, the pernicious health impacts of the Crisis are not merely biological in character – the deadly result of an easily transmissible pathogen run rampant. Nor are they simply the inadvertent product of collective individual irrationality and recklessness in flouting government directives to wear masks and isolate. Rather, the global health disaster engendered by the spread of the SARS-CoV-2 virus cannot be understood removed from the wide-reaching institutionalization and deepening of pro-market *neoliberal* programs in place since the 1970s (Primrose *et al.* 2020; Luisetti 2022; Sparke and Williams 2022; Wamsley and Benatar 2023).

Four decades of neoliberal efforts to restructure socio-ecological spheres through a narrowly economistic lens have, ultimately, intensified the scope of the pandemic in at least three ways. First, the *commodification of healthcare systems* – reorienting them from public goods to profit-making domains – lessened both the accessibility and quality of healthcare services. States have been left ill-equipped to handle a public health crisis on the scale of COVID-19, with hospital capacity scaled back, essential healthcare components privatized or outsourced, and austerity imposed on health budgeting, particularly following the Global Financial Crisis of 2007/08 (Schrecker and Bambra 2015; Labonté and Stuckler 2016; Fouskas and Gokay 2020; Navarro 2020).

Second, diminished public investment in infrastructure, equipment, vaccine research and development, and medicines has occasioned states to cede ground on *preventative medicine*, instead relying on pharmaceutical companies to devise strategies for a pathogenic response. Typically, the for-profit imperatives of the pharmaceutical sector have made it less inclined to invest in non-remunerative research and development on infectious diseases or preventive medicine in general. Unless the state has been willing to bestow guaranteed revenues (such as those available under

DOI: 10.4324/9781003017110-1

so-called 'Operation Warp Speed' in the United States), the development of more profitable *post facto* treatments remained the focus of industry (Harvey 2020; Anderson 2023). Third, neoliberalism has left populations broadly vulnerable to the epidemic, by negatively influencing the *social determinants* of human health. By aggravating economic inequality, making work increasingly precarious, and undermining the quality and affordability of public services (such as public housing, childcare, and aged care), significant portions of the population faced higher risk in relation to the pathogen and possessed fewer resources to cope with its consequences (Navarro 2020; Bambra *et al.* 2021; Davy and Dickinson 2023).[1]

These outcomes correspond with the longer-term structural dynamics of global capitalism, which are marked by systemic contradictions. In particular, sustained capital accumulation depends on the conditions of social reproduction, such as birthing and raising children, caring for friends and family, and preserving household and community networks. These very same necessities, however, tend to be undermined by the systemic compulsion of capitalism toward perpetual accumulation (Fraser 2016, 2022). Accordingly, while health and healthcare might be use values *par excellence*, they are of limited interest to capital unless they can be converted into exchange value, or otherwise configured to the pursuit of expanding accumulation (Doyal 1979; Baer 1982; Leys 2009). Indeed, prior to the outbreak of the GCC, the rapid globalization of the corporate agri-food regime clearly contributed to the precipitous emergence and rapid dissemination of pathogens through its ongoing disruption and commodification of local socio-ecological processes (Wallace 2016, 2020; Akram-Lodhi 2021; Waitzkin 2021). Similarly, in the midst of the pandemic, capitalist states were frequently willing to risk the spread of infection and heightened mortality rates as a means to maintain a minimum level of accumulation. Advice from public health officials around quarantine measures was often rebuffed to keep the non-essential economy open and/or enable resumption of regular production and consumption practices (Knott 2020; Leake *et al.* 2020).

It is hard, in this context, to avoid the conclusion that death, disease, and ill-health are inexorably interrelated with their *political-economic* context (Bambra 2011; Chernomas and Hudson 2013). Both individual and population health are structured by the complex interactions between ideas, interests, and institutions that are, in turn, inexorably interrelated with the material conditions in which societies produce, distribute, exchange, consume, and reproduce. These political-economic processes shape the capacity of the human body to reach its full potential, and the ability of society to prevent disease and cure illness. Accordingly, they influence all elements of human health – from food consumption and occupational health and safety, to inequality, healthcare, and housing, and even the biophysical conditions in which humans live (Doyal 1979; Leys 2009; Marya and Patel 2021).

Indeed, it was precisely this premise with which we hoped to engage when originally proposing the present book to Routledge in June 2019 – less than six months before the initial outbreak of SARS-CoV-2 in Wuhan. Prior to the crisis, a suite of complex challenges already confronted the enduring health and well-being of humanity: persistent occupational health and safety disasters; declining mental health standards in myriad social spheres; uneven access to quality healthcare services; and ongoing concerns with the spread of HIV/AIDS in sub-Saharan Africa, to name but a few. As with the pandemic, these 'health' or 'healthcare' matters cannot be understood outside of their political-economic context. Rather, contemporary capitalism, particularly the extension of its neoliberal form, has proven to be a pivotal factor in constituting these phenomena (Schrecker and Bambra 2015; Sell and Williams 2020; Sparke 2020). Accordingly, while scholarly and political attention to the efficacy of healthcare systems has burgeoned over the course of the pandemic, our purpose in preparing this volume was to compile a series of critical reflections on these abiding political-economic determinants and their health-related implications.

Among the explosion of valuable politically-minded health studies that have arisen in the last decade or so, there are simply no extensive samplings of the critical political economy of health and healthcare that might be of wide service to academics and practitioners alike. The *Handbook* aims to redress this lacuna by taking stock of established and cutting-edge theoretical approaches to the field; the political-economic dimensions of key contemporary issue-areas and their manifestation in geographically varied settings; and a plethora of alternative health and healthcare configurations for a post-neoliberal (even post-capitalist) world. All of this has been done with an open – somewhat agnostic – view of the boundaries of political economy, as a means to open the volume as much as possible to the diverse perspectives and empirical foci comprising the field. In doing so, our intention is to revitalize scholarly interest in the political economy of health and healthcare by demonstrating its epistemological pertinence for comprehending a range of pressing social concerns. Equally, we aspire to exhibit the strategic relevance of political economy as a field of study for scholars and activists committed to transforming the world in more progressive, even radical, directions. Most obviously, this is manifest in multiple chapters establishing healthcare as a site of political contestation: between commercial forces seeking to commodify it further, and other movements striving to retain it as a public good and reduce extant gross inequalities of access. In both respects – as an invitation to intellectual controversy and stimulus for political activity – we hope that the book contributes to 'illuminat[ing] the world in which we live so that we may act in it intelligently and effectively' (Baran and Sweezy 1966: 27–8).

The contours of political economy

Before reflecting on its novel contribution to critical accounts of matters relating to health and healthcare, it is first necessary to delineate briefly the contours of political economy as a field of social inquiry. Political economy constitutes a critical social science, examining the complex constellation of interrelated factors that determine the material basis of human societies, both individually and collectively. Pertinently, this use of the term distinguishes it from its common deployment to refer to the normative study of government policies, as distinct from the study of 'economics' as the study of market functions (*e.g.* Little 2002). It also remains distinct from the 'economics imperialism' of particular traditions of neoclassical economics – such as the 'public choice' theories of James M. Buchanan and others at the Virginia School (see: Candela 2018) – which use these principles to examine public policy processes (Fine and Milonakis 2009; Madra and Adaman 2010). Accordingly, as understood in this book, political economy is not concerned with broadening the topics to which neoclassical economic tools are applied – in this case, to the study of health and healthcare (*e.g.* Furton *et al.* 2022). Rather, it constitutes a more complex approach to understand real-world economic issues. In this endeavor, it builds on a rich historical legacy, stretching back at least to the Physiocrats and Adam Smith in the Eighteenth Century, through scholars such as David Ricardo, Karl Marx, Thorstein Veblen, John Maynard Keynes, Joan Robinson, and John Kenneth Galbraith. While diverging in their conceptual and ideological orientations, these figures commonly sought to comprehend the progress and dynamics of society through the study of accumulation, growth, and distribution processes (Stilwell 2002, 2023; Stilwell *et al.* 2022b).

More concretely, political-economic inquiry may be understood – somewhat taxonomically – as grounded in at least four methodological commitments (Stilwell 2019). First, political economy entails *critical engagement with mainstream economic thought*, centered on a neoclassical theory of hyper-rational individuals each seeking to maximize their utility and interacting in self-equilibrating markets. Such abstract and unrealistic accounts are devoid of social and historical analysis, particularly due to their methodological individualism and implied separation between politics and economics (Hodgson 2001; Lawson 2015). As such, they provide little explanatory insight into the complexity and unpredictability of real-world economic systems, especially that of capitalism (Arnsperger and Varoufakis 2008; Fine 2015; Westra 2021). Second, political economists make the case for adopting *alternative theoretical traditions* that articulate more realistic and holistic accounts of economic processes as a means to comprehend their real-world complexity. Various 'schools' have developed in this regard, ranging from Marxism and institutionalism, to feminism and ecological economics (see: Lee 2009; Stilwell *et al.* 2022a).

Third, political economy embarks from the ontological proposition that real-world phenomena do not fit neatly into boxes labeled 'economy', 'society', 'politics', and so forth. In turn, practitioners seek to foster constructive *transdisciplinary* interchanges with other social scientific disciplines – such as geography, psychology, and sociology – and utilize insights from them in order to foster an *interdisciplinary* approach to the study of economic issues (Fine and Milonakis 2009; Crespo 2017). Fourth, and finally, because it recognizes that economic issues are inexorably entwined with socio-ecological concerns and political judgments, political economy recognizes that questions of *ideology* inevitably pervade the study of these matters (Myrdal 1969; Fine 1980; Heilbroner 1989; Jo 2022). Accordingly, contrary to the positive-normative distinction commonly deployed within neoclassical economics (see: Grivaux and Badiei 2022), it is futile to present the discipline as somehow 'value-free' (Davis 2022). Instead, the objective is to make these ideologies explicit and subject to scrutiny.

In practice, because political economy has been extended in distinct directions by different schools, its commitments have commonly engendered a broader scope of inquiry than that found in neoclassical economics. The latter attempts to replicate the formalism and universalism of the natural sciences, such that it narrowly focuses on questions of allocative efficiency and stability in markets (Mirowski 1991). Conversely, political economy adopts a more critical and social scientific epistemology, thereby opening up more complex lines of research that analyses the interrelations between economic, political, social, cultural, historical, and ecological dynamics.

Two interrelated lines of substantive investigation may be identified in this regard (Munro 2004: 146–7). First, political economy explores the complex provisioning processes through which goods, services, income, and wealth are *produced*, *distributed*, *exchanged*, and *consumed* within historically specific socio-economic systems, such as capitalism or communism (Lee 2009; Jo and Todorova 2017; Stilwell *et al.* 2022b). It also examines the manner in which this provisioning process occurs within both commodified and non-commodified social spheres (for instance, within the home, family, or community), thereby highlighting the necessary nexus between *reproduction* of human life and preservation of socio-economic existence (Bhattacharya 2017; Mezzadri *et al.* 2022). Political economy addresses how the organization of these processes is structured by constellations of ideas, interests, and institutions, and the resulting winners and losers engendered by this formation – particularly through exploring the operation of power therein (Stilwell 2002; Spies-Butcher *et al.* 2012). Second, political economy simultaneously explores the systemic implications of such provisioning processes. It considers how their specific societal configurations, along with the imperatives arising from them, generate (often-contradictory) dynamics and power relations (such as those of class). These, in turn, influence the direction of virtually all other socio-ecological structures – from family life and institutions of governance, to our collective functioning within extant biophysical arrangements (Moore 2015; Ferguson 2020). Thereby, it deliberates on the broader repercussions of these processes for the material reproduction of both humanity and the ecological systems we inhabit (Jo and Todorova 2017).

Reconsidering the prevailing study of health and healthcare

The chapters in this book elaborate on this agenda as a means to comprehend, and revitalize scholarly interest in, the complex drivers and social implications of contemporary issues of health and healthcare. Over the course of recent decades, health and healthcare have been subject to intellectual curiosity, scrutiny, and political contestation (*e.g.* People's Health Movement *et al.* 2022). Such discussions have provoked their fair share of ethical and political conundrums, and it is an understatement to say that very little has been academically or practically settled in this broad arena (Birn *et al.* 2017; Parker and García 2018). How should 'health' and 'healthcare' be defined? Who should be the primary focus of analysis when dealing with human health? How much health is enough? What kinds of social mechanisms help generate healthy societies? Which social actors and institutions should be involved in delivering healthcare, and which should not? These are but a few of the questions that immediately spring to mind when reflecting on the intricate domains of health and healthcare, and a wealth of corollary and subsidiary issues could easily accompany them.

Of course, it is possible to approach these matters from multiple conceptual and disciplinary perspectives, all of which contribute to our understanding of certain elements of them (Collyer 2015). In this respect, health and healthcare are prisms through which concerns relating to identity, economics, politics, sociology, science, and philosophy are refracted, rendering them rich and perplexing fields of study. Nevertheless, conventional explanations for health and morbidity within scholarly and policy discourse have, until recently, largely fallen into one of two broad traditions: *biomedical* and *behavioral* (for critical surveys, see: Chernomas and Hudson 2013: 4–5; Birn *et al.* 2017: 90–2).

The former approach conceives of health as a primarily individual and biological phenomenon, in which the human body is the locus and source of ill-health, subject to biomedical manipulation and/or interventions. From this perspective, health is comprehended predominantly as the lack of disease, rather than as a more holistic (social, psychological, cultural) state of well-being. Concretely, illness and disease are deemed the product of a combination of 'natural' factors – genes and germs – and treatment focuses on restructuring individual biology, largely through pharmaceuticals, surgery, or genetic intervention (Clarke *et al.* 2003; Yuill *et al.* 2011: 7–10). Conversely, behavioral approaches examine health and illness as a function of individual or household behavior and beliefs, such that poor health is typically imputed to poor decisions or lack of volition. Accordingly, normative recommendations center on utilizing a combination of education, counseling or incentive-based measures to eliminate, regulate, or circumvent self-destructive activities, as a means to engender desirable health outcomes (Cockerham 2005; Baum and Fisher 2014). In different ways, both the biomedical and behavioral approaches decontextualize health from its broader socio-political environment, instead attributing poor health to the individual human body and/or mind while formulating corresponding remedial measures targeting these spheres (Birn *et al.* 2017: 90–4; Rocca and Anjum 2020).

More recently, however, an alternative approach has sought to transcend this methodological individualism and, in doing so, has become increasingly popular within mainstream public health scholarship and political discourse. The *social determinants of health* (SDH) approach (*e.g.* Marmot and Wilkinson 2005; WHO 2008) recognizes that health outcomes stem from myriad social factors beyond healthcare alone, and are not reducible to the products of economically organized medical science. Alternatively, in seeking to discern the complex determinants of human health, this tradition highlights the importance of indicators of socio-economic status (SES), such as income, wealth, and education (Braveman *et al.* 2011; Braveman and Gottlieb 2014). The now extensive literature in this area predominantly isolates such indicators as a means to demonstrate their causal association with negative and/or positive health outcomes, thereby implying that securing the correct balance of SES indicators would precipitate more favorable societal and/or global health consequences (Birn *et al.* 2017: Chapter 7).

Undoubtedly, SDH approaches have heightened our analytical and public awareness of injustices surrounding health and health delivery – a fact that was plainly evident during successive COVID waves, as the relations between inequality and ill-health became increasingly stark (Bambra *et al.* 2021). Without pre-existing, broad institutional acceptance of the association of SES with health status among public health institutions, researchers, hospitals, and international organizations, discussions concerning inequality and COVID would not have occurred with such potency within media and governmental circles (WHO 2021; Bonner 2023). Nevertheless, despite this important contribution in identifying a broad nexus of social factors shaping health outcomes, the SDH literature tends to disregard the 'upstream' social conditions and power structures that adversely affect health (Navarro 2009; Schofield 2015). That is, the tradition largely fails to progress further up the causal chain to address how the social determinants of poor health (such as inequality) are, themselves, determined by structural factors, such as class or the systemic imperative of capitalism toward perpetual capital accumulation. As David Coburn (2004: 44) saliently notes with regard to SDH, 'inequality or [socioeconomic status] simply refer to individuals or families who are higher or lower on some characteristic without any real social relationships between these, and without any necessary antagonism between those lower or higher'.

Hence, while recognizing the significance of SDH studies in refocusing scholarly and political attention on social factors as the fulcrum of health and healthcare studies, the *political-economic* orientation of this collection seeks to shift how we comprehend associations between SES and health. It places the locus of causality not so much on socio-economic *status*, but rather on the embodied *structural forces*, *power*, and *political struggles* that bring about the proximate status of SES indicators in the first place (Labonté and Ruckert 2019; Sell and Williams 2020; Waitzkin *et al.* 2020). As formulated across this volume, the *political economy of health* is concerned with critically analyzing the historically specific nexus of political-economic structures, processes, and social relations that constitute conditions in which people live and work, and thereby engender particular individual and societal patterns of health, illness, and well-being (Krieger 2011; Chernomas and Hudson 2013). Concomitant to this, the *political economy of healthcare* addresses the impact of these political-economic forces on the production, distribution, and consumption of health services, and the manner in which the latter reflects the power relations of the societies within which medical institutions operate (Waitzkin 1978; Baer 1982).

In short, the capacity of individuals and societies to enjoy a healthy life is not solely attributable to biomedical factors, individual lifestyles, or the presence of particular socio-economic indicators. Rather, all of these are shaped by systemic political-economic dynamics and social relations that determine the environment in which we function (Mooney 2012; Marya and Patel 2021). In the context of antagonistic class relations within capitalism, political economy stresses the degree to which capital utilizes its structurally advantageous position to effect political and organizational outcomes that bring about or maintain the inequalities taxonomized by SDH researchers (Navarro 2002; Navarro and Muntaner 2004). While the latter appositely points to the social nature of health injustice – for example as arising from factors such as uneven access to affordable social housing, poor education, income and wealth inequality, or inadequate welfare systems – political economy insists that the latter is neither incidental nor accidental. Rather, class power and class struggle – however subtly arranged, regulated, or reinforced – are largely responsible for the inequalities we now recognize more broadly as affecting health and well-being (Coburn 2010).

To illustrate, many recent studies of mental health have usefully avoided biologically deterministic explanations of problems such as anxiety and depression, by instead locating their social determinants in factors such as employment instability, discrimination, inequality, adverse life experiences, poor education, familial instability, and isolated or destitute residential and working conditions (*e.g.* Compton and Shim 2015; Alegría *et al.* 2018). Yet, as Jana Fey's contribution to this volume reveals, the proliferation of such factors must be comprehended as, at least partly, having been propelled by efforts from capital and capitalist state institutions to neoliberalize the governance of multiple spheres of social life over recent decades. As a means to secure ongoing capital accumulation, however, these endeavors have undermined the social conditions for mental health – whether through the commodification of desire and leisure, codifying increasingly precarious working conditions and homeownership, or introducing multiple rounds of fiscal austerity (Matthews 2019). Thus, as Vicente Navarro (2009: 423) pithily quips: '[i]t is not *inequalities* that kill people [...] it is *those responsible for these inequalities* that kill people'.

In idiosyncratically developing this agenda across their respective chapters, the contributions to this *Handbook* stand on the shoulders of giants in the field – from Louis-René Villermé, Rudolf Virchow, and Friedrich Engels, to Lesley Doyal, Howard Waitzkin, Vicente Navarro, Julian Tudor-Hart, and Gavin Mooney – to analyze the complex political-economic determinants of myriad contemporary health and healthcare issues. In doing so, as with political-economic analysis more broadly, there is also a strong tendency among chapters to develop their accounts through eschewing the traditional division of labor erected between disciplines within the social sciences (see also: Navarro 1976: viii). Instead, the volume brings together an array of authors seeking to demonstrate the saliency of political economy for comprehending contemporary health and healthcare practices by embracing interdisciplinary insights from diverse scholarly domains, such as history, epidemiology, political science, anthropology, and sociology. The resulting studies present wide-ranging and critical reflections on the pernicious effects of neoliberalism and capitalism on health, while also demonstrating the need to rethink the political means to redress these concerns.

Structure of the volume

In articulating this agenda, the chapters in this volume are apportioned across five distinct sections. *Part one* features chapters reflecting on the political economy of health and healthcare from different theoretical traditions. The objective of this section is not to provide a meta-theoretical framework for the *Handbook* as a whole. Indeed, the volume interprets political economy as an irreducibly pluralist endeavor, characterized by multiple, overlapping schools of thought. Accordingly, as a means to enable readers to engage with and juxtapose ideas from each, this opening section introduces and critically reflects on the contribution of multiple contemporary schools – both mainstream and more critical – within the political economy of health and healthcare (see also: Mooney 2009; Davis and McMaster 2017). Each chapter focuses on an individual theoretical approach: (neoclassical) health economics, the economics of conventions, Marxism, post-Keynesianism, feminism, new materialism, and behavioral economics.

Building on these conceptual insights, *parts two and three* examine the political-economic character of a variety of long-standing health and healthcare issues from around the globe. Each chapter reflects critically on the form and implications of these issues, by investigating their relation to developments in contemporary capitalism and, in particular, the contemporary extension of neoliberalism. The *Constitution of the World Health Organization* (WHO 1948: 1) proclaims that '[t]he enjoyment of the highest attainable standard of health is one of the most fundamental rights of every human being'. Moreover, '[g]overnments have a responsibility for the health of their peoples which can be fulfilled only by the provision of adequate health and social measures'. From this perspective, by means of their capacity to influence both the social determinants of health and prevailing healthcare system, states should play a key role in securing the health and well-being of its citizens as a basic right. Nevertheless, as demonstrated by the chapters in these sections, the increasingly pervasive influence of neoliberalism as a rationality of governance over the preceding four decades has seen states largely abrogate this obligation. Instead, widespread neoliberal policies and governance mentalities have undermined the socio-ecological conditions determining health, while cultivating and institutionalizing commodified healthcare primarily as a site of capital accumulation (see also: Sparke 2020). Put simply, the present political-economic context has generated many noxious consequences for human health and well-being.

Part four is organized around exploring the interplay of these dynamics in determining health trends and the direction of healthcare systems in geographically specific environments. Concentrating on a diversity of countries and regions – from sub-Saharan Africa and post-Soviet Eastern Europe, to the European Union and Australia – chapters critically investigate how the vicissitudes of health and healthcare delivery are intertwined with contextually specific historical and contemporary political-economic processes, as well as the broader dynamics of global capitalism. As grimly revealed by the GCC, the interplay of these factors engenders substantial divergences in population health and well-being, as well as the capacity of healthcare systems to prevent and treat illness and disease (Sheehan and Fox 2020; Serikbayeva *et al.* 2021; Jones and Hameiri 2022). Consistent with the preceding two sections, these chapters also collectively reveal a common 'red-thread' running through their case-studies: neoliberalism has fostered a shift from healthcare as a public good to a novel site of capital accumulation *via* its commodification, while simultaneously producing deleterious consequences for the broader social determinants of population health.

Given the multifaceted malaise afflicting health and healthcare outlined over the preceding four sections, it remains prudent to ask: what political-economic conditions are necessary to secure a more positive, equitable course in global population health and well-being, and how can healthcare systems be geared toward this end? Can such outcomes be engendered through reconfiguring capitalism in more progressive directions, or are broader, revolutionary socio-ecological transformations required? In addressing these complex normative questions, *part five* concludes the volume by surveying the opportunities and challenges associated with constructing alternative political economies of health and healthcare that transcend their extant neoliberal, or even capitalist, forms (see also: Deppe 2010; Waitzkin *et al.* 2018; Adler-Bolton and Vierkant 2022). To this end, contributions analyze a range of existing systems that diverge from prevailing institutions and ideologies – such as those of Cuban internationalism and commons-based healthcare arrangements – and the more general lessons for political economy that can be extrapolated from their operation in practice. This final section also includes more speculative accounts of how alternative health and healthcare processes may be restructured – for instance, according to principles of degrowth or post-capitalism – to foster more socially just, inclusive, and effective outcomes. In both cases, chapters unanimously favor extending practices of decommodification and reinstitutionalizing more democratic political practices, upon which fundamentally different health systems might be constructed.

Across each section, in keeping with our commitment to foster renewed interest in the political economy of health and healthcare as a valuable field of study, we have sought to include a diversity of germane perspectives and issues. Nevertheless, some apposite theoretical approaches and topics did not 'make the cut', or only receive brief mention within existing chapters. For instance, the traditions of *institutional economics* (Champlin and Knoedler 2008; Hodgson 2008; Josifidis and Supic 2022) and *social economics* (Davis 2001; Davis and McMaster 2017) present powerful theoretical alternatives to the prevailing neoclassical school informing mainstream 'health economics' and, thus, warrant further elaboration in future research. Moreover, the particular implications of capitalism for the health and healthcare needs of *Indigenous groups* (Saggers and Walter 2007; Ullah 2016) and *queer communities* (Padilla *et al.* 2007; Bell 2020) are germane issues that remain comparatively underexplored within extant political-economic literature.

Moreover, as acutely highlighted during the GCC, capitalism also engenders contradictory political-economic processes that have deleteriously affected population health by perpetuating *racialized* (Laster Pirtle 2020; McClure *et al.* 2020) and *developmental inequalities* (Birn *et al.* 2017; Labonté and Ruckert 2019) within and between countries. Such inequalities have also fed into contemporary problems of *addiction* (Young and Markham 2017; Courtwright 2019), which have been especially pronounced in the ongoing *opioid epidemic* sweeping across the Americas (Pereira 2021; Hansen *et al.* 2023). Finally, as the ecological rhythms of the Earth continue to be detrimentally affected by climate change, the complex interrelations between these and capitalism in determining global *planetary health* (Gill and Benatar 2020; Baer and Singer *forthcoming*) promise to become an increasingly prominent topic in coming decades. Readers interested in further exploring these important themes should consult the illustrative sources for each listed above, in conjunction with the broader reflections on the political economy of health and healthcare explored in this volume.

Looking forward

This *Handbook* was prepared in the midst of yet another capitalist crisis that menaced the continued well-being of societies. In turn, it was submitted in early 2023 when COVID-19 remained a virulent – if less politically deliberated – threat to population health, especially in the context of the continued obstinacy of neoliberalism (Šumonja 2021; Wood *et al.* 2023). The volume, thereby, emerges in a context in which the importance of health for politics, as well as the political-economic character of health, could not be more prescient. Since early 2020, the world has been in the grips of the novel coronavirus, its variants, and now subvariants. With close to 610 million reported cases and 6.5 million deaths at the time of writing, COVID-19 has demonstrated not only the critical importance of public health, but also the general centrality of political-economic issues to health and well-being. Whether considering geographical disparities and resource-poor healthcare settings; unequal access to care; deep relationships between inequality, race, and poor health outcomes; North-South disparities in access to medicines; or the extraordinarily ageist results of austerity, long-term care, and residential outbreaks, the ongoing pandemic has thrust the political-economic character of health and healthcare heavily into the spotlight.

By subjecting the latter to scrutiny with regard to a wide range of issues and within diverse geographical contexts, we hope that this volume facilitates a rejuvenation of debate over the complex social determinants of health. Indeed, we consider the book less a 'handbook' in the conventional sense – as an introductory reference to various topics – and more a 'reader' compiling a range of argumentative pieces, deliberately designed to provoke critical discussion and future scholarly work. That is, we wish for the chapters contained herein to contribute to shifting the epistemological locus of deliberations on health and healthcare from the confines of neoclassical economics and neoliberal policies, toward more capacious formulations of their political-economic character. In the present conjuncture, this task is more salient than ever.

Nevertheless, while necessary, this step alone remains insufficient as a means to achieve more amenable conditions for human health. Renewed scholarly concern with the political economy of health and healthcare as a field of study must be complemented by the involvement of social movements capable of struggling for progressive or radical political alternatives across this terrain (Panitch and Leys 2009; Waitzkin *et al.* 2018). We do not, in this regard, predict any sudden regression of the current neoliberal orientation of health and healthcare due to the publication of this volume. Instead, for scholars and activists seeking to secure transformative health outcomes in a post-GCC era, we tender this *Handbook* as a kind of clarion call for political strategy. As the following chapters demonstrate, the quality of health and healthcare systems remain products of material and ideological determinants that, *themselves*, must be contested and reoriented in order to effect alternative outcomes.

For instance, as Patrick Neveling's contribution reveals, the appalling occupational health and safety (OH&S) conditions confronting workers in the global garment industry have not simply arisen from the actions of negligent individual employers. Rather, they stem from numerous historical institutions, policies, and laws codified by capitalist states that prioritize accumulation over worker safety, as well as globalized commodity chains that both minimize capital investment in technology and circumvent expenditure on OH&S for 'undeserving' workers. Effectively redressing such concerns necessitates locating the capitalist state, the garment industry, and the exploitative dynamics of global capitalism as sites of political contestation (see also: Heino 2013; Lax 2020). The broader implication here is that, while illness and death are an inevitable part of human life, the dynamics of neoliberalism and capitalism accelerate and magnify this reality in avoidable ways. As such, 'the demand for a healthier society is, in itself, the demand for a radically different socio-economic order' (Doyal 1979: 296–7).

In this respect, while its constitutive chapters adopt multiple, sometimes incommensurable political angles on issues of health, the volume as a whole should contribute to the formulation of political strategies centered on what Slavoj Žižek (2017) has called the 'courage of hopelessness'. For Žižek, it is self-defeating to trust in the deceptive optimism of a promised progressive future when confronted by breakdowns in the existing political-economic order. Indeed, 'the light at the end of the tunnel is probably the headlight of another train approaching us from the opposite direction' (Žižek 2017: xii). Conversely, *despairing* at the perpetual failure of techno-managerial and neoliberal reforms within the status quo and, thus, *acknowledging* the gravity of the current conjuncture may foster decisive political action and the pursuit of more radical transformation (see also: Žižek 2023). To paraphrase Romain Rolland's (1920) famous maxim, the necessary optimism of the will for emancipatory political action must first be nourished by a substantial pessimism of the intellect.

The chapters of the *Handbook* contribute to this orientation by explicating (i) the scope and scale of contemporary health and healthcare challenges, *and* (ii) their intimate relation to the routine operation of neoliberal policies and the structural dynamics of capitalism. Hence, the volume challenges critical scholars and activists hoping to address (i) to confront the inherent limitations – the 'hopelessness' – of acquiescing to (ii) as the ultimate horizon for action and, thus, of pursuing incremental political solutions to eventually render the status quo more palatable. In the crisis-ridden conjuncture of contemporary capitalism, the effects of neoliberalism in eviscerating the socio-ecological conditions of health have been recognized and weaponized by Far-Right movements (Stuckler 2017; Falkenbach and Heiss 2021; Labonté and Baum 2021). For instance, the latter have promulgated forms of 'welfare chauvinism' – promising maintenance or augmentation of welfare benefits for core constituencies, while disregarding minorities (Greer 2017). This was notoriously exemplified in 2016 by placards adorning the 'Brexit bus' undertaking to remedy UK health concerns upon leaving the EU by reallocating an additional £350 million each week to the NHS. Analogously, we hope that the contents of the book may prompt progressive and radical social forces to reflect on the need to *embrace* the inescapably dire consequences for health and healthcare propagated by neoliberalism and capitalism. The associated 'despair' arising from recognizing the hopelessness of attempting to 'fix' the status quo via perennial techno-managerial tinkering may, in turn, prompt these movements to channel their efforts toward systemic political-economic change to secure more efficacious and equitable health outcomes.

On this semi-sanguine note, we would like to take the opportunity to acknowledge and express our appreciation to those who have helped bring this undertaking to fruition. Despite the demanding, often gloomy context in which it was conceived and organized over the past few years, it has been a pleasure to work together to prepare the *Handbook*. In this respect, we first wish to thank each other, as co-editors, for the opportunity to develop a project collectively in a research area of substantial social import. We are also sincerely grateful to all chapter authors for their excellent contributions and ongoing commitment to the project, especially when many divided their expertise between academia and working as medical professionals during the GCC. Our heartfelt thanks go out to Andy Humphries at Routledge for his patience, enthusiasm, and sage advice on the volume during its extended compilation and gestation. Thank you, too, to the team at Routledge for their fine work in helping to ensure the book's production was a straightforward and positive experience. Finally, to our families and loved ones, we must extend our warm appreciation for your enduring support while the book was completed – especially given two new additions were born during its production! We hope that this volume will contribute in some small way to revitalizing debate over the complex political economy of health and healthcare so that they and future generations may contribute to a world in which capital accumulation is subordinated to the health and welfare of humanity and the planet.

Note

1 Similarly, despite the GCC manifestly demonstrating the pernicious repercussions of neoliberalism for both population health and healthcare systems, the latter continues to delimit the ideological horizon for public health discourse (Primrose *et al.* 2020). Since the outbreak of the pandemic, mainstream political deliberations have largely disregarded the potential for introducing alternative measures designed to restructure the neoliberal subsumption of social reproduction to capital through reconfiguring existing health systems. Instead, public policy aspirations have remained been oriented toward facilitating the prompt resumption of economic activity *within* extant neoliberal structures (Šumonja 2021; Wallace 2023; Wood *et al.* 2023) – that is within 'the partition of the sensible' (Rancière 1998).

References

Adler-Bolton, B. and Vierkant, A. 2022, *Health Communism: A Surplus Manifesto*, Verso, London.

Akram-Lodhi, A.H. 2021, 'Contemporary pathogens and the capitalist world food system', *Canadian Journal of Development Studies*, 42(1–2), pp. 18–27.

Alegría, M., NeMoyer, A., Falgàs Bagué, I., Wang, Y. and Alvarez, K. 2018, 'Social determinants of mental health: Where we are and where we need to go', *Current Psychiatry Reports*, 20, pp. 1–13.

Anderson, T. 2023, 'From operation warp speed to TRIPS: Vaccines as assets', in Di Muzio, T. and Dow, M. (eds), *COVID-19 and the Global Political Economy: Crises in the 21st Century*, Routledge, London, pp. 122–35.

Arnsperger, C. and Varoufakis, Y. 2008, 'Neoclassical economics: Three identifying features', in Fullbrook, E. (ed), *Pluralist Economics*, Zed Books, London, pp. 13–25.

Badiei, S. and Grivaux, A. 2022, 'The positive and the normative in economic thought: A historical-analytic appraisal', in Badiei, S. and Grivaux, A. (eds), *The Positive and the Normative in Economic Thought*, Routledge, London, pp. 1–24.

Baer, H.A. 1982, 'On the political economy of health', *Medical Anthropology Newsletter*, 14(1), pp. 1–17.
Baer, H.A. and Singer, M. 'Planetary health: Capitalism, ecology and eco-socialism', *Capitalism, Nature, Socialism*. Published online April 2023.
Bambra, C. 2011, *Work, Worklessness, and the Political Economy of Health*, Oxford University Press, Oxford.
Bambra, C., Lynch, J. and Smith, K.E. 2021, *The Unequal Pandemic: COVID-19 and Health Inequalities*, Policy Press, Bristol.
Baran, P.A. and Sweezy, P.M. 1966, *Monopoly Capital*, New York University Press, New York.
Baum, F. and Fisher, M. 2014, 'Why behavioural health promotion endures despite its failure to reduce health inequities', in Cohen, S. (ed), *From Health Behaviours to Health Practices*, Wiley Blackwell, London, pp. 57–68.
Bell, J. 2020, 'Between private and public: AIDS, health care capitalism, and the politics of respectability in 1980s America', *Journal of American Studies*, 54(1), pp. 159–83.
Bhattacharya, T. 2017, *Social Reproduction Theory: Remapping Class, Recentering Oppression*, Pluto Press, London.
Birn, A.E., Pillay, Y. and Holtz, T.H. 2017, *Textbook of Global Health*, Oxford University Press, Oxford.
Bonner, A. (ed.) 2023, *COVID-19 and Social Determinants of Health: Wicked Issues and Relationalism*, Policy Press, Bristol.
Braveman, P., Egerter, S. and Williams, D.R. 2011, 'The social determinants of health: Coming of age', *Annual Review of Public Health*, 32, pp. 381–98.
Braveman, P. and Gottlieb, L. 2014, 'The social determinants of health: It's time to consider the causes of the causes', *Public Health Reports*, 129(suppl. 2), pp. 19–31.
Butcher, B.S., Paton, G.J. and Cahill, D. 2012, *Market Society: History, Theory, Practice*, Cambridge University Press, Cambridge.
Candela, R. 2018, 'Public choice: The Virginia school', in Marciano, A. and Ramello, G.B. (eds), *Encyclopedia of Law and Economics*, Springer, New York, pp. 1712–1720.
Champlin, D.P. and Knoedler, J.T. 2008, 'Universal health care and the economics of responsibility', *Journal of Economic Issues*, 42(4), pp. 913–38.
Chernomas, R. and Hudson, I. 2013, *To Live and Die in America: Class, Power, Health and Healthcare*, Pluto Press, London.
Clarke, A.E., Shim, J.K., Mamo, L., Fosket, J.R. and Fishman, J.R. 2003, 'Biomedicalization: Technoscientific transformations of health, illness, and US biomedicine', *American Sociological Review*, 68(2), pp. 161–94.
Coburn, D. 2004, 'Beyond the income inequality hypothesis: Class, neo-liberalism, and health inequalities', *Social Science and Medicine*, 58(1), pp. 41–56.
Coburn, D. 2010, 'Inequality and health', in Panitch, L. and Leys, C. (eds), *Socialist Register: Morbid Symptoms*, Merlin Press, London, pp. 39–58.
Cockerham, W.C. 2005, 'Health lifestyle theory and the convergence of agency and structure', *Journal of Health and Social Behavior*, 46(1), pp. 51–67.
Collyer, F. (ed.) 2015, *The Palgrave Handbook of Social Theory in Health, Illness and Medicine*, Springer, New York.
Compton, M.T. and Shim, R.S. 2015, 'The social determinants of mental health', *Focus*, 13(4), pp. 419–25.
Courtwright, D.T. 2019, *The Age of Addiction: How Bad Habits Became Big Business*, Harvard University Press, London.
Crespo, R.F. 2017, *Economics and Other Disciplines: Assessing New Economic Currents*, Routledge, London.
Davis, J.B. (ed.) 2001, *The Social Economics of Health Care*, Routledge, London.
Davis, J.B. 2022, 'Economics as a normative discipline: Value disentanglement in an "objective economics"', in Badiei, S. and Grivaux, A. (eds), *The Positive and the Normative in Economic Thought*, Routledge, London, pp. 87–107.
Davis, J.B. and McMaster, R. 2017, *Health Care Economics*, Routledge, London.
Davy, L. and Dickinson, H. 2023, 'COVID-19 and the economy of care: Disability and aged care services into the future', in Di Muzio, T. and Dow, M. (eds), *COVID-19 and the Global Political Economy: Crises in the 21st Century*, Routledge, London, pp. 136–50.
Deppe, H.U. 2010, 'The nature of health care: Commodification versus solidarity', in Panitch, L. and Leys, C. (eds), *Socialist Register: Morbid Symptoms*, Merlin Press, London, pp. 29–38.
Doyal, L. 1979, *The Political Economy of Health*, Pluto Press, London.
Falkenbach, M. and Heiss, R. 2021, *The Populist Radical Right and Health*, Springer, New York.

Ferguson, S. 2020, *Women and Work: Feminism, Labour, and Social Reproduction*, Pluto Press, London.

Fine, B. 1980, *Economic Theory and Ideology*, Edward Arnold, London.

Fine, B. 2015, 'Neoclassical economics: An elephant is not a chimera but is a chimera real?' in Morgan, J. (ed), *What Is Neoclassical Economics? Debating the Origins, Meaning and Significance*, Routledge, London, pp. 194–213.

Fine, B. and Milonakis, D. 2009, *From Economics Imperialism to Freakonomics: The Shifting Boundaries Between Economics and Other Social Sciences*, Routledge, London.

Fouskas, V.K. and Gokay, B. 2020, 'COVID-19 and the bankruptcy of neoliberalism in the context of Global Shift', *Open Democracy*, 5 May, accessed 1 May 2022, <https://www.opendemocracy.net/en/can-europe-make-it/covid-19-and-bankruptcy-neoliberalism-context-global-shift/>.

Fraser, N. 2016, 'Contradictions of capital and care', *New Left Review*, 100(July-August), pp. 99–117.

Fraser, N. 2022, *Cannibal Capitalism: How Our System Is Devouring Democracy, Care, and the Planet and What We Can Do About It*, Verso, London.

Furton, G.L., Rizzo, M.J. and Harper, D.A. 2022, 'The political economy of public health', *Public Choice*, 195, pp. 1–3.

Gill, S.R. and Benatar, S.R. 2020, 'Reflections on the political economy of planetary health', *Review of International Political Economy*, 27(1), pp. 167–90.

Greer, S.L. 2017, 'Medicine, public health and the populist radical right', *Journal of the Royal Society of Medicine*, 110(8), pp. 305–8.

Hansen, H., Netherland, J. and Herzberg, D. 2023, *Whiteout: How Racial Capitalism Changed the Color of Opioids in America*, University of California Press, California.

Harvey, D. 2020, 'Anti-capitalist politics in the time of COVID-19', *Davidharvey.org*, 19 March, accessed 21 July 2021, <http://davidharvey.org/2020/03/anti-capitalist-politics-in-the-time-of-covid-19/>.

Heilbroner, R.L. 1989, *Behind the Veil of Economics: Essays in the Worldly Philosophy*, WW Norton and Company, New York.

Heino, B. 2013, 'The state, class and occupational health and safety: Locating the capitalist state's role in the regulation of OHS in NSW', *Labour and Industry*, 23(2), pp. 150–67.

Hodgson, G.M. 2001, *How Economics Forgot History: The Problem of Historical Specificity in Social Science*, Routledge, London.

Hodgson, G.M. 2008, 'An institutional and evolutionary perspective on health economics', *Cambridge Journal of Economics*, 32(2), pp. 235–56.

Jo, T.-H. 2022, 'Heterodox economics and ideology', in Chester, L. and Jo, T.-H. (eds), *Heterodox Economics: Legacy and Prospects*, World Economics Association Books, Bristol, pp. 204–51.

Jo, T.H. and Todorova, Z. 2017, 'Social provisioning process: A heterodox view of the economy', in Jo, T.-H., Chester, L., and D'Ippoliti, C. (eds), *The Routledge Handbook of Heterodox Economics*, Routledge, London, pp. 29–40.

Jones, L. and Hameiri, S. 2022, 'COVID-19 and the failure of the neoliberal regulatory state', *Review of International Political Economy*, 29(4), pp. 1027–52.

Josifidis, K. and Supic, N. 2022, 'Corporate capital and (de) monopolization of public health in the USA: An institutionalist perspective', *Journal of Economic Issues*, 56(2), pp. 378–86.

Keynes, J.M. 2013 [1923], *A Tract on Monetary Reform*, Cambridge University Press, Cambridge.

Knott, M. 2020, 'Leaked Trump Administration figures project 3000 COVID-19 deaths a day in the US', *Sydney Morning Herald*, 5 May, accessed 21 March 2021, <https://www.smh.com.au/world/north-america/leaked-trump-administration-figures-project-3000-covid-19-deaths-a-day-20200505-p54ps3.html>.

Krieger, N. 2011, *Epidemiology and the People's Health: Theory and Context*, Oxford University Press, Oxford.

Labonté, R. and Baum, F. 2021, 'Right wing politics and public policy: The need for a broad frame and further research comment on "A scoping review of populist radical right parties' influence on welfare policy and its implications for population health in Europe"', *International Journal of Health Policy and Management*, 10(8), pp. 519–22.

Labonté, R. and Ruckert, A. 2019, *Health Equity in a Globalizing Era: Past Challenges, Future Prospects*, Oxford University Press, Oxford.

Labonté, R. and Stuckler, D. 2016, 'The rise of neoliberalism: How bad economics imperils health and what to do about it', *Journal of Epidemiology and Community Health*, 70(3), pp. 312–8.

Laster Pirtle, W.N. 2020, 'Racial capitalism: A fundamental cause of Novel Coronavirus (COVID-19) pandemic inequities in the United States', *Health Education and Behavior*, 47(4), pp. 504–8.

Lawson, T. 2015, 'What is this "school" called neoclassical economics?' in Morgan, J. (ed), *What Is Neoclassical Economics? Debating the Origins, Meaning and Significance*, Routledge, London, pp. 30–80.
Lax, M.B. 2020, 'Falling short: The state's role in workplace safety and health', *New Solutions*, 30(1), pp. 27–41.
Leake, J., Shipman, T., Wright, O. and Lay, K. 2020, 'Coronavirus: 100,000 dead if UK eases lockdown too fast, scientists warn', *The Times*, 10 May, accessed 21 March 2021, <https://www.thetimes.co.uk/edition/news/coronavirus-100-000-dead-if-uk-eases-lockdown-too-fast-scientists-warn-rqqbf956g>.
Lee, F. 2009, *A History of Heterodox Economics: Challenging the Mainstream in the Twentieth Century*, Routledge, London.
Leys, C. 2009, 'Health, health care and capitalism', in Panitch, L. and Leys, C. (eds), *Socialist Register: Morbid Symptoms*, Merlin Press, London, pp. 1–28.
Little, I.M.D. 2002, *Ethics, Economics, and Politics: Principles of Public Policy*, Oxford University Press, Oxford.
Luisetti, F. 2022, 'The neoliberal virus', in Lemm, V. and Vatter, M. (eds), *The Viral Politics of COVID-19: Nature, Home, and Planetary Health*, Springer, New York, pp. 181–200.
Madra, Y.M. and Adaman, F. 2010, 'Public economics after neoliberalism: A theoretical–historical perspective', *The European Journal of the History of Economic Thought*, 17(4), pp. 1079–106.
Marmot, M. and Wilkinson, R. (eds) 2005, *Social Determinants of Health*, Oxford University Press, Oxford.
Marya, R. and Patel, R. 2021, *Inflamed: Deep Medicine and the Anatomy of Injustice*, Penguin, London.
Matthews, D. 2019, 'Capitalism and mental health', *Monthly Review*, 70(8), pp. 49–62.
McClure, E.S., Vasudevan, P., Bailey, Z., Patel, S. and Robinson, W.R. 2020, 'Racial capitalism within public health: How occupational settings drive COVID-19 disparities', *American Journal of Epidemiology*, 189(11), pp. 1244–53.
Mezzadri, A., Newman, S. and Stevano, S. 2022, 'Feminist global political economies of work and social reproduction', *Review of International Political Economy*, 29(6), pp. 1783–803.
Mirowski, P. 1991, *More Heat Than Light: Economics as Social Physics, Physics as Nature's Economics*, Cambridge University Press. Cambridge.
Mooney, G. 2009, *Challenging Health Economics*, Oxford University Press, Oxford.
Mooney, G. 2012, *The Health of Nations: Towards a New Political Economy*, Bloomsbury Publishing, London.
Moore, J. 2015, *Capitalism in the Web of Life: Ecology and the Accumulation of Capital*, Verso, London.
Munro, D. 2004, 'Method in political economy: A comment', *Journal of Australian Political Economy*, 54, pp. 146–7.
Myrdal, G. 1969, 'Social values and their universality', *International Social Work*, 12(1), pp. 3–11.
Navarro, V. 1976, *Medicine Under Capitalism*, Prodist, New York.
Navarro, V. 2002, *The Political Economy of Social Inequalities: Consequences for Health and Quality of Life*, Baywood, New York.
Navarro, V. 2009, 'What we mean by social determinants of health', *International Journal of Health Services*, 39(3), pp. 423–41.
Navarro, V. 2020, 'The consequences of neoliberalism in the current pandemic', *International Journal of Health Services*, 50(3), pp. 271–5.
Navarro, V. and Muntaner, C. 2004, *Political and Economic Determinants of Population Health and Well-Being: Controversies and Developments*, Baywood, New York.
Padilla, M.B., Vásquez del Aguila, E. and Parker, R.G. 2007, 'Globalization, structural violence, and LGBT health: A cross-cultural perspective', in Meyer, I. and Northridge, M.E. (eds), *The Health of Sexual Minorities: Public Health Perspectives on Lesbian, Gay, Bisexual and Transgender Populations*, Springer, New York, pp. 209–41.
Panitch, L. and Leys, C. (eds) 2009, *Socialist Register: Morbid Symptoms*, Merlin Press, London.
Parker, R. and García, J. (eds) 2018, *The Routledge Handbook on the Politics of Global Health*, Routledge, London.
People's Health Movement, Medact, Third World Network, Health Poverty Action, Medico International, ALAMES, Viva Salud and Sama. 2022, *Global Health Watch 6: In the Shadow of the Pandemic*, Bloomsbury Publishing, London.
Pereira, P.J.D.R. 2021, 'Drugs, violence, and capitalism: The expansion of opioid use in the Americas', *Latin American Perspectives*, 48(1), pp. 184–201.

Primrose, D., Chang, R. and Loeppky, R. 2020, 'Pandemic unplugged: COVID-19, public health and the persistence of neoliberalism', *Journal of Australian Political Economy*, 85, pp. 17–28.
Rancière, J. 1998, *Disagreement: Politics and Philosophy*, University of Minnesota Press, Minnesota.
Rocca, E. and Anjum, R.L. 2020, 'Complexity, reductionism and the biomedical model', in Anjum, R.L., Copeland, S. and Rocca, E. (eds), *Rethinking Causality, Complexity and Evidence for the Unique Patient: A Causehealth Resource for Healthcare Professionals and the Clinical Encounter*, Springer, New York, pp. 75–94.
Rolland, R. 1920, 'Review of *The sacrifice of Abraham* by Raymond Lefebvre, *L'Humanité*, 19 March.
Schofield, T. 2015, *A Sociological Approach to Health Determinants*, Cambridge University Press, Cambridge.
Schrecker, T. and Bambra, C. 2015, *How Politics Makes Us Sick: Neoliberal Epidemics*, Springer, New York.
Sell, S.K. and Williams, O.D. 2020, Health under capitalism: A global political economy of structural pathogenesis', *Review of International Political Economy*, 27(1), pp. 1–25.
Serikbayeva, B., Abdulla, K. and Oskenbayev, Y. 2021, 'State capacity in responding to COVID-19', *International Journal of Public Administration*, 44(11–12), pp. 920–30.
Sheehan, M.C. and Fox, M.A. 2020, 'Early warnings: The lessons of COVID-19 for public health climate preparedness', *International Journal of Health Services*, 50(3), pp. 264–70.
Sparke, M. 2020, 'Neoliberal regime change and the remaking of global health: From rollback disinvestment to rollout reinvestment and reterritorialization', *Review of International Political Economy*, 27(1), pp. 48–74.
Sparke, M. and Williams, O.D. 2022, 'Neoliberal disease: COVID-19, co-pathogenesis and global health insecurities', *Environment and Planning A: Economy and Space*, 54(1), pp. 15–32.
Saggers, S. and Walter, M. 2007, 'Poverty and social class', in Carson, B. (ed), *Social Determinants of Indigenous Health*, Allen and Unwin, Crows Nest, pp. 87–107.
Stilwell, F. 2002, *Political Economy: The Contest of Economic Ideas*, Oxford University Press, Oxford.
Stilwell, F. 2019, 'From economics to political economy: Contradictions, challenge, and change', *American Journal of Economics and Sociology*, 78(1), pp. 35–62.
Stilwell, F. 2023, 'The future for political economy: Towards unity in diversity? *Review of Political Economy*, 35(1), pp. 189–210.
Stilwell, F., Primrose, D. and Thornton, T.B. (eds) 2022a, *Handbook of Alternative Theories of Political Economy*, Edward Elgar, Cheltenham.
Stilwell, F., Primrose, D. and Thornton, T.B. 2022b, 'Introduction to the Handbook of Alternative Theories of Political Economy', Stilwell, F., Primrose, D. and Thornton, T.B (eds), *Handbook of Alternative Theories of Political Economy*, Edward Elgar, Cheltenham, pp. 2–15.
Stuckler, D. 2017, 'The dispossessed: A public health response to the rise of the far-right in Europe and North America', *The European Journal of Public Health*, 27(1), pp. 5–6.
Šumonja, M. 2021, 'Neoliberalism is not dead: On political implications of COVID-19', *Capital and Class*, 45(2), pp. 215–27.
Szreter, S. 2005, *Health and Wealth: Studies in History and Policy*, University of Rochester Press, New York.
Ullah, A. 2016, *Globalization and the Health of Indigenous Peoples: From Colonization to Self-Rule*, Routledge, London.
Waitzkin, H. 1978, 'A Marxist view of medical care', *Annals of Internal Medicine*, 89(2), pp. 264–78.
Waitzkin, H. 2021, 'Confronting the upstream causes of COVID-19 and other epidemics to follow', *International Journal of Health Services*, 51(1), pp. 55–58.
Waitzkin, H., Pérez, A. and Anderson, M. 2020, *Social Medicine and the Coming Transformation*, Routledge, London.
Waitzkin, H. and the Working Group on Health Beyond Capitalism. (eds) 2018, *Health Care Under the Knife: Moving Beyond Capitalism for our Health*, New York University Press, New York.
Wallace, R. 2016, *Big Farms Make Big Flu: Dispatches on Influenza, Agribusiness, and the Nature of Science*, New York University Press, New York.
Wallace, R. 2020, *Dead Epidemiologists: On the Origins of COVID-19*, Monthly Review Press, New York.
Wallace, R. 2023, *The Fault in Our SARS: COVID-19 in the Biden Era*, Monthly Review Press, New York.
Wamsley, D. and Benatar, S. 2023, 'Global health, COVID-19 and the future of neoliberalism', in Di Muzio, T. and Dow, M. (eds), *COVID-19 and the Global Political Economy: Crises in the 21st Century*, Routledge, London, pp. 107–21.
Westra, R. 2021, *Economics, Science and Capitalism*, Routledge, London.

Wood, J.D., Ausserladscheider, V. and Sparkes, M. 2023, 'The manufactured crisis of COVID-Keynesianism in Britain, Germany and the USA', *Cambridge Journal of Regions, Economy and Society*, 16(1), pp. 19–29.

World Health Organization. 1948, 'Constitution of the World Health Organization', WHO, accessed 7 April 2022, <https://www.who.int/about/governance/constitution>.

World Health Organization. 2008, *Closing the Gap in a Generation: Health Equity Through Action on the Social Determinants of Health, Final Report of the Commission on Social Determinants Of Health*, World Health Organization, Geneva.

World Health Organization. 2021, *COVID-19 and the Social Determinants of Health and Health Equity: Evidence brief*, World Health Organization, Geneva.

Young, M. and Markham, F. 2017, 'Coercive commodities and the political economy of involuntary consumption: The case of the gambling industries', *Environment and Planning A: Economy and Space*, 49(12), pp. 2762–79.

Yuill, C., Crinson, I. and Duncan, E. 2011, *Key Concepts in Health Studies*, Sage, London.

Žižek, S. 2017, *The Courage of Hopelessness: Chronicles of a Year of Acting Dangerously*, Penguin, London.

Žižek, S. 2023, *Too Late to Awaken: What Lies Ahead When There Is No Future?* Penguin, London.

PART I

Theorizing health and healthcare

2

MAINSTREAM HEALTH ECONOMICS AND THE COVID-19 PANDEMIC

John B. Davis, Geoffrey M. Hodgson, Gerry McCartney and Robert McMaster

As a life-threatening disease, COVID-19 has severely disrupted socio-economic activities and prompted massive state interventions. Medical scientific expertise has simultaneously assumed critical importance as a means to comprehend the properties of the SARS-CoV-2 virus in the search for therapeutic and curative treatments. However, the pandemic also invites us to ask how health economics can contribute to our response and future resilience. Does the pandemic represent a 'health economics moment'? This is one of the questions we investigate in this chapter.

Much of contemporary health economics is derived from neoclassical economics (Forget 2004), and is predicated on the notion that individuals behave as *Homo Economicus* – 'rational economic man' [*sic*] – in instrumentally seeking to maximize their utility (Hodgson 2013; McCloskey 2016). Its advocates view it as an applied field (Culyer and Newhouse 2000; Jones 2012), providing a useful 'toolkit' (*e.g.* Parkin *et al.* 2013) that enhances our understanding of the value of medical procedures and treatments through generating (scientific) evidence of their potential consequences. As discussed further below, this 'toolkit' notion refers to the value neutrality of the techniques applied and, thus, a 'view from nowhere' (Nagel 1986) conception of objectivity in science – one in which the value of scientific ideas is determined by their distance from subjective beliefs. From this perspective, health economics resembles a hammer or screwdriver of no inherent value; its usefulness resides in its functionality.

Health economists contribute to a vast array of health evaluation and priority setting projects frequently funded by public bodies. Moreover, health economics research attracts funding levels disproportionate to other areas of economics.[1] Its methods, analysis, and argumentation influence formulation of both policy and approaches to the provision of medical care. The World Bank (2015) and the World Health Organization (WHO 2014) identify health economics as an important aid in policy framing. These references to health economics, thereby, align with the 'toolkit' notion of Parkin *et al.* (2013). We feel this is a highly contentious claim, especially in the context of COVID-19.

We dispute this for two principal reasons. First, all economics is value-laden, and health economics is no exception. Accordingly, we trace the value structure underlying the latter to its utilitarian orientation. Second, health economics equates agents' comportment with that of *Homo Economicus*, which centers on selfishness and atomistic individualism. This is based on 'I' language, whereas many health issues necessarily invoke 'we' language, with a range of concomitant

DOI: 10.4324/9781003017110-3

normative and ethical implications. Reflecting on these two limitations, we contend that mainstream health economics is frequently inadequate in its examination of health and healthcare issues, such as those presented by the COVID-19 pandemic. Like all approaches, health economics can only offer a partial account of phenomena. That said, we argue that the partiality of the mainstream tradition is incredibly narrow, frequently suggestive of the status of a special case. In developing our critical reflection, we present the basis of an alternative approach emphasizing the importance of language in orienting analysis.

The remainder of the chapter is structured as follows: the next section outlines the pillars of health economics – its 'toolkit'. Following this, we discuss the mainstream (health) economics of contagious disease, before then considering the normative implications and potential shortcomings of this approach. Our aim is to highlight the need for a broader basis for analyzing health and illness. We acknowledge that, in some respects, the COVID-19 pandemic reveals the economy to be one element of a wider healthcare system that is constitutive of the provisioning processes through which societies produce and reproduce.[2] Our view is that mainstream health economics envisions the reverse of this.

The 'toolkit': the three pillars of mainstream health economics

Neoclassical health economics emerged as a distinct field of applied microeconomics in the 1970s following the works of Kenneth Arrow (1963), Selma Mishkin (1962), and Michael Grossman (1972). Arrow and Grossman have been especially influential in shaping the theoretical direction and development of the field (Forget 2004; Mooney 2009; Soares 2015). Arrow contrasts the standard theoretical conception of market exchanges with the characteristics of the demand and supply of medical care – identifying the latter as marked by uncertainty in demand, externalities, and information asymmetries. Grossman's model utilizes a Beckerian approach in conceiving health as a capital stock in which utility-maximizing individuals choose to invest (and consume). Arrow's influence ensured that health economics remains nested in neoclassical welfare economics, while Grossman influenced analysis of the demand for health and medical care, as well as the maximand in some areas of economic evaluation.

Health economics has three analytical pillars: demand, supply, and economic evaluation. Much of its theoretical development occurred in the 1970s and 1980s, with subsequent developments according greater prominence to economic evaluation (Mooney 2009). The remainder of this section outlines the principal aspects of these three pillars.

The demand for health and healthcare

For Grossman (1972), health is defined in a primarily functional way: as freedom from illness, where this impedes an individual's ability to engage in work and/or leisure. Health has both investment and consumption characteristics, although Grossman emphasizes the former. The demand for health is treated as a derived demand, in that it permits the agent to participate in activities that either directly or indirectly contribute to utility. Grossman further distinguishes health from healthcare, where the latter is a derived demand of the former. Therefore, an individual will only demand healthcare as a means to improve their health.

In the model, individuals inherit a stock of health capital, which depreciates during adulthood with age. Over their lifespan, individuals are confronted with a constrained optimization problem in how much to invest in their health stock. This produces a stream of benefits, such as enabling the individual to work and earn income. There is potential for time trade-offs between investing in health, such as through exercise, medical insurance, and in the production of other goods. Grossman argues that with exogenously determined rates of depreciation in health stock, which are correlated with age, an individual must decide whether to continue investing, and the amount of any investment. Lifespan is, therefore, endogenous – subject to an individual's cost-benefit calculation.

The model provides a host of predictions, including that individuals' medical expenditures increase with age as depreciation of the health stock accelerates. Demand for health and medical care is positively correlated with an individual's wage rate and, therefore, their enhanced ability to afford medical treatment. The more educated demand more health, which increases the optimal stock level as education increases the productivity, or efficiency, of investment. Medical care expenditure, however, is negatively correlated with education levels, *ceteris paribus*. Some of these predictions are uncontroversial in that they have empirical and intuitive appeal. Yet, Grossman's logic implies that it is a rational decision for the poor to die at an earlier age than the rich, given the relative costs and expected returns on health investment. That is, there is less incentive for the poor and uneducated to invest in their health![3]

From our perspective, Grossman's argument is important for establishing or reinforcing within health economics three foundational precepts: (1) a conception of health as a stock and as *de facto* focus (Mooney 2009); (2) the Cartesian duality of mind and body; and (3) an instrumental or consequentialist basis for evaluation.

The second is particularly worthy of further reflection, while we postpone discussion of evaluation until later in this chapter. Grossman's argument that the demand for health and healthcare pivots on the stock of health is redolent of the body as a machine. Indeed, there may be a moral equivalent between the body and the machine, given the identical incentive structures between Grossman's approach and the broader literature on human capital (*e.g.* Bhattacharya *et al.* 2014). In contrast, the mind, as the site of calculating optimality, is separated from the body. There is certain insouciance in how Grossman (1972: 238) expresses the process of optimization: '[i]f [depreciation] grows continuously with age after some point in the life cycle, persons would choose to live a finite life'.

Grossman's argument speaks to a biomedical explanation of illness, in that it is analogous to increased capital depreciation, or a broken machine in which the mind calculates the net benefits, or otherwise, of repair (Davis and McMaster 2017). The focus is on the individual's calculation. This, thereby, reduces all relationships to arguments in a utility function, and echoes later work in developing the supply-side of healthcare, to which we turn.

The supply of healthcare

The mainstream literature here analyses a range of areas, including the following: the comparative analysis of healthcare systems, access to treatment and care as part of broader examinations of equity, and provider incentives and behavior. There are also studies of optimal provision, such as healthcare productivity (Burgess 2012), while the 1970s and 1980s witnessed attempts to develop analyses of the hospital as a firm (Harris 1977). Given the argument of the present chapter, we focus on what we feel is the most important aspect of this work: the relationship between physician and patient. We acknowledge that there is extensive and insightful health economics discussion on equity, and on prioritizing healthcare provision toward the most effective interventions and practices, and we allude to this in the context of economic evaluation later in the chapter.

The mainstream approach assumes selfish utility-maximizing agents. That said, a theoretical innovation, which attempts to acknowledge the Hippocratic Oath, concerns interdependent utility functions between physician and patient. Thus, not only does the patient gain utility from any treatment that leads to their recovery from illness, but their physician also benefits (Mooney and Ryan 1993). Indeed, Williams (1998) declared that the physician-patient association represented a 'perfect' agency relationship, in that the physician is driven to act in the interests of their patient. Williams' contention assumes that the utility functions of physicians and patients completely map onto each other.

Given mainstream behavioral tenets, it is difficult to conclude that Williams' argument represents anything other than a special case. Rather, the literature emphasizes potential trade-offs in the utility function of the physician between the self-interest of this agent and that of the patient in the presence of information asymmetries and the influence of the Hippocratic Oath. The health economics version of the classic agency problem revolves around the potential for supplier-induced demand (*e.g.* McGuire 2000, 2011). The issue reduces to the weighting of arguments in the physician utility function. McGuire argues that physicians exercise persuasive powers over their patients and that the direction this takes is sensitive to remuneration structures. Given these underlying assumptions, it is theoretically appealing to presume some manifestation of supplier-induced demand, especially in US studies (Rice 2012), which directs attention to efficient resource allocation. If the institutional governance of physician-patient relations is such that supplier-induced demand is intrinsic, then there is a basis for arguing that there are tendencies to over-provide clinical services.

In short, health economics models the primary relationship in medical care as a principal-agent exchange, where the information advantage of physician-agents is tempered by the interdependence of their utility function with that of their patient-principals. Both are assumed to operate as utility maximizers. Within the approach, the optimization process of the physician is complicated by tensions between selfishness and other-regarding values.

Economic evaluation

Much of the health economics literature concentrates on economic evaluation, and it is this area that most explicitly applies neoclassical welfare theory (Forget 2004). Specifically, Grossman's emphasis on health shapes the maximand adopted in economic evaluation (Mooney 2009). These are the bases of health economists' 'toolkit' (Parkin *et al.* 2013). Evaluation based on the assessment of costs and benefits provides policymakers with the necessary information to allocate scarce resources to ensure efficiency and an optimal outcome (Bhattacharya *et al.* 2014; Birch and Gafni 2006; Chilton *et al.* 2020).

Evaluation attempts to provide a single measure of the benefits of specific medical procedures and treatments. In some evaluation procedures, the aggregated utilities of individual patients associated with a particular treatment provide an overall estimate of benefit, which can then be divided by the cost of the treatment to provide a cost-per-unit health gain (*e.g.* Quality-Adjusted Life Year [QALY[4]]) basis of comparison across treatments and patients.[5] This assessment assumes that private utility maximization (in QALY terms) is all that matters to people. An advantage of QALYs lies in the assessment of mortality and morbidity on a single scale (Drummond *et al.* 2005; Round 2012). Accordingly, assuming the existence of 'trade-offs' between competing needs, this informs decisions on alternative resource allocations, such as which medical treatments should be prioritized.

Yet, it should be noted that QALYs are not necessarily associated with utility maximization: the two are discrete and independent entities. An issue with *some* elements of health economics is that the two are conflated. To some extent, this is reflected in the intermittent debates about the appropriate maximand in evaluation techniques between 'welfarism' and 'extra-welfarism'. With welfarism, evaluation is predicated on the aggregation of subjective assessments of individual 'consumer' (patient) utility associated with a particular treatment protocol. The maximand is, therefore, utility. This is markedly Paretian (Culyer 1989). In contrast, Culyer and others advocate an alternative maximand: health. Valuation no longer solely relies on the subjective judgment of patient-consumers, with expert opinion assuming an important role. While this debate is of importance in that it can potentially affect the design of medical interventions, it is beyond the scope of our focus.

Economic assessment doubtless provides some insight into the complex processes of medical evaluation. We do not dispute this. Nonetheless, we have reservations over the use of the notion of a 'toolkit' and the value neutrality it implies. Rather, we believe that health economics should be explicit about its underpinning value structure. We develop this point in the next section in the context of COVID-19.

The mainstream approach and pandemics

If the 2007–08 financial crisis represented a 'Minsky moment' (McCulley 2009), does the COVID-19 pandemic represent a 'health economics moment'? The pandemic presents obvious public health and economic challenges. Therefore, one may ask: will the 'toolkit' of health economics, as outlined above, contribute to effectively addressing these difficulties?

Prior to COVID-19, the economic literature examining the impact of pandemics was not extensive (Keogh-Brown *et al.* 2010). In the period following the COVID-19 outbreak, economists attempted to address this and contribute to a greater understanding of the economics of pandemics. Macroeconomic simulations are especially prominent in this literature, while others have considered behavioral changes, and optimal treatment and prevention designs. Pre–COVID-19, the engagement between economics and epidemiology related primarily to modeling and predicting changes in behavior following an outbreak of a contagious disease (Bhattacharya *et al.* 2014). In this section, we illustrate some of the mainstream contributions to the study of COVID-19, before discussing the foundational theoretical approach of the pre–COVID-19 literature, which informs mainstream health economics' engagement in the area.

COVID-19, macroeconomics and epidemiology

A functioning economy is predicated on public health and *vice versa*. To reinforce this precept, analyses of COVID-19 have hitherto coalesced around the view that there is either limited or zero trade-off between the economy and proliferation of SARS-CoV-2, or 'between lives and livelihoods' (Ilzetzki and Moll 2020). On this, the examination of non-pharmaceutical interventions (NPIs) – principally 'lockdowns' and physical distancing regulations – has considered the counterfactual of an absence of NPIs (*e.g.* Douglas *et al.* 2020), with Sweden perhaps providing a natural experiment.[6] In surveying economists, Ilzetzki and Moll (2020) find that a majority believed lockdowns do not cause further economic harm than associated with allowing the virus to spread uncontained through the population. In their analysis of the impact of the 1918 Spanish Influenza pandemic on US cities, Correia *et al.* (2022) conclude that those areas affected experienced a marked decline in economic activity. They observe that those cities enacting stricter NPIs early in the pandemic demonstrated little or no adverse impact on 'local economic outcomes', and recovered comparatively quickly post-pandemic.

Earlier work by Keogh-Brown *et al.* (2010) contrasted a simulated impact of various types of pandemics (mild and severe) with the 1918 outbreak. They predicted that a pandemic might result in behavioral changes, such that consumption – especially 'social consumption' (such as hospitality services) – is reduced, and that policy changes associated with a public health response, such as lockdown, have pronounced macroeconomic impacts in depressing growth trajectories. In comparing the contemporary capitalist economy with that impacted by the 1918 pandemic, Keogh-Brown contends that there is greater flexibility in labor supply and higher 'social' consumption that is postponed. Both imply that modern economies have greater vulnerability to falls in activity, albeit of a transient nature. Perhaps the ability of many organizations to restructure their activities online mitigates the impact alluded to by Keogh-Brown *et al.* Indeed, this may be one of the lasting legacies of the COVID-19 pandemic.

Giannitsarou *et al.* (2021) and Kaplan *et al.* (2020) present examples of economic analyses tailored to the COVID-19 pandemic. The former models a second wave of COVID-19, concluding that infection rates are sensitive to the duration of immunity and that 'optimal' NPIs postpone subsequent waves and mitigate prevalence. The latter integrates epidemiological modeling of virus transmission and spread with a heterogeneous agent macroeconomic model. The authors claim this enables analysis of possible distributional impacts of the pandemic and policy responses across the population. The assumption is that the economically precarious are also the most vulnerable in a pandemic. Kaplan *et al.*, thus, conclude that governments encounter a challenging set of policy considerations over distributional consequences.

Kaplan *et al.* is illustrative of attempts to animate epidemiology and economic modeling, and commendably transcend disciplinary silos. Yates (2020) presents another example among those advocating this interdisciplinary approach to overcome the limitations in extant mainstream model design. In the early stages of the pandemic, the UK's Scientific Advisory Group for Emergencies' epidemiological model did not incorporate behavioral responses to changed risk. Macroeconomic modeling employed by central banks also did not factor in virus transmission (Yates 2020). Yet, the feedback between public health and economic behavior seems obvious. Demand is likely to contract for activities such as hospitality where the risk of infection is deemed greatest by consumers and, as consumption declines through voluntary physical distancing, the spread of the virus is likely to decline.

Neoclassical economics, epidemiology and infectious disease

In focusing on behavioral responses to disease, economists' contributions unsurprisingly assume the presence of *Homo Economicus* (Bhattacharya *et al.* 2014; Philipson 2000). A central idea here concerns the 'excess burden of disease'. Thus, estimates are made of the epidemiological 'costs' of disease, such as lost earnings and the disutility of illness, and excess burden, which assesses the costs of disease avoidance and incorporates opportunity costs. Both constitute the total economic cost of disease. With increasingly severe disease, the expectation is that self-interested agents will be motivated to minimize costs and adopt preventive measures, such as physical distancing and the avoidance of activities where disease may be prevalent. This implies that epidemiological costs and the excess burden of disease increase. Yet, with self-protection and decline in infections, epidemiological costs may eventually fall, implying total economic costs will either plateau or increase at a diminishing rate. What is the case for the individual is, via aggregation, assumed to be applicable to society *in toto*. Indeed, this frames disease as a tax: utility-maximizing individuals adopt actions that avoid the costs of this 'tax' up to the point where the benefits of disease prevention equal the estimated costs of it at the margin. This is identical to Grossman's mode of explanation in employing the standard Samuelsonian approach: all economic problems are framed as issues of constrained optimization.

This analytical foundation underpins the investigations of four strands in the mainstream literature (Laxminarayan and Malani 2011). These include the following: (1) the impact on investment decisions and productivity associated with infectious disease; (2) disease prevention, treatment, and individual risk-taking behavior; (3) vaccination as an instrument in disease prevention; and (4) the optimal design of treatment and prevention programs, and the efficient allocation of resources. We consider (2) and (3) in the greatest detail. To some extent, (4) follows from the implications of the economics of (2) and (3), and (1) resonates with the macro simulations outlined above.

Illness is, obviously, a source of disutility. In situations of risk or uncertainty, given diminishing marginal utility, individuals assume risk-averse positions. With infectious disease, where the individual lacks knowledge about potential severity, it is rational for agents to adopt self-protection strategies and actions, such as physical distancing. Behavior changes following the emergence of effective treatments in response to a novel disease, such as COVID-19. This assumption is traced to Peltzman's (1975) study of driving following safety regulations, contending that there is evidence that drivers become less cautious following the mandatory installation and use of various devices, such as seat belts. The diminishing risks of harm influenced driver attitude in terms of speed, and so forth. In effect, there are compensating changes in behavior following the re-evaluation of risk. Analogously, in the case of COVID-19, the development of improved treatments will, *ceteris paribus*, engender declining costs associated with contracting the virus, such that it is no longer rational for an individual to adopt self-protection activities (Laxminarayan and Malani 2011). Indeed, there are many possible trade-offs. Surveying the literature, Laxminarayan and Malani (2011: 192) conclude: '[s]elf-protection both slows the spread of infections and *reduces the return from public interventions to slow disease*' (emphasis added). They indicate that the notion of risk compensation implies individual and state initiatives are substitutes, and not complementary (see also: Philipson 1996, 2000). As the state increases the intensity and range of protective measures, individuals accordingly have less incentive to engage in self-protection.

During the COVID-19 pandemic, an important component of state intervention has centered on vaccination rollouts. Here, mainstream analysis has emphasized the externality properties of the latter, as applied to all scales: individual, organizational, and global, subject to 'contextual' differences (Laxminarayan and Malani 2011: 196). Given the nature of externality (social benefit is generally greater than any benefit accruing to an individual from vaccination), this engenders a 'classic public goods problem' (Laxminarayan and Malani 2011; Philipson 1996, 2000). As an increasing proportion of the population is vaccinated, and the closer society approaches vaccine-induced herd immunity, there is a growing divergence between social and private benefits. The benefits for the last individual (country) are much less than those for disease eradication to all other individuals (countries). This is a variation of the free-rider problem: the individual has an incentive to avoid the disutility associated with treatment, such as vaccination, assuming others will be treated (vaccinated). This is an important source of market failure, with the prediction of a sub-optimal outcome in that there will be an under-consumption of treatment. In the context of COVID-19, while state programs, which offer vaccines free-at-the-point-of consumption, may overcome market failure by reducing the costs of treatment, this may only be partial. If participation is voluntary, a program may yet be subject to the public goods problem. The issue then becomes one of structuring incentives to facilitate an efficient and effective outcome (see the line of argumentation made by Appleby 2020).

Several studies amend underpinning auxiliary assumptions of the mainstream approach. Agüero and Beleche (2017), for instance, report that 'health shocks' can produce persistent behavioral changes that improve health outcomes following a pandemic. Hansen *et al.* (2008) investigate 'anxious' individuals' willingness-to-pay for an influenza vaccine. This group perceives the benefits of a vaccine to be comparatively greater and is willing-to-pay more than the median. Hansen *et al.* accordingly conclude that anxiety distorts decision-making, especially under uncertainty.

Thus, behavioral sensitivities are prominent considerations in the design of optimal prevention and treatment programs. The health economics narrative aligns with new behavioralism in broader mainstream economics, in that discussion centers on individual incentives and trade-offs (*e.g.* Bhattacharya *et al.* 2014). Further, Chilton *et al.* (2020) argue that welfare economics – with its analysis of the 'big trade-offs', such as equity-efficiency – is the most appropriate basis to future-proof society against the costs of subsequent waves of COVID-19 and other viruses. Welfare economics, they argue, moves us away from the 'narrow' perspective that the virus is predominantly a medical issue. Instead, it furnishes an 'interface' between the 'medical and social' through its cost-benefit analysis of consequences. Appleby (2020) reinforces health economics as a 'toolkit' concept, which illuminates trade-offs and cost-benefit ratios associated with a range of possible interventions.

Some normative undercurrents

The preceding two sections described the 'tools within the toolkit', demonstrating that mainstream health economics explanations are predicated on the optimizing agent and the accompanying 'toolkit' is presented as value-neutral. We believe this formulation is naïve and utterly misleading. Accordingly, in this section, we draw out two important normative elements that undermine the value neutrality of the health economics 'toolkit' and question its reliance on the utility-maximizing individual. Specifically, we critically reflect on (1) the centrality of utilitarianism to economic evaluation, and (2) the posited value neutrality of mainstream health economics. As Boulding (1969: 2) argued:

> I am prepared to [...] say that no science of any kind can be divorced from ethical considerations [...] Science is a human learning process which arises in certain subcultures in human society and not in others, and a subculture [...] is a group [...] defined by the acceptance of common values [...] This means that even the epistemological content of science, that is, what scientists think they know, has an ethical component.

Health economics is no different. The 'toolkit' metaphor is highly misleading and even disingenuous. Following the central behavioral assumption of utility maximization, the mainstream approach envisions and privileges a particular type of language – 'I' as opposed to 'we'. Both presume different ethical properties. We argue that public health is configured on the latter rather than the former (Reicher 2021). By ignoring 'we' features, mainstream health economics presents a skewed analysis of public health, in general, and the COVID-19 pandemic, in particular.

A very peculiar 'toolkit': the utilitarianism of mainstream health economics

Utilitarianism is a consequentialist philosophy of right where the value of any action rests solely on outcomes or consequences. Process, duty and virtue have no intrinsic value. Ends justify means. For the utilitarian version of consequentialist reasoning, the greatest good is measured by aggregating the utility of all parties, and the action that provides the greatest overall utility should be pursued. It is well documented that neoclassical economics, especially welfare economics, embraces consequentialist and aspects of utilitarian ethical principles, despite protestations of value neutrality (Sen 1987). Over its history, neoclassicism has embarked on a series of refinements to its underlying utilitarian value frame (DeMartino 2022; Sen 1987). The Paretian welfare test established, in theory, the basis for the protection of those who are harmed because of some action that meets with the utilitarian calculus. The Kaldor-Hicks potential compensation criterion followed, as did a move from cardinal to ordinal utility and preferences.

Yet, unique among applied fields, health economics retains fundamental consequentialist-utilitarianism, in that it remains underpinned by assumptions of cardinal utility (Forget 2004). That is, health economics

> [d]evelops tools used nowhere else in the discipline [...] It measures the cardinal utility of various health states [...] [which] allow(s) economists to add up and divide utilities across interventions and people, and to engage in the kind of welfare analysis – limited to the healthcare sector – that most economists thought impossible
>
> (Forget 2004: 618).

In his analysis of utilitarianism and health economics, Dolan (2001) ascribes utilitarianism to five characteristics: consequentialism; monism; welfarism; preference satisfaction; and sum ranking, where social welfare is deduced from the aggregation of individual utilities (see also: Sen 1987). To illustrate, consider health economics evaluation employing QALYs. According to Dolan, QALYs 'satisfy' two of the five characteristics – consequentialism and monism. In addition, Dolan (2001: 74) argues that it is 'common practice to aggregate QALYs according to sum ranking', though there is nothing intrinsic in the measure that requires it. Benefits may be weighted to reflect the deservingness, or otherwise, of certain dimensions (see: Nussbaum 2000 on cost-benefit analysis). QALYs are, accordingly, consequentialist and not *necessarily* utilitarian. Yet, Dolan concedes that his taxonomy weighs each of the components equally and acknowledges that economic evaluation is frequently conflated with utilitarianism due to the tendency to employ the maximization decision rule, and from the practice that 'most' empirical studies aggregate QALYs according to sum ranking.

Thus, evaluation within health economics potentially departs from the strictures of utilitarianism, but is still consequentialist. Following both Dolan and Forget, such evaluation as 'commonly practiced' (Dolan 2001 75) embraces elements of utilitarianism. This resonates with the trajectory associated with its central tenets. Accordingly, we believe that neoclassical health economics is predicated on a value system that overlooks issues of dignity, duty, and process.

The 'toolkit' notion's mistaken conception of scientific objectivity

That scientific objectivity derives from a 'toolkit' conception of science is the famous, now widely rejected, 'view from nowhere' idea of science (Nagel 1986). The rationale behind this view is that objectivity depends on scientists being independent of their subject matter. The intuition is that practitioners can somehow 'stand outside' what they investigate. However, this is not the view that most scientists who develop tools of investigation hold – instead, assuming that objectivity in science involves a 'view from somewhere' and that scientists inevitably 'stand inside' their subject matter. For example, astronomers are able to investigate a wide range of the electromagnetic spectrum not visible to the human eye, because they have developed an apparatus of specialized telescopes designed to allow them to 'see' non-visible bands of the spectrum. They, thereby, 'see' by determining how to place themselves in a position to do so within their technologies. Consequently, *what* science sees in the world depends on *how* scientists see, where this depends on how they 'stand inside' their subject of investigation.

In health economics, this involves medical practitioners and health economists determining *what* improving health requires by focusing attention on *how* health is understood in the societies they live in – a 'view from somewhere' idea, whereby they 'stand inside' the world they investigate. Thus, to understand *what* health requires in the case of a pandemic, medical practitioners and health economists need to know *how* their strategies for combatting the problem are influenced by their public reception. This, then, requires that they understand the societies in which they live. Tools are not neutral in their effects, but get different uses depending upon who takes them up. The 'view from nowhere' and mainstream health economics 'toolkit' treat societies as monolithic and homogeneous. They develop strategies for combatting disease in a top-down way as if they work in the same way in all societies. To treat diseases such as COVID-19 requires developing technologies appropriate to the social circumstances at hand that, as in the case of the electromagnetic spectrum, make it possible to see the nature of the disease. We characterize an approach that explicitly embraces this 'view from somewhere' perspective as a political economy orientation.

Scientists, then, stand inside their subject matter, and the idea that they could stand outside them distorts their representation and impedes their investigation. The two distortions that the mainstream 'view from nowhere' health economics involves, we have emphasized, are that health economics can be value-neutral and rests on its individualist, utility-maximizing conception of economic agents. Both distortions employ abstract, 'view from nowhere', 'I' language, in contrast to contextualized, 'view from somewhere', 'we' language.

The pronouns 'I' and 'we' are used in ordinary language to represent different points of view – whether a thought or action stems from a single individual or many individuals. Sciences, however, can also represent their investigations and subject matters as stemming from a single individual perspective or from collections of individuals. The 'I' perspective ignores the diversity of views in a science, and represents theories as any single individual would always adopt – a universal 'I' idea and 'view from nowhere' conception of objectivity. It follows that disagreements cannot exist in science, and all agents must act in a utility-maximizing way – defined as 'rational' by mainstream economics. However,

> [i]n its excessive quest for generality, utility-maximizing rational choice theory fails to focus on the historically and geographically specific features of socio-economic systems. As long as such theory is confined to ahistorical generalities, then it will remain highly limited in dealing with the real world.
>
> (Hodgson 2012: 94)

Consider how sciences can also represent their investigations and subject matters as stemming from collections of individuals. A 'we' perspective recognizes that sciences are not socially monolithic and homogeneous, and that scientists have different values and relationships to their investigations and methods (see also: Boulding 1969, 1986). Their theories represent the state of understanding of a scientific community at any one time, and science is the product of how collections of people in scientific communities comprehend how 'we' understand our subjects and methods of investigation. Value differences are central to explaining the foundations on which different scientists' theories depend. It also follows there is always a diversity of ways in which agents can be understood as acting (see also: DeMartino 2022). A political economy orientation, emphasizing context, grasps both health economics itself as socially embedded and the behaviors it investigates as social relationships having many motivations.

To illustrate, consider again the notion of externalities. The mainstream account of vaccinations against infectious disease centers on individual cost-benefit calculations vis-à-vis the binary decision of being vaccinated or not. Yet, the greater the proportion of the population immunized, the less incentive for the unvaccinated to become immunized. The utility maximizer is confronted with the optimization problem *regardless* of circumstances. The only contextual distinction concerns information. With diminishing marginal utility, the assumption is that people are risk-averse. *Ceteris paribus*, a rational individual faced with a lack of information about vaccine efficacy, or risk of harm, is disinclined to accept a vaccination offer (*e.g.* Philipson 2000).

During pandemics, the externalities of individual action can be substantial. A key feature of the SARS-CoV-2 virus is its transmissibility (WHO 2021). Accordingly, COVID-19 has an exponential growth property. Over the course of the pandemic, a scientific consensus emerged that face coverings, especially in crowded or indoor spaces, significantly reduce virus transmission (*e.g.* Han *et al.* 2020; WHO 2021). The most recent Delta variant led to increased infection and transmissibility over previous variants (Centers for Disease Control and Prevention 2021). In indoor settings, without a face covering, one symptomatic person can infect many others, thereby affecting morbidity and mortality.[7] Vaccination greatly reduces, but does not eliminate, symptoms, transmissibility, and illness. This prompts three important points. First, the unintended side-effects of an individual's (in)actions over face coverings create a substantial divergence between private costs and benefits. Wearing a mask, a minor discomfort for the individual, may have an extensive social benefit. The scale of this disjuncture has not yet been explored in mainstream analyses of pandemics. Second, the mainstream account assumes that the individual is the best judge of their welfare. However, during a pandemic – defined by a substantial degree of ignorance and uncertainty – to what extent can this be assumed to remain the case? Third, individual actions with potentially significant social impacts – such as wearing masks – raise moral questions, such as social responsibility and citizenship, which resonate more with a 'we' rather than 'I' framing.

Fundamental to a 'we' perspective on health is the nature of public health. Whereas mainstream health economics is highly individualist in focusing on motivations, a political economy approach emphasizes how people in different societies interact in ways that affects their health. This insight is missing in much of the recent literature on COVID-19 built around the three analytical pillars of mainstream health economics: demand, supply, and economic evaluation. Absent is how health in a society has aggregate characteristics that necessitate understanding the mutually reinforcing nature of individual behaviors and social outcomes (Davis and McMaster 2021). Conversely, a health economics that captures this understanding must adopt a 'we' perspective on health as public health. As Longino (1990: 180) argues: '[s]cientific knowledge is social both in the ways it is created and in the uses it serves'.

Conclusions

At the outset of the chapter, we asked: is COVID-19 health economics' 'moment'? This is a complex question, in that it infers that health economics potentially provides insight into the nature of pandemics and our best responses to them. There have been valuable contributions from economists interrogating macroeconomic effects and in tracing the economic impacts of previous pandemics. Economists have also engaged epidemiologists to improve modeling and predictions. Interestingly, there appears to be a consensus that there is no trade-off between health and 'the economy'. The former, perhaps, is a prerequisite of the latter. We return to this below.

Health economics has concentrated on presenting economic evaluation as an illuminating 'toolkit', and on discussing individual behavioral responses to investigate optimal resource allocation and efficient governance (of vaccines, for example). On both counts, we find that health economics presents a very partial perspective, far from the 'objective' approach its advocates believe they portray. We demonstrated how the three pillars of mainstream health economics sculpt analysis of the ongoing pandemic. Grossman's human capital model utilizes a constrained optimization approach confined to individual utility maximizers. Far from being value-neutral, it reinforces the Cartesian dualism between mind and body. The latter is conflated with a capital 'thing', and illness resembles either a broken or a malfunctioning machine within which the utility-maximizing mind resides. The prediction that the poor have a shorter lifespan than the wealthy is unsurprising, yet the conclusion that this is a consequence of rational decision-making is unsettling. It suggests that, in the context of COVID-19, those in less secure employment and lacking adequate income are making an optimizing decision to subject themselves to greater risks of exposure by continuing to work. Social inequalities are, accordingly, merely differential constraints. Context in the form of, for example, power structures and institutional settings is only another constraint in an optimizing algorithm. This extends to the second pillar of health economics – supply. Here, a principal-agent relationship is employed to study the provision of medical care. Interdependent utility functions hint at a commonality between economic agents – patients and clinicians – suggesting a 'we' perspective. Yet, even here, 'I' continues to trump 'we'. Physicians are subject to trade-offs in their utility, and narrow financial motives can crowd out regard for others.

In general, the 'I' terminology underpinning health economics distorts the 'we' language of health, and the COVID-19 pandemic. The willingness of people to be vaccinated in much of the Global North, where vaccines are readily available, is a testament to the collective 'we' experience of the pandemic, as opposed to the narrower 'I' of the mainstream. Rather than seeing state and individual mitigations in a pandemic as trade-offs, as the mainstream account supposes, we view them as complementary. The state can and should promote a common endeavor, a shared responsibility – a 'we'. One can argue how effectively governments have reacted to the pandemic by assuming the responsibility of leadership, by countering misinformation, and by consistent messaging. Nonetheless, we believe that, in principle, a 'we' frame is far more illuminating and instructive than the 'I' frame in examining health matters.

If anything, the COVID-19 pandemic reinforces the importance of our health: health matters! The consensus among economists that there is no overarching trade-off between health and the economy, perhaps, has greater ramifications than initially seemed apparent. Grossman emphasizes that without health, the prospects of economic activity are limited. This implies that economic activity is conditional on population/public health. Yet, if the latter assumes a 'we' frame, surely it follows that the economy is similarly constituted? In their defense of conventional health economics, Parkin *et al.* (2013) invoked Adam Smith as providing the basis for 'I' in economic analysis, manifest as Max U. For us, this distorts Smith and his complex picture of human motivation, where morality and selfishness are in tension. By following an *anti*-Smithian, utilitarian route that reduces all motivation to subjective 'preferences', or 'utility', mainstream health economics holds that the value of any action rests solely on whether it promotes preferences. We believe that this is harmful to the economics of health, where moral motivation and the 'we' matter. The enduringly explosive nature of COVID-19 infection illustrates this. Smith provides a basis for studying the economy in terms of social provisioning, where interdependent individuals organize to address their material, emotional, and other needs and wants, and to socially reproduce. Accordingly, the economy is embedded in society, not the reverse. The economy, including market exchange, is part of a wider healthcare system.

Notes

1 Health economics contributes to medical decision-making through health technology, assessment and may be seen as a counterweight to industry-led attempts to maximize revenue streams from healthcare services (see: Kristiansen and Mooney 2004).

2 We follow Boulding (1986) and Power (2004) in describing social provisioning as processes in which interdependent individuals organize to address their needs and wants and to socially reproduce. Market exchange is part of this. For instance, Boulding (1986: 10) writes: 'Modern economics has gone wholly towards the view of economic life as society organized by exchange and has largely lost sense of it being a process of provisioning of the human race, or even the whole biosphere'.

3 There have been various developments and refinements of particular aspects of the model, including those relating to the depreciation of health capital, longevity and uncertainty, education and health, and the household production of health, among others (see: Zweifel 2012). Health economists regard Grossman's demand for health as pivotal to the establishment and subsequent development of the field (Lindgren 2017).

4 The QALY measure combines two dimensions: improvement (if any) in health status (quality), and expected duration of any recovery, such as treatment resulting in an increased lifespan (Dolan 2001; Round 2012).

5 Some health economists advocate nuanced employment of QALY-type measures to capture expected utility. However, this is not extended to consideration of willingness-to-pay, which may be associated with, for example, 'non-health-enhancing aspects of the process of care', which yield utility. Contingent valuation techniques, such as discrete choice experiments, are increasingly evident in the literature. These differ from QALY calculations that do not include information on/from individuals on their desire for health/healthcare, or their individual trade-off decisions, but are based on studies measuring health end-points to determine the capacity to benefit from an intervention.

6 Sweden did not follow most other European countries in imposing NPIs, opting instead for voluntary physical distancing. At the time of writing, the contraction in Swedish national income was greater than its Scandinavian neighbors and its death toll comparatively higher (*e.g.* Boyle 2021; Conyon *et al.* 2020).

7 A recent case study in the USA illustrates this. In May 2021, a symptomatic elementary school teacher infected students (12 of the 22 tested in their class) over two days of exposure. This led to secondary infections in the rest of the school and in the wider community (Lam-Hine *et al.* 2021).

References

Agüero, J.M. and Beleche, T. 2017, 'Health shocks and their long-lasting impact on health behaviors: Evidence from the 2009 H1N1 pandemic in Mexico', *Journal of Health Economics*, 54, pp. 40–55.

Appleby, J. 2020, 'Tackling COVID-19: Are the costs worth the benefits?', *British Medical Journal*, 369, p. m1496.

Arrow, K.J. 1963, 'Uncertainty and the welfare economics of medical care', *American Economic Review*, 53, pp. 941–73.

Bhattacharya, J., Hyde, T., and Tu, P. 2014, *Health Economics*, Palgrave Macmillan, Basingstoke.

Birch, S. and Gaffni, A. 2006, 'Decision rules in economic evaluation', in Jones, A.M. (ed), *The Elgar Companion to Health Economics*, Edward Elgar, Cheltenham, pp. 492–502.

Boulding, K.E. 1969, 'Economics as a moral science', *American Economic Review*, 59, pp. 1–12.

Boulding, K.E. 1986, 'What went wrong with economics?' *The American Economist*, 30, pp. 5–12.

Boyle, R.J. 2021, 'Sweden's pandemic approach: The costs of keeping the economy open during the pandemic', 8 July, accessed 14 July 2021, <https://www.northerntrust.com/united-kingdom/insights-research/2021/weekly-economic-commentary/sweden-pandemic-approach>.

Burgess, J.F. 2012, 'Productivity analysis in healthcare', in Jones, A.M. (ed), *The Elgar Companion to Health Economics*, Edward Elgar, Cheltenham, pp. 359–369.

Centers for Disease Control and Prevention 2021, 'Delta variant: What we know about the science', 11 August, accessed 30 August 2021, <https://www.cdc.gov/coronavirus/2019-ncov/variants/delta-variant.html>.

Chilton, S., Nielsen, J.S. and Wildman, J. 2020, 'Beyond COVID-19: How the "dismal science" can prepare us for the future', *Health Economics*, 29, pp. 851–3.

Conyon, M.J., He, L. and Thomsen, S. 2020, 'Lockdown and COVID-19 deaths in Scandinavia', 22 July, accessed 21 December 2021, <https://papers.ssrn.com/sol3/papers.cfm?abstract_id=3616969>.

Correia, S., Luck, S. and Verner, E. 2022, 'Pandemics depress the economy, public health interventions do not: Evidence from the 1918 flu', 22 August, accessed 28 September 2022, <https://papers.ssrn.com/sol3/papers.cfm?abstract_id=3561560>.Culyer, A.J. 1989, 'The normative economics of healthcare finance and provision', *Oxford Review of Economic Policy*, 5, pp. 34–58.

Culyer, A. and Newhouse, D. (eds) 2000, *Handbook of Health Economics* (Vols 1 and 2), Elsevier, Amsterdam.

Davis, J.B. and McMaster, R. 2017, *Health Care Economics*, Routledge, London.

Davis, J.B. and McMaster, R. 2021, A contextualist approach to health economics, 15 July, accessed 21 July 2021, <https://papers.ssrn.com/sol3/papers.cfm?abstract_id=3887616>.

DeMartino, G.F. 2022, *The Tragic Science: How Economists Cause Harm (Even as They Aspire to do Good)*, University of Chicago, Chicago.

Dolan, P. 2001, 'Utilitarianism and the measurement and aggregation of quality-adjusted life years', *Healthcare Analysis*, 9, pp. 65–76.

Douglas, M., Katikireddi, S., Taulbut, M., McKee, M. and McCartney, G. 2020, 'How can we protect against the wider health impacts of the COVID-19 pandemic response?' *British Medical Journal*, 369, p. m1557.

Drummond, M., Sculpher, M.J., Torrance, G.W., O'Brien, B.J. and Stoddart, G.L. 2005, *Methods for the Economic Evaluation of Healthcare Programmes* (Third Edition), Oxford University Press, Oxford.

Forget, E.L. 2004, 'Contested histories of an applied field: The case of health economics', *History of Political Economy*, 36, pp. 617–37.

Giannitsarou, C., Kissler, S. and Toxvaerd, F. 2021, 'Waning immunity and the second wave: Some projections for SARS-CoV-2', *American Economic Review: Insights*, 3(3), pp. 321–38.

Grossman, M. 1972, 'On the concept of health capital and the demand for health', *Journal of Political Economy*, 80, 223–55.

Han, E., Tan, M.M.J., Turk, E., Sridhar, D., Leung, G.M., Shibuya, K., Asgari, N., Oh, J., Garcia-Basterio, A.L., Hanefeld, J., Cook, A.R., Hsu, L.Y., Teo, Y.Y., Haymann, D., Clark, H., McKee, M. and Legido-Qigley, H. 2020, 'Lessons learnt from easing COVID-19 restrictions: An analysis of countries and regions in Asia-Pacific and Europe', *The Lancet* (Health Policy), 396, pp. 1525–34.

Hansen, D.G., Halvorsen, P.A. and Kristiansen, I.S. 2008, 'Willingness-to-pay for a statistical life in times of a pandemic', *Health Economics*, 17, pp. 55–66.

Harris, J.E. 1977, 'The international organization of hospitals: Some economic implications', *Bell Journal of Economics* 8(2), pp. 467–482.

Hodgson, G.M. 2012, 'On the limits of rational choice theory', *Economic Thought*, 1, pp. 94–108.

Hodgson, G.M. 2013, *From Pleasure Machines to Moral Communities: An Evolutionary Economics Without Homo Economicus*, University of Chicago Press, Chicago.

Ilzetzki, E. and Moll, B. 2020, 'Lockdowns and UK economic performance', *London School of Economics*, 25 November, accessed 1 January 2021, <https://voxeu.org/article/lockdowns-and-uk-economic-performance>.

Jones, A.M. (ed.) 2012, *The Elgar Companion to Health Economics*, Edward Elgar, Cheltenham.

Kaplan, G., Moll, B. and Violante, G.L. 2020, 'The great lockdown and the big stimulus: Tracing the pandemic possibility frontier for the US', 1 September, accessed 1 January 2021, <https://benjaminmoll.com/wp-content/uploads/2020/08/PPF.pdf>.

Keogh-Brown, M.R., Wren-Lewis, S., Edmunds, W.J., Beutels, P. and Smith, R.D. 2010, 'The possible macroeconomic impact on the UK of an influenza pandemic', *Health Economics*, 19, pp. 1345–60.

Kristiansen, I. and Mooney, G. (eds) 2004, *Evidence-Based Medicine in its Place*, Routledge, London.

Lam-Hine, T., McCurdy, S.A., Santora, L. Duncan, L., Corbett-Detig, R., Kapusinzky, B. and Wills, M. 2021, 'Outbreak Associated with SARS-CoV-2 B.1.617.2 (Delta) variant in an elementary school – Marin County, California, May-June 2021', *Morbidity and Mortality Weekly Report*, 70, pp. 1214–19.

Laxminarayan, R. and Malani, A. 2011, 'Economics of infectious diseases', in Glied, S. and Smith, P.C. (eds), *The Oxford Handbook of Health Economics*, Oxford University Press, Oxford, pp. 189–205.

Lindgren, B. 2017, 'Foreword to the 2017 edition', *The Demand for Health: A Theoretical and Empirical Investigation*, Grossman, M., Columbia University Press, New York, pp. xi–xxvi.

Longino, H. 1990, *Science as Social Knowledge: Values and Objectivity in Scientific Inquiry*, Princeton University Press, Princeton, NJ.

McCloskey, D.N. 2016, 'Max U vs. Humanomics: A critique of neo-institutionalism', *Journal of Institutional Economics,* 12, pp. 1–27

McCulley, P.A. 2009, 'The shadow banking system and Hyman Minsky's economic journey', 26 May 2009, accessed 14 July 2021, <https://www.pimco.com/en-us/insights/economic-and-market-commentary/global-central-bank-focus/the-shadow-banking-system-and-hyman-minskys-economic-journey/>.

McGuire, T.G. 2000, 'Physician agency', in Culyer, A.J. and Newhouse, J.P. (eds), *The Handbook of Health Economics*, Vol. 1A, North-Holland, Amsterdam, pp. 461–536.

McGuire, T.G. 2011, 'Physician agency and the payment for primary care', in Glied, S. and Smith, P.C. (eds), *The Oxford Handbook of Health Economics*, Oxford University Press, Oxford, pp. 602–623.

Mishkin, S.J. 1962, 'Health as an investment', *Journal of Political Economy*, 70(Part 2: Investment in Human Beings), pp. 129–57.

Mooney, G. 2009, *Challenging Health Economics*, Oxford University Press, Oxford.

Mooney, R and Ryan, M. 1993, 'Agency in health care: Getting beyond first principles', *Journal of Health Economics* 12(2), pp. 125–135.

Nagel, T. 1986, *The View from Nowhere*, Oxford University Press, Oxford.

Nussbaum, M.C. 2000, 'The costs of tragedy: Some moral limits of cost-benefit analysis', *The Journal of Legal Studies* 29(S2), pp. 1005–1036.

Parkin, D., Appleby, J. and Maynard, A. 2013, 'Economics: The biggest fraud ever perpetrated on the world? Comment', *The Lancet*, 382, 12 October, pp. e11–e15.

Peltzman, S. 1975, 'The effects of automobile safety regulations', *Journal of Political Economy*, 83, pp. 677–726.

Philipson, T.J. 1996, 'Private vaccination and public health: An empirical examination for US measles', *Journal of Human Resources*, 31, pp. 611–30.

Philipson, T.J. 2000, 'Economic epidemiology and infectious diseases', in Culyer, A.J. and Newhouse, J.P. (eds), *The Handbook of Health Economics*, Vol. 1A, North-Holland, Amsterdam, pp. 1761–1799.

Power, M. 2004, 'Social provisioning as a starting point for feminist economics', *Feminist Economics*, 10, pp. 3–19.

Reicher, S. 2021, 'Whatever Johnson says, we can't defeat COVID with "personal responsibility" alone', *The Guardian*, 6 July, accessed 14 July 2021, <https://www.theguardian.com/commentisfree/2021/jul/06/boris-johnson-policy-pandemic-restrictions>.

Rice, T. 2012, 'The physician as the patient's agent', in Jones, A.M. (ed), *The Elgar Companion to Health Economics*, Edward Elgar, Cheltenham, pp. 271–279.

Round, J. 2012, 'Is a QALY still a QALY at the end of life?' *Journal of Health Economics*, 31, pp. 521–7.

Sen, A. 1987, *On Ethics and Economics*, Blackwell, Oxford.

Soares, R.R. 2015, 'Gary Becker's contributions to health economics', *Journal of Demographic Economics*, 81, pp. 51–7.

Williams, A. 1998, 'If we are going to get a fair innings, someone will need to keep the score!' in Barer, M., Getzen, T. and Stoddart, G. (eds), *Health, Healthcare and Health Economics*, Wiley, New York, pp. 319–330.

World Health Organization. 2021, 'Coronavirus disease: Advice for the public', December, accessed 1 January 2022, <https://www.who.int/emergencies/diseases/novel-coronavirus-2019/advice-for-public/when-and-how-to-use-masks>.

Yates, T. 2020, 'Without joined up thinking about COVID and the economy, Britain is just guessing', 30 September, accessed 14 July 2021, <https://www.theguardian.com/commentisfree/2020/sep/30/covid-economy-britain-guessing-eat-out-policy>.

Zweifel, P. 2012, 'The Grossman model after 40 years', *European Journal of Health Economics*, 13, pp. 677–82.

3

THE ECONOMICS OF CONVENTIONS AND HEALTHCARE

Philippe Batifoulier and Nicolas Da Silva

Without adequate health, it is difficult, if not impossible, to participate in socio-economic and democratic life. The COVID-19 crisis has served as a potent reminder of the exceptional nature of health in this regard. As exemplified by the temporary stay-at-home strategies implemented by governments around the world, the threat posed by the SARS-CoV-2 virus to citizens' health led to the suspension of large segments of economic and social life. For neoclassical economists and many political figures, public health measures such as lockdowns constituted a utilitarian calculation, in which governments were compelled to choose between economic activity and health or, at least, determine an equilibrium point between these objectives (*e.g.* Gourinchas 2020; WSJ Editorial Board 2020). That is, this formulation assumed a trade-off between health and economy: while stay-at-home orders were acknowledged as potentially able to flatten COVID mortality and morbidity curves, they could only do so at the cost of simultaneously undermining economic growth and potentially sending the economy into recession. Neoclassical economics thereby reduced potentially countless courses of political measures to a delimited range of choices, which were then to be weighed against each other, while also acceding to utilitarianism as the only possible ethical standard for evaluating such actions (Eyal 2020).

This particular case illustrates a broader normative problem underpinning neoclassical economics: namely, the manner in which it rarely seeks to question the type of economy or economic policy that would best protect population health. Instead, the tradition engages in a form of economization (Çalişkan and Callon 2009), whereby 'activities, behaviors and spheres or fields are established as being economic' (Çalişkan and Callon 2009: 370). Specifically, neoclassical economics advances the rational and individualistic figure of *Homo Economicus* to all spheres of socio-economic life to frame them as amenable to the foundational neoclassical problem: how to maximize the utility of a given actor under a given set of constraints. In this formulation, both humans and institutional agencies are comprehended as rational business units, which evaluate costs against benefits and, accordingly, compute decisions with an eye to maximizing their self-interest (Brown 2015).

While the extension of this economistic logic to many areas of socio-economic life has been problematic, health is perhaps the sphere in which this transposition is most inconsistent and ethically problematic. In particular, this is because lives are not reducible to prices. Moreover, if there is a pecuniary cost, it is that of health protection – without which economic activity is vulnerable.

DOI: 10.4324/9781003017110-4

For instance, if an economistic metric had been deployed in a manner similar to that applied during the COVID-19 pandemic, the systems of social protection implemented in France in 1945 – the welfare systems designed to protect citizens against the financial consequences of social risks, such as those arising from illness, maternity, and old age – would not have existed in a country ruined by war. This is the case with many social protection systems around the world. It was the ethical imperative to protect health itself that triggered the state to finance pervasive access to care and allowed the population to benefit from medical discoveries (such as penicillin).

In contrast to the prevailing neoclassical tradition, political-economic analysis articulates a markedly different conceptual framework with which to comprehend and evaluate health and healthcare systems. Accordingly, the present chapter makes the case that both are guided by competing values, rather than reducible to the economistic logic of the market alone. These values are not individual preferences but, rather, are collectively held by multifarious actors and social groups. Moreover, such values do not function as external constraints or exogenously given drivers of social activity in a particular situation. Instead, they are endogenous to the coordination processes between actors and, thus, can be associated with the concept of *conventions* – that is collective representations that guide the judgment of individuals (Favereau 1985). Departing from the neoclassical tradition, we make the case that actors do not make decisions on the basis of rational self-interest, but do so in situations of uncertainty on the basis of conventions. In articulating this case, we rely on the conceptual framework of the French school of the 'economics of conventions' (EoC) (Boltanski and Thevenot 2006; Diaz-Bone and Favereau 2019), which allows us to consider healthcare and health policy as strongly normative issues. Critical political-economic analysis cannot ignore the latter because health is a domain in which a plurality of social values, habits, deontological and professional rules, and ethics are omnipresent and, when codified as conventions, function to determine the social direction of health processes.

Hence, in this chapter, we present a political economy of health that takes seriously the plurality of values in healthcare. This articulation is developed across two parts. In the first, we examine the EoC tradition from its origins to its development in the field of healthcare. In the second, based on a discussion on the concepts of marketization and industrialization, we propose a conventionalist way of thinking about neoliberal policy in healthcare and health in capitalism.

From mainstream health economics to the economics of conventions

The French institutionalist approach of the EoC constitutes a transdisciplinary movement in the social sciences. Health issues are some of the most actively researched topics in the tradition, which addresses a wide range of topics such as professional ethics, doctor-patient interaction, health democracy, inequalities, industrialization, funding priorities, health insurance, hospital management, liberal medicine, digitization and quantification of health, and health capitalism (Batifoulier 1992; Batifoulier and Diaz-Bone 2021; Batifoulier 2022). In examining these matters, the EoC explicitly challenges mainstream health economics by comprehending health itself as an irreducibly social phenomenon: providing a theory of the plurality of values that are mobilized during patient-doctor encounters, as well as during the formulation and implementation of health-related policies. The EoC in the field of healthcare has also expanded conceptions of normativity to propose a finer mapping of coordination and regulation processes. To elucidate these insights, the first section below reviews the EoC's primary conceptual acumen, derived primarily from Keynesian economics and Boltanski and Thevenot's (2006) pragmatic sociology. The second section then contrasts the subjective figure of *Homo Economicus* populating neoclassical economics with the *Homo Conventionalist* underpinning the EoC in order to demonstrate the plurality of values marking healthcare and their implications for the tradition. In doing so, we rely first on Arrow's recognition of the fundamental role of social conventions in healthcare, and then on the concept of 'order of worth' to understand the diversity of values informing the healthcare field.

The economics of conventions: conceptualizing a plurality of values

The EoC constitutes a conceptual tradition that explores the significance of judgments made by individuals in their social interactions with others (Desrosières 2011). In this respect, the tradition develops an intuition initially formulated by Keynes in Chapter 12 of his *General Theory* (2007 [1936]). For Keynes, unemployment arises due to deficient effective demand, which is chiefly composed of investment by firms. If interest rates are high, investment will correspondingly be low, which has pernicious repercussions for employment. For Keynes, however, interest rates are largely determined by behavior in financial markets by speculators and other investors who share a common expectation about the state of economic affairs. In turn, Keynes' thesis is that these investors' evaluation of future returns on their investment is based on a 'pure convention'. This reasoning is illustrated by Keynes' famous analogy of a newspaper beauty contest, in which entrants are asked to select the six most attractive faces from a large group of photographs, with those picking the most popular faces then eligible for a prize. Rather than choosing the face that s/he believes is most beautiful, Keynes argued that participants wishing to maximize their chances of winning a prize would consider common perceptions of attractiveness, and then make their selections based on this inference from their knowledge of public perception. Assuming that each participant adopts similar reasoning, then a convention is held to stabilize expectations among all entrants.

In this respect, conventions are effective means of coordinating human activities that produce social order. However, even if they can sometimes be explicitly identified, there is no established formulation of a convention. Its genesis is often unknown and, if not, knowledge of its history has no effect on its application. Moreover, a convention is arbitrary in the sense that there are other ways of coordinating behaviors (Favereau 1995). This arbitrariness, like the vagueness of the definition, is not an obstacle to its application, even if compliance with the convention is not supported by legal sanctions. From the small decisions of everyday life and the conventions of the language studied by the philosopher David Lewis (1969), to larger economic decisions, one cannot coordinate his or her behavior with that of another person without having any idea of the collective of which they are both constitutive.

Since the way of judging (others, the situation, oneself in the situation) is not unique but plural, coordination cannot be defined as a given (or a law) of nature. The notion of convention, thus, serves as a support to denaturalize coordination, and to put forward a plurality of values that guide the judgments of individuals. Therefore, coordination cannot be conceived without the constraint of legitimacy. Individuals decide, conform, or denounce the rules according to their preconceived representation of acceptable behavior. There is no coordination of behavior without coordination of *representations* of behavior. This analysis leads to a conception of institutions defined as a set of rules that are always interpreted by a convention. It is, thus, conventions that confer consistency to institutions.

These conventions are normative references. There are not as many normative references as there are persons; otherwise, we would fall back into the world of preferences underpinning neoclassical economics. Instead, there are a small number of shared references that can be called conventions, which are shared representations held by a collective. One of the gains made by the EoC, in this respect, is to have highlighted a diversity of representations. Boltanski and Thévenot (2006), for instance, identify six conventions or 'orders of worth' (*ordre de grandeur*), which constitute organized principles of evaluation and are linked to political philosophies. Each of these conventions is directed toward a particular expression of justice or the common good, including a particular 'principle of evaluation' or justificatory regime. The theory focuses on the plurality of forms of justice.

This framework of orders of justification was developed to understand when a conception of the common good, based on one principle of justification, is criticized according to criteria based on another. According to the 'civic order of worth' (or civic convention), for example, all individuals should have access to human rights to promote the general interest. The 'market order', in contrast, endorses everyone to behave as an agent of the market to improve wealth creation (Boltanski and Thévenot 2006). Yet, such orders are not restricted to this dichotomy between market and general interest. Other orders of worth matter, such as the 'industrial order' (increasing efficiency and expertise), or the 'domestic' order of worth (doing good for family and relatives). According to Boltanski and Thévenot (2006), these orders of worth are linked to political philosophies: Rousseau for the civic order, Smith for the market order, Saint Simon for the industrial order, and Bossuet for the domestic order.

For the EoC, to justify and develop itself, the market order needs to refer to values. It has normative foundations. Conversely, criticizing the development of the market order in healthcare is also based on values and relies on other conventions. It is this dynamic of justification and criticism that underpins health systems, which is why values are regarded as the basic institutional foundations to be comprehended when studying the specific plurality of these systems' empirical normative realities. The EoC studies the tensions between several normative orders as one of the driving forces of institutions and social processes. With this conceptual framework in mind, we are able to take into account the plurality of possible representations of health and healthcare, and the concomitant impossibility of reducing these to a universal and invariable conception, as presented within mainstream health economics.

From Arrow's critique to health economics of conventions

The EoC offers a fruitful conceptual approach to challenge neoclassical analyses. This is particularly the case in the field of health economics. One can usefully recall the reflection of Mark Blaug (1998: S65) that 'health economics would seem to be a perfect topic for heterodox dissent' and 'is a field which must make the average neoclassical economist squirm because it challenges his or her standard assumptions at every turn'. This is reminiscent of Kenneth Arrow's (1963: 949) prior deliberation on the limits of neoclassical theory for analyzing healthcare, in which he observes that the doctor is not a 'barber':

> It is clear from everyday observation that the behavior expected of sellers of medical care is different from that of business men [*sic*] in general. These expectations are relevant because medical care belongs to the category of commodities for which the product and the activity of production are identical. In all such cases, the customer cannot test the product before consuming it, and there is an element of trust in the relation. But the ethically understood restrictions on the activities of a physician are much more severe than on those of, say, a barber. His behavior is supposed to be governed by a concern for the customer's welfare which would not be expected of a salesman. In Talcott Parsons's terms, there is a 'collectivity-orientation,' which distinguishes medicine and other professions from business, where self-interest on the part of participants is the accepted norm.

In this excerpt, Arrow insists on two characteristics that are important for understanding the activity of doctors and, more broadly, of health professionals. On the one hand, the activity of healthcare is a service and not a product, which is why it is impossible to test the product before consuming it. Healthcare is a trust good and/or an experience good. On the other hand, Arrow insists on the ethical dimension of healthcare activity: professionals cannot simply act to maximize his or her personal interest. The activity of healthcare involves a 'collectivity-orientation'. The challenge for the economist, then, is to understand which values go beyond the pursuit of individual interest and guide behavior. What are the values that structure the world of healthcare?

Mainstream health economics does not ignore the issue of medical ethics (and, more generally, the role of values in the health system). However, it conceptualizes ethical rules as merely means to satisfy the self-interests of doctors. From this perspective, the patient, just like profit or leisure, is an object that can increase or decrease the utility of doctors. Medical ethics, accordingly, is reduced to an internalization of the utility function of patients into the utility function of doctors. The resulting 'caring externality' is a special type of market externality, in which altruism and ethics are conflated (Davis and McMaster 2017). As argued by Bloche (2001: 1100):

> Health economists admire Arrow's article for its path-breaking analysis of market failure resulting from information asymmetry, uncertainty and moral hazard. But his suggestion that anticompetitive professional norms can compensate for the market failures is at odds with economists' more typical treatment of professional norms as monopolistic constraints on contractual possibility.

Davis and McMaster (2007) and Batifoulier and Da Silva (2014) have demonstrated the paradox, contradictions, and absurdity of this strategy, which is based on a dogmatic position about values, conceiving of the doctor as comparable to the figure of *Homo Economicus* deployed by neoclassical economics to comprehend all other economic processes. The introduction of ethics in the utility function of the physician leads to contradictory public policy recommendations: should economic incentives be used for the doctor and the 'barber'?

More heterodox health economists, in contrast, seek to introduce a more non-instrumental conception of values into their analyses (Hodgson 2009). Specifically, the EoC seeks to address the political dimension of health systems through explicitly considering the plurality of values in healthcare. Healthcare is heavily value-laden, and accordingly, we need a theory to understand both the importance and plurality of these values. Mainstream economics is not free from values, though its values are only consistent with the promotion of efficiency and individual responsibility, and recognition of individual sovereignty, based on the notion of the utility-maximizing individual. To understand that values in healthcare are not reducible to that of individual self-interest, the EoC has articulated a notion of convention as a social and collective representation. Provision of healthcare, in turn, is a matter of confronting different sets of values – both in theory and in practice.

Specifically, there is an incongruity between different ways of providing healthcare, which can be understood through the notion of convention. From this perspective, conventionalist approaches to healthcare attempt to clarify what constitutes a 'good' doctor, 'good' care, a 'good' hospital, a 'good' health funding system, or how to determine and set priorities in healthcare (for different applications, see: Batifoulier and Diaz-Bone 2021). Table 3.1 summarizes different normative conceptions in healthcare. It shows that health cannot be reduced to a single normative conception, where the only legitimate values are those of efficiency, competition, self-interest, and individual sovereignty. Instead, several competing sets of values, or conventions, exist.

In the table above, a distinction is made between six orders of worth or convention, which are defined by a 'higher common principle' based on the values held by individuals in this particular

Table 3.1 Plurality of orders of worth in healthcare

Order of worth	*Higher common principle*	*Qualified healthcare*	*Qualified policy in healthcare*	*Important persons in healthcare*
Market	- Competition - Self-interest	- Commodification - Market competitiveness	- Free market	- Consumers
Civic	- General will - Collective action	- Collective welfare - Solidarity	- Welfare policy - Solidarity union	- Public communities - Representatives
Industrial	- Efficiency - Performance	- Technical efficiency	- Industrialization of medicine	- Experts - 'Welfare elite'
Domestic	- Proximity, - Neighborhood - Tradition	- Reputation - Trustworthiness	- Family doctor - Regular physician	- Relatives - Chain of personal dependencies
Frame	- Popularity - Audience - Public recognition	- Passion - Enthusiasm	- Promotion of notoriety and celebrity - Charismatic	- People with signs of public esteem
Inspired	- Imagination - Inspiration	- Innovation - Creativity	- Medical research policy	- Medical scientist - Researcher

order of worth. There is no single order of worth linked to a healthcare sphere, but a set of multiple orders. For this reason, health is not considered as a specific order of worth or an autonomous sphere of justice. In any situation, the orders of worth can be equally invoked as moral arguments to legitimize or criticize healthcare.

Each order of worth sustains a specific set of qualified things (objects and policy) in order to build a coherent common world, in which particular qualities are attributed. There is a plurality of values acting as a conception of what is 'good' in healthcare. For instance, a diploma or degree in medicine, and all the associated policies of certification and accreditation belong to the industrial order of worth and are supports that confer legitimacy on the quality of a medical or surgical act. In the market order of worth, in contrast, we focus more on pecuniary concerns so that determining whether a given medical procedure constitutes 'value for money' is prioritized when reflecting on its standing.

Extending Boltanski and Thévenot (2006) to study welfare state, the Welfare Conventions Approach (WCA) introduces another set of conventions, such as the philanthropic convention (emphasizing the moral duty to help the most vulnerable), the Fordist convention (full employment), or the entrepreneurial convention (to turn everyone into an entrepreneur). The aim is to consider the 'governmentality' of welfare as disputes (Rose and Miller 1992). Welfare (and health policy) is a matter of disagreement that can be traced to such welfare conventions.[1] Drawing inspiration from the WCA, the remainder of this chapter conceptualizes health policies as moral disputes between 'orders of worth' (Hanrieder 2016; Batifoulier *et al.* 2019).

Health policy under neoliberalism

Based on the preceding account, this section contends that the EoC provides the basis for an original perspective on healthcare systems and health policies through its focus on the confrontation between multiple principles of justice. Specifically, we show how this theoretical approach analyzes the changing character of health and healthcare processes that have prevailed during the neoliberal era since the late-1970s. After discussing the phenomena of marketization and industrialization in healthcare, we then demonstrate how the neoliberal transformation of values in the field of healthcare has precipitated the development of a novel form of health capitalism.

Marketization and industrialization of healthcare

After the Second World War, healthcare systems were constructed in opposition to market logic. In most OECD countries, the consequences of the War reinforced the tendency toward public organization of healthcare – either by the state itself or through professional organizations. The priority was to extend access to healthcare by citizens in a civic convention driven by the injunction of solidarity. Concurrently, healthcare professionals (doctors and others) benefited from the growth of the healthcare sector – not only through higher incomes, but also through greater freedom in the structure of their work. Since the late-1970s, however, public policy has changed its objective and, under the influence of neoliberal ideology, began to favor the marketization and industrialization of care – orders of worth that subsequently became dominant.

The marketization of healthcare is a phenomenon widely considered in the academic literature. In all countries, states have institutionalized economic incentives to modify the behavior of healthcare actors (professionals, patients, insurers, manufacturers, and so forth). Whether on the supply or demand side, where solidarity once prevailed, the market order of worth now predominates (Saltman 2002; Maarse 2006; André *et al.* 2016). This process can take many forms and does not only refer to the transition of public property to private property. The state can privatize certain sectors of healthcare – for example by selling public hospitals to private companies – but it can also introduce market logics into the public service. This has been manifest, for instance, in the corporatization of public hospitals, whereby competition and efficiency have been codified as the primary yardsticks for determining their operating procedures (Simonet and Katsos 2020). Privatization also concerns the financing of healthcare: in many countries, the share of public financing is decreasing in favor of private financing (households and private insurance) (*e.g.* Duckett 2020).

Such transformations have been implemented not merely to reduce public spending, but also to reflect a particular conception of 'good' care – understood as being delivered most efficiently and effectively by commercial institutions. While marketization policies may have clashed, and still clash, with the ethics of many health professionals and values of patients, they have gradually contributed over the years to modifying the values of these actors (Monneraud 2009). Recalling Arrow's metaphor from above, even if a doctor is not a barber, s/he tends to become one. If the patient is not a consumer, s/he tends to become one. From this perspective, commodification is not a rationalization: it is one principle of justice among others. According to the EoC, to posit that the market convention dominates is not to suggest that it is the only possible convention. There are many other, equally legitimate forms. Therefore, the dominant position of a convention is not a matter of legitimacy *per se*, but rather reflects the operation of power has having previously established its hegemonic position. That is, a convention does not prevail because it is supposedly more 'legitimate', but because it was supported and entrenched by powerful political-economic actors (Batifoulier *et al.* 2019; Vahabi *et al.* 2020).

In addition to marketization, the evolution of health systems during the neoliberal period has been characterized by the industrialization of healthcare (Da Silva 2021, 2022). The quality of healthcare provided by professionals is not an objective datum, but depends on how 'good' care is understood by individuals and within society more broadly. In other words, there is a plurality of conventions of 'quality' healthcare. The health professions (and in particular doctors) have been built around the necessary autonomy of professionals in patient-caregiver relationships

(Freidson 1988). Patients expressing a distinctive need must be cared for by professionals capable of understanding this singularity and adapting their knowledge to each case. Following Boltanski and Thévenot, a 'good' doctor is one who cultivates a close relationship with her/his patient (domestic convention) and who is capable of creativity and innovation (inspired convention). This inspired/domestic convention of quality of healthcare was at the heart of the development of post-war health systems.

However, from the 1970s, this convention of quality of healthcare was criticized on multiple grounds. First, the criticism of medical autonomy was challenged by patients themselves in a movement against medical paternalism (Barbot and Dodier 2002). Historically, while physicians enjoyed significant power over patients (high asymmetric information), with the development of chronic diseases like AIDS, patients have begun to inform themselves and challenge medical power. The resulting patient empowerment has engendered a reduction in the autonomy of physicians in their work. Second, in the context of the unprecedented development of medical knowledge production, evidence-based medicine contributed to relativizing the place of the physician in the provision of healthcare. It is a method of prioritizing medical knowledge that places the randomized clinical trial at the top of the hierarchy (Sackett *et al.* 1996). In other words, there has been a deepening of the division of medical labor. Third, the development of new public management and mainstream health economics has led to critical reflections on the autonomy of health professionals in their activity.

Such criticisms collectively inspired health system reform and contributed to the development of another convention of healthcare quality: the industrial convention. According to this convention, proximity to the patient and creativity are not qualities but defects. The 'good' healthcare professional must not adapt to the unique circumstances or distinctiveness of the patient; instead, they should apply impersonal guidelines.[2] This transformation has required the reform of healthcare institutions. It implies the organization of medical research grounded in evidence-based medicine to produce generalizable standards; certification and dissemination of these standards by health agencies; information systems capable of shedding light on the 'black box' of patient-caregiver relationships; incentives that encourage the adoption of these standards; and sanctions for deviant practices. Table 3.2 summarizes the differences between the industrial convention in healthcare and the inspired/domestic convention (Da Silva 2022).

Transformations in the methods of funding providers are probably the easiest way to understand the current hegemony of the industrial convention in healthcare. In hospitals and primary care services, the major health systems have introduced incentives based on an industrial conception of the quality of care. The promotion of pay-for-performance schemes in primary care is exemplary here. The objective of this method of remuneration is to circumvent asymmetries of information between patient and doctor by remunerating doctors according to a quantifiable productivity indicator. The 'Quality Outcome Framework' in Great Britain and the 'Remuneration on public health objectives' in France are striking examples (Roland and Guthrie 2016). In hospitals, the introduction of diagnostic-related groups works on a similar principle (Fetter 1980). In this instance, healthcare activities defined *a priori* as particular and incommensurable with others are grouped under homogeneous categories in order to modify the pricing methods of provider establishments. In both cases, quality of care is no longer defined as the adaptation of the professional to the health needs of patients, but as the application of a protocol defined beforehand for each type of patient. Quality is no longer concerned with proximity and inspiration, but is primarily oriented around performance. Such industrialization trends concern not only hospitals and primary care, but also the entire healthcare and care sector: nursing, nursing homes, home services (disability and aging), and telemedicine and the digitalization of health (for a survey, see: Da Silva 2022).

Table 3.2 Two conventions of quality of healthcare labor

	Inspired/domestic convention	*Industrial convention*
Definition of disease	Qualitative break with the normal state	Quantitative break with the normal state
Subject of the activity	Patient/disease pair	Disease
Problem of healthcare to be solved	Distinctiveness and complexity	Heterogeneity of practices
Subject of healthcare	Individual patient	Average patient
Specificity of knowledge	Based on experience	Based on standards
Task of professionals	Adapt to the case	Assign cases
Definition of quality	Professional	Evidence-based medicine
Professional ethics	Act on behalf of the patient	Act in accordance with standards
Institution of trust	Professional ethics	Certification agencies

Values and the development of health capitalism

This industrial vision of quality has buttressed reform of hospitals in Western countries around the establishment of activity-based pricing and, more broadly, so-called 'new public management' reforms. Industrialization also accords with a market order for which care must be cost-effective. So, a 'good' doctor in a 'good' hospital should be both a skilled doctor and a professional who procures funds for the institution.

However, there are other definitions of what constitutes 'good' care, each of which is equally legitimate because they are linked to other orders of worth. Patients value the 'domestic order of worth', where healthcare is accessible with a quick medical appointment. Patients also value doctors available in proximity to their home. In many ways, patients thereby repudiate the domination of a market-industrial convention. However, neoliberal policies prioritize this order of worth by defining what is more and less valuable. This power of valorization (Eymard-Duvernay 2016) is crucial to understand contemporary healthcare reforms. Power is here associated with the ability to rank values. One convention can dominate another, but not in the sense of legitimacy because all conventions are equally legitimate. It is the actors who promulgate the market-industrial convention that are dominant, rather than the convention in itself.

Against the domination of the market-industrial convention, during the COVID-19 crisis, caregivers often promoted other values and sought to recapture power by removing the hospital managers whose role was to force health professionals to adapt their work to industrial logic. In the name of the health imperative and general interest (civic convention), the force of tradition (domestic convention), and the imagination in power (inspired convention), they organized measures to combat the prevailing shortage of personnel, masks, and respirators that hindered effective public health responses to the pandemic. Medical practices have also been transformed to adapt to the influx of patients, such as through new ways of working (*e.g.* telemedicine), or through total dedication to medical work by choosing to live apart from one's family.

A broader appeal to a plurality of values has also emerged from the crisis. The pandemic revealed how criticism of the market-industrial status quo, formed on the basis of a plurality of alternative healthcare values, could disrupt the normal course of business to the point of temporarily halting economic activity. Nevertheless, the appropriation of such critical reflections is the basis of the new dynamics of capitalism. The EoC offers an important conceptual framework through which to comprehend this dynamic.

Capitalism indisputably damages health. The unemployment, poverty, and economic insecurity engendered by capitalism impact on health (Freudenberg 2021). Unequal societies are also a cause of health deprivation (Wilkinson and Pickett 2010). More broadly, all the failures of capitalism can be interpreted in terms of deteriorating health: bodies bear the scars of the contradictory dynamics of the system (Marya and Patel 2021). Accordingly, in order to preserve population health, capitalism should be destabilized. Yet, capitalism remains resilient and even continues to expand more deeply into health processes through the actions of private insurers, for-profit hospitals, the corporate healthcare industry, and pharmaceutical firms that commodify healthcare to make a profit. This was grossly exemplified during the COVID-19 pandemic, which not only caused suffering, death, bankruptcy, and unemployment for many, but has also produced a small number of new billionaires and further augmented the wealth of many existing billionaires (Popcevski 2022).

The EoC helps to explain why capitalism continues to survive and thrive in this manner, without ignoring the myriad critical reflections leveled against the system. Indeed, conventions (order of worth) are not only resources of justification, but also supports for criticism. As the conventionalist analysis of Boltanski and Chiapello (2005) has shown, capitalism needs criticism and enemies in order to renew itself. It endogenizes certain critical reflections, as well as some of the values and normative principles they express, to transform itself and quash visions of the system as detrimental to health. For instance, the centrality of healthcare values offers a new vector of development for capitalism, which seeks to disarm arguments that the economic activities of corporate and other for-profit actors are harmful to health via an ideology that justifies further engagement with the system. This ideology offers attractive life prospects and not just material benefits. Health is essential for a 'good life'. Therefore, capitalism now promises a healthy life that can save people from diseases and epidemics, such that securing this objective necessitates reinforcing and supporting the system. Underpinning this logic is a form of 'healthism' (Conrad 1992), in which health is equated with the 'value of values', an allegory of all that is good in life. Initially associated with the medicalization of society, healthism in the language of capitalism relies on the cult of the healthy body to change human behavior by elevating (capitalist-led) health to a central value.

The resulting novel focus on health within the system has sought to generate new ways of life to promote the well-being of citizens. Health capitalism must generate increased quality of life and life expectancy – with recent trends in transhumanism constituting the culmination of a general tendency of the system when it is interested in health issues (Thomas 2022). In the context of reclaiming the centrality of health, the pharmaceutical industry, for-profit hospitals, and health insurance have promoted entrepreneurial behavior, less as a means to heal disease than to heal *life* itself. By relying on perfect health as an 'ethical compass', health capitalism seeks not only to repair a dysfunction and make the disease disappear, but also to propose new life habits and lifestyle conditions to everyone. This logic then infuses all aspects of socio-economic life: technological innovation, digitalization and the internet of things, the business of well-being in companies and stress management, the support of sports activities as a way of surpassing oneself, and the protection of the environment to preserve human health (Cooper 2008).

This health-based capitalism is oriented around patient empowerment and makes citizens market players. Yet, it affords no place for the reduction of inequalities. The narrative of 'good health' targets the richest and the most worried with the concern of the healthy body. That is, this recentralization of health is oriented toward those most receptive to messages of well-being, and to the maintenance of their health capital and the healthy body – namely, the wealthiest and most privileged segments of the population. The pool of potential customers for these new markets is, therefore, smaller but more consumer-oriented. The objective is not to maximize the number of customers, but to deepen the demand of *certain* consumers through meeting their need for personalization and distinctiveness. The business model is based on high prices for those who can afford to pay higher costs for additional quality, and who benefit from products that are not accessible to everyone. Accordingly, this narrative is far removed from the struggle against social inequalities in health (Žižek 2018).

Conclusion

Because patients and doctors are *a priori* conceived as *Homo Economicus*, neoclassical economics holds that they must be made responsible in the only effective way: via financial incentives that will activate their self-interest. However, with regard to health, patients are a long way removed from this abstract figure, who has no problems of birth and survival or of passions associated with fear of illness and death, because s/he is immortal. Simultaneously, while doctors are, of course, sometimes able to act in an opportunistic manner, medical ethics is more than a means to satisfy their self-interest. Morality, social values and professional ethics are central to the health sector. Unlike neoclassical economics, the political economy of health and healthcare acknowledges such values as inherent to economic analysis and seeks to analyze their plural forms and performative implications in practice.

In this chapter, we have examined how the French school of the EoC accords importance to the plurality of these values in order to consider different normative conceptions of health and healthcare. Accordingly, a value-free analysis of health policy is unfeasible. In practice, the EoC examination of a plurality of values is not only a means to criticize neoliberalism. It is also a way to understand its expansion in health and healthcare processes, because neoliberal policy also requires moral justifications. Debating about the political economy of health is, thus, not analogous to deliberating on any other economic practice. Of course, health is an important part of financialized capitalism. Yet, health can also generate new ways of life that attempt to secure the well-being of citizens.

The conventionalist approach illuminates this reflection in two ways. First, contemporary forms of health capitalism involve competing conceptions of the common good that can be analyzed with the pluralist framework of the EoC to comprehend its several orders of justification (market order, industrial order, domestic order, and so forth). Second, health constitutes a new spirit of capitalism, supported by a novel moral reasoning. Emphasizing concern for the self and the healthy body, the affirmation of health as 'good in itself' shows that capitalism cannot evolve without integrating the claim for good health. Yet, the system can only do so in limited and contradictory ways that, in turn, remain oriented around advancing the interests of a wealthy and powerful minority. The EoC, thereby, provides a powerful means for comprehending the conventions legitimizing capitalism, while pointing to the need to transcend its political-economic confines in order to secure broader health and healthcare objectives.

Notes

1 Similarly, the work of Chiapello and Knoll (2020) seeks to disentangle the diverse rationalities that give social problems their particular form, and offers ways to frame social problems through identifying dedicated causes and solutions.

2 Evidence suggests that health professionals regret having to treat diseases rather than patients, which leads to the promotion of evidence-based medicine rather than patient-centered medicine (Bensing 2000).

References

André, C., Batifoulier, P., and Jansen-Ferreira, M. 2016, 'Healthcare privatization processes in Europe: Theoretical justifications and empirical classification', *International Social Security Review*, 69(1), pp. 3–23.

Arrow, K.J. 1963, 'Uncertainty and the welfare economics of medical care', *American Economic Review*, 53(5), pp. 941–73.

Barbot, J, and Dodier, N. 2002, 'Multiplicity in scientific medicine: The experience of HIV-positive patients', *Science, Technology, and Human Values*, 27, pp. 404–40.

Batifoulier, P. 1992. 'Le rôle des conventions dans le système de santé', *Sciences Sociales et Santé*, 10(1), pp. 5–44.

Batifoulier, P. 2022, 'Health, conventions and society', in Diaz-Bone, R. and de Larquier, G. (eds), *Handbook of Economics and Sociology of Conventions*, Springer, Berlin, pp. 1–23.

Batifoulier, P. and Da Silva, N. 2014, 'Medical altruism in mainstream health economics: Theoretical and political paradoxes', *Review of Social Economy*, 72(3), pp. 261–79.

Batifoulier, P., Da Silva, N. and Duchesne, V. 2019, 'The dynamics of conventions: The case of the French Social Security System', *Historical Social Research*, 44(1), pp. 258–84.

Batifoulier, P. and Diaz-Bone, R. (eds) 2021, 'Conventions, health and society – Convention theory as an institutionalist approach to the political economy of health', *Historical Social Research*, Special issue 46(1).

Bensing, J. 2000, 'Bridging the gap: The separate worlds of evidence-based medicine and patient-centered medicine', *Patient Education and Counseling*, 39, pp. 17–25.

Blaug, M. 1998, 'Where are we now in British health economics?' *Health Economics*, 7(S1), pp. S63–78

Bloche, M.G. 2001, 'The market for medical ethics', *Journal of Health Politics, Policy and Law,* 26(5), pp. 1099–112.

Boltanski, L. and Chiapello, E. 2005, *The New Spirit of Capitalism*, Verso, New York.

Boltanski, L. and Thévenot, L. 2006, *On Justification: Economies of Worth*, Princeton University Press, New Jersey.Brown, W. 2015, *Undoing the Demos: Neoliberalism's Stealth Revolution*, Zone Books, New York.

Çalışkan, K. and Callon, M. 2009, 'Economization, part 1: Shifting attention from the economy towards process of economization', *Economy and Society*, 38(3), pp. 369–98.

Chiapello, E. and Knoll, L. 2020, 'The welfare conventions approach: A comparative perspective on social impact bonds', *Journal of Comparative Policy Analysis: Research and Practice*, 22(2), pp. 100-15.

Conrad, P. 1992, 'Medicalization and social control', *Annual Review of Sociology*, 18, pp. 209–32.

Cooper, M. 2008, *Life as Surplus: Biotechnology and Capitalism in the Neoliberal Era*, University of Washington Press, Seattle.

Da Silva, N. 2021, 'The industrialization of "liberal medicine" in France: A labor quality conventions approach', *Historical Social Research*, 46(1), pp. 85–111.

Da Silva, N. 2022, 'The industrialization of healthcare and its critics', in Diaz-Bone, R. and de Larquier, G. (eds), *Handbook of Economics and Sociology of Conventions*, Springer, Berlin, pp. 1–25.

Davis, J. and McMaster, R. 2007, 'The individual in mainstream health economics: A case of persona non-grata', *Healthcare Analysis,* 15(3), pp. 95–210.

Davis, J. and McMaster, R. 2017, *Healthcare Economics*, Routledge, New York.

Desrosières, A. 2011, 'The economics of convention and statistics: the paradox of origins', *Historical Social Research*, 36(4), pp. 64–81.

Diaz-Bone, R. and Favereau, O. 2019, 'Perspectives of economics of convention on markets, organizations, and Law: An introduction', *Historical Social Research*, 44(1), pp. 25–51.

Duckett, S. 2020, 'The consequences of private involvement in healthcare – The Australian experience', *Healthcare Policy*, 15(4), pp. 21–5.

Eyal, G. 2020, 'Beware the trolley zealots', *Sociologica*, 14(1), pp. 21–30.

Eymard-Duvernay, F. 2016, 'Valorisation: Les pouvoirs de valorisation – L'accroissement de la capacité éthique, sociale et politique des acteurs', in Batifoulier, P., Bessis, F., Ghirardello, A., de Larquier, G. and Remillon, D. (eds), *Dictionnaire des Conventions*, Presses Universitaires du Septentrion, Villeneuve d'Ascq, pp. 291–5.

Favereau, O. 1995, 'L'économie des conventions: Politique d'un programme de recherches en sciences sociales', *Actuel Marx*, 17, pp. 103–13.

Fetter, R., Shin, Y., Freeman, J., Averill, R., Thompson, J. 1980, 'Case mix definition by diagnosis related groups', *Medical Care*, 18, pp. 1–53.

Freidson, E. 1988, *Profession of Medicine: A Study of the Sociology of Applied Knowledge*, University of Chicago Press, Chicago.

Freudenberg, N. 2021, *At What Cost: Modern Capitalism and the Future of Health*, Oxford University Press, New York.

Gourinchas, P.O. 2020, 'Flattening the pandemic and recession curves', in Baldwin, R.E. and Weder B (eds), *Mitigating the COVID economic crisis – Act fast and do whatever*, pp. 31–39.

Hanrieder, T. 2016, 'Orders of worth and the moral conceptions of health in global politics', *International Theory*, 8(3), pp. 390–421.

Hodgson, G. 2009, 'Towards an alternative economics of healthcare', *Health Economics, Policy and Law,* 4, pp. 99–114.

Keynes, J.M. 2007 [1936], *The General Theory of Employment, Interest and Money*, Kessinger Publishing, LLC, Whitefish, MO.

Lewis, D. 1969, *Convention: A Philosophical Study*, Harvard University Press, Cambridge.

Marya, R. and Patel, R. 2021, *Inflamed: Deep Medicine and the Anatomy of Injustice*, Farrar, Straus and Giroux, New York.

Maarse, H. 2006, 'The privatization of healthcare in Europe: An eight-country analysis', *Journal of Health Politics, Policy and Law*, 31(5), pp. 981–1014.

Monneraud, Lise. 2009. The dominant economic(s) prism in health reforms: From economic constraint to economic paradigm", *Central European Journal of Public Policy,* 3, pp. 22–49.

Popcevski, N. 2022, 'The billionaire boom: Capital as power and the distribution of wealth', in Di Muzio, T. and Dow, M. (eds), *COVID-19 and the Global Political Economy*, Routledge, New York.

Roland, M. and Guthrie, B. 2016, 'Quality and outcomes framework: What have we learnt?' *British Medical Journal*, 354, p. i4060.

Rose, N. and Miller, P. 1992, 'Political power beyond the state: Problematics of government', *The British Journal of Sociology,* 43(2), pp. 173-205.

Sackett, D., Rosenberg, W., Gray, M., Haynes, B. and Richardson, S. 1996, 'Evidence based medicine: What it is and what it isn't', *British Medical Journal,* 7023(312), pp. 71–2

Saltman, R. 2002, 'Regulating incentives: The past and present role of the state in healthcare systems', *Social Science and Medicine*, 11(54), pp. 1677–94.

Simonet, D. and Katsos, J.E. 2020, 'Market reforms in the French healthcare system: Between regulation and yardstick competition', *Public Money and Management*, 42(3), pp. 1–8.

Thomas, A., 2022, 'Transhumanism and advanced capitalism: Elitist logics and dangerous implications', in Jorion, P. (ed), *Humanism and its Discontents*, Palgrave Macmillan, Cham, pp. 151–80.

Vahabi, M., Batifoulier, P. and Da Silva, N. 2020, 'A theory of predatory welfare state and citizen welfare: The French case', *Public Choice*, 182, pp. 243–71.

Wilkinson, R. and Pickett, K. 2010, *The Spirit Level: Why Equality Is Better for Everyone*, Penguin, London.

WSJ Editorial Board 2020, 'The lockdown's destruction', *Wall Street Journal*, 30 July, accessed 19 September 2022, <https://www.wsj.com/articles/the-lockdowns-destruction-11596150889>.

Žižek, S. 2018, *Like a Thief in Broad Daylight: Power in the Era of Post-Human Capitalism*, Penguin, London.

4

UNDERSTANDING MARX ON HEALTH

Toward a class-based approach

Raju Das[1]

Illness is only partly a matter of biology – whether biology involves viruses or biological impairment in the human body. Biology does affect human health, albeit mediated by social processes. The latter are rightly stressed in the social determinants (or social dimensions) of health (SDH) approach – a topic on which there is a growing literature that is not only academic (Marmot and Wilkinson 2005), but also policy-oriented. According to the US government, social determinants of health include economic stability, education access and quality, healthcare access and quality, neighborhood and built environment, and social and community context. Similarly, the Government of Canada (2007: n.p.) suggests:

> Social determinants of health refer to a specific group of social and economic factors within the broader determinants of health. These relate to an individual's place in society, such as income, education or employment. Experiences of discrimination, racism and historical trauma are important social determinants of health for certain groups such as Indigenous Peoples, LGBTQ and Black Canadians.

Recognizing the fact that better health cannot be promoted merely by pills and vaccines, but rather has social dimensions, is admirable. Yet, it is necessary to adopt a more critical perspective on SDH themselves. It is not enough to suggest that health has many (disparate) social (or non-biological or non-medical) dimensions. There is a need to unpack the nature of the 'social' itself in SDH, in order to emphasize what can be called the *class dimensions of health*. Specifically, the class character of the social, in order to emphasize that is the *capitalist* 'social' – must be at the center of discussion on SDH. However, this is not the case in the extant literature on the topic. Indeed, in an opinion piece for the *British Medical Journal*, Freudenberg (2021: n.p.) notes:

> Mounting evidence suggests that key features of 21st century capitalism add to the global burden of disease [...] within and among nations [...] Despite these links between dominant political and economic structures and health, health professionals are often reluctant to use

DOI: 10.4324/9781003017110-5

the word capitalism when analyzing the world's current health problems and proposing solutions.

Some of the scholars who are developing critical perspectives on health (*e.g.* Navarro 2009; Muntaner *et al.* 2015; Raphael *et al.* 2019; Flynn 2021; Raphael and Bryant 2023) do discuss relations between capitalism and health. However, they posit that capitalism is one of many determinants influencing health, albeit a major one. This intervention is welcome, though it remains deficient because of its pluralism: the full power of capitalism to produce adverse health outcomes is not considered. That is, such accounts fail to recognize that the social dimensions of health other than capitalism are *also* influenced by capitalist class relations and economic development.

Investigation of the social relations of capitalist production and exchange is the focus of Marx's *Capital*, especially *Volume One*. As part of this analysis, Marx provides useful insights into an important aspect of workers' lives: health. These insights must be carefully analyzed. According to Marx (1887: 181), in capitalist society, workers' health is severely compromised: 'the capitalist mode of production [...] has seized *the vital power* of the people by the very root' [emphasis added]. To the extent that Marx *does* talk about health, however, his approach remains relatively narrow, in that he is almost solely concerned with the dynamics of employment/unemployment and wages. Accordingly, Marx largely abstracts from other social determinants that are shaped by capitalism, including corporate production of food and medicine, and inadequate government investment in healthcare (Braveman *et al.* 2011). Therefore, there is a need to develop a broader class-based approach to health.

In making this case, the remainder of this chapter is divided into two sections. First, in re-articulating Marx's thoughts about the impacts of multiple aspects of capitalist production on workers' health, I focus on: the value of labor power as a commodity relative to wages, employment precarity, and the resultant low income; length of the working day; physical conditions at the site of production; and the despotic control over workers exercised by capitalists. Second, I supplement these reflections with other insights from Marx (especially from his social theory) and from contemporary Marxists, as a means to develop a broader class-based approach. In particular, my focus here is on social relations, alienation, the state, social oppression, environmental damage, and working-class power – *all of which* are, more or less, shaped by capitalist class society.

Preliminary steps toward a class dimension of health approach: Marx's insights in *Capital*

The value of labor power, wages, precarity, and low income

Labor power is the physical and mental ability to produce useful goods and services. Good health is partly an aspect of labor power. It is also a condition for the sale and purchase of labor power: an ill worker cannot offer herself/himself in the labor market. Labor power is bought and sold in a comparable manner to other commodities. The cost of labor power – that is wages – should be equal to the cost of its production (and reproduction):

> If the owner of labor-power works to-day, to-morrow [they] must again be able to repeat the same process in the same conditions as regards *health and strength.* [Their] means of subsistence must therefore be sufficient to maintain [them] in [their] normal state as a laboring individual.
>
> (Marx 1887: 121; emphases added)

Yet, in reality, wages fall *below* the value of labor power for millions of people. This is why they cannot meet their needs, including the need for food or healthcare. This situation, which can be called 'super-exploitation', makes people fall ill:

> The minimum limit of the value of labor-power is determined by the value of the commodities, without the daily supply of which the laborer cannot renew [their] *vital energy*, consequently by the value of those means of subsistence that are *physically indispensable*. If the price of labor-power [...] falls below its value [...] under such circumstances it can be maintained and developed only in *a crippled* [or, unhealthy] *state*.
>
> (Marx 1887: 122, emphases added)

Assuming that the resources needed, directly or indirectly, for good health (*e.g.* food, drinks, medicine, hospital facilities, and doctor's advice) are available mainly as commodities, if wages fall below the value of labor power, people cannot access these commodities. They cannot, therefore, lead a healthy life.

The working-class is not homogenous: it includes skilled and unskilled labor. However, in some cases, this distinction prevents a segment of the working-class 'from exacting equally with the rest the value of their labor-power' (Marx 1887: 140). Those who perform dangerous work, which can adversely affect their health, are often not paid as skilled workers. For example, 'although the labor of a fustian cutter demands great bodily exertion, and is at the same time unhealthy, yet it counts only as unskilled labor' (Marx 1887: 140). If a given type of work demands above-average amount of bodily and mental exertion, and yet is considered unskilled or less skilled, then the resultant low wage does not cover the full cost of the reproduction of labor power. This situation can contribute to illness.

People's income and, therefore, their ability to access the resources needed for good health depend not only on wages, but also on employment – specifically, the number of hours worked.[2] Common people have no or little access to productive resources, so they must rely on wage-labor; yet, whether or not they are hired depends on capital's need for them, rather than their own need. Capital's need constantly changes with fluctuations in the economy, which thereby inevitably causes a situation of employment precarity. For instance, other things constant, if a rise in investment leads to augmented wages that, in turn, reduce profit, this may engender a slow-down in investment or capital resorting to technical change to reduce its reliance on wage-labor. Accordingly, '[t]he rise of wages [...] is confined within limits that not only leave intact the foundations of the capitalistic system, but also secure its reproduction on a progressive scale' (Marx 1887: 436). Capital resorts to technological change (or geographical relocation) and, thus, increases unemployment/under-employment in a given place. This adversely influences health, as this reserve army of labor 'is made up of generations of human beings *stunted, short-lived*, swiftly replacing each other, plucked, so to say, before maturity' (Marx 1887: 181).

Low wages, unemployment, and under-employment may lead to poverty, which is an important social determinant of health. The poverty of the working-class and affluence of the bourgeoisie are internally linked (Das and Mishra 2023). They are, in fact, two sides of the same coin: 'in the selfsame relations in which wealth is produced, poverty is produced also' (Marx 1887: 496). Relations of competition among capitalists lead to technical changes which, in turn, cause unemployment, under-employment, and employment precarity. The latter drives down wages, too. Further, relations of capitalist exploitation, or super-exploitation, can cause extremely low wages. Unequal distribution of income and consumption items in capitalist society also leads some people to go hungry, while others live rather comfortably. If wages fall *much* below the value of labor power, people may even go hungry. In capitalism, '[e]verything [...] depends upon making hunger permanent among the working class', because the hunger of some is expected to force others (the non-hungry) to work harder (Marx 1887: 452). Such hunger can be considered as a prelude to illness. The half-starved souls' ability to fight infection, pollution, and other unfavorable conditions in the workplace and elsewhere (discussed below) is compromised. In capitalism, 'the increase of the death-rate through [illnesses such as] tuberculosis, scrofula, etc., increases in intensity with the deterioration of the physical condition of the population, [and this deterioration is due to] poverty' (Marx 1887: 498).

Long hours of work

Just as wages are expected to be sufficient to pay for normal expenses, the length of the working day should be reasonable to ensure that the worker gets enough rest. However, workers are forced to work longer than their body-mind complex can normally tolerate. Long working days ruin workers' physical and mental/spiritual health. Capital 'usurps the time for growth, development, and healthy maintenance of the body' (Marx 1887: 179). For the capitalists:

> It is not the *normal maintenance* of the labor-power which is to determine the limits of the working day; it is the greatest possible daily expenditure of labor-power, no matter how *diseased,* compulsory, and *painful* it may be, which is to determine the limits of the laborers' period of repose.
>
> (Marx 1887: 179)

Long working days, wherein workers are forced to incur an 'extra expenditure of labor time' (Marx 1887: 163), lead workers to physical and mental exhaustion, yet the time for rest is limited:

> [Capital] reduces the *sound sleep* needed for the *restoration, reparation, refreshment of the bodily powers* to just so many hours of torpor as the revival of an organism, absolutely *exhausted,* renders essential.
>
> (Marx 1887: 179, emphases added)

Social intercourse and support for familial relations, which require time, can contribute to happiness and better mental health. Yet, by forcing men and women to work long hours, capital does not allow them to have the time 'for the fulfilling of social functions and for social intercourse' (Marx 1887: 178–9). Moreover, having to work long hours does not allow 'free labor at home within moderate limits for the support of the family' (Marx 1887: 272).

Capitalist production is ordinarily based on the law of equal exchange of commodities. Marx (1887: 163) explains the law by positing that '[a]part from natural *exhaustion* through age' and related factors, workers 'must be able on the morrow to work with the same normal amount of *force, health and freshness* as to-day' (emphases added). When the working day is excessively prolonged, however, 'the price of labor-power may fall below its value' (Marx 1887: 371). This is because the expenses that workers must incur in order to deal with the extra wear and tear are not included in the price of labor power (wage):

> Up to a certain point, the increased wear and tear of labor-power, inseparable from a lengthened working day, may be compensated by higher wages. But beyond this point the wear

> and tear increases in geometrical progression, and every condition suitable for the normal reproduction and functioning of labor-power is suppressed.
>
> (Marx 1887: 371)

In other words, with working-life artificially shortened due to overwork, during the course of working for, say, ten years, a worker contributes value via their labor power equivalent to 30 years, yet they are only paid for ten years' work. Clearly, this will adversely affect workers' health. Marx (1887: 163) explains the process by using the worker's voice:

> I will [...] husband my sole wealth, labor-power [which will not exist without good health], and abstain from all foolish waste of it. I will each day [...] put into action only as much of it as is compatible with its normal duration, and *healthy development*. By an *unlimited extension* of the working day, you may in one day use up a quantity of labor power greater than I can restore in three. What you gain in labor I lose in substance. The use of my labor-power and *the spoliation of it* are quite different things [...] That is against our contract and the law of exchanges.
>
> (emphases added)

Through prolonging the working day, other things constant, longer working hours will engender greater surplus value and, therefore, profit. Accordingly, '*in its blind unrestrainable passion, its were-wolf hunger for surplus labor*' (Marx 1887: 179), capital as a whole does not care about 'the *physical and mental degradation*, the premature death, the torture of over-work' (Marx 1887: 181, italics added).

Capital as a whole is reproduced through capitalist competition, which also affects workers' health adversely: driven by competitive pressure to reduce the costs of production, every capitalist is forced to extract as much work as possible from their workers. The excessive prolongation of the working day 'does not [...] depend on the good or ill will of the individual capitalist. Free competition brings out the inherent laws of capitalist production, in the shape of external coercive laws having power over every individual capitalist' (Marx 1887: 181).

In fact, as we have seen, capitalism's law of exchange itself puts *no limit* to how long the worker is made to work. According to this law, 'the consumption of the commodity belongs not to the seller who parts with it, but to the buyer, who acquires it' (Marx 1887: 163). Therefore, the capitalist tries to consume and squeeze out as much labor power as possible. This inevitably harms workers' health. Indeed, '[c]apital is reckless of *the health or length of life* of the laborer, unless under compulsion from society' and 'cares nothing for *the length of life* of labor-power' (Marx 1887: 179).

The hidden abode of production

An important aspect of capitalist society is its 'hidden abode of production' (Marx 1887: 123): the workplace where value and surplus value are produced, and where surplus value is appropriated. The physical conditions of the workplace are often characterized by 'unhealthiness and unpleasantness' (Marx 1887: 170). In some workplaces, '[e]very organ of sense is injured in an equal degree by artificial elevation of the temperature [or lack of proper heating during cold weather], by the dust laden atmosphere, by the deafening noise' and so on (Marx 1887: 285–6).

In every form of society, there is a need to economize the means of production. However, under capitalism, this occurs at the expense of workers' health. For instance, a large number of workers and a large quantity of means of production (*e.g.* machines) are often cramped into a small space in an enterprise without adequate ventilation and light. Marx (1894: 58) makes this point in *Capital, Volume Three*:

> It is well known to what extent economy of space, and thus of buildings, crowds laborers into close quarters. In addition, there is also economy in means of ventilation. Coupled with the long working-hours, the two cause a large increase in diseases of the *respiratory organs, and an attendant increase* in the death-rate.
>
> (emphases added)

What this effectively means is that 'consumption [tuberculosis] and other *lung diseases* among the workpeople are necessary conditions to the existence of capital' (Marx 1887: 315, emphases added). The cramped space of work with adverse effects on health, thus, has a logic: if the amount of space per workers and/or per unit of product is reduced, more profit is produced, other things constant:

> In line with its contradictory and antagonistic nature, the capitalist mode of production proceeds to count the *prodigious dissipation of the laborer's life and health*, and the lowering of his living conditions, as an economy in the use of constant capital and thereby as a means of raising the rate of profit.
>
> (Marx 1894: 55, emphases added)

If workers succeed in forcing capitalists to shorten the working day, the latter respond by resorting to 'an intensification of the labor as is injurious to *the health of the workman* and to his capacity for work' (Marx 1887: 283, emphases added). Capital seeks to fill all potential pores by making workers work every single minute: 'steal[ing] the time required for the consumption of *fresh air and sunlight*' and 'higgl[ing] over a meal-time', such that it does not allow people to eat their meals peacefully.

For many, work is also often not often enjoyable. Because it is not easy to remain attentive while performing disagreeable work, one commits mistakes, and this leads to accidents and injuries. There are, thus, potential mental health implications of the capitalist nature of work: work in capitalist enterprises 'exhausts the nervous system to the uttermost', and 'it does away with the many-sided play of the muscles, and confiscates every atom of freedom, both in bodily and intellectual activity' (Marx 1887: 284–5).

Many workers die, fall ill, or become disabled due to accidents and injuries at work. In conjunction with the performance of unpleasant work, as just mentioned, there are other reasons for this. Accidents happen because workplaces are cramped. Marx talks about the 'danger to life and limb among the thickly crowded machinery which, with the regularity of the seasons, issues its list of the *killed and wounded* in the industrial battle' (Marx 1887: 286, emphases added). Many accidents happen because workers, including child workers, lack adequate training. There is also a tendency in capitalism toward an increase in the speed of machines in order to increase output and profit, which increases the likelihood of accidents.

A major reason for accidents at work is that capitalists often fail to pay adequate attention to safety rules, because doing so costs money and eats into profit. As if anticipating the current neoliberal form of capitalism, Marx (1894: 55) holds that workers are subjected to the capitalist tendency toward the neglect of '*safety rules in production processes pernicious to health, or, as in mining, bound up with danger*' (emphases added). This 'disregard for safety measures to ensure the security, comfort, and health of laborers' results in 'the casualty lists containing *the wounded and killed* industrial workers' (Marx 1887: 57, emphases added). When workers are disabled due to accidents, they are less likely to be hired than those who are not, leading to their income shrinking, which inexorably affects their health.

Class dimensions of health: a broader Marxist approach

Dialectical methodological considerations

As Marx himself demonstrates, capitalist relations of production and exchange are harmful to people's health. Yet, there is a need to go beyond an approach to health that is rooted in the labor market and production. This broader approach must be informed by a stratified ontology that Marx (1973 [1857]: 237) advocates in *Grundrisse*, where the concrete must be seen as 'the concentration of many determinations, hence unity of the diverse', and where the 'many determinations' exist at multiple *levels* (of abstraction). This means that concrete *outcomes* are *produced* as *effects* of *mechanisms* that exist by virtue of underlying *social relations*.

Accordingly, if health is a concrete aspect of the multi-layered reality of life, then its social determinants must be seen as existing at different levels, some of which are more abstract/general – that is one-sided – than other levels. At a more concrete level, the social determinants of health include processes that the existing SDH literature has rightly emphasized – such as adequate income and economic inequality. Yet, these concrete determinants are to be seen as being determined, in turn, by more general determinants: namely, by capitalist social relations and mechanisms (*i.e.* the capitalist political-economic system, including production and state policies). These determinants are, more or less, *internal* aspects of capitalist society because it cannot exist without these relations and mechanisms. Hence, the structures of capitalism make it too powerful to be considered as merely *one* among many social determinants.

Capitalist class relations of production and exchange

Moving from method to political economy, one can suggest that Marx's broader approach to health is actually implicit in *Capital, Volume One.* This is indicated by his comment that: '[a]ccumulation of wealth at one pole is [...] at the same time accumulation of *misery, agony of toil, slavery, ignorance, brutality, mental degradation*, at the opposite pole' (Marx 1887: 451). Embedded in this insightful remark are two main elements of his implicit broader approach, the elements to which he does pay explicit attention, as discussed above. These are as follows: (i) capitalist *social relations* give rise to the *mechanisms* of the organization of work, production, and accumulation of value (*e.g.* commodification of necessities; reliance on wage-work; insecure employment; exploitation; capitalist competition; economic inequality) which, in turn, produce (ii) certain *effects* on workers (*e.g.* inadequate income due to low wages and/or insecure employment; unsafe physical conditions in the workplace; and long hours of work). These two processes, consequently, engender adverse impacts on workers' health. In terms of health, then, there is a hierarchy of concepts: social relations of capitalism → mechanisms → effects on workers → effects on workers' health. Therefore, economic inequality and attendant economic deprivation (both relative and absolute) are a major cause of ill-health. According to Marx, workers produce wealth for capitalists, but workers do not enjoy that wealth to meet their needs. Resources do exist for people to enjoy good health, but they are not held under workers' control to enable this principle to be realized.

It bears repetition that Marx's implicit broader approach to health includes his explicitly narrow approach contained in *Capital, Volume One*. The latter is actually supported by more recent work, which examines, for example, how '[t]he physical aspects of work – the traditional domain of occupational health and safety – represent [a] [...] pathway through which work influences health' (Braveman *et al.* 2011: 385–7). Recent research also suggests that working overtime has been associated with injury, illness, and mortality and that many people who do not earn enough to cover basic necessities (the working poor) are less likely to have health-related benefits (Collins *et al.* 2004; Braveman *et al.* 2011). Particularly relevant here is Engels' concept of social murder, which is indicative of the violence inflicted by capitalists upon the human body (Das 2018). This refers to avoidable death caused by capitalism:

> Many [die] [...] of starvation, where long-continued want of proper nourishment [calls] forth fatal illness, when it [produces] such debility that causes which might otherwise have remained inoperative brought on severe illness and death. The English working-men [correctly] call this 'social murder'[...] [whereby the bourgeoisie] has placed the workers under conditions in which they can neither retain health nor live long; that it undermines the vital force of these workers gradually, little by little, and so hurries them to the grave before their time [...] [S]ociety knows how injurious such conditions are to the health and the life of the workers, and yet does nothing to improve these conditions. That it knows the consequences of its deeds; that its act is, therefore, not mere manslaughter, but murder.
>
> (Engels 1845: 33, 87)

Capitalist production of natural and built environments

In capitalism, the incessant pursuit of wealth in its abstract form and for its own sake adversely affects natural and built environments and, thus, also the human body. The circulation between nature and society is disturbed, as the profit-driven system dominated by private capital upsets 'the metabolic interaction between man [*sic*] and the earth [...] by destroying the circumstances surrounding that metabolism' (Marx 1887: 637). More is taken from nature than is invested into it, leading to a decline in natural fertility. Reduced fertility requires an increased use of chemicals in food production. So, people in cities (and in villages) depend on chemicalized food, which harms health. The concomitant rural-urban distinction is a major trait of capitalist class society: capitalist production of the built environment delinks the city from the village:

> Capitalist production, by collecting the population in great centers, and causing an ever-increasing preponderance of town population [...] disturbs the circulation of matter between man and the soil, *i.e.*, prevents the return to the soil of its elements consumed by man in the form of food and clothing; it therefore violates the conditions necessary to lasting fertility of the soil. By this action it destroys at the same time the *health of the town* laborer and the intellectual life of the rural laborer.
>
> (Marx 1887: 637)

This process, termed the 'metabolic rift' by Foster and others (Foster and Burkett 2016), has implications for the health of common people as both workers and consumers.

The built environment that capitalism produces is not conducive to good health. For example, low-income people cannot afford decent dwellings, while housing inequality is also unhealthy.

Marx (1887: 458) says that: 'the greater the centralization of the means of production, the greater is the corresponding heaping together of the laborers, within a given space', and 'the swifter capitalistic accumulation, the more miserable are the dwellings of the working-people'. If a given space is needed for the construction of an efficient built environment or for the residential needs of the affluent people, then the poor are denied – they are dispossessed of – access to that space:

> 'Improvements' of towns, accompanying the increase of wealth, by the demolition of badly built quarters, the erection of palaces for banks, warehouses [...] the widening of streets for business traffic, for the carriages of luxury, and for the introduction of tramways [...] drive away the poor into even *worse and more crowded hiding places*.
>
> (Marx 1887: 458, emphases added)

Crowded neighborhoods are not conducive to good health. Living in overcrowded areas is a major cause of the spread of infectious diseases and for other health conditions. '[P]overty robs the workman of the conditions most essential to his [*sic*] labor, of space, light and ventilation' (Marx 1887: 305).

Capitalist alienation

Implicit in Marx's theory of health is the fact that 'social relations' matter. A specific implication of this idea, I would argue, is that alienation matters, although Marx does not explore the connection. Alienation is experienced when people do not have control over the means of production, over how productive work happens, or over the wealth (value) produced. One is also separated from fellow human beings with whom there is a relation of competition, not solidarity (Marx 1844; Sayers 2011). Workers' performance of labor is controlled by capital. The main aim of such control is to maximize their work effort and minimize their resistance. Workers must work under 'the authority' of the capitalist, and '[t]he control of the capitalist [over workers] [...] is despotic' (Marx 1887: 231). Capital indeed subjects workers to 'a *barrack discipline*, which [...] fully develops the [...] labor of overlooking, thereby dividing the workpeople into operatives and overlookers, into private soldiers and sergeants of an industrial army' (Marx 1887: 286, emphases added). There are definite implications of the barrack discipline and the regime of despotic control in the workplace for mental health of workers, although Marx fails to explicitly explore this. It cannot be enjoyable working when there is a constant danger of someone looking over one's shoulder. To the extent that a strict labor control regime weakens the potential for resistance in the workplace, this must contribute to a sense of helplessness which, in turn, negatively influences mental health.

More broadly, if health is impacted by social conditions, then alienation must affect health and, especially, mental health (Bramel and Friend 1982; Yuill 2005; Crinson and Yuill 2008; Oversveen 2021). Modern neuroscience holds that cultivation of loving-kindness and generosity toward fellow human beings promotes physical and mental health (Davidson and Begley 2012), but capitalism promotes alienation from fellow human beings and is, therefore, clearly unhealthy. The detailed theoretical and empirical study of the health impact of alienation in capitalist society is an urgent task. There is, indeed, a need to link two literatures – that on alienation and that on SDH – more adequately than has been done.

Alienation can occur outside of work-life. There are also relevant social relations outside of work/production, including in the family. For example, one implication of overwork is that, once again to quote Marx (1887: 178–9), there is no time 'for the fulfilling of social functions and for social intercourse'. Here, Marx is hinting at the importance of social intercourse for good health.

Recent research also suggests that a lack of nourishing relations can have an adverse impact on health (Umberson and Montez 2010). There is also the fact that families as large social aggregates of closely linked people, which could provide a limited basis for solidarity (and childcare), are weakening or collapsing, without an alternative social site (*e.g.* a commune) taking its place. The family as an institution, which used to be an 'extra-economic' realm – one that is beyond the considerations of the cash nexus and competition – has, indeed, been changing: '[t]he bourgeoisie has torn away from the family its sentimental veil and has reduced the family relation to a mere money relation' (Marx and Engels 1848: 16). The gradual collapse of large-scale families (*e.g.* extended families), in the absence of an alternative communal life based on solidarity and love, cannot but have an adverse impact on people's health. Family interactions have allowed people to share their struggles and sorrows and, thus, provided psychoanalytic assistance; big families have been a site for the care of the ill (which has happened at the expense of unpaid labor primarily completed by women). Marx also stresses the importance of care for children inside the family (although he assumes – mistakenly – that this caring work has to be performed by mothers). If caregivers have to work outside of the home, this can cause 'the neglect and maltreatment' of children, expressed as '*insufficient nourishment, unsuitable food*' and children's experience of estrangement (Marx 1887: 273, emphases added). Relatedly, when parents must be away at work and when alternative childcare is not available, children's mental and physical health is likely to be compromised.

Special oppression in capitalist society

Marx does not ignore racial and gender oppression, but he does not write about them in a systematic and detailed manner (Das 2022b). To the extent that he does (Brown 2012; Anderson 2022), he does not explore the implication of gender or racial inequality in capitalism for health. The burden of reproductive work carried out by women and children can affect their health. Similarly, oppressed racial groups might suffer disproportionately from illnesses (see: Aspholm 2020). Moreover, the effects of the social relations and mechanisms of capitalism on workers' health and their access to healthcare are impacted by discrimination on the basis of relations such as gender, race, ethnicity, and religion.

Implicit in Marx's theory is also a theory of discrimination against people with disability (Das 2022b). In his value theory, '[t]he labor objectified in value [of commodities] is labor of an average social quality, it is an expression of average labor-power' (Marx 1887: 227). This means that an impaired/disabled worker's labor does not count as average labor, which underpins value. As noted above, an impaired worker may be unemployed or under-employed, or when employed, they may not receive the average wage, thereby reducing their income, which will have adverse implications on their health. There is an additional aspect that Marx seems to ignore, on which recent scholarship has shed light (Slorach 2011). Those workers who have a degree of physical and mental disability are subjected to discrimination from 'employers wishing to avoid paying the additional costs of hiring a disabled worker, whether in the form of workstation adaptations, interpreters, readers, environmental modifications or liability insurance' (Slorach 2011: n.p.). Such discrimination may have adverse health implications.

The capitalist state and working-class power

The state is central to Marx's social theory and political economy. In the general interest of the capitalist class, and because of popular pressure from below, the state does introduce policies to help common people, but there are strong limits to what the state can do because of its class and capitalist character (Marx 1887; Das 2022a). The state's class character has adverse implications for workers' health. The withdrawal of state intervention from the health sector, including the privatization of the public sector provisioning of healthcare, and state-led promotion and subsidization of corporatization and monopolization in the health industry, cannot but have adverse effects on health. Similarly, the pro-corporate priorities of contemporary capitalist states – such as support for weapons manufacturers with its big military budgets, or corporate welfare (tax-breaks and subsidies for capital) – reduce its ability to promote the conditions necessary for healthy living. This requires not only better healthcare, but also mitigation of climate change and epidemics. Therefore, a critical examination of what the state can and cannot do to improve health (as well as the environment, which has implications for health) is an important task.

Workers' agency is a part of Marx's broader approach to health because it is an important part of his social theory and political economy. Workers' health is not entirely a function of capitalists' needs. Ordinary people's struggles for good health matter. Men and women demand good health because it is in their own interest. There are at least three practical implications of Marx's thinking about health in relation to workers' agency.

First, if information/knowledge is power, then workers must demand that governments collect social statistics on health (and other aspects of wellbeing). Governments should periodically establish 'commissions of inquiry into economic conditions', including 'into the exploitation of women and children' and 'into housing and food' (Marx 1887: 7).

Second, while 'the natural tendency of capitalist exploitation' (Marx 1887: 57) hurts workers' health, well-funded countermeasures in the form of government policies can be instituted to weaken the effects of this tendency and, thus, enhance workers' health status, to some extent. For instance, Marx (1887: 343) recognizes that '[t]he protection afforded by the Factory Acts against dangerous machinery has had a beneficial effect'. In turn, he discusses the 'fact that the number of accidents, though still very high, has decreased markedly since the inspection system was established' in the English context of his time (Marx 1887: 57).

Third, workers have to fight for the measures that ensure good health. Historically, '[t]heir formulation [...] and proclamation by the State, were the result of a long struggle of classes' (Marx 1887: 187). This view applies to more contemporary times, too. As Greer (2018) notes, the disappointing public health performance of the United States is, at least partly, related to its low and declining rates of unionization.

A healthy workforce is one of the long-term interests of the capitalist class that the state is expected to meet. However, one cannot assume that the capitalist state will automatically introduce measures in the interest of workers' health or that, if it does, it will implement them fully. Hence, workers must actively fight for better living standards, including health, to force the state to grant some concessions. Of course, Marx would argue that until wage-labor itself is abolished, and until workers democratically control the production process and productive resources to meet their own needs in an ecologically sustainable way, workers' health will suffer. He is correct.

Conclusion

What can be called Marx's political economy of health centers on wage-labor and the production of value. If a worker cannot produce surplus value, they are not needed or hired by capital, so they are denied access to the required means of subsistence, including food, shelter, and healthcare. Even if they are hired, they may not receive adequate compensation. If one does not have adequate income from wage-work due to low wages, unemployment, or under-employment, one does not have the money to meet basic needs such as health. Moreover, poor working conditions and a harmful physical environment produced by capitalism also ruin health. Clearly, health is an important part of the value of labor power and the process of the production of value. Therefore, health is an important part of Marx's political economy and, indeed, of his class theory as such (Das 2017).

However, Marx's approach to health informed by his theory of capitalist *production* – primarily in *Capital, Volume One* – is narrowly based. This articulation abstracts from processes beyond the workplace, or the hidden abode of production of value and surplus value. Yet, his overall social theory – including a stratified ontology and focus on the importance of social relations, as well as his political economy of capitalism – points toward a much broader approach to workers' health. Such an approach is only implicit, however. This broader Marxist approach to health – one that places emphasis on the class dimensions of health that are based in, and that are also outside of, capitalist commodity production – needs to be uncovered and further developed. This chapter has only indicated how this can be done. Such a task is necessary not only to better understand the social dimensions of health, but also to produce the knowledge that is necessary to promote a socialist political movement of common people for better health.

Notes

1 This chapter draws heavily on Das (2023).

2 Of course, this formulation abstracts from other sources of income, such as self-employment and state benefits.

References

Anderson, K. 2022, 'Revisiting Marx on race, capitalism, and revolution', *Monthly Review*, 73(10), pp. 40–8.

Aspholm, R. 2020, 'To talk about racial disparity and COVID-19, we need to talk about class', *Jacobin*, August 15, accessed 12 January 2023, <https://jacobinmag.com/2020/08/racial-disparity-covid-19-coronavirus>.

Bramel, D. and Friend, R. 1982, 'The theory and practice of psychology', in Ollman, B. and Vernoff, E. (eds), *The Left Academy: Marxist Scholarship on American Campuses*, McGraw-Hill, New York, pp. 166–201.

Braveman, P., Egerter, S. and Williams, D. 2011, 'The social determinants of health: Coming of age', *Annual Review of Public Health*, 32, pp. 381–98.

Brown, H. 2012, *Marx on Gender and the Family*, Brill, Boston

Collins, S., Davis, K., Doty, M. and Ho, A. 2004, *Wages, Health Benefits, and Workers' Health*, Commonwealth Fund, New York.

Crinson, I. and Yuill, C. 2008, 'What can alienation theory contribute to an understanding of social inequalities in health?' *International Journal of Health Services*, 38(3), pp. 455–70.

Das, R. 2017, *Marxist Class Theory for a Skeptical World*, Brill, Leiden.

Das, R. 2018, 'Anti-materialism, capitalism, and violence against the human body: Some preliminary comments', *Monthly Review* Online, accessed 21 January 2023, <https://mronline.org/2018/04/20>.

Das, R. 2022a, *Marx's Capital, Capitalism, and Limits to the State: Theoretical Considerations*, Routledge, London.

Das, R. 2022b, 'Social oppression, class relation, and capitalist accumulation', in Fasenfest, D. (ed), *Marx Matters*, Brill, Leiden, pp. 85–110.

Das, R. 2023, 'Capital, capitalism and health', *Critical Sociology*, 49(3), pp. 395–414.

Das, R. and Mishra, D. (eds) 2023, *Global Poverty*, Brill, Leiden.

Davidson, R. and Begley, S. 2012, *The Emotional Life of Your Brain,* Penguin Books, London.

Engels, F. 1845, The Conditions of the English Working Class, accessed 27 November 2022, <https://archive.org/details/conditionworkingclassengland>.

FAO (Food and Agriculture Organization). 2022, Zero Hunger Challenge, accessed 1 December 2022, <http://www.fao.org/zhc/hunger-facts/en/>.

Flynn, M. 2021, 'Global capitalism as a societal determinant of health: A conceptual framework', *Social Science and Medicine*, 268, p. 113530.

Foster, J. and Burkett, P. 2016, *Marx and the Earth: An Anti-Critique*, Brill, Leiden.

Freudenberg, N. 2021, 'Why do we ignore capitalism when we examine the health crises of our time?' accessed 27 January 2023, <https://blogs.bmj.com/bmj/2021/05/06/why-do-we-ignore-capitalism-when-we-examine-the-health-crises-of-our-time/>.

Government of Canada. 2007, 'Social determinants of health and health inequalities', accessed 21 December 2022, <https://www.canada.ca/en/public-health/services/health-promotion/population-health/what-determines-health.html>.

Greer, S. 2018, 'Labor politics as public health: How the politics of industrial relations and workplace regulation affect health', *European Journal of Public Health*, 28(3), pp. 34–7.

Marmot, M. and Wilkinson, H. 2005, *Social Determinants of Health*, Oxford University Press, Oxford.

Marx, K. 1844, Economic and Philosophic Manuscripts, accessed 9 January 2023, <https://www.marxists.org/archive/marx/works/1844/manuscripts/preface.htm>.

Marx, K. 1887, Capital, Volume One, accessed 9 January 2023, <https://www.marxists.org/archive/marx/works/download/pdf/Capital-Volume-I.pdf>.

Marx, K. 1894, Capital, Volume Three, accessed 9 January 2023, <https://www.marxists.org/archive/marx/works/download/pdf/Capital-Volume-III.pdf>.

Marx, K.1973 [1857], *Grundrisse*, Pelican Books, London.

Marx, K. and Engels, F. 1848, The Communist Manifesto, accessed 9 January 2023, <https://www.marxists.org/archive/marx/works/download/pdf/Manifesto.pdf>.

Muntaner, C., Ng, E., Chung, H. and Prins, S.J. 2015, 'Two decades of neo-marxist class analysis and health inequalities: A critical reconstruction', *Social Theory and Health*, 13(3–4), pp. 267–87.

Navarro, V. 2009, 'What we mean by social determinants of health', *International Journal of Health Services*, 39(3), pp. 423–41.

Oversveen, E. 2021, 'Capitalism and alienation: Towards a Marxist theory of alienation for the 21st century', *European Journal of Social Theory*, 25(3), pp. 440–57.

Raphael, D., Bryant, T. and Rioux, M. 2019, *Staying Alive: Critical Perspectives on Health, Illness and Health Care*, Canadian Scholars' Press, Toronto.

Raphael, D. and Bryant, T. 2023, 'Socialism as the way forward: Updating a discourse analysis of the social determinants of health', Critical Public Health, 33(4), pp. 387–394.

Sayers, S. 2011, *Marx and Alienation*, Palgrave Macmillan, New York.

Slorach, R. 2011, 'Marxism and disability', *International Socialism Journal*, 129, accessed 7 December 2022, <https://isj.org.uk/marxism-and-disability/>.

Umberson, D. and Montez, J. 2010, 'Social relationships and health: A flashpoint for health policy', *Journal of Health and Social Behavior*, 51(1), pp. S54–66.

Yuill, C. 2005, 'Marx: Capitalism, alienation and health', *Social Theory and Health*, 3, pp. 126–43.

5
FEMINIST POLITICAL ECONOMY, HEALTH AND CARE

Tamara Daly

In the National Gallery of Victoria, Australia, hangs a 1954 painting of a Melbourne streetscape by the artist John Brack. It depicts an unending stream of office workers leaving financial district jobs on Collins St. during the 5p.m. rush, immediately or eventually for home. Considered iconic for the period, the painting evokes drudgery with its monochromatic tone and depiction of the workers' stern faces. Gazing at it from a contemporary standpoint, I am struck by the homogeneity of the workers. It is a class of male, white-collar workers, all wearing suits, with only a few that present as female. The stream of workers is white, appears able – there is not a wheelchair or cane in sight – and middle-aged, with only some seemingly older or younger.

It is from such popular and academic depictions of workers that feminist political economy (FPE) has critically evaluated 'malestream' political economy (PE): *against* the homogeneity of class analysis; and *for* an epistemological turn (i) toward gender and class, inclusive of social reproduction, and (ii) toward race, sexuality, ability, immigration, age, and interlocking with other social locations. This FPE privileging of gender, along with other social locations, has yielded rich insights into the nature of social relations as a means to discern who benefits from political-economic processes, and under what particular contexts and conditions. Often, women's work – in both its paid and unpaid forms – is undervalued and unseen. Armstrong and Armstrong (2010) term it 'The Double Ghetto'. Likewise, in Brack's painting, workers are headed from work to somewhere, to be fed and cared for, to be cleaned, and to be made ready for work the next day. Like the painting, the broader political economy literature either dismisses or assumes this social reproductive work, as it is beyond the prevailing analytical 'frame', and therefore unseen. Conversely, FPE seeks to engage with this largely invisible, unpaid social reproductive work that *necessarily* supports the mode of production and that is performed mostly by females. This is the work that enables household income to be transformed into goods and services of the kind that can sustain all members of that household. Accordingly, Luxton and Braedley (2010: 14) refer to this as comprising 'the processes necessary to enable workers to show up on the job'.

FPE is an international field but, as Luxton (2006: 11) argues, its Canadian 'development and deployment' has been of notable importance, in part due to its influence on the politics of the women's movement. However, Canadian feminist political economy (C-FPE) has been under-recognized in the international literature, and this chapter seeks to make clear some of its pertinent contributions to the study of health and healthcare in Canada and beyond. There are a variety of

DOI: 10.4324/9781003017110-6

political economy schools and traditions, and no single chapter can address all of them. Therefore, my focus centers on a rich debate raised by C-FPE from within an especially strong antecedent of political economy that emerged in the late-1960s within Canadian political economy (C-PE) (Vosko 2002: 59) and that continues today. In presenting this chapter, I thereby write proximally: while influenced by, and immersed in, the context of broader FPE debates, C-FPE is my training, intellectual grounding, and point of reference.

This chapter has two aims. It situates this Canadian variant of FPE alongside, but distinct from, C-PE. It also outlines what C-FPE contributions have made to the study of health and social care. The chapter is organized as follows. The first section broadly articulates C-PE as a particular stream of political economy. The next section focuses on the distinctive path of C-FPE, along with some of its key intellectual contributions. The chapter then turns to address some of the distinctive contributions of C-FPE to comprehending healthcare, and how it fills gaps in the existing literature on the topic. By doing so, I argue that health and care work is a rich empirical space within which to further refine and expand the FPE framework. The final section summarizes the chapter's main points.

Canadian political economy

Like those writing in the broader field of political economy, the Canadian approach is critical, comparative, interdisciplinary, often socialist, and historical. Wallace Clement and Glen Williams (1989) argue that a renewed interest on political economy in the country came with the release of *The Watkins Report* (1968). It proffers a socialist and Canadian nationalist approach to the resource extraction economy (Cohen 2020) and, according to Clement (1989), reinvigorated the work of Canadian economic historian Harold Innis' staples thesis. This was followed by Kari Levitt's (1970) critical reflections of the multinational corporation. Research originating from these streams flourished and was complemented by analyses of the relationship between Canada and the UK and between Canada and the United States – *viz.* both types of welfare states and types of capitalism. As a participant in the early debate, Drache (1978: 5) succinctly summarize the contemporary field of political economy as 'the study of society as an integrated whole', along with 'social relations as they relate to the economic system of production'. Many of the field's important ideas are outlined in the iconic journal, *Studies in Political Economy (SPE)*, first published in 1979, as well as a bevy of important books written by many key authors.

The field of political economy that developed in Canada is not uniform in either method or analytical approach (Cohen 2020), but critically focuses on the prevailing social formation – especially the outcomes of how politics and economics are enmeshed – and on power and resource distribution. It provokes insightful questions about which classes materially benefit and under what conditions, as well as investigating the impacts arising from the dynamics of the prevailing capitalist mode of production. Studies grapple with tensions between structure and agency, ideas and material conditions, the role of states and markets, and class relations. Importantly, C-PE locates tensions and contradictions by separately, and then cohesively, analyzing the 'whole' in ways that consider historical and socio-cultural contexts.

While relying on multiple forms of data – including qualitative, quantitative, and archival – political economy analyses differ from positivist, purely quantitative, or solely economic analyses. The latter tend to focus on statistical significance, relationships between independent and dependent variables, and theoretical assumptions about how economies function by identifying ways in which social reality is complex, context-dependent, and evolving. C-PE analyses, in contrast, are usually comparative – between nations, groups, systems, or sub-sectors. Moreover, it addresses questions concerning how types of welfare states operate; how sectors of the economy perform; the changing nature of (neoliberal) capitalism and shifts to standard employment relations; work and the labor process; whether services are for-profit or public and with what result; where income inequality exists and for whom; and what is included in state services and who is eligible to receive them. Many studies query the spectrum between universalism and individualism, and emphasize equality and redistribution as outcomes of primary importance.

Some of these insights were outlined in the book, *The New Canadian Political Economy* (Clement and Williams 1989). It called on future books and articles to be 'multi-faceted and diverse' (Clement 1997: 7) and, importantly, to integrate 'women, gender, sexuality, race and class as well as other systemic discriminations, such as age and ability' (Luxton 2006: 13). By 1989, insights from far and adjacent fields were infusing fresh approaches and new methodological space into C-PE. However, as Luxton (2006) strongly argues, even by the mid-2000s – and despite casting a wider tent – C-PE had only incorporated limited C-FPE insights, had largely resisted gender as a key analytical category, and marginalized feminism within it.

Canadian *feminist* political economy: a distinctive approach

C-FPE developed a strong and distinctive voice over the course of the past half-century. Some presuppositions are shared with C-PE: analysis of the 'whole'; taking context seriously; the enmeshment of politics and economics; and a focus on power and its uneven distribution. What is distinctive are C-FPE contributions to conceptualizing who and what the 'whole' includes: ranging from who and what gets valued, to what remains invisible, and how uneven distribution is experienced when thinking about gender, class, race, and other locations. Importantly, an entire volume of *Studies in Political Economy* (Volume 30, Issue 1) was dedicated to the past and future of FPE, even while the broader field of C-PE was still grappling with how to incorporate feminist insights more fully. The volume was, as Armstrong and Connelly (1989: 5) argue, 'about feminist praxis; about the theoretical assumptions that are reflected in women's struggles to improve their conditions and about the implications of these activities for theory'.

While remaining in conversation with C-PE, C-FPE began developing as a distinctive field by situating gender as central to its analysis, alongside other advances in feminism. Vosko (2002: 55) delineates four overlapping scholarly phases that had produced 'gender-sensitive political economy research'. First, starting around the mid-1970s, and developing during the early to mid-1980s, C-FPE scholarship focused on correcting the analytic exclusion of gender from class analysis (Armstrong and Armstrong 1983; Connelly 1983; Luxton 1983; MacDonald 1984; Cohen 1987; MacDonald and Connelly 1989). It documented the sex/gender division of labor in households (Luxton 1980; Armstrong and Armstrong 1985), and sex segregation in paid work and wage inequities (Luxton 1980; Armstrong and Armstrong 1983; Connelly 1983). Key reflections demonstrated the necessary relations between surplus production and social reproduction, and the types of unpaid work that enabled workers to attend paid employment.

Second, by the mid-1980s, scholars shifted to an abstract level of analysis to debate what, where, and how to locate paid and unpaid work by women in the capitalist social formation, with two camps emerging (Vosko 2002). One camp identified the primacy of ideology, and the other, the sexual division of labor at all levels but, most importantly, at the level of the mode of production (Hamilton 1978; Armstrong and Armstrong 1983; Luxton 1983). Pat Connelly (1983) offered an important path from the theoretical impasse: rejecting biological framings of gender, along with approaches adding women to class or class to gender, in favor of conducting historically and geographically situated examinations of women's household and paid labor to accord analytical weight to both ideology and materiality. Likewise, Jane Jenson (1986) called for the specificity of history and place, as well as the need for empirical and applied contributions. She notes that describing the ways in which the capitalist state might contribute to gender-based oppression does not explain why, when, or how it happens, and that any theory of the state must address its relative analytic autonomy. Jensen's interjection focused attention on the capitalist social formation, especially the constitutive importance of struggle and resistance.

Debates shifted again from the mid-1980s (Vosko 2002) in a third phase, to critically reflect on disciplinary approaches in fields such as economics (MacDonald 1984), and apply the framework to specific sectors, such as fisheries (MacDonald and Connelly 1989), the content and context of nursing work (Das Gupta 1996), and long-term care (Aronson and Neysmith 1997). This phase included an epistemological shift from a singular focus on the mode of production toward the multiplicity of women's experiences in everyday life (Luxton and Findlay 1989; Smith 1989) and women's intersecting social locations (Armstrong and Connelly 1989). Radical feminist research pushed the field toward further analytical clarity, especially in relation to its critical reflections on the failure to theorize race (Bannerji 1991).

By the mid-1990s, C-FPE moved further toward its fourth phase, with analyses of interlocking systems of domination and intersectional theorizing (Vosko 2002). Studies began to articulate the deep interrelations between gender, race and ethnicity, class, sexuality, and age (Arat-Koc 1997). C-FPE scholars had been, as Luxton (2006) explains, influenced and engaged in debates with liberal and socialist feminists. Moreover, its conceptual work continues to engage with intersectional feminism (Ferguson 2016): both to situate gender as a central analytical precept and to engage with race and ethnicity.

Because of this sustained momentum, there are multiple ways in which C-FPE makes distinctive analytical contributions. First, scholars often disaggregate their investigations to provide critical insights into specific labor markets or sub-sectors, while also introducing the household and assessing social relations. This enables practitioners to determine the conditions within which people live and work, as a means to produce intersectional analyses that reveal social relations centered on 'gendered class' (*e.g.* Macdonald and Connelly 1989), 'raced gender' (*e.g.* das Gupta 1996), 'gender, raced, migrant, health status' (*e.g.* Doyal and Anderson 2005), and 'aged gender' (*e.g.* Estes 2004).

Second, C-FPE shifts analytical focus from production alone (Bezanson and Luxton 2006; Bezanson 2010), to consider its complex interplay with social reproductive work – that which sustains us as humans, is often performed without pay, and is considered less valuable than productive, paid labor. As Bezanson (2010: 107) notes, social reproduction is the 'daily and generational reproduction of the population' and 'is concerned with the dynamics that produce and reproduce people in material, social, and cultural ways'. Furthermore, '[i]t speaks to the ways in which states act to mediate and stabilize social relations in particular historical periods in order to ensure economic and social stability'. That those who identify as female – regardless of class or race – undertake most social reproductive work underscores the need for gendered analysis, and the persistence of a gendered division of labor. Particularly since the mid-2000s, this insight has allowed C-FPE to consider not only broad social relations such as gender and class, but also others such as race, age, and disability as important and interlocking forms of social oppression. For instance, as Vosko *et al.* (2009) show, industrial and occupational sex segregation persists not only with earnings differences between men and women, but it also remains evident across race, immigrant, and ethnicity lines.

Third, because of the centrality of social reproduction in its analysis, C-FPE identifies the undervalued role of care, whether paid or unpaid (Luxton 1980; Armstrong *et al.* 2008). It shows how most paid care work is not only gendered, but also racialized and classed work. Analogously, it is traditionally considered naturalized to women and assumed that all women know how to do it, such that it does not require special skills. As a result, C-FPE studies point out how, like unpaid care work, paid care work is generally invisible, undervalued, poorly recognized, and poorly remunerated (Baines *et al.* 2016). This enables C-FPE to see the blurry boundaries that exist between types of work, and between productive and social reproductive work – including liminal work that exists between formal and informal, and paid and unpaid, healthcare work (Daly *et al.* 2015; Daly and Armstrong 2016). The blurriness of the boundaries in healthcare – as a sector and as work – makes it an especially rich analytical space, and C-FPE has made multiple contributions to it, as the next section shows.

Canadian feminist political economy as an entry-point to health and care

This section outlines C-FPE assumptions and findings, using examples from the field of health and care. Health is a dynamic, rich, and complex field of study of particular diseases, bodies, remedies, devices, techniques, and approaches, among other matters. It is also inexorably interdisciplinary, with multiple constructions of knowledge competing, co-creating and debating in health studies, crossing from bench science through biomedical and clinical approaches to social sciences, humanities, and the arts. Its scale ranges from the sub-cellular level, to the micropolitics of the tableside, bedside, or clinic, to meso-level organizational arrangements, to the macro-level politics of transnational trade and multi-country treaties and assemblies. It spans from the study of individuals to groups and populations, as well as social locations that structure each. Studying health and care involves multi-methods of design and data analysis, including experimental, intervention, and case study, using qualitative, quantitative, and mixed methods. Its investigation often includes place as an important factor, as health is produced in households without pay, and by the voluntary sector, market, and state.

C-FPE scholarship makes important contributions to how we understand healthcare and health systems. Below, I discuss broad C-FPE assumptions as they apply to analyses of health and care. Next, I present findings from studies within health and care that confirm, refute, refine, and extend the fields of political economy, health services, and policy research.

Blurry boundaries

For C-FPE scholars, the 'whole' of health is analytically located both inside and outside health systems, and involving often-contradictory interactions within the social formation. Inside health systems, these interactions result from: inelastic demand for healthcare; health professions that fix ill-health but are unable to prevent poor health outcomes; significant market failures requiring governments to fund and/or deliver services; weaknesses in universal policies and healthcare knowledge systems that cover some illnesses, body parts, or groups better than others. In conjunction, they also stem from gender regimes that structure poor recognition, and push the performance, of unpaid healthcare work in paid workspaces.

Outside of health systems, and at the level of the social formation, C-FPE scholars consider how health is impacted by factors comprising the capitalist system. The latter include the following: national and global markets, and the drive for surplus value, that produce ill-health due to unhealthy working conditions and lack of comprehensive labor market protections; income inequality and insecurities of housing and food; and governmental adoption of new public management measures. These elements are complemented by gender regimes that legitimize some workers over others by reifying inequities of pay and position for care work – such as that carried out by teachers, and daycare, social care, and healthcare workers – so that the skills and time invested in this work remain underappreciated, despite its centrality to the reproduction of capitalism (Coburn 2004).

Access to health and receipt of care are often separated analytically. Within such framings, the former is considered a feature of health services or as arising from broader social determinants, and the latter, the purview of social care and social reproduction, and the work of the voluntary sector or of families (Baines *et al.* 2016). Conversely, this dichotomy creates what C-FPE scholars see as a false separation between health and care, and a limited notion of what work should be considered within the context of health and care. For instance, across the extensive health policy literatures, and in top healthcare journals, health and care 'tasks' are often studied as distinct areas, with 'health' occupying the professional side and all other tasks deemed to be non-professional, less skilled, and referred to as 'care'. The provision of health involves work performed by *professionals* such as doctors, nurses, therapists, dentists, and others with diagnostic capabilities. This is the most visible and highly paid work, though all the professions earn less and have less autonomy and legal responsibility than do doctors. Conversely, C-FPE positions all health *and* care as 'work': whether it is performed for pay or voluntarily, regardless of where it occurs (including hospitals and clinics, communities, day programs, residential or communal living, and private dwellings), and includes within its ambit a broad range of professional, para-professional, lay, and ancillary tasks. For instance, it incorporates informal, unpaid work conducted in households and other private spaces by patients and families (Barken *et al.* 2016), as well as privately hired workers (Daly and Armstrong 2016) – all of whom may be delegated duties normally performed by healthcare professionals.

Whether to limit what is included as part of publicly funded systems, or to demarcate clearly 'scientific' from other types of work, it is also important to note the socially constructed boundaries around health and care that remain intact in most of the extant health literature. As a highly technical field, as well as one that involves skills that are tacit and less easily measured, formal healthcare work organization is complicated, jurisdictional, and located in gendered relations and the politics of austerity. For instance, regarding what counts as 'healthcare', the illustrative example of fire trucks increasingly being called first to attend to 'medical' scenes is highly instructive. As Braedley (2006) shows, a shift to fire personnel performing healthcare work reveals not only the fragility of the health and social care economy, but also the masculinized character of public sector work.

C-FPE studies, thus, reveal complicated and blurry divisions of labor: defining who does, what work tasks, and under what conditions across both formal, paid healthcare work (Armstrong *et al.* 2008), and informal, unpaid work in households and other private spaces.

Multi-scalar orientation

C-FPE operates at multiple scales. More than some other critical framings, C-FPE scholars study inequality not only at individual and organizational scales, but also in terms of market and state relations. Among C-FPE healthcare scholars, the field of health presents a special case: unlike many goods and services, demand for health is inelastic – we all need care regardless of our ability to pay – and on the supply side, the provision of health is a high barrier-to-entry field requiring large capital investments and an ever-changing professionalized knowledge base. States, in westernized welfare regimes, correct the market failures often associated with unequal access to healthcare, using a variety of welfare state models to fund, deliver, and administer its systems, including universalism.

Social relations, social reproduction, and 'relational' health and care work

C-FPE analysis complicates how, at each scale, unequal gender and race relations are constructed and reproduced, what skills are undervalued, and in what ways care work is (in)visible. These ontological considerations are often neglected in many health field analyses. For instance, the work of care is normally less visible and is often invisible. It is performed by those who are delegated tasks from professionals: *para-professionals*, such as care aides; *ancillary workers* (*e.g.* food services, laundry, cleaners, maintenance); *lay folks*, who are unpaid and related by blood or relationship to care recipients; and *administrators*, including managers (Armstrong *et al.* 2008). International comparisons also show how this division of labor differs depending on how the work is organized. A much stricter and hierarchical division – privileging healthcare over social care and the further marginalization of ancillary work – exists in neoliberal workplaces like nursing homes in Canada, compared with the more holistic understanding informing the Swedish model of long-term care (Daly and Szebehely 2012). Such work is afforded low value, as it is viewed as traditionally 'women's work' (Armstrong *et al.* 2008), thus revealing complex gender relations.

Conversely, C-FPE comprehends health work, care work, and ancillary work as integrally related. That is, the tradition proffers a wider view of what healthcare entails by comprehending all care work as *relational*: between those doing the work and those receiving the care (Armstrong and Braedley 2013). This formulation highlights the imperative of comprehending the needs of the recipient and worker together, rather than privileging the patient alone, as in medical models such as 'patient-centered care' (Daly 2013). Importantly, this insight derives from the ways in which C-FPE centers unpaid social reproductive work as *essential* to productive labor (Baines and Armstrong 2019). It assesses how some non-professional work that is central to healthcare – such as cleaning, laundry, and food services (Armstrong and Day 2017, 2020; Lowndes *et al.* 2018) – has been rendered subordinate and invisible relative to paid, professional tasks (Armstrong *et al.* 2008).

Focused studies of long-term residential care offer insight into how this relationality is assumed. While most of the literature focuses on the patient/client or recipient of residential care and their outcomes, C-FPE sees both health and care work in this sector as relational work that involves interactions between those providing and receiving care. Accordingly, Armstrong and Daly (2004: 9) argue that 'good quality care requires good working conditions', while poor working conditions make it difficult to produce high-quality healthcare outcomes. Paradoxically, health settings are more prone to unhealthy working conditions, with violence, illness, and injury high compared with jobs normally deemed dangerous (Armstrong *et al.* 2009; Banerjee *et al.* 2012; Daly *et al.* 2012). Simultaneously, burnout among unpaid care providers is typically high because of too few supports and an excessively heavy burden being placed on family care providers (Daly 2007). Conversely, the provision of safe, well-remunerated, and positive working conditions is conducive to superior health outcomes. For instance, previously successful pay equity gains for healthcare workers in British Columbia, a province of Canada, not only have reflected the success of healthcare unions in securing these advances (Cohen and Cohen 2006), but also afford a means to improve conditions for residents of long-term care.

In this respect, C-FPE presents a critical materialist feminist perspective on health that is entrenched within, but also critical of, political economy. As Scott-Dixon (2009: 41) argues, health approaches must:

> Grasp health and physical experiences as shaped by structural relations of power and inequality; understand bodies as socially located – positioned within broader contexts of interaction between institutions and social networks; and view improving health outcomes as a meaningful model of political intervention.

Correspondingly, the C-FPE frame prompts reflections on a range of material political-economic concerns. These include the following: the structural oppressions that produce poor health outcomes or consequences; who lacks access to services and where gaps exist; what communities, work, and issues are at the margins of study and access to health; how some services and groups are marginalized; what differences exist in health outcomes for different groups; and the tensions and contradictions, power relations, and interlocking systems of oppression (social locations) structuring peoples' chances at good health. Health equity is deeply rooted in the C-FPE approach, by focusing on which groups' chances are impacted by unequal health access, under what political, economic and social contexts, and what organizational, household and other institutional conditions are core to the analysis.

There is a long history of broader FPE scholarship investigating how access to health systems is produced by, and contributes to, reproducing inequity. This inequity derives from poor health outcomes being disproportionately experienced by those already impoverished or politically marginalized – due to extant gender relations (Doyal 1979, 1995, 2000), or complex and interlocking systems of oppression, such as gender, migrant, racial, and disease status (Doyal and Anderson 2005). Likewise, C-FPE adopts a *health equity* lens by locating power inequities within aggregated social relations, and then disaggregating when particular groups experience worse conditions, access to services, or outcomes. Universal or 'equal' approaches assume that when high-quality healthcare is available to all, it will meet the needs of everyone, regardless of class, gender, ethnicity, or other barriers. Feminists critically analyze the standardized approach within healthcare, which often normalizes health to men and male bodies. As one study of women's health services concludes: *viz.* heart attacks and other high-priority areas of medicine, women present with different symptoms that are under-recognized, have different access to intensive-care beds in hospitals as they are thought to be less ill, and have less support through to rehabilitation as they usually remain responsible for social reproduction even when ill (Daly *et al.* 2008).

In contrast, a health equity approach assumes that some groups will require more services, or ones delivered differently to attend to specific needs and others that can redress systemic barriers like poverty (Daly *et al.* 2008). With this framing, C-FPE draws attention to the importance of exploring structures, working and living conditions, and contexts that create unequal conditions, access, and outcomes for some groups. C-FPE scholars often ask questions about equity by employing case studies to account for interlocking systems of oppression. Their analyses privilege gender, age, racialization, class, citizenship/migration status, sexual identity and orientation, health, disability, and place (Armstrong *et al.* 2008; Scott-Dixon 2009; Daly 2013; Grigorovich 2015; Daly and Armstrong 2016; Storm *et al.* 2017; Daly and Rioux 2019).

To do so, C-FPE scholars assume that the social, economic, and political determinants of health structure the opportunities for people to make choices. As a result, C-FPE scholars explore and explain health inequities by asking questions including the following: how is society constructed to include and exclude certain people from accessing health? Who decides about who gets what health benefits (*i.e.* which groups/nations/places) and under which conditions? Within this tradition, class remains an important way to understand the dynamics of inequality because health outcomes are tied to market relations.

However, C-FPE health scholarship – with its attention to social reproduction within households – also offers some consideration of care work *and* material embodiment through documenting and exploring the sexed, gendered, and racialized experiences of people (Daly *et al.* 2008). In such analyses, both sex and gender are privileged because – unlike many other goods or services – health is embodied. Furthermore, analyses of health and health systems that locate sex and gender in relation to class, to race, and to other oppressive systems are considered (Daly *et al.* 2008; Scott-Dixon 2009; Grigorovich 2015), including the manner in which place matters (Brassolotto 2016), but always in ways that are complicated by the tensions between structures and agency. As Armstrong *et al.* (2001) argue, echoing Marx, people make choices but cannot choose the conditions within which they make them. Consequently, C-FPE scholars demonstrate how the complexity of peoples' lives extends beyond the social relations of gender and class in ways that intersect and interlock with other forms of structural oppression. These complex social relations impact access to, and quality of, care – as exemplified by the challenges experienced by elderly Lesbian adults receiving home care due to their sexuality and the privacy of home spaces (Grigorovich 2015).

Public and private responsibility

In conducting its investigations, C-FPE also addresses issues revolving around the role of the state, market, voluntary sector, and household in producing funding, delivering, managing, and otherwise being responsible for the maintenance of good health; and how data and information are collected and used by the state and market as sources of power and control.

Because health is often the largest public sector budget item, it is a stable and secure quasi-market space within those states that adopt the neoliberal market principles of new public management and state austerity (Armstrong and Baines 2021). Despite state involvement in healthcare to address demand and correct supply, C-FPE scholars point out the ways in which both access to health and the outcomes of health interventions remain inequitable in outcome, and unequal in distribution. C-FPE examines market contradictions in multi-scalar ways, by attending to how neoliberalism and capitalism are experienced in everyday life (Braedley and Luxton 2010). Consequently, analysis of health market players reveals the deleterious effects of the privatization of key parts of the system. For instance, in long-term care, privatization has perniciously affected ownership, costs, and space to provide care, and reoriented management toward prioritizing profit and shifting costs to individuals (Armstrong and Armstrong 2019). Other studies reveal how policy shifts favoring commercial and private providers in home care (Daly 2007), or in long-term care (Daly 2015), have seen public funds intended for care channeled into private profits.

In addition, for C-FPE, health data, knowledge, and information are not considered neutral. Rather, they are deemed inexorably political and an important locus of power through which some of the 'relations of ruling' (Smith 1996) should be understood. Data systems that aggregate health system encounters to produce quality metrics have been shown to have negative consequences for frontline care work, as well as how good workplace and health outcomes are measured. The data systems often detract from frontline work (Armstrong *et al.* 2016) by taking attention from actual care work in favor of *measuring* care, and then produce worse working conditions with unclear benefits alongside poorer caring conditions with detrimental care quality outcomes (Daly 2019; Daly *et al.* 2020). The sheer volume of data collected by the state to manage and govern healthcare is significant, but this data tends to encapsulate what can easily be counted as opposed to true accountability for how public dollars are being used to produce good health outcomes and working conditions (Daly 2019). This failure results in weak accountability for public sector funding (Choiniere 2011; Choiniere *et al.* 2016). It also serves to change the nature and form of regulation adopted from one that supports professional decision-making toward more prescriptive forms of counting and rule violation (Daly *et al.* 2016).

In C-FPE analyses, standardized health data, knowledge, and information are, thus, considered political and imbued with power. Furthermore, public funding of health with private data about organizations' performance, including labor practices related to good working conditions, health outcomes, and maintenance of good spaces, creates poor public accountability (Daly 2019).

Conclusion: contributions and change

C-FPE is a distinctive approach and makes several key contributions by building on the assumptions that gender, racialization, and other social relations exist within and alongside capitalist relations. By analyzing social reproduction alongside productive labor, C-FPE makes distinctive contributions that place the structures of capitalist, patriarchal, and colonial systems into the frame. In turn, deploying its acumen to study health and healthcare provides a powerful set of tools to conceptualize issues that impact people's everyday lives: revealing the relations that limit agency (the choices), structure opportunities (the chances), further construct power relations (the conditions), and define and delimit outcomes (the consequences). C-FPE analyses explore unequal power from gender, racialization, class, disability, and Indigenous relations in concert with how capitalist systems affect and are affected by health. Furthermore, understanding how social relations produce interlocking systems of oppression, and differing chances – situational advantages and disadvantages and different outcomes – is critically important. Finally, identifying how care work is organized in the market, including how it is (under)valued, mirrors the invisible and undervalued role of unpaid social reproductive work carried out in households in gendered, racialized, and classed ways.

This chapter not only highlighted some of the ways in which C-FPE has made distinctive abstract analytical contributions, but also outlined a stream focused on the study of health and care. The studies reviewed highlight the intersecting, multi-scalar, and comparative approaches of C-FPE to comprehending international trends in the funding, delivery, and administration of healthcare; the gendered division of paid and unpaid work; and what counts as health and care work. The chapter discussed key contributions of the tradition toward thinking through the parameters and impacts of precarious work; the ways in which privatization of funding and delivery affects access to healthcare; the role of privatization; and the political nature of health data.

One of the key precepts of C-FPE is making a difference and aiming for social justice in a way that assumes that the world can change to produce greater equality and improved outcomes. The starting point is identifying which questions to ask, and which stories are important. This is a multifaceted conversation between those with expertise in 'doing' and those who can bring skills of theory and analysis. C-FPE scholars locate expertise in the study's participants (Smith 1999), not the researchers, thereby shifting the locus of power. It also sees peoples' experiences as important sources of data. C-FPE does not dismiss personal experiences as biased and subjective data; instead, scholars embrace it particularly for the ways in which it contributes to an understanding of experiences of how power is exercised through myriad, complex political and social relations (Daly and Lowndes 2018). Training the next generation of practitioners to shift socially constructed systems and re-work organizations, as well as the next generation of scholars to conduct the research, is an incredibly important way to make a difference. Additionally, for C-FPE scholars, reflexivity is a central part of the work when learning with and from others.

A final point, then, is that C-FPE believes that research should be used to bring about change (Armstrong and Lowndes 2018), and must be conducted, produced, and shared in ways that benefit those who do the work and have the experiences. While including academic forms of sharing knowledge and information, a central consideration is the way in which information is shared with broader publics and those who make decisions on their behalf. One team has found success with 'bookettes', or short books that tell stories and bring together vignettes about promising practices that can be implemented to improve working conditions and healthcare (Reimagining long-term care n.d.; Baines and Gnanayutham 2018). In other contributions, digital stories and blog posts have enabled scholars to share findings in ways that reach wider audiences, including the public, practitioners, and policymakers (Imagine Aging n.d.). Through such initiatives, as Luxton (2006: 11) argues, C-FPE has made significant contributions to understanding social reproduction, and also advancing 'political strategies for human liberation'.

References

Arat-Koc, S, 1997, 'From "Mothers of the Nation" to migrant workers: Immigration policies and domestic workers in Canadian history", in Bakan, A. and Stasiulis, D. (eds), *Not one of the Family: Foreign Domestic Workers in Canada*, University of Toronto Press, Toronto, pp. 53–79.

Armstrong, H., Daly, T and Choiniere, J. 2016, 'Policies and practices: The case of RAI-MDS in Canadian long-term care homes', *Journal of Canadian Studies*, 50(2), pp. 348–67.

Armstrong, P. and Armstrong, H. 1983, 'Beyond sexless class and classless sex: Towards feminist Marxism', *Studies in Political Economy*, 10(1), pp. 7–43.

Armstrong, P. and Armstrong, H. 1985, 'Political economy and the household rejecting separate spheres', *Studies in Political Economy*, 17(1), pp. 167–77.

Armstrong, P. and Armstrong, H. 2010, *The Double Ghetto: Canadian Women and Their Segregated Work*, Oxford University Press, Ontario.

Armstrong, P. and Armstrong, H. 2019, *The Privatization of Care: The Case of Nursing Homes*, Routledge, New York.Armstrong, P. and Baines, D. 2021, 'Privatizations, hybridization and resistance in contemporary care work', in Baines, D. and Cunningham, I. (eds), *Working in the Context of Austerity*, Bristol University Press, Bristol, pp. 97–110.

Armstrong, P., Armstrong, H. and Coburn, D. 2001, 'The political economy of health and care', in Armstrong, P., Armstrong, H. and Coburn, D. (eds), *Unhealthy Times: Political Economy Perspectives on Health and Care in Canada*, Oxford University Press, Toronto, pp. vii–x.

Armstrong, P. Armstrong, H. and Scott-Dixon, K. 2008, *Critical to Care: The Invisible Women in Health Services*, University of Toronto Press, Toronto.

Armstrong, P. Banerjee, A. Szebeheley, M. Armstrong, H. Daly, T. and Lafrance, S. 2009, *They Deserve Better: The Long-term Care Experience in Canada and Scandinavia*, Canada Centre for Policy Alternatives, Ottawa.

Armstrong, P. and Braedley, S. 2013, *Troubling Care: Critical Perspectives on Research and Practices*, Canadian Scholars Press, Toronto.

Armstrong, P. and Connelly, P. 1989, 'Feminist political economy: An introduction', *Studies in Political Economy*, 30(1), pp. 5–12.

Armstrong, P. and Daly, T. 2004, *There Are Not Enough Hands*, CUPE, accessed 9 January 2023, <https://archive.cupe.ca/updir/CUPELTC-ReportEng1.pdf>.

Armstrong, P. and Day, S. 2017, *Wash, Wear and Care*, McGill-Queen's University Press, Montreal.

Armstrong, P. and Day, S. 2020, 'Clothing matters: Locating wash, wear, and care', *Studies in Political Economy*, 101(1), pp. 1–16.

Armstrong, P. & Lowndes, R. (eds) 2018, *Negotiating tensions in long-term residential care: Ideas worth sharing*. Canadian Centre for Policy Alternatives, Montreal.

Aronson, J. and Neysmith, S.M. 1997, 'The retreat of the state and long-term care provision: Implications for frail elderly people, unpaid family carers and paid home care workers', *Studies in Political Economy*, 53(1), pp. 37–66.

Baines, D. and Armstrong, P. 2019, 'Non-job work/unpaid caring: Gendered industrial relations in long-term care', *Gender, Work, and Organization*, 26(7), pp. 934–47.

Baines, D., Charlesworth, S. and Daly, T. 2016, 'Underpaid, unpaid, unseen, unheard and unhappy? Care work in the context of constraint', *Journal of Industrial Relations*, 58(4), pp. 449–54.

Baines, D. and Gnanayutham, R. 2018, 'Rapid ethnography and a knowledge mobilization project: Benefits from Bookettes', in Armstrong P. and Lowndes, R. (eds), *Creative Teamwork: Developing Rapid, Site-Switching Ethnography*, Oxford University Press, New York, pp. 156–70.

Banerjee, A., Daly, T., Armstrong, P., Szebehely, M., Armstrong, H. and LaFrance, S. 2012, 'Structural violence in long-term residential care for older people: Comparing Canada and Scandinavia', *Social Science and Medicine*, 74(3), pp. 390–8.

Bannerji, H. 1991, 'But who speaks for us? Experience and agency in conventional feminist paradigms', in Bannerji, H., Carty, L., Delhi, K., Heald, S. and McKenna, K. (eds), *Unsettling Relations: The University as a Site of Feminist Struggles*, The Women's Press, Toronto, pp. 67–108.

Barken, R. Daly, T. and Armstrong, P. 2016, 'Family matters: The work and skills of family/friend carers in long-term residential care', *Journal of Canadian Studies*, 50(2), pp. 321–47.

Bezanson, K. 2010, 'Child care delivered through the mailbox: Social reproduction, choice, and neoliberalism in a theo-conservative Canada', in Luxton, M. and Braedley, S. (eds), *Neoliberalism and Everyday Life*, McGill-Queen's University Press, Montreal, pp. 90–112.

Bezanson, K. and Luxton, M. 2006, *Social Reproduction: Feminist Political Economy Challenges Neoliberalism*, McGill-Queen's University Press, Montreal.

Braedley, S. 2006, 'Someone to watch over you: Gender, class and social reproduction', in Luxton, M. and Bezanson, K. (eds), *Social Reproduction: Feminist Political Economy Challenges Neo-Liberalism*, McGill-Queen's University Press, Montreal, pp. 215–30.

Braedley, S. and Luxton, M. 2010, *Neoliberalism in Everyday Life*, McGill-Queen's University Press, Montreal.

Brassolotto, J. and Daly, T. 2016, 'Scarcity discourses and their impacts on renal care policies, practices, and everyday experiences in rural British Columbia', *Social Science and Medicine*, 152, pp. 138–46.

Choiniere, J.A. 2011, 'Accounting for care: Exploring tensions and contradictions', *Advances in Nursing Science*, 34(4), pp. 330–44.

Choiniere, J.A., Doupe, M., Goldmann, M., Harrington, C., Jacobsen, F.F., Lloyd, L., Rootham, M. and Szebehely, M. 2016, 'Mapping nursing home inspections and audits in six countries', *Ageing International*, 41(1), pp. 40–61.

Clement, W. 1989, 'Mel Watkins and the foundation of the new Canadian political economy', in Clement, W. and Williams, G. (eds), *The New Canadian Political Economy*, McGill-Queens University Press, Montreal, pp. 16–35.

Clement, W. 1997, 'Introduction: Whither the new Canadian political economy?' in Clement, W. (ed) *Understanding Canada: Building on the New Canadian Political Economy*, McGill-Queens University Press, Montreal, pp. 3–18.

Clement, W. and Williams, G. 1989, *The New Canadian Political Economy*, McGill-Queen's University Press, Montreal.

Coburn D. 2004, 'Beyond the income inequality hypothesis: Class, neo-liberalism, and health inequalities, *Social Science and Medicine*, 58(1), pp. 41–56.

Cohen, M.G. 1987, *Free Trade and the Future of Women's Work: Manufacturing and Service Industries*, Garamond Press, Toronto.

Cohen, M.G. 2020, 'An alternative Canada? Mel Watkins' nationalism, socialism, and contributions to the new Canadian political economy', *Studies in Political Economy*, 101(2), pp. 265–72.

Cohen, M.G. and Cohen, M. 2006, 'Privatization: A strategy for eliminating pay equity in health cares', in Bezanson K. and Luxton, M. (eds), *Social Reproduction*. McGill-Queen's University Press, Montreal, pp. 117–44.

Connelly, P. 1983, 'On Marxism and feminism', *Studies in Political Economy*, 12(1), pp. 153–61.

Daly, T. 2007, 'Out of place: Mediating health and social care in Ontario's long-term care sector', *Canadian Journal on Aging*, 26(Suppl.1), pp. 63–75.

Daly, T. 2012, 'The politics of women's health equity: Through the looking glass', *Canadian Woman Studies*, 29(3), pp. 84–95.

Daly, T. 2013, 'Imagining an ethos of care within policies, practices and philosophy', in Armstrong, P. and Braedley, S. (eds), *Troubling Care*, Canadian Scholar's Press, Toronto, pp. 33–46.

Daly, T. 2015, 'Dancing the two-step: Deterrence-oriented regulation = ownership consolidation in Ontario's long-term care sector', *Studies in Political Economy*, 95(1), pp. 29–58.

Daly, T. 2019, *Public Funds, Private Data: A Canadian Example, The Privatization of Care: The Case of Nursing Homes*. Routledge Press, New York.

Daly, T., Armstrong, P., Armstrong, H., Braedley, S. and Oliver, V. 2008, *Contradictions: Health Equity and Women's Health Services in Toronto*, Wellesley Institute, accessed 9 January 2023, <https://www.wellesleyinstitute.com/wp-content/uploads/2011/11/Contradictions-report.pdf>.

Daly, T., Armstrong, P. and Lowndes, R. 2015, 'Liminality in Ontario's long-term care facilities: Private companions' care work in the space "betwixt and between"', *Competition and Change*, 19(3), pp. 246–63.

Daly, T., and Armstrong, P. 2016, 'Liminal and invisible long-term care labour: Precarity in the face of austerity', *Journal of Industrial Relations*, 58(4), pp. 473–90.

Daly, T, Choiniere, J. and Armstrong, H. 2020, 'Code work: RAI-MDS, measurement, quality and work organization in long-term residential care in Ontario', in Mykhlovskiy, E., Armstrong, P., Armstrong, H. and Choiniere, J. (eds), *Health Matters*, University of Toronto Press, Toronto, pp. 75–91.

Daly, T. and Lowndes, R. 2018, 'Feminist political economy and flexible team interviewing' in Armstrong, P. and Lowndes, R. (eds), *Creative Teamwork: Developing Rapid, Site-Switching Ethnography*, Oxford University Press, New York, pp. 63–80.

Daly, T., Struthers, J. Müller, B. Taylor, D., Goldmann, M., Doupe, M. and Jacobsen, F. 2016, 'Prescriptive or interpretive regulation at the frontlines of care work in the "three worlds" of Canada, Germany and Norway', *Labour/Le Travail*, 77(Spring), pp. 36–71.

Daly, T. and Szebehely, M. 2012, 'Unheard voices, unmapped terrain: Comparing care work in long-term residential care for older people in Canada and Sweden', *International Journal of Social Welfare*, 21, pp. 139–48.

Das Gupta, T. 1996, 'Anti-black racism in nursing in Ontario', *Studies in Political Economy*, 51(1), pp. 97–116.

Doyal, L. 1979, *The Political Economy of Health*, Pluto Press, London.

Doyal, L. 1995, *What Makes Women Sick: Gender and the Political Economy of Health*, Rutgers University Press, New Jersey.

Doyal, L. 2000, 'Gender equity in health: Debates and dilemmas', *Social Science and Medicine*, 51(6), pp. 931–9.

Doyal, L. and Anderson, J. 2005, '"My fear is to fall in love again"; How HIV-positive African women survive in London', *Social Science and Medicine*, 60(8), pp. 1729–38.

Drache, D. 1978, 'Rediscovering Canadian political economy', in W. Clement and D. Drache (eds.), A Practical Guide to Canadian Political Economy. James Lorimer, Toronto, pp. 1–45.

Estes, C.L. 2004, 'Social security privatization and older women: A feminist political economy perspective', *Journal of Aging Studies*, 18(1), pp. 9–26.

Ferguson, S. 2016, 'Intersectionality and social-reproduction feminisms', *Historical Materialism*, 24(2), pp. 38–60.

Grigorovich, A. 2015, 'Negotiating sexuality in home care settings: Older lesbians and bisexual women's experiences', *Culture, Health and Sexuality*, 17(8), pp. 947–61.

Hamilton, R. 1978, *The Liberation of Women*, Allen and Unwin, London.

Imagine Aging. n.d., 'Digital stories', accessed 9 January 2023, <https://imagine-aging.ca/>.

Jenson, J. 1986, 'Gender and reproduction or babies and the state', *Studies in Political Economy*, 20(1), pp. 9–46.

Lowndes, R., Daly, T. and Armstrong, P. 2018, '"Leisurely dining": Exploring how work organization and informal care shape residents' dining experiences in long-term care', *Qualitative Health Research*, 28(1), pp. 126–44.

Luxton, M. 1980, *More Than a Labour of Love: Three Generations of Women's Work in the Home*, Women's Press, Toronto.

Luxton, M. 1983, 'Two hands for the clock: Changing patterns in the gendered division of labour in the home', *Studies in Political Economy*, 12(1), pp. 27–44.

Luxton, M. 2006, 'Feminist political economy in Canada and the politics of social reproduction', in Luxton, M. and Bezanson, K. (eds), *Social Reproduction: Feminist Political Economy Challenges Neo-Liberalism*, McGill-Queen's University Press, Montreal, pp. 11–44.

Luxton, M. and Findlay, S. 1989, 'Is the everyday world the problematic? Reflections on Smith's method of making sense of women's experience', *Studies in Political Economy*, 30(1), pp. 183–96.

MacDonald, M. 1984, 'Economics and feminism: The dismal science', *Studies in Political Economy*, 15(1), pp. 151–78.

MacDonald, M. and Connelly, M.P. 1989, 'Class and gender in fishing communities in Nova Scotia', *Studies in Political Economy*, 30(1), pp. 61–85.

Re-imagining long-term care. n.d., 'Publications', accessed 9 January 2023, <https://reltc.apps01.yorku.ca/publications#Ideas%20worth%20sharing>.

Rioux, M. and Daly, T. 2019, 'Constructing disability and illness', in Raphael, D., Bryant, T. and Rioux, M. (eds), *Staying Alive: Critical Perspectives on Health, Illness, and Health Care*, Canadian Scholars Press, Toronto, 3rd edn, pp. 305–24.

Scott-Dixon, K. 2009, 'Public health, private parts: A feminist public-health approach to trans issues', *Hypatia*, 24(3), pp. 33–55.

Smith, D.E. 1989, 'Feminist reflections on political economy', *Studies in Political Economy*, 30(1), pp. 37–59.

Smith, D.E. 1996, 'The relations of ruling: A feminist inquiry', *Studies in Cultures, Organizations and Societies*, 2(2), pp. 171–90.

Smith, D.E. 1999, *Writing the Social: Critique, Theory and Investigations*, University of Toronto Press, Toronto.

Storm, P., Braedley, S. and Chivers, S. 2017, 'Gender regimes in Ontario nursing homes: Organization, daily work, and bodies', *Canadian Journal on Aging*, 36(2), pp. 196–208.

Vosko, L. 2002, 'The past (and futures) of feminist political economy in Canada: Reviving the debate', *Studies in Political Economy*, 68(1), pp. 55–83.

Vosko, L., Macdonald, M. and Campbell, I. 2009, *Gender and the Contours of Precarious Employment,* Routledge, New York.

Watkins, M. 1968, *Foreign Ownership and the Structure of Canadian Industry: Report*, Privy Council Office, Queen's Printer, Ottawa.

World Health Organization. n.d., 'Social determinants of health', accessed 2 February 2023, <https://www.who.int/health-topics/social-determinants-of-health#tab=tab_1>.

6

POST-KEYNESIAN ECONOMICS AND HEALTHCARE

Steven Pressman

Healthcare is one of the largest and fastest-growing categories of government spending, and a major reason many governments struggle to deal with large budget deficits. In the future, spending on health relative to GDP will rise further as populations age and people require more medical attention, and as new discoveries make expensive treatments possible that are not imaginable today. On the contrary, the economic health of countries requires that its citizens are accorded adequate healthcare and its workers are healthy. An effective healthcare system is also necessary to prevent and control health crises, as well as their most pernicious political and economic effects.

The COVID-19 pandemic put a spotlight on the trade-off between health issues and economic prosperity. To prevent the Coronavirus from spreading, and to save lives, many countries were compelled to place temporary restrictions on gatherings and business operations. This, in turn, led to many business failures, loss of jobs and incomes, and reduced economic activity. Subsequent efforts to revive economic activity by lifting restrictions resulted in a rapid spread of the Coronavirus.

In addition to healthcare, decent and affordable health insurance is essential to secure favorable health outcomes. Those lacking insurance do not know whether healthcare will be available or affordable when necessary. Even for those with insurance, healthcare expenses can quickly wipe out lifetime savings. This is why healthcare is a leading cause of rising household debt (excluding mortgage debt) and personal bankruptcy in the US (Scott and Pressman 2015).

Despite its importance, post-Keynesian economists have tended to shy away from health economics – with the notable exception of Dunn (2006). Two recent reference works – King (2012) and Harcourt and Kriesler (2013) – lack entries on health. The only mention of health or healthcare in either book concerns its impact on household debt. One reason for such neglect is that post-Keynesians focus on macroeconomics rather than microeconomics; within the former, they concentrate on effective demand, while avoiding the supply-side of the economy. To address this lacuna, the present chapter sets out a post-Keynesian approach to health economics, with particular emphasis on the US. The next section discusses the socio-economic importance of healthcare. Section two, 'The standard approach to healthcare economics' summarizes the neoclassical approach to health economics. Section three, 'The post-Keynesian approach' explains the main tenets of post-Keynesian economics and their relevance to health; then the fourth section, 'Toward

DOI: 10.4324/9781003017110-7

a post-Keynesian healthcare policy', applies these principles to healthcare policy-including those implemented to deal with the COVID-19 pandemic and its economic consequences.

The healthcare problem

Healthcare is often a matter of life and death. Accordingly, the demand for healthcare is substantial and enduring. This is one way healthcare differs from other goods and services. There are others. Healthcare providers possess the necessary knowledge for diagnosis and treatment; consumers do not. Further, many procedures and treatments are very expensive – some can run into the millions of dollars. Without health insurance, they are not affordable.

Furthermore, when health insurance is optional – as it is in the US – this creates a number of problems. Those more likely to need the insurance (the elderly and sickly) will buy it, while many who are healthy will take their chances. This makes the cost of health insurance rise to the point that it becomes greater than the ability of many people to afford it. Even countries with government-provided health insurance face a cost problem. In this case, the cost problem is political: what potentially life-saving measures will citizens be allowed to have and at what cost (where the cost is higher taxes paid by everyone)?

This would be of minor concern if countries received a good return on their healthcare expenditures. In the US, this is not the case. It spent 18.8 percent of its GDP on healthcare during 2020, compared to 9.7 percent in other OECD nations.[1] Yet, by most measures, the US healthcare system performs worse than that in other developed nations. Given both its affluence and large expenditures on healthcare, the US should have relatively high life expectancy. In fact, it ranks near the bottom of the list among developed nations (Kamal 2019). Infant mortality, a good indicator of the quality of national healthcare, measures the percentage of newborns dying before completing their first year of life. In 2019, the US ranked 51st in the world, with an infant mortality rate of 5.8 – much higher than the world leaders, Japan (2) and Norway (2.5), and even far behind Belarus (3.6) and Cuba (4.4).[2]

In addition, the US does not perform better than other Anglo-Saxon countries on health outcomes such as five-year cancer survival rates, breast and cervical cancer screening rates, and asthma mortality rates (Hussey *et al.* 2004). It performs worst when it comes to medical and medication errors, next-to-worst in terms of physician time and accessibility, and worst for efficiency (duplicate tests, medical records not reaching specialists in time, and so forth) compared to four other developed nations (Davis *et al.* 2004). More recently, the US placed dead last in the Commonwealth Fund (Schneider *et al.* 2021) ranking of the healthcare systems of 11 developed nations based on 72 indicators (focusing on efficiency, equity, access, and outcomes, and then combining them to get an overall quality ranking).

Despite spending so much money on healthcare, many Americans lack health insurance – 45 million people, or 16 percent of the US population, in 2006. The *Affordable Care Act* ('Obamacare') subsequently cut the uninsured rate by nearly half over the next decade. After then rising due to Republican restrictions following their 2016 election victory, the expansion of Obamacare during the Coronavirus pandemic cut the uninsured rate again to 8.3 percent in 2021.[3] When this provision ends in 2023, the percentage of those in the US without health insurance is sure to rise. Finally, even the many Americans with health insurance face coverage gaps, which can lead to bankruptcy because of a life-threatening disease. This is rather mind-boggling, as the purpose of insurance is to eliminate such risks. Private health insurance in the US does *not* do this. It limits annual and lifetime benefits. Likewise, Medicare currently contains no limits on out-of-pocket expenses, has large gaps in prescription drug coverage, and does not cover long-term care services such as nursing homes or home health aides.

The standard approach to healthcare economics

Most economists recognize these problems with the US healthcare market. Neoclassical economists contend that for markets to work, they must be competitive, consumers must be rational and knowledgeable, and market externalities must be few and minor. Yet, these conditions do not hold in the case of healthcare. Markets are oligopolistic, consumers are neither rational nor knowledgeable, and significant externalities exist (Arrow 1963) – including infectious diseases like the Coronavirus.

In order to address these problems, one solution offered by neoclassical economists involves making healthcare markets more competitive. Competition can be increased by allowing more practitioners, and reducing regulations on practicing medicine or selling drugs (Friedman and Kuznets 1946). However, this solution raises another problem: healthcare consumers are unable to judge the quality of care they receive or the effectiveness of the broad array of possible medical interventions. Most neoclassical economists ignore such human foibles.

Neoclassical economists also hold that externalities can be reduced by health insurance. However, insurance creates other problems. It increases the risk of moral hazard by creating incentives for people to be less careful. People are more likely to smoke, shun exercise, and eat poorly because they will not have to pay for the consequences of this behavior. There is also an adverse selection problem. The young and those in good health are less likely to purchase insurance (believing they will not need it), while those with health issues will likely purchase insurance. This increases the cost of insuring people, and leads to financial problems for those who miscalculate their future need for healthcare. It also leads people to opt out of carrying health insurance. Arrow (1963) explained how these concerns would be mitigated with high co-payments and deductibles. Individuals would then have incentives to reduce bad behaviors because the health-related problems will be costly. Extinguishing bad behavior also mitigates, to some extent, the problem of adverse selection, as the relatively healthy will not save as much from doing without health insurance, and they will be more likely to purchase it, reducing the cost of insuring everyone.

Finally, what is missing in the neoclassical approach is a solution to the problems of monopolistic insurance and pharmaceutical companies, consumers who lack the knowledge possessed by doctors, and externalities. The neoclassical approach also ignores the problem of the incongruity between the great demand for potentially life-saving healthcare, and the inability of most people to afford such care when high deductibles and co-payments are required by their healthcare insurance.

The post-Keynesian approach

In contrast to the market-based orientation of neoclassicism, post-Keynesian economics seeks to expand and develop the ideas of John Maynard Keynes, best known for his work on the macroeconomic causes of economic slumps. Keynes (1936) saw economic growth as a means to create jobs and end the Great Depression, and he advocated increasing demand to achieve this end. Keynes also wanted people to live good lives by enjoying more leisure, the arts, and culture (Carter 2020). An economic slump makes this impossible, so jobs and adequate income are necessary. Furthermore, for Keynes (1936: 372), the 'outstanding faults of the economic society in which we live are its failure to provide for full employment and its arbitrary and inequitable distribution of wealth and incomes'. Inequality leads to less consumption, hurting economic growth, and employment. It also has social costs, including greater health problems, which preclude living a good life.

Building on the conceptual insights of Keynes, this section sets out four tenets that can be used to underpin a post-Keynesian approach to health and healthcare policy: (1) uncertainty (rather than risk) in decision-making; (2) income effects trumping substitution effects; (3) focusing on historical time rather than equilibrium; and (4) imperfect competition as the norm in developed capitalist economies.

Uncertainty in decision-making

Post-Keynesian economics stresses the importance of uncertainty rather than calculable risk in making decisions. Uncertainty means the future is unknowable, while knowing the past provides only limited insights into the future (O'Donnell 1990; Rosser 2001). As Keynes (1937: 214) remarked: 'The sense in which I am using the term ['uncertainty'] is that in which the prospect of a European war is uncertain, or the price of copper [...] twenty years hence, or the obsolescence of a new invention'. Facing uncertainty, as opposed to risk, we cannot calculate the probabilities of possible future outcomes, and individual choice cannot stem from maximizing utility. As a result, people obey rules and norms, follow what others do, and rely on habits when making decisions.

Uncertainty pervades healthcare. It begins with the individual patient, who may not be clear about his or her symptoms. It continues due to differences among patients and how their emotional state, as well as their physical state, affects how they feel and how they respond to treatments (Meyer *et al.* 2021). This creates uncertainty in diagnosing a disease, in selecting a way to treat the disease, and in observing the results of any treatment (Han *et al.* 2011). In addition, the effect of any treatment is uncertain. A particular drug may be a miracle cure for one patient, do nothing for another patient, and have severe negative side-effects for yet another patient.

Income effects trumping substitution effects

When people are unable to assess probabilities, incentives have little effect. This is why income effects dominate substitution effects for post-Keynesian economists. That is, economic incentives matter less to people than having income to be able to purchase things. Thus, post-Keynesians reject Say's Law, which assumes that supply will automatically create its own demand, and does not allow for long-run unemployment because labor supply will lead inexorably to labor demand. Instead, for post-Keynesians, demand creates its own supply and fluctuations in demand determine the unemployment rate (Keynes 1936: Chapter 2).

This has two implications for health economics. First, people must have sufficient income to purchase adequate health insurance and receive healthcare, or the government must ensure this happens. A second implication concerns income inequality. Following Keynes, post-Keynesian economists have emphasized that inequality creates demand problems (Cynamon and Fazzari 2015; Stockhammer 2015). Yet, inequality also generates health problems because it creates stress that, in turn, leads to health problems. A substantial empirical literature demonstrates this (Wilkinson 1992, 1996; Shively 2000; Marmot 2004; Thoits 2020; O'Connor *et al.* 2021). Wilkinson (1992) showed that inequality was more important than average income in determining the health of a national population and good health outcomes. Kaplan *et al.* (1996) found that income inequality closely tracks death rates in US states and cities. This relationship has been found in many other studies, employing different data sets and time-periods, and using numerous control variables (Wilkinson 1996; Pickett and Wilkinson 2015). Great inequality partially explains why the US has low life expectancy and high infant mortality, while spending so much on healthcare.

Focusing on historical time rather than equilibrium

The relationship between inequality and health dovetails with the post-Keynesian emphasis on historical time rather than equilibrium (Setterfield 1995). History matters for healthcare in many ways. There is the previously mentioned issue of how stress leads to worse health. In addition, growing up poor and lacking adequate nutrition, or living in a polluted environment, will generate health problems. We cannot return to the past and fix this. Nor can we undo things that lead to health problems. Bad experiences and habits early in life cannot be reversed (Dunn 2006: 282). Those whose mother lacked prenatal care, or who smoked and consumed alcohol while pregnant, will experience greater health problems throughout their life. Children who do not exercise, and who eat fatty foods and sweets, will more likely develop diseases as they age and will require more healthcare. Not knowing the future, and not being able to restart one's life when health problems arise, requires preventing things that lead to future health problems.

Imperfect competition as the norm

Healthcare markets are not the competitive markets of standard economic theory where the consumer is sovereign. In fact, consumers generally pay little or nothing for their healthcare if they have good insurance in the US. Moreover, insurance companies determine which doctors people can see and what treatments are covered, while doctors determine the type of insurance they will accept. Consumers cannot see any doctor they want and cannot search for lower prices or higher quality doctors unless they are wealthy enough to be able to pay in full for the cost of the service. Very few consumers fall into this category.

In addition, both drug firms and insurance companies have substantial monopoly power. In the former case, this arises because of patents. In the latter case, it arises because the national government or an insurance company determines what care is available or covered by the insurance, and what price it will pay doctors. This generates monopoly profits that sustain market power through advertising to consumers, financial incentives to physicians, contributions to politicians, and anti-competitive practices that deter other firms from entering the market (Vaithianathan 2006).

John Kenneth Galbraith (1967) argued that large corporations manage demand in order to mitigate uncertainties in the market, along with those associated with large R&D expenditures. Given large costs and great uncertainty when developing new drugs, it is only natural that firms will seek to develop market power and influence consumers. As a result, pharmaceutical companies do not compete based on price, where substitution effects come into play. Instead, they seek to control market demand by targeting the psychological needs of consumers and distinguishing their drugs from other drugs on the market. In the US, they can advertise directly to consumers, who then pressure their doctor to prescribe the promoted medication (Spurgeon 2000).

Considerable evidence indicates that pharmaceutical companies are effectively monopolistic marketing firms. Their marketing expenditures are more than double their R&D expenditures (Reinhardt 2004: 108), with a large fraction of pharmaceutical R&D expenses going to Phase IV studies of drugs already on the market. Once a drug is approved by the US Food and Drug

Administration (FDA), doctors can prescribe it for anything. Phase IV studies are designed to learn about possible additional uses of an approved drug. 'Research expenses' for this are mainly payments made to doctors to prescribe a drug for new uses, with results then reported back to the company (Angell 2004: 39, 157–64). Other 'research' likewise supports marketing efforts more than attempts to improve health outcomes. Drugs are often tested against placebos rather than existing medications known to be effective; tests exclude certain groups of people, minimizing possible side-effects of the drug; and firms control dosages when comparing their drug to an existing one (Abramson 2004: 101–4). These tests are performed primarily to gain approval of a drug and help market it (Angell 2004; Kassirer 2004).

Toward a post-Keynesian healthcare policy

These four post-Keynesian tenets lead to different policy implications than those that follow from neoclassical economic theory. This section looks at three issues: cost containment, coverage, and policy responses to the COVID-19 pandemic.

Cost containment

Neoclassical health economists, following Arrow (1963), usually assume that consumers are rational and knowledgeable. To keep healthcare costs under control, they propose high co-payments and deductibles as a way to rein-in healthcare spending. However, this approach is unlikely to be effective. It discourages cost-effective preventive services, leading to more expensive interventions in the future (Zweifel and Manning 2000; Dunn 2006). It also flies in the face of what we know about human behavior. Behavioral economics teaches us that people tend to avoid problems and bad news. They grudgingly see doctors, despite the long-term costs of doing so. They require financial incentives and reminders in order to have regular checkups and to take care of health problems before they become more debilitating and costly. High deductibles and co-payments *discourage* people from engaging in behavior that promotes good health (Thaler and Sunstein 2009) and reduces healthcare costs in the long-run.

Adopting standard cost-containment methods to circumvent moral hazard and adverse selection is problematic for another reason: it disproportionately hurts low-income groups. Co-payments and high deductibles redistribute the costs of financing healthcare from the healthy and wealthy to the sick and non-wealthy, who often cannot afford to have their healthcare expenditures comprise a large fraction of their total spending. This also worsens inequality because deductibles are like a regressive tax (such as poll tax or head tax). As a result, besides affecting the behavior of low-income individuals unable to pay the tax, it will lead to worse health outcomes for those at the bottom of the income distribution range.

A more effective system would *encourage* behaviors such as annual checkups and routine care by making these services free. It would support free or inexpensive early intervention programs for children and pregnant women (nutritional education and food supplements for low-income women) that have been shown to improve children's mental and physical development (Evans *et al.* 1994: 19–20). These programs save money in the long-run because it is cheaper to provide assistance early in life than to deal with the long-term consequences of not doing so. Accordingly, such measures fall under the rubric of Keynes' (1936: 378) 'socialization of investment' – the government providing socially necessary services as a means to increase people's quality of life over the long-term.

Coverage

Following along this line, post-Keynesian economists recognize the difference between wants and needs (Lavoie 1994), and see healthcare as a fundamental human need, along with food, clothing, and shelter. Post-Keynesians see healthcare, like access to a job, as a basic right (Dunn 2006). There are many ways to achieve this. Firms could be required to provide health insurance to their employees, with the government insuring those without jobs. One downside to this solution is that it would discourage hiring, since firms would be required to provide health insurance for new employees, and firms that reduce their workforce the most will gain a competitive advantage. Alternatively, the government can insure all citizens. Most developed countries in the world have chosen this option. Through Medicare and Medicaid, the US government has insured its elderly and indigent populations, and the Veterans Administration (VA) insures military veterans. Everybody else must buy personal insurance, or receive it through their employer. Obamacare made it more affordable for people to purchase insurance, but the lack of health insurance in the US remains a problem. It is mainly an income problem. The uninsured cannot afford coverage, even when heavily subsidized (Agarwal *et al.* 2017).

From a post-Keynesian perspective, one advantage of government insurance is that it can be financed with general tax revenues. This is more progressive than insurance financed by employers, with the cost then passed on to workers in the form of lower wages or larger employee contributions to their health insurance premiums. With employer-provided insurance, everyone pays the same amount for insurance, regardless of their income level. This is effectively a regressive tax, where the poor pay larger fractions of their income for health insurance than the rich. When the government finances healthcare, progressive individual income tax rates and a progressive corporate income tax ensure that the rich will pay more for their insurance than middle-class and poor individuals.

From a post-Keynesian perspective, the best option for the US would be to move toward universal healthcare with a single-payer system operated by the government. This alternative has low administrative costs. Medicare spends US$132 per person on administration, while private US insurance companies spend US$700 (Frakt 2018). Single payers can also negotiate with drug companies for lower costs. Both the VA and Medicaid already do this and receive steep discounts; Medicare has taken a first step in this direction by capping the cost of insulin for diabetics. Another advantage of single-payer systems is that governments can charge different co-payments and deductibles based on individual income (Seidman 1990). Since the government already has information on household income through individual income tax returns, this is easy to do. Low-income households would pay little or nothing for their healthcare, while high-income households would pay substantially more than middle-income households.

While single-payer solves many healthcare problems, it does not address the root cause of the US healthcare crisis. We noted above that the US was an outlier in the world economy: it spends a great deal of money on healthcare, but has worse health outcomes than other developed nations. This likely stems from the great income inequality in the US. A post-Keynesian healthcare policy will, thus, require dealing with income inequality because of its impact on health. This necessitates a more progressive tax and spending policy. Keynes supported this for demand-related reasons (Pressman 1997), but another reason for such a policy is that people would begin life with better health: those at the bottom of the distributional pyramid would have more income to purchase healthcare, while greater equality would also reduce the stress that arises from inequality. This would benefit people at all income levels, since national health expenditures would be lower, and because better health and better healthcare minimize the negative consequences of severe pandemics.

Rejecting high co-payments and deductibles as a means of reducing healthcare expenditures, a post-Keynesian approach would focus on controlling spending and costs through government regulation. Most important, independent regulatory agencies and price controls are required, while conflicts of interest in the healthcare system need to be eliminated. Gifts from pharmaceutical companies to doctors should not be allowed, as such gifts affect the drugs that doctors prescribe (Aleksanyan 2021). The FDA must be made independent of drug companies; currently, they are paid by pharmaceutical companies wanting approval to sell drugs (Harris and Berenson 2005). Government bodies making important decisions about public health and safety should not be supported by pharmaceutical companies, and individuals making key policy decisions should not benefit financially from their decisions.

Finally, advertising by pharmaceutical companies to consumers should not be permitted. Neoclassical economists regard advertising as benign, believing it merely informs consumers (Nelson 1974). Yet, pharmaceutical companies typically hide the dangers of drugs from consumers and the FDA, extol the virtues of drugs with few or no benefits, and use advertising to generate fear so that consumers will pressure their doctor to prescribe expensive medications (Moynihan and Cassels 2005). In contrast, for post-Keynesians, marketing is not designed to inform consumers; rather, it aids the planning goals of firms and manipulates consumers (Galbraith 1967). Thus, a post-Keynesian healthcare policy would insist on banning pharmaceutical advertising to US consumers, similar to the ban existing in virtually all developed nations.[4] Drug companies should not seek to influence consumers or the decisions made by doctors, and doctors should not face conflicts of interest when prescribing medication or diagnostic testing.

Post-Keynesian economists also support price controls as a means of controlling inflation. Galbraith (1952) argues that large companies already control prices, and it is not hard for the state to control prices that are already controlled. When governments afford drug companies a monopoly on new medications, the former should be able to negotiate lower prices and limit monopoly profits. The market is already distorted. Price controls put the power of the government against the power of large drug companies. The US is the only developed nation that does not control drug prices. In Canada, prices cannot exceed the median price in seven other developed nations when first introduced; thereafter, it can only increase with inflation. As a result, drug prices in Canada are around one-half to two-thirds that of US prices (Angell 2004: 219–20). Similar results hold for other developed countries. On average, US prescription drug prices are more than double the prices in France, in Germany, in Japan, and in the UK (Mulcahy *et al.* 2021). The result is that much US healthcare spending ultimately goes to senior executives and shareholders of pharmaceutical companies because the government does not counter the market power of Big Pharma. This worsens inequality in the US, which then indirectly worsens health outcomes.

COVID-19

Finally, it is worth reflecting on the potential contribution of post-Keynesian health economics in the context of the ongoing COVID-19 pandemic. Several characteristics of the Coronavirus make it particularly dangerous. As is now well-established, it is highly contagious; many infected people have no symptoms; and the probability of dying is relatively high for those infected with the virus, especially for the elderly. In economic terms, this is a classic externality. During the pandemic, and before an effective vaccine protected a large part of the population, many people went about their daily business of buying and selling goods, and continued to interact with others, which imposed significant personal and social costs (infections, healthcare expenses, lost wages, and even death) on those not participating in these transactions. Some of this behavior stemmed from the need to work and be paid; some came from an irrational belief that COVID-19 was not a problem; and some was due to human instincts to interact with others. Whatever the cause, such externalities require a government response.

Shutdowns initially kept the Coronavirus from spreading and worsening the public health crisis. However, more was necessary. Post-Keynesian economists support government controls on prices to promote the public good (Galbraith 1952), something that would have helped mitigate the high inflation that resulted when economies reopened. For the same reason, they would support mask and social distancing mandates, and controls on the extent to which businesses can stay open. The big trade-off is between public safety and keeping businesses open so that people have jobs and incomes. Navigating this trade-off is the role of public policy.

Government played a big role in propping-up demand through spending policies that helped many families pay their bills. Unemployment insurance is, at best, a stop-gap measure, but it is necessary. In developed countries with generous unemployment insurance programs, only two-thirds of the unemployed are covered, and they receive around two-thirds of their previous income. In less generous countries, such as the US, less than 30 percent of those unemployed receive unemployment insurance and the benefits are just one-third of previous wages (O'Leary and Wandner 2020: 17). This is not enough to subsist, nor enough to keep people inside and prevent them from infecting others. In the US, one solution to this problem was expanded unemployment benefits. The March 2020 *CARES Act* provided an additional US$600 per week in unemployment benefits to recipients, and expanded eligibility to include gig workers and the self-employed. Still, millions of Americans in need of work to obtain income did not qualify for this aid.

Besides the income problems facing individuals, there were concerns for the solvency of small firms that could not access capital markets and had limited access to loans from financial institutions. When shutdowns and social distancing make some businesses unprofitable, the government must help – otherwise, many firms will go under, slowing down future economic recovery. Large entertainment events, such as football games and concerts, posed great health risks given the characteristics of COVID-19. For public safety, plane and train travel, as well as entertainment venues, had to keep many seats open and unsold. Restaurants needed to operate at half capacity or less, especially since people could not wear masks while eating.

Providing firms with money increases the chance that they will survive a pandemic and people can return to their previous jobs. The Paycheck Protection Program (PPP), part of the *CARES Act*, helped somewhat. It enabled small businesses to borrow ten weeks of usual expenses. Loans were forgiven if firms maintained their payroll and kept their employees. However, the PPP had many problems. Money went to firms (like the LA Lakers) that were not struggling, and to small businesses owned by private equity firms, wealthy individuals, or larger businesses (Chetty *et al.* 2022). Also, there was considerable fraud. Many firms took the PPP money but did not use it to pay workers. Some workers were paid less than they were previously making, with the firm pocketing the difference. Nevertheless, the big problem was that, despite the PPP, many workers were laid off and lost their employment connection, making an economic revival in the US more difficult once vaccinations reduced the dangers from COVID-19.

The UK developed a more post-Keynesian approach, and a more successful economic strategy. By directly aiding *both* workers and firms, they avoided the sorts of problems that plagued the PPP (Durrant *et al.* 2021). The Coronavirus Job Retention Scheme gave money to furloughed workers retained as employees, paying them as much as 80 percent of their usual wages. Low-income workers were also eligible for an additional monthly payment, up to the equivalent of US$500. Workers remained connected to their jobs. Firms survived because their largest expense (payroll) was largely covered by the government. The plan maintained flexibility for firms, in that they could bring workers back when conditions allowed. Importantly, aid went to workers and not companies, and it went only to workers employed by companies facing economic problems due to the pandemic. Thriving liquor store employees got no government aid, while employees of struggling pubs received a good deal of assistance. The different unemployment picture in the two countries reveals the British success here. In the UK, unemployment increased gradually in 2020, from 4 percent pre-pandemic to 4.9 percent in October. US unemployment, in contrast, almost doubled from 3.5 percent to 6.7 percent over the same period, after peaking at nearly 15 percent in April.

A final problem due to COVID-19 is that it increased income and wealth inequality (Daly *et al.* 2020). Many US households had enormous debt before the Coronavirus struck. COVID-19 led to the loss of jobs and incomes, which worsened inequality. The policy response – governments providing money to individuals and sustaining employment – certainly helped. Moreover, a moratorium on repaying college debt helped indebted households in the short-run. However, the wealthy did best of all during the pandemic. Monetary policy cut interest rates to zero, helping the rich, whose wealth portfolio is weighted toward stocks that rose sharply due to the low interest rates. This did not help the large majority of working-class and middle-class households that own little stock (Batty *et al.* 2021; Ferreira 2021) and remain deeply in debt. To spur spending, and keep economies growing as the Coronavirus pandemic subsides, one post-Keynesian remedy would provide debt relief to working-class and middle-class households. This can be done by liberalizing bankruptcy laws, or having the government write down some college loan debt in return for some sort of public service (Scott and Pressman 2015).

Conclusion

Post-Keynesian economics seeks to advance the economic insights of Keynes. Its two main contributions to health economics are as follows: (i) an emphasis on the macroeconomic determinants of health, which include ensuring that people have jobs and good health insurance, and (ii) a focus on income inequality, both as a factor in determining demand and as a factor contributing to health problems. For post-Keynesians, income equality is understood as bolstering consumption and employment. However, it also improves health outcomes. Post-Keynesian economics offers two primary macroeconomic policy measures to secure these objectives: first, greater government investment when business firms are unwilling to invest (with an emphasis on provision of healthcare and meeting health needs); and second, more progressive government tax policies – such as higher top individual income tax rates, corporate income taxes, and inheritance taxes – to improve income distribution, increase consumer spending, and bolster economic growth. Finally, as this chapter argues, post-Keynesian economics offers some microeconomic policy measures that would improve health outcomes. Most prominently, this may include universal health insurance with a single payer, cost controls on pharmaceuticals, and limits on advertising drugs.

Notes

1 See: <https://stats.oecd.org/>.
2 See: <https://worldpopulationreview.com/countries/infant-mortality-rate-by-country/>.
3 See: <https://www.pgpf.org/blog/2022/11/nearly-30-million-americans-have-no-health-insurance>.
4 Only New Zealand and the US allow this practice.

References

Abramson, J. 2004, *Overdosed America*, Harper Collins, New York.
Agarwal, R., Mazurenko, O. and Menachem, N. 2017, 'High-deductible health plans reduce health care cost and utilitization, including use of needed preventive services', *Health Affairs*, 36, pp. 1762–8.
Aleksanyan, Y. 2021, *Pharmaceuticals, Physicians and Money*, Ph.D. dissertation, Colorado State University.
Angell, M. 2004, *The Truth About the Drug Companies*, Random House, New York.
Arrow, K. 1963, 'Uncertainty and the welfare economics of medical care', *American Economic Review*, 53, pp. 941–73.
Batty, M., Deekan, E. and Volz, A. 2021, 'Wealth inequality and COVID-19: Evidence from the distributional financial accounts', *FEDS Notes*, Board of Governors of the Federal Reserve System, Washington, DC.
Carter, Z. 2020, *The Price of Peace: Money, Democracy, and the Life of John Maynard Keynes*, Random House, New York.
Chetty, R., Friedman, J., Hendren, N. and Stepner, M. 2022, 'The economic impacts of COVID-19: Evidence from a new public database built using private sector data', *NBER Working Paper 27431*.
Cynamon, B. and Fazzari, S. 2015, 'Inequality, the great recession, and slow recovery', *Cambridge Journal of Economics*, 40, pp. 373–99.
Daly, M., Buckman, S. and Seitelman, L. 2020, 'The unequal impact of COVID-19: Why education matters', *FRBSF Economic Letter*, 29 June, pp. 1–5.
Davis, K., Schoen, C., Schoenbaum, S.C., Audet, A-M.J., Doty, M.M. and Tenney, K. 2004, *Mirror, Mirror on the Wall: Looking at the Quality of American Health Care through the Patient's Lens*, Commonwealth Fund, New York.
Dunn, S. 2006, 'Prologomena to a post-keynesian health economics', *Review of Social Economy*, 64, pp. 273–99.
Durrant, T., Pope, T., Lilly, A., Guerin, B., Shepheard, M., Nickson, S., Schuller, J.-A., Mullens-Burgess, E. and Dalton, G. 2021, *Whitehall Monitor 2021*, Institute for Government, London.
Evans, R., Barer, M. and Marmor, T. 1994, *Why Are Some People Healthy and Others Not? The Determinants of the Health of Populations*, Aldine de Gruyter, New York.
Ferreira, F. 2021, 'Inequality in the time of Covid-19', *Finance and Development*, 58, pp. 20–3.
Frakt, A. 2018, 'Is Medicare for all the answer to sky-high administrative costs?' *New York Times*, 15 October.
Friedman, M. and Kuznets, S. 1946, *Income from Independent Professional Practice*, NBER, New York.
Galbraith, J.K. 1952, *A Theory of Price Control*, Harvard University Press, Cambridge, MA.
Galbraith, J.K. 1967, *The New Industrial State*, Houghton Mifflin, Boston.
Han, P., Klein, W. and Arora, N. 2011, 'Varieties of uncertainty in health care: A conceptual taxanomy', *Medical Decision Making*, 31, pp. 828–38.
Harcourt, G. and Kriesler, P. (eds) 2013, *The Oxford Handbook of Post-Keynesian Economics* Oxford University Press, Oxford.
Harris, G. and Berenson, A. 2005, '10 voters on panel backing pain pills had industry ties', *New York Times*, 25 February, pp. A1, A20.
Hussey, P.S., Anderson, G.F., Osborn, R., Feek, C., McLaughlin, V., Millar, J. and Epstein, A. 2004, 'How does the quality of care compare in five countries?' *Health Affairs*, 23(3), pp. 89–99.
Kamal, R. 2019, 'How does us life expectancy compare to other countries?' Accessed 27 June 2020, <https://www.healthsystemtracker.org/chart-collection/u-s-life-expectancy-compare-countries/#item-start>.
Kaplan, G., Pamuk, E., Lynch, J., Cohen, R. and Balfour, J. 1996, 'Income inequality and mortality in the United States', *British Medical Journal*, 312, pp. 999–1003.
Kassirer, J. 2004, *On the Take: How Medicine's Complicity with Big Business Can Endanger Your Health*, Oxford University Press, New York.
Keynes, J.M. 1936, *The General Theory of Employment, Interest and Money*, Macmillan, London.
Keynes, J.M. 1937, 'The general theory of employment', *Quarterly Journal of Economics* 51, pp. 212–23.
King, J. (ed.) 2012, *The Elgar Companion to Post-Keynesian Economics*, 2nd ed., Edward Elgar, Cheltenham.
Lavoie, M. 1994, 'A Post-Keynesian approach to consumer choice', *Journal of Post Keynesian Economics*, 16, pp. 539–62.
Marmot, M. 2004, *The Status Syndrome: How Social Standing Affects Our Health and Longevity*, Times Books, New York.

Meyer, A., Giardina, T., Khawaja, L. and Singh, H. 2021, 'Patient and clinician experiences of uncertainty in the diagnostic process: Current understanding and future directions', *Patient Education and Counseling*, 104, pp. 2606–15.
Moynihan, R. and Cassels, A. 2005, *Selling Sickness: How the World's Biggest Pharmaceutical Companies Are Turning Us All into Patients*, Nation Books, New York.
Mulcahy, A.W. Whaley, C.M., Gizaw, M., Schwam, D., Edenfield, N. and Becerra-Ornelas, A.U. 2021, *International Prescription Drug Price Comparisons*, RAND, Santa Monica.
Nelson, P. 1974, 'Advertising as information', *Journal of Political Economy*, 82, pp. 729–54.
O'Connor, D., Thayer, J. and Vehara, K. 2021, 'Stress and health: A review of psychobiological processes', *Annual Review of Psychology*, 72, pp. 663–88.
O'Donnell, R. 1990, 'An overview of probability, expectations, uncertainty and rationality in Keynes' conceptual framework', *Review of Political Economy*, 2, pp. 253–66.
O'Leary, C. and Wandner, S. 2020, 'An illustrated case for unemployment insurance reform', *Upjohn Institute Working Paper 19–317*, W.E. Upjohn Institute for Employment Research, Kalamazoo.
Pickett, K. and Wilkinson, R. 2015, 'Income inequality and health: A causal review', *Social Science and Medicine*, 128, pp. 316–26.
Pressman, S. 1997, 'Consumption, income distribution and taxation: Keynes' fiscal policy', *Journal of Income Distribution*, 7, pp. 29–44.
Reinhardt, U. 2004, 'An information infrastructure for the pharmaceutical market', *Health Affairs*, 23, pp. 107–12.
Rosser, J.B. 2001, 'Alternative Keynesian and Post-Keynesian perspectives on uncertainty and expectations', *Journal of Post Keynesian Economics*, 23, pp. 545–66.
Schneider, E., Shah, A., Doty, M., Tikkanen, R., Fields, K. and Williams III, R. 2021, *Mirror, Mirror 2021: International Comparison Reflects Flaws and Opportunities for Better U.S. Health Care*, Commonwealth Fund, New York.
Scott, R. and Pressman, S. 2015, 'Inadequate household deleveraging: Income, debt, and social provisioning', *Journal of Economic Issues*, 49, pp. 483–92.
Seidman, L. 1990, *Saving for America's Economic Future*, M.E. Sharpe, Armonk, NY.
Setterfield, M. 1995, 'Historical time and economic theory', *Review of Political Economy*, 7, pp. 1–27.
Shively, C. 2000, 'Social status, stress and health in female monkeys', in Tarvol, A. and St. Peter, R.F. (eds), *The Society and Population Health Reader – A State and Community Perspective*, New Press, New York, pp. 278–89.
Spurgeon, D. 2000, 'Doctors feel the pressure from direct to consumer advertising', *Western Journal of Medicine*, 172, p. 60.
Stockhammer, E. 2015, 'Rising inequality as a cause of the present crisis', *Cambridge Journal of Economics*, 39, pp. 935–58.
Thaler, R. and Sunstein, C. 2009, *Nudge*, Penguin, New York.
Thoits, P. 2020, 'Stress and health: Major findings and policy implications', *Journal of Health and Social Behavior*, 51, pp. S41–S55.
Vaithianathan, R. 2006, 'Health insurance and imperfect competition in the health care market', *Journal of Health Economics*, 25, pp. 1193–1202.
Wilkinson, R. 1992, 'Income distribution and life expectancy', *British Medical Journal*, 304, pp. 165–8.
Wilkinson, R. 1996, *Unhealthy Societies: The Afflictions of Inequality*, Routledge, London.
Zweifel, P. and Manning, W. 2000, 'Moral hazard and consumer incentives in healthcare', in Culyer, A. and Newhouse, J. (eds), *A Handbook of Health Economics*, Elsevier, London, Vol. 1, pp. 409–59.

7

NEW MATERIALISMS AND THE (CRITICAL) MICROPOLITICAL ECONOMY OF HEALTH

Nick J. Fox

New materialism is a portfolio term that has been applied to a range of ontological approaches in the social sciences and humanities that have in common a '(re)turn to matter' (Diener 2020: 45; Fox and Alldred 2017: 15-22). These approaches reprise aspects of Indigenous/First Nation ontologies that acknowledge continuities between natural and social worlds (Rosiek *et al.* 2020; Sundberg 2014), while challenging cultural and linguistic approaches in Western social theory (Chibber 2017). They supply an active engagement with materiality and bodies, and model power and resistance within a messy, heterogeneous and emergent social world (Braidotti 2011: 137; Grosz 1994; Saldanha 2006).

This ontology has been applied to a growing range of topics (Fox and Alldred 2017), including health (Duff 2014; Fox 2011; Potts 2004). From such a perspective, health and illness are considered as relational, processual and emergent, rather than as an essential quality of an individual body: an assemblage (Fox 2011: 366) of physical, biological, social, cultural and political forces. This analysis has implications for care and for well-being more generally (Coffey 2022; McLeod 2017). Despite this growing body of work – which includes the application of new materialist ontology to social stratifications by gender (Lorraine 2008) and race (Colebrook 2013), and the analysis of capitalist social relations by theorists such as Deleuze and Guattari (1984, 1988), DeLanda (2006) and Massumi (2015: 83–91) – it has not as yet translated into a political economy of health inequalities. This chapter outlines the potential for a new materialist critical political economy of health, building on recent work that has addressed the more-than-human production of inequalities (Fox and Alldred 2021; Fox and Powell 2021).

However, the new materialisms concern themselves with ontological entities such as assemblages and affects that diverge from the conventional focus of political economy studies upon societal structures, systems and social classes (Coburn 2004; Scambler 2007). Scholars such as Latour (2005: 130–1) and Massumi (2015: 87–8) have questioned critical approaches that 'explain' the social world in terms of 'deep' social structures, focusing instead on the 'affects' (capacities to affect or be affected) within the events and interactions that occur in workplaces, markets and other quotidian dynamics of social life (Connolly, 2013: 404; Massumi, 2015: 87–91). Furthermore, the new materialisms acknowledge the wide range of human and non-human materialities that produce and reproduce the social and natural world (Bennett 2010; Coole and Frost 2010; Fox and Alldred 2017). These features of the approach require a 'micropolitical' re-thinking of the social

DOI: 10.4324/9781003017110-8

relations of capitalism, with the potential to supply a critical understanding of how the events of the everyday produce socio-material dis/advantage and social divisions.

The next section outlines key features of new materialist ontology, and the 'ethological' approach of Deleuze (1988) that supplies the conceptual framework for a 'critical micropolitical economy' (CMPE). I re-read Marx's analysis of the social relations of capitalism in terms of the post-anthropocentrism, relationality and ontological monism that are features of the new materialisms (Connolly 2013: 399; Fox and Alldred 2018b). I illustrate the CMPE by analyzing the inequalities that emerged during the COVID-19 pandemic, before concluding with an assessment of the opportunities afforded by a new materialist approach.

The new materialisms

Despite the breadth of approaches comprising the 'new materialisms', they share some core features. First, they each emphasize questions of matter (Coole and Frost 2010: 2; Haraway 1992: 65). However, the matter addressed by the new materialisms is not an inert substrate for human activity, but relational and emergent (Coole and Frost 2010: 28); 'lively' (Bennett 2010); and 'affective' (having a capacity to affect or be affected) or agentic (Connolly 2013: 400). Moreover, 'materiality' is broadly defined to include not only bodies, physical stuff, spaces and places, but also human concepts/constructs and human epiphenomena such as memory or imagination – all of which can *affect materially* (Barad 2007: 152; Braidotti 2013: 3, Fox and Alldred 2019). This focus shifts social studies of health and illness from an emphasis on their discursive production toward a re-engagement with health and well-being as materially embodied and embedded (Cluley 2020: 286; Fox and Alldred 2017: 132–4; McLeod 2017: 8).

Second, the new materialisms acknowledge a material world that does not comprise stable entities with fixed, essential attributes, but a *relational* and uneven world that emerges in unpredictable ways around actions and events (Potts 2004: 19), as different human and non-human materialities interact. This relationality requires that we ask of a body or any other materiality not what it *is*, but what it can *do* in a specific context (Buchanan 1997). This has the effect of de-stabilizing supposedly unitary phenomena such as 'human', 'woman', 'truth' and 'power' (Braidotti 2011: 130; Colebrook 2013; Deleuze and Guattari 1988: 275). In the modern period, biomedicine has considered 'health' and 'illness' as inherent attributes of an organic body (Fox 2011: 359), leading to individualized treatment, and an emphasis on personal responsibility (McLeod 2017: 11). New materialist ontology undermines this ontology of an essential and prior body, seeing bodies, health and illness as emergent and entangled within socio-material networks or assemblages comprising both human and non-human matter (Deleuze and Guattari 1988: 90; Fox 2012: 64–70).

Third, the new materialisms cut across many social science dualisms (Braidotti 2011: 129), including the mind/matter, human/non-human and culture/nature dualities that underpinned humanism (van der Tuin and Dolphijn 2010: 155). This is not, however, a move to universalism or a unitary perspective on materiality. Instead, it opens up a multiplicity and diversity that exceeds and overwhelms the dichotomies it replaces (Deleuze 2001: 95). This transversality puts in question other social theory dualisms including animate/inanimate, reason/emotion, surface/depth, and (significantly for this chapter) micro/macro and structure/agency (Braidotti 2013: 4–5; Coole and Frost 2010: 26–7; van der Tuin and Dolphijn 2010: 157). This ontology acknowledges bodies, health and illness as 'socio-material' and 'more-than-human': processually and endlessly emergent from the intersections of physical, biological, social, cultural, economic and political forces, but irreducible to any one of these realms (Fox 2011: 366; McLeod 2017: 158).

To establish a 'new materialist' approach to the political economy of health, I shall focus on one strand: Deleuze's (1988) 'ethological' ontology of matter. Central to ethology is the study of *affects* – defined as 'capacities for affecting and being affected', and of how these affects diminish or strengthen a body's or a thing's power to act (Deleuze 1988: 125–6). In this ontology, matter – both 'human' and 'non-human' – is not defined by form, substance or fixed attributes, but simply by its *capacities*. Capacities are not inherent, but emerge relationally when one body or thing interacts with (affects) other similarly contingent and ephemeral bodies, things and ideas (DeLanda 2016: 143–4; Deleuze 1988: 123; Deleuze and Guattari 1988: 261).

Deleuze and Guattari (1988: 22) describe these contextual arrangements of bodies and things as *assemblages*. Assemblages emerge in unpredictable ways around actions and events (Bennett 2005: 445; Deleuze and Guattari 1988: 88), 'in a kind of chaotic network of habitual and non-habitual connections' (Potts 2004: 19), drawn together by their constituents' capacities to affect or be affected (Deleuze 1988: 124). It follows that the *micropolitics* of affects within assemblages (Deleuze and Guattari 1988: 216) is key to unlocking how the world and everything in it is produced, from moment to moment.

Ethology's focus upon affects and capacities requires 'health' to be understood *micropolitically,* in terms of the everyday affective and relational engagements between bodies and the material world (Duff 2014: 53; Fox 2011). 'Health' needs to be understood relationally: as the 'actual measurable capacity to form new relations' (Buchanan 1997: 82) and a 'quantum of a body's power of acting' (Duff 2014: 75). Furthermore, it is not the body itself, but the assemblages within which a body participates, that is 'healthy' (Buchanan 1997: 82). This perspective underpins the remainder of this chapter, as I develop a micropolitical economy of health.

Challenges for a critical (micro)political economy of health

The political economy of health and healthcare has traditionally been inclined toward a critical or Marxist analysis of the social relations of capitalism (Coburn 2004; Doyal and Pennell 1979; Navarro 2009; Scambler 2007, 2012). Political economy in this register has often been characterized by a top-down notion of power vested in a sovereign state; an understanding of the social relations of capitalism as structural; economic inequalities baked into these social relations; and health inequalities produced by a constellation of material factors acting on bodies positively or negatively (Scambler 2007).

New materialist ontology does not map directly or neatly on to this framing. The monism underpinning new materialist perspectives (Connolly 2010: 178) dispenses with any idea of a foundation or 'other level' or reality beyond the everyday (van der Tuin and Dolphijn 2010: 155). This leaves no space ontologically for structures, systems or mechanisms, a top-down conception of power (Fox and Alldred 2018b: 318), or the 'micro/macro' distinction sometimes drawn in both social theory and economics between interpersonal encounters and the legal and governance processes of 'the State' deemed to shape societies and economic systems (DeLanda 2006: 4–6).

A further divergence concerns the association between 'social class' and health inequalities in rich and poor nations, generally ascribed by sociologists and epidemiologists to material deprivation (Bambra *et al.* 2020; Marmot and Bell 2012; Navarro 1976; Townsend and Davidson 1982). An ethological approach problematizes the aggregation of disparate bodies into two, five or seven discrete 'classes' based on attributes such as occupation, income or the more complex mix of assets postulated by neo-Bourdieusian scholars (Savage *et al.* 2013: 223). Instead, asking what a body can do addresses capacities as emergent and contingent.

Finally, critical political-economic models of health inequalities have postulated a cause/effect relationship between the social relations of capitalism and inequality, usually based on some version of the structural, top-down model outlined above. The new materialisms supplant this model with an understanding of social production as a micropolitical and emergent process deriving from the affective flows in assemblages of matter. This acknowledges that a flow of affect requires both a capacity to affect *and* a capacity to be affected: in this relational perspective, it is no longer appropriate to designate one component of an assemblage as independent and another as a dependent variable (Massumi 2015: 94–5).

Toward a (micro)political economy of health

To articulate a critical political economy of health from an ethological perspective, I apply the three core aspects of new materialist ontology outlined above: relationality, post-anthropocentrism and monism. I illustrate these with examples from recent health research with a bearing on political economy, to inform a subsequent micropolitical analysis of the social relations of capitalism, inequalities, and a new materialist perspective on power and resistance.

First, ethology replaces an essentialist understanding with a relational ontology that acknowledges that what a body can do derives from context-specific capacities (Delanda 2016: 2). These emerge when the affects (capacities to affect or be affected) between a body or thing and other matter draw them into assemblage (Massumi 2015: 94). The flows of affect in a particular assemblage consequently establish the micropolitics of what the bodies and other matter can do. Changes to the composition of an assemblage will lead to alterations in capacities, opening up or closing down possibilities for action. These latter may, in turn, establish relative advantages or disadvantages (henceforth, 'dis/advantages') – as discussed below.

To illustrate, a study (Fox 2017) of digital health technologies (DHTs) – ranging from the *Fitbit* fitness monitor to implantable medical devices – used a relational analysis to assess the micropolitics of DHT/body assemblages. The affects within these assemblages included not only the capacities of the devices to monitor vital signs or physiologically intervene (for instance, delivering a shot of insulin or defibrillation electric shocks). Rather, they also assembled bodies variously with the commercial interests behind devices, the privatization of healthcare, biomedicine and public health surveillance (Fox 2017: 143–6). These latter affects placed constraints on what bodies using these technologies could do, potentially translating into specific physical, psychological or social dis/advantage, such as dependence on health professionals, or a loss of corporeal autonomy as devices instigated physiological or biochemical interventions. However, the study also suggested how DHT assemblages might be intentionally 're-engineered' to substitute constraining micropolitics with a 'citizen health' micropolitics that opened up new political opportunities by networking users, monitoring and flagging environmental hazards, and building coalitions to improve public health (Fox 2017: 146–7).

Second, the monism of new materialist ontology makes everyday events the sole arena wherein social, economic and political forces are deployed to produce and reproduce social divisions and inequalities (Edwards 2010: 283; Latour 2005: 130–1). Consequently, assemblages cut across a conventional 'micro/macro' dualism, linking bodies to 'macro' social, political and economic phenomena (DeLanda 2006: 17). Analyzing an event (*e.g.* a factory worker using a machine to process raw materials, an interaction between shopper and assistant at a supermarket till, or a marketing campaign that promotes highly processed foodstuffs) requires acknowledging that the components of the assemblage producing this event include both immediate human and non-human matter, and a wider range of affective matter. These include corporations, commerce, finance, local, national and international government, policies, laws, health and welfare services, and abstract (but still materially affective) concepts such as citizenship, governance and community.

This crosscutting analysis was applied in a recent study of obesity and weight loss (Fox *et al.* 2018). Analysis of interview data revealed the wide range of affective materialities in the 'becoming-fat' assemblage of overweight and obese bodies, and the 'becoming-slimmer' assemblage of those trying to lose weight. These included not only food, fat, physical environments, food producers and processing industries, food retailers, diet regimens and weight loss clubs, but also wider social, cultural and economic formations such as global food trade, market exchange and agri-business (Fox *et al.* 2018: 111). These material components variously affected bodies during everyday encounters, such as during a shopping trip to a supermarket or exercising in a gym. Critically, this analysis found that the only difference in the make-up of the 'becoming-fat' and 'becoming-slimmer' assemblages (apart from slimming clubs and low-fat food options in the latter) was the desire of slimmers to lose weight. Micropolitically, this desire was pitted against powerful forces in the assemblage deriving from agri-business, food processing, delivery and retail industries, which promoted processed and high-fat foods at lower prices than 'healthier' alternatives (Fox *et al.* 2018: 122–3). This micropolitical analysis enabled insight into how 'macro' socio-economic phenomena such as industrial food production, and retail and marketing businesses interacted with the 'micro' processes of weight gain and dieting (Fox *et al.* 2018: 123–4).

Finally, micropolitical analysis must acknowledge the affective capacities of *all* matter in the events that produce social and natural worlds (*cf.* Barad 2007: 226–30). This aspect of ethology addresses an aspect of human interactions with the material world that – as noted earlier – is downplayed in contemporary political economy approaches. It is founded on the acknowledgment that all matter is affective. Accordingly, it may contribute significantly to the micropolitics of everyday encounters, to relative advantage or disadvantage and, thus, to health inequalities.

The significance of such non-human material interactions has been revealed in recent research (Fox and Gavrilyuk, 2022) on workplace interactions between bodies and non-human matter. This disclosed great material disparities between the daily work of different workers, leading to sustained advantage or disadvantage. For example, in the cases examined, teachers or senior managers were accommodated in spacious, high-quality, well-regulated and amenable workspaces, with comfortable furnishings, information and communication technology, and other resources needed for them to work productively and creatively. In contrast, manual work was physically demanding, while these workers' encounters with the raw materials, machinery of production and weather could make workplaces inefficient, uncomfortable and occasionally debilitating (see also: Fernandes 1977). In place of roomy offices and executive dining rooms, there were noisy work-floors, cramped meeting places and canteens, and utilitarian sanitation.

These three building blocks of a new materialist political-economic approach enable analysis of the social, political and economic forces summarized by the term 'capitalism' (the same might be done with terminology such as 'patriarchy', 'democracy', 'colonialism' and 'neoliberalism'). In line with the relational premise of ethology, I shall not attempt to define what capitalism is, but instead ask: what does it actually do?

What does capitalism do?

In Volume 1 of Capital, Marx (2011 [1867]: 185) supplied part of the answer to this question: capitalism transforms human labor-power (capacity to labor) into capital. This is achieved via two relational transactions. The first is a production transaction (in ethological terms: an affective movement) that exchanges wages for the labor required to add value to a commodity (Marx 2011

[1867]: 186–7). The second transaction/affective movement takes place in a market environment of some sort (ranging from physical markets to commodity exchanges to online retail), where this added-value commodity is exchanged for the money/material resources that provide the capitalist with a return (surplus value or profit) on her/his investment (Marx 2011 [1867]: 168).

The relational analysis of capitalism set out in *Capital* is directly translatable into the monist perspective of new materialism. Yet, rather than treating capitalism as an abstraction or a structural social relation (Scambler 2007: 299), it can be analyzed by exploring emblematic examples of these production and market affects in action: within concrete manifestations such as a factory and a marketplace (DeLanda 2006: 17–18). Further work is needed, however, to overcome the anthropocentric focus of *Capital:* for Marx (2011 [1867]: 202–4), the non-human matter (NHM) – including the means of production – in this affect-economy was no more than a substrate for the social relations that generate surplus value. Nevertheless, exploring the more-than-human assemblages of these settings can reveal how both bodies and NHM are affective within these event-assemblages.

For instance, a factory production assemblage can be summarized as comprising at least (and in no particular order): a worker; raw materials; means of production (buildings, tools, technology, knowledge); wages; other workers; managers; and a boss (owner or shareholders). More specifically, a production affect-economy assembles together NHM (raw materials, physical means of production, wages) and human matter (workers, boss, management). As well as supplying the material means for workers to gain a wage and bosses to create value-added commodities, this arrangement of matter establishes new capacities in the raw materials as they are transformed into value-added products. For example, a 'blast furnace assemblage' establishes new capacities as it transforms iron ore into cast iron or steel for construction, cutlery and weapon manufacture. Meanwhile, as noted earlier in this section, daily interactions with the work environment (treated by Marx simply as the means of production) may affect humans in multiple ways, producing physical, psychological and social dis/advantage.

Similarly, at its simplest, a market-event may be summarized as an assemblage comprising at least (and in no particular order): a commodity; trader A; customer B; competitor traders; competitor customers; money/material resources; and a market environment. To elaborate, the affect-economy of a market assembles commodities for trade, traders and customers within a specific place and time. While – as Marx noted – the exchange of commodity and money between trader and customer enables the value added to the commodity to be realized, from a more-than-human perspective, commodities gain new capacities (and lose others) in this process. For instance, steel processed into cutlery gains capacities to cut, spear and scoop food, while losing its more general capacity as a raw material. It also affects competitor traders and customers in the immediate market environment, establishing a benchmark for the exchange-value of similar products, thereby sustaining the underlying dynamic of a market economy (Prey 2012: 265).

These two more-than-human events capture the arrangements of bodies and NHM in the phenomena denoted by the shorthand: 'capitalism'. In practice, these assemblages will contain further relations and affects, including trade unions, accountants and book-keepers, the infrastructure of shopping centers and trading estates, financial institutions, credit cards, and laws and their enforcement by 'the state' – such as safety and employment law, regulatory frameworks governing production and consumption, and fiscal policies.

This ethological micropolitical analysis also supplies insight into how the concrete transactions/affective movements entailed in production and market assemblages endure. The micropolitics in each of these assemblages produces both intended and unintended capacities in their human and non-human components. In the production assemblage, the decision by workers to sell their labor-power, though in principle voluntary, ties the worker into dependency on a wage, precluding alternative means to subsist such as self-employment or communal/co-operative production. Furthermore, as noted above, the work environment may produce differential physical, psychological and social dis/advantage in manual, non-manual and professional staff, including through its impacts on health and well-being. While condemning the disadvantaged to grim daily routines, more pleasant conditions may be a 'perk' for relatively advantaged workers and, at least theoretically, act as a source of aspiration for others to advance as a means to ameliorate their daily material circumstances.

The market assemblage, meanwhile, acts micropolitically to establish monetary exchange-values for a growing range of matter, encompassing most goods and services produced by human labor. This establishes money as a transactional medium between humans, further reducing alternatives to wage-labor such as barter, tithing, while also generating wealth inequalities both between owners of the means of production and labor, and between higher- and lower-waged workers. In this way, the micropolitics of the physical marketplace extends beyond its immediate boundaries, establishing a positive feedback loop of affects that sustain and develop concrete and abstract markets, in due course establishing what would be described in structural sociology as a 'market economy'.

These micropolitics suggest why production and market assemblages sustain and proliferate over time, and how capitalist micropolitics produce social inequalities (including health inequalities) via the inevitable production of dis/advantage in those who are drawn into production and market assemblages. Furthermore, it suggests how 'power' is to be understood in this monist political economy. Without 'another level' to the social world, power can no longer be considered as extraneous or 'top down'. Instead, it is integral to the assemblages that produce events in everyday life (Barad 2007: 94), and comprises nothing more, nor less, than the interactions between assembled relations as they affect and are affected (Braidotti 2013: 188–9; Patton 2000: 52). Expressions of power (and resistance) are the outcomes of micropolitical material forces and intensities operating within events (Fox and Alldred 2018b).

Simultaneously, 'power' is necessarily transient and fluctuating – a momentary production of an affect between matters. Regularities or continuities in power (for instance, management authority over workers) depend upon repeated assertions of an assemblage micropolitics. These micropolitical patternings in time and space may have provided the semblance of overarching social structures or systems (for instance, 'patriarchy' or 'capitalism), but this regularity is illusory: power can have continuity only so long as it is replicated in the next event, and the one after that, and may quickly evaporate when assemblage micropolitics change (Fox and Alldred 2018b).

Capitalism, tiny dis/advantages and health: insights from a pandemic

The previous conceptual framework disclosed that the myriad affective interactions between materialities produce relational, context-specific, and emergent capacities and incapacities in bodies, and the consequent opportunities and constraints upon what they can do. Some of these opportunities or constraints may be trivial, producing only transitory dis/advantage. For instance, a taxi-driver's pay will depend upon productivity: bad weather or a breakdown will temporarily constrain the number of customers transported in a day. This single loss of income is unlikely to produce enduring disadvantage or ill-health. However, if this disruption is repeated, the ensuing material constraints can – over a month, year or lifetime – establish enduring disadvantage relative to workers paid a fixed salary. Such material disadvantage may, over time, produce relative material deprivation, with physical, psychological or social sequelae.

This drip feed of myriad opportunities and constraints generated by the micropolitics in events can be considered as the 'thousand tiny dis/advantages' of daily life.[1] How, then, might such tiny dis/advantages affect health and well-being? As noted earlier, new materialist theorists have argued that 'health' should not be understood as an individual attribute, but as relational, reflecting how engagements with the material world establish a body's performative capacities. Findings from recent research (Fox and Powell 2021) found that – on a range of indicators – those in good health had notably and statistically significantly higher levels of positive capacities and lower levels of negative capacities than poor-health respondents. This suggests that health disparities are intertwined (possibly inextricably) with the differential production of socio-material dis/advantage in contemporary societies. In effect, 'health' and 'dis/advantage' are part of the same phenomenon: the quotidian and unending production of positive and negative capacities as bodies interact with both human and non-human matter (Fox and Powell 2021).

The connection between the everyday micropolitics of capitalist production and markets, tiny dis/advantages and health outcomes can be explicated further by applying the CMPE approach to the socio-economic and ethnic disparities revealed during the COVID-19 pandemic. Public health studies have documented wide divergences/inequalities in infection prevalence and death rates from the virus. Age-adjusted death rates of those living in the most deprived areas are more than twice those of those in the least deprived areas (Blundell *et al.* 2020: 19–20), while black Britons' death rates from COVID-19 are almost three times those of white men (Office for National Statistics 2020).

Beyond these headline figures, other data can inform a CMPE assessment of how everyday participation in production and market assemblages contributes to these disparities. Occupational differences in COVID-19 death rates are striking: working-age men in manual (semi- or unskilled), caring and leisure occupations had a death rate over three times that of professional and technical workers (ONS 2021). Throughout the pandemic, coronavirus 'hot spots' have emerged. For example, meat-processing plants in Australia, the UK, the US and elsewhere have been sources of localized community outbreaks (Dyal *et al.* 2020). In their review of cases, Middleton *et al.* (2020) suggest that these plants are sources of widespread transmission because of the physical and socio-economic circumstances of meat processing. The cool, humid conditions in these plants retain live viruses for longer on hard surfaces; the work produces dense aerosols of animal debris that may transmit the virus between staff; noisy working conditions require workers to speak loudly or shout, thereby augmenting the potential for airborne transmission; and crowded workplaces limit potential for social distancing. Other risky working environments such as food packaging and 'sweat-shop' garment manufacturers have also been implicated as COVID hot spots (Middleton *et al.* 2020: 1; O'Connor 2020).

Earlier, I set out the production and market components of a 'capitalism-assemblage' comprising human and non-human elements. During the COVID-19 pandemic, a further component has been added to this assemblage: the virus itself. This has its own affective capacities: a capacity for a protein spike on its surface to inject RNA into a host cell; the capacity of this RNA to hijack the host cell's genetic mechanisms to replicate copies of the virus; and a capacity to remain viable in aerosols and droplets, and on hard and soft surfaces (Fehr and Perlman 2015). While the capitalism-assemblage continues to generate its outputs and surplus value, it is simultaneously hijacked by the coronavirus to its own ends: to pass from human body to body using the channels of globalized production and commerce, international travel and urbanization. In effect, it becomes a *pandemic-assemblage*, whose micropolitics have enabled the global dissemination of the virus (Fox 2022).

A CMPE perspective reveals how the micropolitics of capitalist production and markets produce these transmission hot spots and occupational divergences. A demand for cheap food and cheap clothing has driven down profit margins so that manufacturers will depend upon low-paid and precarious labor (often drawn disproportionately from ethnic minority groups) and poor working and living conditions (Dyal *et al.* 2020; Middleton *et al.* 2020: 1). All these 'tiny disadvantages' increase the chances of COVID-19 infection and, hence, dissemination within such environments. More broadly, the tiny dis/advantages experienced by workers in manual and public-facing jobs will be most affected by the viral affects in the pandemic-assemblage. In contrast, many workers in non-manual and professional jobs have working conditions that do not carry the same exposure, and many have been able to work from home during the pandemic (ONS 2021).

Typically, the public health response to these disparities has been individualized: based on voluntary and mandatory measures to alter COVID-risky behaviors. In contrast, a CMPE analysis acknowledges that the pandemic is a consequence of the micropolitics of capitalist and globalized production and market assemblages, in which the virus is inextricably caught up. The 'baked-in' inequalities of capitalist production and market assemblages shape the likelihood of contact with the coronavirus in the everyday encounters associated with different types and patterns of work. Meanwhile, the relative health status and prevalence of underlying medical conditions in different socio-economic and ethnic groups further shape the severity and rates of death arising from infection.

Conclusion

I have suggested in this chapter how a new materialist ontology can establish a *critical* (micro) political economy approach to health that utilizes the relational, monist and post-anthropocentric perspective of the new materialisms. This ontology has sometimes been criticized within the social sciences for apparently undercutting a capacity for a 'political' analysis of events and, in particular, denying opportunities to assert the negative consequences of the structures or systems reified by terms such as 'capitalism', 'patriarchy', 'neo-liberalism' (Rekret 2018: 55).

In contrast, the analysis here suggests that an ethological ontology of assemblage, affect/capacity and micropolitics can sustain a critical response, although its monism requires a substantive shift in how 'capitalism' and these other conventional terms are understood. To reiterate: in this ontology, the 'social relations of capitalism' are re-thought as material affects (capacities to affect or be affected) within the assemblages of human and non-human matter that constitute the events of the everyday. These affects include the social forces conventionally designated as power (or as social structural). The micropolitics of these events/assemblages produce opportunities and constraints on what constituent components can do, and consequent tiny advantages and disadvantages. Accretions of these tiny dis/advantages may, in due course, establish more lasting patterns of inequality.

What then is the value of a critical new materialist political economy approach? First, an ethological ontology offers the benefit of simplicity. Three concepts (affect, assemblage and micropolitics) establish the framework for the CMPE. Similarly, its monism removes the need for potentially complex and occasionally convoluted explanations (Martin and Lee 2015: 717) of how indirectly observable social structures or mechanisms affect the everyday production of the social world and human history. Second and consequently, the CMPE is empirically oriented. The focus of social inquiry is upon complex affective flows that transcend 'micro'/'macro' distinctions. Assemblages, affects and micropolitics events may be studied via a mix of established social research methods of data collection, including observation, interviews, surveys and even social experiments (Fox and Alldred 2018a). Nor is this CMPE limited to assessment of the capitalist-assemblage: other political and economic assemblages (for instance, command economy, feudalism, despotism) may also be subjected to critical scrutiny using the same conceptual framework and analytical methodology.

Third, it enables – and indeed requires – assessment of the affective capacities of the breadth of matter. It thereby cuts across the culture/nature dualism that has privileged human agency and, thus, limited political-economic insight into phenomena such as climate change, agricultural sustainability and health that do not neatly fit within either of these distinct categories. The 'vital materialism' applied in the CMPE acknowledges that matter is central to production and market assemblages, affecting human bodies materially in multiple ways. The illustration of how the affects of COVID-19 have transformed capitalism into a 'pandemic-assemblage' offers a new insight into how the non-human interacts with the granularity of human activities.

These insights provide the basis for a novel research agenda that can explore the everyday material production of dis/advantage in contemporary societies, including dis/advantages leading to health inequality. This agenda can delve into the complexities of interactions between bodies, politics and economics at the level of the everyday event (whether an event is a consumer doing their weekly shopping or a meeting of world leaders to discuss climate change), supplying greater insight into how capitalist production and market assemblages generate dis/advantage and inequality. Concomitantly, this agenda also offers the potential for critical political-economic interventions: to alter the affects and micropolitics in these events, thereby ameliorating disadvantage and reducing inequalities.

Note

1 This formulation references new materialist scholarship that has replaced discrete 'gender' and 'race' categories with 'a thousand tiny sexes' (Grosz 1993) or 'tiny races' (Saldanha 2006).

References

Bambra, C., Riordan, R., Ford, J. and Matthews, F. 2020, 'The COVID-19 pandemic and health inequalities', *Journal of Epidemiology and Community Health*, 74, pp. 964–8.

Barad, K. 2003, 'Posthumanist performativity: Toward an understanding of how matter comes to matter', *Signs: Journal of Women in Culture and Society*, 28(3), pp. 801–31.

Barad, K. 2007, *Meeting the Universe Halfway*, Duke University Press, Durham.

Bennett, J. 2005, 'The agency of assemblages and the North American blackout', *Public Culture*, 17(3), pp. 45–65.

Bennett, J. 2010, *Vibrant Matter*, Duke University Press, Durham.

Blundell, R., Dias, M.C., Joyce, R. and Xu, X. 2020, 'COVID-19 and Inequalities', *Fiscal Studies*, 41(2), pp. 291–319.

Braidotti, R. 2011, *Nomadic Theory*, Columbia University Press, New York.

Braidotti, R. 2013, *The Posthuman*, Polity, Cambridge.

Buchanan, I. 1997, 'The problem of the body in Deleuze and Guattari, Or, what can a body do?' *Body and Society*, 3(3), pp. 73–91.

Chibber, V. 2017, 'Rescuing class from the cultural turn', *Catalyst*, 1(1), pp. 27–55.

Cluley, V. 2020, 'Becoming-care: Reframing care work as flesh work not body work', *Culture and Organization*, 26(4), pp. 284–97.

Coburn, D. 2004, 'Beyond the income inequality hypothesis: Class, neo-liberalism, and health inequalities', *Social Science and Medicine*, 58(1), pp. 41–56.

Coffey, J. 2022, 'Assembling wellbeing: Bodies, affects and the "conditions of possibility" for wellbeing', *Journal of Youth Studies*, 25(1), pp. 67–83.

Colebrook, C. 2013, 'Face race', in Saldanha, A. and Admans, J.M. (eds), *Deleuze and Race*, Edinburgh University Press, Edinburgh, pp. 35–50.

Coole, D.H. and Frost, S. 2010, 'Introducing the new materialisms', in Coole, D.H. and Frost, S. (eds), *New Materialisms: Ontology, Agency, and Politics*, Duke University Press, London, pp. 1–43.

Connolly, W.E. 2010, 'Materialities of experience', in Coole, D.H. and Frost, S. (eds), *New Materialisms: Ontology, Agency, and Politics*, Duke University Press, London, pp. 178–200.

Connolly, W.E. 2013, 'The "new materialism" and the fragility of things', *Millennium*, 41(3), pp. 399–412.
DeLanda, M. 2006, *A New Philosophy of Society*, Continuum, London.
DeLanda, M. 2016, *Assemblage Theory*, Edinburgh University Press, Edinburgh.
Deleuze, G. 1988, *Spinoza: Practical Philosophy*, City Lights, San Francisco.
Deleuze, G. and Guattari, F. 1984, *Anti Oedipus: Capitalism and Schizophrenia*, Athlone, London.
Deleuze, G. and Guattari, F. 1988, *A Thousand Plateaus*, Athlone, London.
Deleuze, G. 2001. *Pure Immanence: Essays on a Life*, Zone Books, Princeton, NJ.
Diener, S. 2020, 'New Materialisms', *The Year's Work in Critical and Cultural Theory*, 28(1), pp. 44–65.
Doyal, L. and Pennell, I. 1979, *The Political Economy of Health*, Pluto Press, London.
Duff, C. 2014, *Assemblages of Health*, Springer, Dordrecht.
Dyal, J.W., Grant M.P., Broadwater, K., Bjork, A., Waltenburg, M.A., Gibbins, J.D., Hale, C., Silver, M., Fischer, M., Steinberg, J., Basler, C.A., Jacobs, J.R., Kennedy, E.D., Tomasi, S., Trout, D., Hornsby-Myers, J., Oussayef, N.L., Delaney, L.J., Patel, K., Shetty, V., Kline, K.E,. Schroeder, B., Herlihy, R.K., House, J., Jervis, R., Clayton, J.L., Ortbahn, D., Austin, C., Berl, E., Moore, Z., Buss, B.F., Stover, D., Westergaard, R., Pray, I., DeBolt, M., Person, A., Gabel, J., Kittle, T.S., Hendren, P., Rhea, C., Holsinger, C., Dunn, J., Turabelidze, G., Ahmed, F.S., deFijter, S., Pedati, C.S., Rattay, K., Smith, E.E., Luna-Pinto, C., Cooley, L.A., Saydah, S., Preacely, N.D., Maddox, R.A., Lundeen, E., Goodwin, B., Karpathy, S.E., Griffing, S., Jenkins, M.M., Lowry, G., Schwarz, R.D., Yoder, J., Peacock, G., Walke, H.T., Rose, D.A. and Honein, M.A. 2020, 'COVID-19 among workers in meat and poultry processing facilities – 19 States', *Morbidity and Mortality Weekly Report*, 69(18), pp. 557–61.
Edwards, J. 2010, 'The materialism of historical materialism', in Coole, D.H. and Frost, S. (eds), *New Materialisms: Ontology, Agency, and Politics*, Duke University Press, London, pp. 281–98.
Fehr, A.R. and Perlman, S. 2015, 'Coronaviruses: An overview of their replication and pathogenesis', *Methods in Molecular Biology*, 1282, pp. 1–23.
Fernandes, L. 1997, *Producing Workers*, University of Pennsylvania Press, Philadelphia.
Fox, N.J. 2011, 'The ill-health assemblage: Beyond the body-with-organs', *Health Sociology Review*, 20(4), pp. 359–71.
Fox, N.J. 2012, *The Body*, Polity, Cambridge.
Fox, N.J. 2017, 'Personal health technologies, micropolitics and resistance: A new materialist analysis', *Health*, 21(2), pp. 136–53.
Fox, N.J. 2022 'Coronavirus, capitalism and a 'thousand tiny dis/advantages': A more-than-human analysis', *Social Theory and Health*, 20, pp. 107–20.
Fox, N.J. and Alldred, P. 2017, *Sociology and the New Materialism*, Sage, London.
Fox, N.J. and Alldred, P. 2018a, 'Mixed methods, materialism and the micropolitics of the research-assemblage', *International Journal of Social Research Methodology*, 21(2), pp. 191–204.
Fox, N.J. and Alldred, P. 2018b, 'Social structures, power and resistance in monist sociology: (New) materialist insights', *Journal of Sociology*, 54(3), pp. 315–30.
Fox, N.J. and Alldred, P. 2019, 'The materiality of memory: Affects, remembering and food decisions', *Cultural Sociology*, 13(1), pp. 20–36.
Fox, N.J. and Alldred, P. 2021, 'Bodies, non-human matter and the micropolitical production of sociomaterial dis/advantage', *Journal of Sociology*, 58(4), pp. 499–516.
Fox, N.J., Bissell, P., Peacock, M. and Blackburn, J. 2018, 'The micropolitics of obesity: Materialism, markets and food sovereignty', *Sociology*, 52(1), pp. 111–27.
Fox, N.J. and Gavrilyuk, T. 2022. 'The more-than-human production of material dis/advantage: A Russian case study', *International Social Science Journal*, 72(246), pp. 1033–51.
Fox, N.J. and Powell, K. 2021, 'Non-human matter, health disparities and a thousand tiny dis/advantages', *Sociology of Health and Illness*, 43(3), pp. 779–95.
Grosz, E. 1993, 'A thousand tiny sexes: Feminism and rhizomatics', *Topoi*, 12(2), pp. 167–79.
Grosz, E. 1994, *Volatile Bodies*, Indiana University Press, Bloomington.
Haraway, D. 1992, 'Otherworldly conversations; terran topics; local terms', *Science as Culture*, 3(1), pp. 64–98.
Latour, B. 2005, *Reassembling the Social: An Introduction to Actor Network Theory*, Oxford University Press, Oxford.
Lorraine, T. 2008, 'Feminist lines of flight from the majoritarian subject', *Deleuze Studies*, 2(Suppl), pp. 60–82.
Marmot, M. and Bell, R. 2012, 'Fair society, healthy lives', *Public Health*, 126(Supplement 1), pp. S4–S10.

Martin, J.L. and Lee, M. 2015, 'Social structure', in Wright, J.D. (ed), *International Encyclopedia of the Social and Behavioral Sciences, Volume 22*, Elsevier, Oxford, pp. 713–18.
Marx, K. 2011 [1867], *Capital, Volume 1*, Dover, New York.
Massumi, B. 2015, *Politics of Affect*, Polity, Cambridge.
McLeod, K. 2017, *Wellbeing Machine*, Carolina Academic Press, Durham.
Middleton, J., Reintjes, R. and Lopes, H. 2020, 'Meat plants – A new front line in the COVID-19 pandemic', *British Medical Journal*, 370, p. m2716.
Navarro, V. 1976, *Medicine Under Capitalism*, Prodist, New York.
Navarro, V. 2009, 'What we mean by social determinants of health', *International Journal of Health Services*, 39(3), pp. 423–41.
O'Connor, S. 2020, 'Leicester's dark factories show up a diseased system', *Financial Times*, 3 July.
Office for National Statistics (UK). 2020, 'Coronavirus (COVID-19) roundup: Deaths and health', 4 August 2020, accessed 30 August 2020, <https://www.ons.gov.uk/peoplepopulationandcommunity/healthandsocialcare/conditionsanddiseases/articles/coronaviruscovid19roundupdeathsandhealth/2020-06-26>.
Office for National Statistics (UK). 2021, 'Coronavirus (COVID-19) related deaths by occupation, England and Wales: deaths registered between 9 March and 28 December 2020', 25 January, accessed 30 January 2021, <https://www.ons.gov.uk/peoplepopulationandcommunity/healthandsocialcare/causesofdeath/bulletins/coronaviruscovid19relateddeathsbyoccupationenglandandwales/deathsregisteredbetween9marchand28december2020>.
Patton, P. 2000, *Deleuze and the Political*, Routledge, London.
Potts, A. 2004, 'Deleuze on Viagra (Or, what can a Viagra-body do?)', *Body and Society*, 10(1), pp. 17–36.
Prey, R. 2012, 'The network's blindspot: Exclusion, exploitation and Marx's process-relational ontology', *TripleC*, 10(2), pp. 253–73.
Rekret, P. 2018, 'The head, the hand, and matter: New materialism and the politics of knowledge', *Theory, Culture and Society*, 35(7–8), pp. 49–72.
Rosiek, J.L., Snyder J. and Pratt, S.L. 2020, 'The new materialisms and indigenous theories of non-human agency: Making the case for respectful anti-colonial engagement', *Qualitative Inquiry*, 26(3–4), pp. 331–46.
Saldanha, A. 2006, 'Reontologising race: The machinic geography of phenotype', *Environment and Planning D: Society and Space*, 24(1), pp. 9–24.
Savage, M., Devine, F., Cunningham, N., Taylor, M., Li, Y., Hjellbrekke, J., Le Roux, B., Friedman, S. and Miles, A. 2013, 'A new model of social class? Findings from the BBC's Great British class survey experiment', *Sociology*, 47(2), pp. 219–50.
Scambler, G. 2007, 'Social structure and the production, reproduction and durability of health inequalities', *Social Theory and Health*, 5(4), pp. 297–315.
Scambler, G. 2012, 'Health inequalities', *Sociology of Health and Illness*, 34(1), pp. 130–46.
Sundberg, J. 2014, 'Decolonizing posthumanist geographies', *Cultural Geographies*, 21(1), pp. 33–47.
Townsend, P. and Davidson, N. 1982, *Inequalities in Health*, Penguin, Harmondsworth.
van der Tuin, I. and Dolphijn, R. 2010, 'The transversality of new materialism', *Women: A Cultural Review*, 21, pp. 153–71.

8

A LOPSIDED REFLATION

The limited contribution of behavioral economics to the political economy of obesity

David Primrose

Except among ardent scholars of literary surrealism, Tommaso Landolfi's (1963) short story, *Gogol's Wife*, has been largely consigned to the dusty corners of university library shelves. Given its offbeat narrative, this is hardly surprising. Briefly, the tale presents itself as a chapter derived from a long-lost biography of the enigmatic Nineteenth Century Russian author, Nikolai Vassilevitch Gogol, as recounted by his Boswell-like biographer, Foma Paskalovitch. After stating at the outset that he possesses previously unknown details concerning Gogol's mysterious private life, Paskalovitch reveals how he learnt that Gogol's 'wife' was actually a life-size rubber balloon named Caracas, who exhibited the physical profile of a woman. Claiming to be the only person besides Gogol to have seen Caracas, Paskalovitch chronicles how the latter developed her own personality, spoke when asking to use the toilet, and even inexplicably contracted syphilis. The account concludes by describing the disturbing events of the couple's silver anniversary, during which Gogol becomes enraged, inserts a bicycle pump into Caracas, and inflates her until she explodes, before throwing the rubber remains into the fire.

With its Kafkaesque narrative, *Gogol's Wife* often makes for unnerving reading and, indeed, is sometimes just downright weird. Particularly striking in Paskalovitch's exposition, though, is his befuddlement over Caracas' physical transformations alongside her seemingly consistent disposition: 'I cast some doubt on the propriety of considering Caracas as a unitary personality; nonetheless I myself could not quite [...] free myself of the impression that [...] this was fundamentally the same woman' (Landolfi 1963: 9). Depending on the level of air pressure filling out her anatomy, Caracas could be fashioned into vastly different feminine appearances – each unique, since she could not revert to prior shapes once deflated. Gogol also ornaments Caracas with different wigs and shades of makeup according to his desires. Periodically, Gogol falls in love with a particular form and preserves it until his affection fades. He then deflates the balloon and begins anew. According to Paskalovitch, these efforts to modify Caracas reflect Gogol's anxious endeavor to obscure common personality traits across her different forms that increasingly infuriate him and, thus, make the balloon more superficially appealing. Thus, he ruminates 'how can I have stated above that it was Nikolai Vassilevitch's will which ruled that woman? In a certain sense, yes, it is true; but it is equally certain that she became no longer his slave but his tyrant' (Landolfi 1963: 3).

DOI: 10.4324/9781003017110-9

This chapter contends that Gogol's interminable rejuvenation of Caracas' appearance is comparable to attempts by behavioral economists (BE)[1] to revitalize the seemingly limp and lifeless foundations of neoclassical economics (NCE) – in this case, when applied to questions of health.[2] Focusing on BE scholarship addressing the drivers of burgeoning global obesity, the chapter demonstrates that the tradition selectively incorporates acumen from psychology primarily to refashion NCE. That is, rather than deploying such interdisciplinary insights to cast the rancid corpse of neoclassicism into the fire *holus bolus*, BE introduces them to lopsidedly 'reflate' the latter via superficial modifications to its problematic conceptual and normative core – particularly its account of individual decision-making as axiomatically hyper-rational. Through this symbiotic relationship with NCE, BE reproduces – albeit, in novel forms – many of its inadequacies, while also engendering pertinent new limitations, which function to reduce the complex social determinants of obesity to narrow economic problems of 'irrational' individual choice. Accordingly, *pace* self-representations of the tradition as iconoclastically 'misbehaving' (Thaler 2015) within the economics discipline, the chapter concludes that behavioralism fails to provide the basis for more a more capacious critical political economy of obesity.

This case is developed across four sections. First, the chapter briefly introduces the contours of contemporary global obesity, and outlines neoclassical efforts to conceptualize its causes and offer ameliorative policy recommendations. Second, it overviews BE reflections on obesity, which explicitly posit themselves against the conceptual and normative limitations of such neoclassical formations. Third, while recognizing the advancements of BE on the latter, the analysis critically reflects on its limitations for informing a critical political economy of obesity. It does so along three primary axes, noting its (i) continuities with NCE; (ii) deterministic formulation of individual agency; and (iii) constricted social ontology. The chapter concludes by reflecting on the need to articulate a more holistic political economy of global obesity than that offered by BE, with particular attention accorded to transcending the individualizing orientation of the tradition when articulating political measures to redress this issue.

Global obesity and neoclassical economics

According to the World Health Organization (WHO 2021), obesity constitutes the accumulation of abnormal or excessive levels of fat that engenders substantial health risks. Specifically, an individual with a body mass index (BMI) exceeding 25 is categorized as 'overweight', while a BMI over 30 leads one to be deemed 'obese'.[3] Utilizing this definition, it has become axiomatic within mainstream public health scholarship and political discourse, since at least the mid-1990s, that the global political economy is confronting a burgeoning obesity 'epidemic' (James 2008).[4] Indeed, the contemporary evidence that international obesity rates have reached crisis levels is damning. According to the latest WHO (2021) estimates, the proportion of the global population classified as obese has nearly tripled since 1975, with over 1.9 billion adults now overweight (39 percent of the global population over 18 years of age), including 650 million deemed obese (13 percent). Moreover, with the exception of those in sub-Saharan Africa and Asia, the majority of the world's population now resides in countries where health problems associated with excess weight and obesity lead to more deaths than complications arising from being underweight. Finally, 340 million children and adolescents between 5 and 19 years of age, and 39 million children under five years old, are overweight or obese. In this respect, obesity now constitutes a substantial public health challenge in both the Global South and North (WHO 2000, 2021). Such trends are associated with an increased risk of chronic conditions such as type 2 diabetes, hypertension, and coronary artery disease (Kopelman 2007), thereby engendering a considerable loss of wellbeing and an increased burden on public health systems (Cawley and Meyerhoefer 2012).

To comprehend the drivers of this global health predicament and help inform appropriate policy responses, neoclassical economists have sought to conceptualize its roots in deliberate increased caloric consumption and reduced physical activity by individuals (see: Cawley 2011; Huckfeldt *et al.* 2012; Capps *et al.* 2018). In doing so, these theorists have formulated explanations using microeconomic theory, centered on modeling the 'rational' decision-making processes of individuals in their food consumption and exercise choices. For neoclassicism, all individuals axiomatically approach decision-making in a universally hyper-rational manner[5] – formalized in the notion of 'constrained optimization', whereby actors seek to maximize (or minimize) an objective according to particular constraints (such as budgets or time). This, in turn, engenders common responses through utility-maximizing behavior (*cf.* Hollis and Nell 1975; Davis 2011). Within this account, individuals – embodied in the subjective avatar of *Homo Economicus*, or 'rational economic man' – possess stable, well-defined, coherent preference sets, manifesting in their choices. They are, thereby, not cognitively impeded in assessing given alternatives, nor hindered by problems of self-control that would impair the identification and pursuit of optimal choices. These attributes equip individuals to pursue their self-interest and realize subjective preferences through market interactions – which, in turn, provide information and incentives to bolster choices, thereby maximizing individual utility and social welfare (the sum of individual utilities) (*cf.* Sen 1977).

Utilizing this conceptual framework, neoclassical theorists have explained rising obesity levels by modeling the consumption decisions of utility-maximizing individuals (see: Finkelstein and Hoerger 2010; Huckfeldt *et al.* 2012; Capps *et al.* 2018). Specifically, obesity is grasped as an outcome of hyper-rational choices, reflecting individuals' readiness to compromise – given proper incentives – their future health for present gratification associated with uninhibited food consumption and less exercise.[6] For instance, assuming that food consumption decisions are motivated by (i) maximizing immediate utility from eating, at the lowest time and pecuniary costs, and (ii) eating in a manner likely to preserve their health capital, individuals weigh immediate pleasures and costs against future rewards and pain through a discount factor, such that their behavior is time-consistent. For any given individual, the optimal amount of food consumption, physical activity, and other diet-related behaviors transpire when the marginal benefit of the last unit consumed (such as the last bite of food taken) equals its marginal cost. Thus, certain individuals will favor unhealthy foods over healthy alternatives, up to the point where the marginal satisfaction derived from consuming the former corresponds to the discounted marginal dissatisfaction of declining future health or bulkier bodily dimensions (Etilé 2019).

Given the difficulties experienced by many individuals in maintaining a healthy weight, NCE holds that the optimal decision for many individuals may be to engage in a lifestyle that leads to excess weight. Put differently, rational, utility-maximizing individuals – having balanced all relevant costs and benefits – believe it is simply too economically costly to weigh less. In turn, they purposively choose a lifestyle that leads to accumulating excess weight (Philipson and Posner 2003; Lakdawalla and Philipson 2009). Thus, many neoclassical accounts posit that technological developments have led to relative price changes since the 1970s – especially falling food prices and declining time costs associated with food production due to the increasingly pervasive adoption of microwaves and food processors. These have, in turn, incentivized rational decisions favoring greater food consumption and weight gain (Cutler *et al.* 2003; Finkelstein and Zuckerman 2008; Lakdawalla and Philipson 2009).

This formulation engenders three generic forms of policy response to address obesity. First, for some (*e.g.* Murphy 2006), obese individuals are obese by choice – having rationally determined that curtailing food consumption or escalating exercise would not vindicate the benefits of subsequent weight loss. Accordingly, public health policies are unnecessary (Philipson and Posner 2008): obesity and other diet-related diseases are individual concerns such that, *a priori*, the market will efficiently supply remedial health inputs.[7] For instance, deteriorating individual health stemming from increased junk-food consumption will engender increases in subjective value accorded to weight- and diet-control behavior, thereby raising demand for exercise, functional food, and dieticians (*cf.* Etilé 2019). For others, public policy may be used to endow consumers with superior information and/or modify relative prices (*e.g.* via taxes) to incentivize healthier eating patterns or promote exercise. Therein, the former measure is justifiable even in lieu of externalities (obese individuals detrimentally affecting others), in that providing better information to consumers possessing only imperfect information should bolster their welfare. The latter measure is only warranted in the presence of externalities, as altering prices in their absence will undermine economic welfare (see: Finkelstein and Hoerger 2010; Cawley 2011).

Behavioral economic interventions into obesity

The neoclassical account above is premised on representing individuals as hyper-rational economic subjects. In this formulation, individuals do not make systematic errors in their decision-making, imperfect self-control does not impede their ability to realize their preferences, and they inexorably act in their own self-interest. Conversely, BE has sought to utilize insights from cognitive psychology to rebuff the presupposition that individuals always make decisions in a manner analogous to *Homo Economicus*. Instead, the tradition seeks to 'increase the explanatory and predictive power of economic theory by providing it with more psychologically plausible foundations' (Angner and Loewenstein 2012: 642; *cf.* Heidl 2016).

Specifically, behavioralism advances empirical evidence derived from economic experiments to conceptualize more interdisciplinary, realistic accounts of actual economic behavior as deviating from hyper-rational precepts due to myriad psychological and contextual considerations beyond the explanatory scope of NCE (Earl 2022: Chapter 1; Foster and Frijters 2023). While sharing with the latter the assumption that individuals formulate optimal choices based on their preferences between available options (Laibson and List 2015), BE does not present a logico-deductive theory of choice engendering *Homo Economicus*. Instead, real-life economic decision-making is inexorably defined by its *boundedly rational* character (Thaler 2015: 23–4): instrumental in its orientation toward constrained optimization, yet refracted through psychological dynamics and elements in their social milieu that would be immaterial to the neoclassical subject (Camerer and Loewenstein 2004). In turn, these considerations – cynically labeled by Thaler (2015: 9) as 'supposedly irrelevant factors' – engender systemic sub-optimal behavioral outcomes, or 'anomalies' (Thaler 1987), diverging from *Homo Economicus*. Thus, individual decision-makers do not consistently order preferences, poorly judge probabilities, fail to address risk 'rationally', regularly commit multiple reasoning errors and, more generally, make decisions guided by cognitive biases, heuristic shortcuts, habits, and social context (Bickley and Torgler 2023).

In articulating this explanation, BE frequently posits that the human brain comprises 'dual systems' of thought – 'automatic' (System 1) and 'reflective' (System 2) – the properties of which shape real-world decision-making (Kahneman 2003; Thaler and Sunstein 2008). Within this framework, decision-making is theorized as a process in which each system concentrates on addressing differing cognitive and deliberative tasks. System 1 is formulated as rapid, instinctual, and emotional and, thus, capable of managing straightforward precepts and stimulation beyond contemplation. In contrast, System 2 is deemed better at handling concepts and deliberative behaviors considered rule-bound, deductive, and logical, as it is described as controlled, effortful, and neutral (Kahneman and Frederick 2002). While neoclassicism assumes that individuals possess complete access to, and utilize, the latter, BE draws on empirical evidence to theorize that the former underpins decision-making in practice. Individuals depend on the automatic system because they are boundedly rational: possessing limited capacity to attend to, process, and recall the contextual information necessary to make a 'rational' choice. Thus, rather than processing complete information in System 2 in a manner corresponding to *Homo Economicus*, individuals have recourse to biases and heuristics, while choices are also shaped by the form in which information is presented (framing effects) (Roberto and Kawachi 2016). Such factors operate in System 1 to simplify and distort information, thereby leading actors to seemingly expedient – albeit not always prudent – choices based on this imperfect information (Kahneman 2003).[8]

BE extends this conceptual framework to identify and theorize why, despite recognizing the adverse health effects of poor diets, smoking, weight gain, and lack of exercise, obese individuals continue to engage in these behaviors (*e.g.* Epstein and Saelens 2000; Downs and Loewenstein 2011; Bragg and Elbel 2017). While acknowledging other factors hindering adoption of optimal health choices – such as insufficient time, financial resources, or personal motivation – BE prioritizes conceptualizing processes operating *beyond* individuals' conscious awareness that engender sub-optimal choices deviating from *Homo Economicus* (Pastore *et al.* 2020). Following Chance *et al.* (2016), at least five such factors may be identified as leading to obesity, in spite individuals' instrumental orientation toward constrained optimization.

First, *individuals are cognitively geared toward impulsive choices* (Chapman and Elstein 1995). As noted above, BE conceptualizes decision-making as arising from interactions between 'dual processes' within the brain. When determining whether to eat ice-cream, for instance, System 1 engenders an approving automatic impulse because it operates rapidly in response to salient emotional stimuli. Conversely, deliberating on the sugar and calorie content of the ice-cream relative to its potential gratification necessitates engaging System 2. Because healthy choices such as eating broccoli or regularly running are often less intuitively appealing than eating ice-cream, System 1 tends to favor the latter unhealthy option. While System 2 esteems healthy choices benefiting individuals in the long-run, it requires effort to be engaged and, thus, is often not utilized for apparently trivial, quotidian decisions such as those relating to food or exercise (Pfeffer and Strobach 2022). Accordingly, System 1 is privileged, thereby leading to impulsive decisions (Cobb-Clark *et al.* 2022).

Second, *individuals are often too preoccupied to reach rational choices*. When actors undertake multiple tasks simultaneously, or are distracted by concerns such as material impoverishment, the limited cognitive processing power of the brain is overwhelmed by competing influences (Mani *et al.* 2013). This, in turn, begets a form of 'cognitive overload', such that the brain is unable to engage System 2 to regulate the more impulsive preferences favored by System 1 (Mullainathan and Shafir 2013). When placed under stress or confused, individuals are consequently more likely to engage in less reasoned, impulsive behavior – such as eating pre-packaged biscuits rather than preparing fruit salad while editing a book – without considering the potential longer-term consequences of doing so (Ward and Mann 2000).

Third, due to the cognitive drain on finite cognitive resources associated with making System 2 decisions, *individuals are often marked by limited willpower* (Hagger *et al.* 2010). Once their limited pool of mental faculties – or self-control – has been temporarily depleted, individuals may revert to simpler, System 1 decision-making processes. Constantly resisting the impulse to eat easily accessible sweets at work while dieting, for instance, diminishes individuals' capacity to resist the next impulse, such as eating cake at a later birthday party (Baumeister *et al.* 1998; Hofmann *et al.* 2012). Due to the plethora of food choices confronting individuals when already cognitively depleted by hunger or fatigue, short-term desire and external influences – such as the framing effects of food advertisements – easily overwhelm efforts at self-control and leads to sub-optimal food and exercise choices (de Haan and van Veldhuizen 2015).

Fourth, *individuals exhibit present-biased preferences*. That is, individual thinking tends to overemphasize immediate costs while discounting long-term benefits – a process known as 'hyperbolic discounting' (Laibson 1997; O'Donoghue and Rabin 2000). Such preferences can create difficulties when attempting to diet and exercise, or even lead individuals to refrain from these pursuits altogether, by exaggerating their immediate costs relative to their future benefits. For example, spending time preparing a fruit salad over eating a bag of chips is costly now, while the potential future benefit (avoiding health problems associated with excess consumption of trans-fats and salt) lies in the future, such that individuals may tend toward the unhealthy option (Richards and Hamilton 2012). Furthermore, individuals expect that they will adopt healthier decisions in the future; albeit, when the future arrives, unhealthy decisions are again made by their present-biased orientation. For instance, in one experiment, employees who had just eaten lunch were asked to nominate which snack they wished to receive the following week: fruit or junk-food. Most chose the fruit. Yet, upon delivery, the record of the planned choices was 'lost', and employees were again asked to choose their snack, leading to only 20 percent preferring the fruit (Read and van Leeuwen 1998).

Fifth, *individuals often make decisions automatically*, particularly in response to contextual influences. Contrary to the NCE assumption that individuals inexorably choose food options to maximize their utility, regardless of how the options are presented, BE demonstrates that presentation of options influences decision-making. Individuals often stick with extant or default options, even when superior, healthier alternatives are available – known as the 'status quo bias' (Kahneman 2003). For instance, restaurant meals often come with a 'default' setting, such as side dish, unless it is deliberately unselected when ordering. By functioning as an external cue influencing how much consumers eat and when to cease, such default larger portion sizes encourage increased caloric intake (Wansink 2004). Similarly, repeated cues over time can trigger consistent behavior that solidifies into habits that are hard to break. For example, especially when experiencing cognitive overload from activities such as working or watching television, individuals may mindlessly repeat learned unhealthy behaviors such as finishing the food on one's plate, or snack during commercial breaks (Wansink 2016).

Such BE reflections on obesity evidently challenge the hyper-rational axioms of NCE theory, and present an alternative conception of the subject to that represented in *Homo Economicus*. This is encapsulated by Thaler and Sunstein's (2008: 24) dichotomy between the 'Econs' of neoclassicism and the 'Humans' inhabiting reality. While the former constitute hyper-rational utility maximizers replete with a given utility function, the latter are more shambolic in their decision-making – more akin to the Homer Simpson 'lurking somewhere in each of us' than to *Homo Economicus*. Even when strategic and purposeful, humans make repeated miscalculations in pursuing their health objectives, and are influenced by external factors. Accordingly, *Homo Sapiens* are cognitively incapable of approximating *Homo Economicus*. As discussed in the concluding section, this conclusion also has pertinent implications for formulating novel policy measures to redress obesity.

The shortcomings of behavioral economics for the political economy of obesity

Nevertheless, the tradition offers only limited acumen for formulating a more capacious political economy of obesity in three primary respects.

Continuities with neoclassical economics

BE scholarship on obesity frequently juxtaposes its own conceptual research on the topic with the problematic presuppositions informing neoclassical accounts (*e.g.* Chance *et al.* 2016; Bragg and Elbel 2017). Behavioralism is held to engender greater 'realism': analyzing the psychological underpinnings of decision-making by real-world individuals, and examining how this diverges from the axiomatically hyper-rational *Homo Economicus*. Concomitantly, contra the monist and deductively derived methodology of neoclassicism, BE fuses interdisciplinary insights from psychology with economic analysis to nourish a more complex account of food and exercise choices (Bickley and Torgler 2023).

However, beyond the confines of the orthodoxy, such 'innovations' appear less groundbreaking. In practice, BE remains constrained by its continued subsumption within neoclassicism: deploying psychology to *buttress* the orthodoxy rather than nourish interdisciplinary, non-neoclassical accounts of health decision-making (Tzotzes and Milonakis 2021). This is explicable by considering BE as constitutive of a broader epistemological trend within economics: that of 'reverse economics imperialism' (see: Fine and Milonakis 2009). This entails NCE bolstering itself and expanding its scope via importing tools sequestered from disciplines such as psychology, sociology, and politics, and then incorporating them within its conceptual contours (Crespo 2017). Framed in this way, BE has participated in such imperialistic practices through selectively utilizing psychology to revise and augment, rather than transcend, neoclassicism (Davis 2013, 2018). This, in turn, engenders two primary shortcomings.

The first is *limited increases in descriptive realism*. Amalgamating psychology within neoclassicism undermines BE's posited objective of explaining empirical evidence deviating from hyper-rationality. Rather than necessitating 'wholesale rejection' of NCE 'based on utility maximization, equilibrium, and efficiency' (Camerer and Loewenstein 2004: 3), behavioral anomalies discovered through experiments 'are used as inspiration to create alternative theories that *generalize existing models*' (Camerer and Loewenstein 2004: 7, emphasis added). That is, BE holds that bolstering its psychological foundations will improve neoclassicism *on its own terms* through enabling increasingly sophisticated theory, superior predictions, and more comprehensive policy recommendations (Rabin 2002).

The result is an incongruous methodology. Behavioralism holds that psychological experimental results will advance economic analysis when filtered through models allowing for phenomena diverging from hyper-rationality. Yet, 'domesticating' (Davis 2008: 363) psychological insights within neoclassicism does not engender greater realism. Instead, BE generalizes the axiom that all behavior is oriented around constrained optimization, while incorporating slight modifications to account for biases, dysfunctions, and heuristics that lead to unhealthy food and exercise choices (White 2017) – what Tzotzes and Milonakis (2021: 179) term 'rationalizing irrationality'. For example, in explaining obesity as arising from a present bias informing individuals' decision-making, Richards and Hamilton (2012) and Courtemanche *et al.* (2015) affix hyperbolic discount functions – disproportionately weighting individuals' concern for short-term gratification over long-term health costs arising from overeating – to an otherwise-neoclassical utility function. Similarly, to account for individuals' decisions to participate in physical activity, Humphreys *et al.* (2015) incorporate habit formation, time-inconsistent preferences, naivety, and projection bias into an orthodox model of individual choice. In such cases, introducing novel psychological parameters merely produces more complex optimization problems to solve. Thus, rather than conceptualizing *actual* decision-making processes, such BE accounts remain dependent on Friedman's (1953) instrumentalist 'as-if' defense to justify *increasingly unrealistic* formulations. To produce sophisticated behavioral obesity models, individuals are assumed to behave *as if* solving more elaborate constrained optimization problems (Berg and Gigerenzer 2010).

A second, related limitation entails BE deploying interdisciplinary insights to *normatively buttress Homo Economicus as the ideal economic subject*. While the tradition rejects this representation as capturing the cognitive capacities of actual human beings, it endures as the archetype for 'rational' cognition and healthy choices, and a potentially realizable subject to be procured through policy (Infante *et al.* 2016). As Thaler (2015: 251) remarks, '[w]ithout the [NCE] rational framework, there are no anomalies from which we can detect misbehavior', such that 'the real point of behavioral economics is to highlight behaviors that are in conflict with the standard rational model' (Thaler 2015: 261). In turn, rather than discarding *Homo Economicus holus bolus*, BE remains symbiotically linked to this hyper-rational subjectivity: 'I mostly advocate for thinking like an Econ' (Thaler 2015: 72).

Specifically, BE retains *Homo Economicus* as a normative model of economic subjectivity because it remains within the foundational *theoretical humanist problematic* of neoclassicism. That is, the tradition investigates the institutional conditions of possibility for securing a market-based social order to reconcile the competing interests of instrumentally rational, self-interested subjects – in this case, *given these subjects are characterized by cognitive limitations* (Primrose 2017). For neoclassicism, behavior approximating *Homo Economicus* provides the subjective microfoundation for markets to reconcile individual and aggregate rationality in a Pareto-efficient manner (see: Madra 2017). BE explains such predictions of functioning markets as faltering due to psychological factors hindering individuals' cognitive capacities relative to *Homo Economicus*, which thereby engender 'irrational' behavior. Accordingly, it bestows central ontological status to the hyper-rational subject in determining the economy as a whole, in that deviations are responsible for market imperfections. For instance, Camerer and Fehr (2006: 47) contend that behavior deviating from hyper-rationality occludes welfare-maximizing outcomes, while sufficient subjects approximating *Homo Economicus* 'may cause aggregate outcomes to be close to the predictions of a [neoclassical] model that assumes that everyone is rational and self-regarding'. Remedial policies fostering more hyper-rational individual choices are, therefore, required to ensure that markets function effectively (as discussed below).

Hence, contrary to the NCE formulation of efficient markets – presupposing individuals as capable of hyper-rationally pursuing health decisions to maximize their long-term utility – BE comprehends obesity as a market failure correlating with sub-optimal, 'irrational' dietary and exercise choices by individual consumers (Karnani *et al.* 2016). As Thaler and Sunstein (2008: 7) posit, '[w]e do not claim that everyone who is overweight is necessarily failing to act rationally, but we do reject the claim that all or almost all Americans are choosing their diet optimally'. Individual 'cognitive failures' – psychologically determined decision-making 'deviations' from *Homo Economicus* that hinder individuals from effectively comprehending and responding to economic incentives – prompt instrumental, yet boundedly rational, choices that may satiate myopic actors' short-term utility, though fail to satisfy their longer-term health interests (Downs and Loewenstein 2011). Such behavior, in turn, is held as responsible for markets failing to secure Pareto-efficient outcomes: begetting both negative 'externalities' (such as increased public health expenditures to redress proliferating obesity; see: Karnani *et al.* 2016) and 'internalities' (such as detrimentally affecting individuals' future health; see: Herrnstein *et al.* 1993; O'Donoghue and Rabin 2006).

Thus, while dismissing hyper-rationality 'as a positive or descriptive theory' (Angner and Loewenstein 2012: 668) of economic decision-making because real individuals do not resemble *Homo Economicus*, BE pathologizes the former as 'anomalous' to, or 'deviating' from, this norm (Mehta 2013). The implicitly phallogocentric character of the 'dual processes' ontology discussed above exemplifies this pathologization (Primrose 2017). Challenging the universalist presumptions of hyper-rationality, and explicitly theorizing emotional processes previously denigrated as 'feminine' or 'soft', appears to address calls by feminist political economists to transcend the modernist reason-emotion dualism (Hewitson 1999). Rather than examining emotion and intuition to articulate a more holistic account of decision-making, however, these are denigrated relative to 'rational' qualities (Clouser 2016). Reliance on System 1 when making food and exercise consumption decisions leads to 'irrational' behavior, as biases and heuristics engender 'faulty' perceptions about choice effects, preferences detrimental in the long-term, or choosing damaging options despite 'rationally' preferring otherwise.

In short, such psychological dynamics alienate obese individuals from their latent hyper-rational preferences, leading to sub-optimal health choices (Infante *et al.* 2016). BE, consequently, frequently deploys psychological labels to substantiate negative value assessments about the *moral* character of boundedly rational individuals, and articulate it as subordinate to the normative ideal of *Homo Economicus* (Mehta 2013). For instance, behavioralism juxtaposes 'hot' (emotional, impulsive) to 'cold' (self-controlled, reflexive) systems in processing external sensory cues (Metcalfe and Mischel 1999), with poor food and exercise decisions arising when the former overwhelms the latter (*e.g.* Gilbert et al. 2002; Nordgren *et al.* 2009). Analogously, the tradition distinguishes between those aware of their self-control problems – such as a tendency to overeat – as 'sophisticated individuals', and those who are not as 'naïve individuals' (*e.g.* O'Donoghue and Rabin 2006; Ruhm 2012). This reasoning, conceptualizing observed deviations from hyper-rationality as resulting from psychological deficiencies, effectively presupposes *Homo Economicus* as normatively correct.

Deterministic conceptions of individual agency

BE reflections on obesity also offer *biologically deterministic* accounts of individual subjects, through under-theorizing social phenomena and their contribution to configuring behavior. Instead, the tradition proceeds by recourse to universal psychological characteristics deemed *intrinsic to human beings as individuals*: explaining 'irrational', unhealthy behavior as due to psychology. This generates impoverished conceptions of agency arising from biologically derived cognitive limitations.

Behavioral accounts of pervasive 'irrationality' undoubtedly better represent real health behavior than *Homo Economicus*. To contest the descriptive realism of hyper-rationality, behavioralism employs insights from cognitive psychology – examining the functioning of the cognitive apparatus informing all human beings (Angner and Loewenstein 2012; for a survey, see Petracca 2017). In turn, it analyses common mistakes made by individuals *as members of the same species* when theorizing systemic 'irrationality' (Frerichs 2019). That is, humans are deemed irrational and fallible *by nature*: '[t]hey are not *homo economicus [sic]*; they are *homo sapiens*' (Thaler and Sunstein 2008: 7, emphases added). Thus, 'irrational' dietary and exercise choices are molded by *psychologically determined 'processing errors'*: being prone to biases and judgmental 'faults', human cognitive processing capabilities are limited relative to *Homo Economicus*, thereby engendering 'poor' decisions and sub-optimal behavior (Pedwell 2017).

Yet, this formulation is not linked to a more holistic account of the psycho-social complexity of decision-making. Accepting cognitive 'limitations' as *a priori* hard-wired in humans, behavioralism downplays the institutionally embedded character of so-called 'irrational' qualities themselves (Streeck 2010). For instance, as noted above, the tradition frequently attributes causal primacy for obesity to individuals' biases toward 'hyperbolic discounting' when making food consumption decisions – exaggerating the short-term costs of healthy alternatives while discounting their long-term advantages, such that they eat excessively processed and calorific foods (*e.g.* Scharff 2009). Nevertheless, BE underplays how such 'reckless' food choices are institutionalized within broader socio-cultural processes, and why individuals internalize them over time (Fine *et al.* 2002; Mahoney 2015). To illustrate, individuals' observed tendency to prioritize short-term food consumption preferences is, arguably, constitutive of the dynamics of subject formation promulgated by neoliberal governmentality: appealing to the passions of individuals as citizen-consumers, able to contribute to society via purchasing and consuming the products (including food) of global capitalism (Guthman 2009). In lieu of such considerations, behavioralism exhibits a 'naturalist bias': focusing on supposedly universal qualities of human nature, while leaving unexplored the historically contingent foundations of consumption behavior in contemporary capitalism (Frerichs 2019).

Circumscribed conceptions of the 'social'

Finally, the BE of obesity articulates only limited insights into the broader social context of individual decision-making. In particular, the tradition *adopts a thin social ontology*. Proponents claim to complicate, or even transcend, the abstract methodological individualism of neoclassicism by conceptualizing the 'messy' sociality of individual health decisions (*e.g.* Foster and Frijters 2023). Behavioralists have promulgated 'socially embedded' accounts of individuals (Davis 2015), whereby 'the degree of rationality bestowed to the agents depends on the context being studied' (Thaler 2000: 134). That is, strong external influences configure actors' behavior, as the factors that affect intuitive decisions are highly dependent on the environment in which behavior occurs. For instance, framing effects and reference dependence inform individual decision-making *viz.* food consumption, reflecting the anchoring of choice in particular circumstances, thereby engendering hyperbolic time discounting (individuals tend to undervalue the future) (Richards and Hamilton 2012).

The corresponding notion of the 'social' here is significantly circumscribed, however. BE focuses on investigating decision-making processes from the perspective of individuals, while largely disregarding the need to conceptualize the complex social context within which such decisions are made. Accordingly, first, the tradition renders a limited conception of *environment*, defined as individuals' immediate physical space. Put differently, individual behavior 'is not guided by what they are able to compute, but by what they happen to see at any given moment' (Kahneman 2003: 1469). Second, there is a restricted conception of *social norms*, conceptualized quantitatively as how the majority of agents operate in a given context (Davis 2013). This examines norms as given, rather than theorizing their social construction (Pedwell 2017). The result is a thin social ontology and instrumental treatment of social phenomena – dealing with the latter only to the extent that they affect individual capacity to process information (Frerichs 2019). In turn, assuming economic conduct corresponds to essentialized conceptions of human nature – as largely psychologically determined – leaves subjectivity and preferences themselves largely unexplored (Davis 2011; White 2017).

The BE of obesity, thereby, excludes three rudimentary insights recognized in other critical social sciences (Leggett 2014). First, agents are not conceptualized as unevenly distributed within extant social structures *prior* to decision-making (Frerichs 2019). Yet, myriad studies demonstrate how obesity is determined by political-economic factors beyond individuals' immediate choice environment, such as capitalist systems of food production and distribution (Fine 1998; Bayliss and Fine 2020: Chapter 5). These include, for instance, production structures that beget high profit margins from processed foods, considerable political power wielded by the food and drinks industry, sizable marketing of highly processed and calorific commodities, inequalities in accessing healthy food options and exercising opportunities, and evolving contemporary practices of mobility (Winson 2013; Clapp 2020). Indeed, even where some recognition is accorded to the impact of factors such as poverty in augmenting the 'cognitive load' of impoverished individuals – thereby engendering sub-optimal food choices and leaving them more susceptible to junk-food marketing (*e.g.* Zimmerman and Shimoga 2014) – these social drivers themselves remain occluded from consideration. Rather than critically examining the structural reasons for impoverished communities being afflicted with disproportionate levels of obesity and diet-related disease (Otero 2018), analytical primacy centers on explaining – and rectifying – the psychological drivers of boundedly rational, unhealthy individual decision-making *within* their given destitute context. The perpetuation of poverty-induced obesity is, thus, naturalized in psychological deficiencies promulgating 'irrational' behavior.

Second, and relatedly, while highlighting interfaces between subjects and their immediate environment, BE disregards the contingency of the latter on historical decisions, contestation, and power relations (Strauss 2009). Guthman (2011), for instance, contextualizes growing obesity within the broader exercise of political-economic power by capital, in conjunction with state-implemented neoliberal reforms, in restructuring the global agri-food system in recent decades as a means to overcome limits to accumulation. Hence:

> Fast and convenient food has been a triply good fix for American capitalism. It entails the super-exploitation of the labor force in its production, it provides cheap food to support the low wages of the food and other industries by feeding their low-wage workers, and it absorbs the surpluses of the agricultural economy, soaking up [...] the excesses of overproduction to keep the farm sector marginally viable
>
> (Guthman 2011: 177).

Accordingly, purchasing inexpensive, calorie-rich food cannot be reduced to an 'irrational' individual choice, as this disregards how the 'current policy environment is a result of political choices, not consumption choices' (Guthman 2011: 194).

Third, BE fails to develop an ontologically thick account of social norms, with the latter conceptualized merely as the aggregation of individual choices (*e.g.* McFerran 2016). It consequently underplays how ideational structures prefigure and influence norms, such as those manifest as ideological messages or traditional values (Žižek 2012 [1994]; Pedwell 2017). Extending on the case of hyperbolic discounting and neoliberalism discussed above, for example, BE deems public health messages on the health risks associated with overeating and a sedentary lifestyle to have been disregarded by obese individuals due to their present bias, in conjunction with factors such as low willpower (*e.g.* Hunter *et al.* 2018). Nevertheless, this focus on restrained food consumption fundamentally conflicts with pervasive, entrenched socio-cultural injunctions in contemporary capitalism – manifest in platforms ranging from corporate advertising to governmental injunctions – impelling consumption as the locus of neoliberal citizenship (Guthman 2009; Cargill 2015).

In disregarding such reflections, BE ignores the broader systemic features and psycho-social dynamics of capitalism when comprehending the complex drivers of obesity. In turn, it posits *reductionist accounts* of this phenomenon. Echoing NCE, behavioralism remains underpinned by methodological individualism (Dold *forthcoming*): confining the study of complex political-economic phenomena to formulating naturalistic explanations of individual decision-making processes through psychological reductionism (Frerichs 2019). In particular, obesity is narrowly conceived as an *economic problem* of individual 'irrational behavior' engendered by actors' limited capacity to comprehend and respond to economic incentives in markets. As noted above, myopic individuals are presumed to prioritize short-term pleasure derived from consuming junk-food and maintaining a sedentary lifestyle over the long-term benefits of a balanced diet. Individual cognition is, thereby, pathologized as responsible for undesirable 'internalities' and 'externalities', while naturalizing structural determinants of ill-health in global capitalism associated with class, inequality, and corporate power (Holt-Giménez 2017: esp. Chapter 5; Clapp 2020).

Wink, wink, nudge, nudge – do no more?

Behavioral reflections on obesity usefully highlight the narrowness and deficiencies of neoclassical accounts of the phenomenon centered on presumptions of hyper-rationality. Contrary to the latter, BE introduces insights from psychology to demonstrate that choices about food and exercise are not undertaken by atomistic subjects akin to *Homo Economicus* – 'lightning calculator[s] of pleasures and pains' (Veblen 1898: 398–9). Rather, such decisions are made by boundedly rational individuals influenced by external factors, and who may repeatedly miscalculate in pursuing their health objectives. Nevertheless, as articulated above, the potential of BE to contribute to comprehending the political economy of obesity remains circumscribed by its enduring subsumption within NCE and axiomatic focus on individual hyper-rationality. Accordingly, the tradition is unable to provide more holistic understandings of health decision-making, nor the broader social forces beyond individuals' immediate choice environment that determine health. Returning to the outré tale of *Gogol's Wife*, BE reflections on obesity thereby offer less fundamentally novel economic accounts of obesity, than another effort to postpone discarding neoclassicism (see: Madra 2017): introducing marginal psychological modifications to adorn it with a more palatable outward appearance, while remaining within the bounds of mainstream epistemological 'respectability'. Such efforts to reflate neoclassicism lopsidedly, rather than abandoning its remains to the fire, ultimately contribute little to a critical political economy of obesity.

Yet, this reading of BE also points to its shortcomings as a foundation for informing *political measures* to help redress obesity.[9] As outlined above, contrary to its hypostatization in NCE, BE recognizes that the hyper-rationality of *Homo Economicus* does not represent real individual decision-making. Accordingly, policy measures depending on channeling individuals toward healthier choices via incentives within competitive markets will be limited in effectiveness (Chance *et al.* 2016). In turn, BE transcends the limited remedial role for the state within NCE; instead, advocating that this institution adopt a more explicit public health function in correcting for pervasive market failures that produce poor health outcomes (Karnani *et al.* 2016; *cf.* Leggett 2014). The policy should ameliorate – or circumvent – the cognitive limitations and pernicious social influences engendering individuals' 'irrational' food and exercise consumption choices within markets. This is especially so given the latter 'not only provide us with what we want, as long as we can pay for it', but 'also tempt us into buying things that are bad for us, whatever the costs' (Akerlof and Shiller 2015: n.p.). The most prominent policy rationale elaborating this case is that of 'libertarian-paternalism' (LP): promulgating minor amendments to the immediate institutional environment (the 'choice architecture') wherein individuals instrumentally pursue their interests, to 'nudge' their behavior in more 'rational', welfare-enhancing directions, albeit without curtailing their freedom to choose (Thaler and Sunstein 2008).

In acknowledging the systemic character of boundedly rational individual decision-making, prompting pervasive anomalous behavior deviating from individuals' own self-interest, BE thereby advocates that such 'anomalies' be harnessed to 'nudge' subjects toward healthier choices. In doing so, the tradition continues to position *Homo Economicus* as the normative *ideal* for decision-making, as well as a subjective condition *potentially realizable* through policy (Primrose 2017). Grounded in the logic of what Hausman (2012: 102) labels 'preference purification', BE seeks to reconstruct the preferences that *would* have informed the decision-making of hyper-rational individuals had their cognition not been 'obstructed' by psychological factors, while establishing realization of such reconstructed preferences as a normative benchmark for policy-making (Infante *et al.* 2016). That is, commencing from the pathologization of bounded rationality (as outlined above), BE initiatives attempt to recreate the preferences of *Homo Economicus* through isolating this norm from distorting psychological influences. In turn, the tradition designs policies to enable boundedly rational individuals to make decisions in accordance with these preferences *as if* they were *Homo Economicus* by circumventing 'any factor that significantly alters the behavior of [real] Humans, even though it would be ignored by [hyper-rational] Econs' (Thaler and Sunstein 2008: 8).

This epistemological foundation begets a circumscribed policy agenda to tackle obesity, centered on the unhealthy *individual* as an 'irrational' subject requiring correction, while retaining an asocial and ahistorical conception of this subject as neither enabled nor constrained by social structures beyond their immediate choice environment (Strauss 2009; Pedwell 2017).[10] More specifically, BE abstracts obesity from the 'messiness' of its multiple political-economic determinants. Instead, as noted above, it is depoliticized as a primarily *economic problem* of individuals' inexorably limited capacity to comprehend and respond to economic incentives which, in turn, begets 'poor', unhealthy choices within markets (Thaler and Sunstein 2008: 8). Consequently, the objective of policy is less redressing obesity *per se*, than correcting for decision-making 'anomalies' held to precipitate this problem: proposing measures augmenting individuals' capacity to 'rationally' respond to economic incentives in markets in a manner akin to *Homo Economicus* (Primrose 2017).

The potential role of the state in redressing obesity is, correspondingly, reduced to yet another factor among a plurality that influences individual health behavior (Leggett 2014). By isolating 'irrational' decision-making by individual citizen-consumers as driving obesity, the locus of state responsibility shifts from implementing holistic public health initiatives, toward developing micropolitical interventions to steer individuals toward more 'rational' self-government within a given context (Fox and Klein 2020). Smith and Toprakkiran (2019), for instance, demonstrate that the plethora of nudge policies instigated to address obesity in the United Kingdom has buttressed extant neoliberal governance regimes by framing this complex socio-ecological problem as one of individual 'responsibilization'. However, in lieu of more capacious public health measures transforming the psycho-social and broader political-economic drivers of obesity existing *prior to* and *following* the event space of a particular nudge, amendments to individuals' proximate choice environment often fail to secure healthy habits that endure beyond this particular context (Pedwell 2017)

Finally, the behavioralist pathologization of individual bounded rationality occludes consideration of policy measures to remedy individual and social dysfunction through redressing the overlapping material sources of poor health. Rather, as noted above, the BE of obesity naturalizes the structural determinants of obesity in contemporary capitalism associated with the prevailing global corporate agri-food regime, class, inequality, and corporate power (Guthman 2011; Winson 2013; Otero 2018). Absent historically specific considerations of the latter, the politics of obesity is framed as a *technical* matter: requiring mobilization of micro-level strategies to bolster individuals' capacity to make 'better choices' (Thaler and Sunstein 2008: 8), and realize their presumed latent (hyper-)rational preferences for healthier options *within* their extant political-economic conditions (Santos and Rodrigues 2014; Mahoney 2015). These measures range, for instance, from shifting the position of sweets at supermarket checkouts below eye level, to introducing innovations to restructure individuals' relations with food such as tray-less cafeterias and advanced ordering of meals (Downs and Loewenstein 2011; Chance *et al.* 2016). By framing such nudge initiatives as universal, 'catch-all' solutions to 'society's major problems' (Thaler and Sunstein 2008: 9) that do not necessitate 'changing the existing social and political structures' (Banerjee and Duflo 2011: 271), BE steers clear of contesting and reconfiguring the historically specific structural roots of poor nutrition or lack of exercise in the dynamics of capitalism. Rather, it fosters a largely decontextualized, economistic emphasis on buttressing individuals' rational consumption behavior via marginally amending their proximate choice environment (Fine *et al.* 2016).

As a means to both comprehend and attempt to alleviate global obesity, BE evidently follows its neoclassical forerunner in remaining markedly deficient. Political economists seeking to grasp this phenomenon would be better served by re-engaging with, and extending, other critical traditions discussed within this volume, while casting out behavioralism to join Caracas and neoclassicism amidst the proverbial flames.

Notes

1 Behavioralism encompasses both 'old' and 'new' strands (Sent 2004). The former, pioneered by Simon (*e.g.* 1955) and developed within the 'frugal heuristics' approach (*e.g.* Gigerenzer 2015), supplants atomistic hyper-rationality with holistic, evolutionary accounts of rationality and individuality. The 'new' school – arising from Tversky and Kahneman (1973, 1974) – retains the atomistic neoclassical conception of individuals, albeit revised to embed agents within an ahistorical and non-developmental social ontology. This newer iteration constitutes the mainstream of behavioral research (Heukelom 2014), and is the most politically influential – manifest in the institutionalization of governmental 'nudge' research units around the world (Whitehead *et al.* 2017). Accordingly, this chapter focuses on the latter strand to assess the extent to which this tradition marks a genuine break with neoclassicism (see: Madra 2017).

2 The arguments in this chapter are developed in relation to the behavioral tradition more broadly in Primrose (2017, 2022).

3 It is beyond the scope of this chapter to engage in debates over the appropriate means to measure obesity. However, for pertinent critical reflections on this theme, see: Guthman (2011) and Otero (2018).

4 While not germane to the present discussion, see Schorb (2022) for a useful account of why it is problematic to refer to burgeoning global obesity levels as an 'epidemic'.

5 In order to distinguish it from the philosophical principle of 'rationality' – holding that actions and opinions should be grounded in reason – this chapter designates the NCE conception of rationality as 'hyper-rationality' (Shaikh 2016: 78). This step circumvents the neoclassical practice of juxtaposing the latter as 'perfect' and real-world cognition as 'imperfect', as well as similar practices within BE scholarship (as discussed below).

6 This explanation echoes the earlier, unsettling account of Becker and Murphy (1988), in which they contend that heroin produces sufficient dopamine that, for some individuals, developing an addiction to the drug constitutes a rational decision in which the utility secured outweighs its immense health and pecuniary costs.

7 Indeed, some neoclassical theorists posit that, in spite of its obvious implications for long-term health, rising obesity normatively justifies the 'free-market' processes they attribute to contemporary capitalism. For instance, Cutler *et al.* (2003: 116) posit that '[w]e suspect that most people are better off from the technological advances of mass food preparation, even if their weight has increased'. Similarly, Finkelstein and Zuckerman (2008: 104) assert that 'increasing rates of obesity are a natural response to a changing world' and, thus, 'may be more an indicator of the success, as opposed to a failure, of markets' to supply the goods and services increasingly demanded by consumers.

8 This is a necessarily brief and partial overview of BE. For more in-depth considerations of the conceptual intricacies of the tradition and its history, see: Heukelom (2014); and Earl (2022).

9 It is not possible to address the plethora of political limitations afflicting BE in this chapter. However, for particularly discerning political-economic reflections on this theme – especially in relation to neoliberalism – see: Leggett (2014); McMahon (2015); Fine *et al.* (2016); and Pedwell (2017).

10 This limitation has recently been recognized in contributions by some prominent BE practitioners themselves, such as that of Chater and Loewenstein (forthcoming).

References

Akerlof, G.A. and Shiller, R.J. 2015, 'The dark side of free markets', *The Conversation*, 21 October, accessed 14 July 2022, <https://theconversation.com/the-dark-side-of-free-markets-48862>.

Angner, E. and Loewenstein, G. 2012, 'Behavioral economics', in Mäki, U. (ed), *Handbook of the Philosophy of Science*, Elsevier, Amsterdam, pp. 641–90.

Baumeister, R.F., Bratslavsky, E., Muraven, M. and Tice, D.M. 1998, 'Ego depletion: Is the active self a limited resource?', *Journal of Personality and Social Psychology*, 74(5), pp. 1252–65.

Bayliss, K. and Fine, B. 2020, *A Guide to the Systems of Provision Approach*, Palgrave Macmillan, London.

Becker, G.S. and Murphy, K.M. 1988, 'A theory of rational addiction', *Journal of Political Economy*, 96(4), pp. 675–700.

Berg, N. and Gigerenzer, G. 2010, 'As-if behavioral economics: Neoclassical economics in disguise?', *History of Economic Ideas*, 18(1), pp. 133–66.

Bickley, S.J. and Torgler, B. 2023, 'Behavioural economics, what have we missed? Exploring "classical" behavioural economics roots in AI, cognitive psychology, and complexity theory', in Altman, M. (ed), *Handbook of Research Methods in Behavioural Economics*, Edward Elgar, Cheltenham, pp. 32–59.

Bragg, M.A. and Elbel, B. 2017, 'Using behavioral economics to improve dietary intake: Alternatives to regulation, bans, and taxation', in Hanoch, Y., Barnes, A. and Rice, T. (eds), *Behavioral Economics and Healthy Behaviors*, Routledge, London, pp. 90–105.

Camerer, C.F. and Fehr, E. 2006, 'When does "economic man" dominate social behavior?' *Science*, 311(5757), pp. 47–52.

Camerer, C.F. and Loewenstein, G. 2004, 'Behavioral economics: Past, present, future', in Camerer, C., Loewenstein, G. and Rabin, M. (eds), *Advances in Behavioral Economics*, Princeton University Press, Princeton, pp. 3–52.

Capps, O., Ishdorj, A., Dharmasena, S. and Palma, M.A. 2018, 'Economic ramifications of obesity: A selective literature review', *The Routledge Handbook of Agricultural Economics*, Routledge, London, pp. 70–83.

Cargill, K. 2015, *The Psychology of Overeating*, Bloomsbury, London.

Cawley, J. 2011, 'The economics of obesity', in Cawley, J. (ed), *The Oxford Handbook of the Social Sciences of Obesity*, Oxford University Press, New York, pp. 120–37.

Cawley, J. and Meyerhoefer, C. 2012, 'The medical care costs of obesity: An instrumental variables approach', *Journal of Health Economics*, 31(1), pp. 219–30.

Chance, Z., Dhar, R., Hatzis, M., Huskey, K., Roberto, C.A. and Kawachi, I. 2016, 'Nudging individuals toward healthier food choices with the 4 P's framework for behavior change', in Roberto, C.A. and Kawachi, I. (eds), *Behavioral Economics and Public Health*, Oxford University Press, New York, pp. 177–202.

Chapman, G.B. and Elstein, A.S. 1995, 'Valuing the future: Temporal discounting of health and money', *Medical Decision Making*, 15(4), pp. 373–86.

Chater, N. and Loewenstein, G. forthcoming, 'The i-frame and the s-frame: How focusing on individual-level solutions has led behavioral public policy astray', *Behavioral and Brain Sciences*, 46(E147), pp. 1–60.

Clapp, J., 2020, *Food*, Polity Press, Cambridge.

Clouser, R. 2016, 'Nexus of emotional and development geographies', *Geography Compass*, 10(8), pp. 321–32.

Cobb-Clark, D.A., Dahmann, S.C., Kamhöfer, D. and Schildberg-Hörisch, H. 2022, 'Self-control and unhealthy body weight: The role of impulsivity and restraint', *Melbourne Institute Working Paper No. 02/22*, January, accessed 19 September 2022, <https://melbourneinstitute.unimelb.edu.au/publications/working-papers/search/result?paper=4010996>.

Courtemanche, C., Heutel, G. and McAlvanah, P. 2015, 'Impatience, incentives and obesity', *The Economic Journal*, 125(582), pp. 1–31.

Crespo, R.F. 2017, *Economics and Other Disciplines*, Routledge, London.

Cutler, D.M., Glaeser, E.L. and Shapiro, J.M. 2003, 'Why have Americans become more obese?', *Journal of Economic perspectives*, 17(3), pp. 93–118.

Davis, J.B. 2008, 'The turn in recent economics and return of orthodoxy', *Cambridge Journal of Economics*, 32(3), pp. 349–66.

Davis, J.B. 2011, *Individuals and Identity in Economics*, Cambridge University Press, Cambridge.

Davis, J.B. 2013, 'Economics imperialism under the impact of psychology: The case of behavioral development economics', *Oeconomica*, 3(1), pp. 119–38.

Davis, J.B. 2015, 'Bounded rationality and bounded individuality', *Research in the History of Economics and Methodology*, 33, pp. 75–93.
Davis, J.B. 2018, 'Behavioral economics and the positive-normative distinction: Sunstein's *Choosing Not to Choose* and behavioral economics imperialism', *Revue Ethique et Economique*, 15(1), pp. 1–15.
De Haan, T. and Van Veldhuizen, R. 2015, 'Willpower depletion and framing effects', *Journal of Economic Behavior and Organization*, 117, pp. 47–61.
Dold, M. 2023, 'Methodological individualism in behavioral economics', in Bulle, N. and Di Iorio, F. (eds), *Palgrave Handbook of Methodological Individualism, Volume I*. Palgrave MacMillan, New York.
Downs, J.S. and Loewenstein, G. 2011, 'Behavioral economics and obesity', in Cawley, J. (ed), *The Oxford Handbook of the Social Sciences of Obesity*, Oxford University Press, Oxford, pp. 138–57.
Duflo, E. and Banerjee, A. 2011, *Poor Economics*, PublicAffairs, New York.
Earl, P.E. 2022, *Principles of Behavioral Economics*, Cambridge University Press, Cambridge.
Epstein, L.H. and Saelens, B.E. 2000, 'Behavioral economics of obesity: Food intake and energy expenditure', in Bickel, W. and Vuchinich, R.E. (eds), *Reframing Health Behavior Change With Behavioral Economics*, Routledge, London, pp. 293–311.
Etilé, F. 2019, 'The economics of diet and obesity: Public policy', *Oxford Research Encyclopedia of Economics and Finance*, Oxford University Press, New York.
Fine, B. 1998, *The Political Economy of Diet, Health and Food Policy*, Routledge, London.
Fine, B., Heasman, M. and Wright, J. 2002, *Consumption in the Age of Affluence*, Routledge, London.
Fine, B., Johnston, D., Santos, A.C. and Van Waeyenberge, E. 2016, 'Nudging or Fudging: The World Development Report 2015', *Development and Change*, 47(4), pp. 640–63.
Fine, B. and Milonakis, D. 2009, *From Economics Imperialism to Freakonomics*, Routledge, London.
Finkelstein, E.A. and Hoerger, T.J. 2010, 'Can fiscal approaches help to reduce obesity risk?', in Crawford, D., Jeffery, R.W., Ball, K. and Brug, J. (eds), *Obesity Epidemiology*, Oxford University Press, pp. 368–79.
Finkelstein, E.A. and Zuckerman, L. 2008, *The Fattening of America*, Wiley, New Jersey.
Foster, G. and Frijters, P. 2023, 'Realeconomik: Using the messy human experience to drive clean theoretical advance in economics', in Altman, M. (ed), *Handbook of Research Methods in Behavioural Economics*, Edward Elgar Publishing, Cheltenham, pp. 80–103.
Fox, N.J. and Klein, E. 2020, 'The micropolitics of behavioural interventions: A new materialist analysis', *BioSocieties*, 15(2), pp. 226–44.
Frerichs, S. 2019, 'Bounded sociality: Behavioural economists' truncated understanding of the social and its implications for politics', *Journal of Economic Methodology*, 26(3), pp. 243–58.
Friedman, M. 1953, 'The Methodology of Positive Economics', in *Essays in Positive Economics*, University of Chicago Press, Chicago, pp. 3–43.
Gigerenzer, G. 2015, *Simply Rational*, Oxford University Press, New York.
Gilbert, D.T., Gill, M.J. and Wilson, T.D. 2002, 'The future is now: Temporal correction in affective forecasting', *Organizational Behavior and Human Decision Processes*, 88(1), pp. 430–44.
Guthman, J. 2009, 'Neoliberalism and the constitution of contemporary bodies', in Rothblum, E. and Solovay, S. (eds), *The Fat Studies Reader*, New York University Press, New York, pp. 187–96.
Guthman, J. 2011, *Weighing In*, University of California Press, Berkeley.
Hagger, M.S., Wood, C.W., Stiff, C. and Chatzisarantis, N.L. 2010, 'Self-regulation and self-control in exercise: The strength-energy model', *International Review of Sport and Exercise Psychology*, 3(1), pp. 62–86.
Hausman, D.M. 2012, *Preference, Value, Choice, and Welfare*, Cambridge University Press, Cambridge.
Heidl, S. 2016, *Philosophical Problems of Behavioural Economics*, Routledge, London.
Herrnstein, R.J., Loewenstein, G.F., Prelec, D. and Vaughan Jr, W., 1993, 'Utility maximization and melioration: Internalities in individual choice', *Journal of Behavioral Decision Making*, 6(3), pp. 149–85.
Heukelom, F. 2014, *Behavioural Economics*, Cambridge University Press, Cambridge.
Hewitson, G. 1999, *Feminist Economics*, Edward Elgar, Cheltenham.
Hofmann, W., Baumeister, R.F., Förster, G. and Vohs, K.D. 2012, 'Everyday temptations: An experience sampling study of desire, conflict, and self-control', *Journal of Personality and Social Psychology*, 102(6), pp. 1318–35.
Hollis, M. and Nell, E.J. 1975, *Rational Economic Man*, Cambridge University Press, Cambridge.
Holt-Giménez, E. 2017, *A Foodie's Guide to Capitalism*, New York University Press, New York.
Huckfeldt, P.J., Lakdawalla, D.N. and Philipson, T.J. 2012, 'Economics of obesity', in Jones, A.M. (ed), *The Elgar Companion to Health Economics*, Edward Elgar, Cheltenham, pp. 70–80.

Humphreys, B.R., Ruseski, J.E. and Zhou, L. 2015, 'Physical activity, present bias, and habit formation: Theory and evidence from longitudinal data', *SSRN*, 12 August, accessed 14 July 2022, <https://ssrn.com/abstract=2643049>.

Hunter, R.F., Tang, J., Hutchinson, G., Chilton, S., Holmes, D. and Kee, F. 2018, 'Association between time preference, present-bias and physical activity: Implications for designing behavior change interventions', *BMC Public Health*, 18, pp. 1–12.

Infante, G., Lecouteux, G. and Sugden, R. 2016, 'Preference purification and the inner rational agent: A critique of the conventional wisdom of behavioural welfare economics', *Journal of Economic Methodology*, 23(1), pp. 1–25.

James, W.P.T. 2008, 'WHO recognition of the global obesity epidemic', *International Journal of Obesity*, 32(7), pp. S120–6.

Kahneman, D. 2003, 'Maps of bounded rationality: Psychology for behavioral economics', *American Economic Review*, 93(5), pp. 1449–75.

Kahneman, D. and Frederick, S. 2002, 'Representativeness revisited: Attribute substitution in intuitive judgment', in Gilovich, T., Griffin, D. and Kahneman, D. (eds), *Heuristics and Biases*, Cambridge University Press, Cambridge, pp. 49–81.

Karnani, A., McFerran, B. and Mukhopadhyay, A. 2016, 'The obesity crisis as market failure: An analysis of systemic causes and corrective mechanisms', *Journal of the Association for Consumer Research*, 1(3), pp. 445–70.

Kopelman, P. 2007, 'Health risks associated with overweight and obesity', *Obesity Reviews*, 8, pp. 13–7.

Laibson, D. 1997, 'Golden eggs and hyperbolic discounting', *The Quarterly Journal of Economics*, 112(2), pp. 443–78.

Laibson, D.I. and List, J.A. 2015, 'Principles of (behavioral) economics', *American Economic Review*, 105(5), pp. 385–90.

Lakdawalla, D. and Philipson, T. 2009, 'The growth of obesity and technological change', *Economics and Human Biology*, 7(3), pp. 283–93.

Landolfi, T. 1963, *Gogol's Wife and Other Stories*, New Directions, New York.

Leggett, W. 2014, 'The politics of behaviour change: Nudge, neoliberalism and the state', *Policy and Politics*, 42(1), pp. 3–19.

Madra, Y.M. 2017, *Late Neoclassical Economics*, Routledge, London.

Mahoney, C. 2015, *Health, Food and Social Inequality*, Routledge, London.

Mani, A., Mullainathan, S., Shafir, E. and Zhao, J. 2013, 'Poverty impedes cognitive function', *Science*, 341(6149), pp. 976–80.

McFerran, B. 2016, 'Social norms, beliefs and health', in Roberto, C.A. and Kawachi, I. (eds), *Behavioral Economics and Public Health*, Oxford University Press, New York, pp. 133–60.

McMahon, J. 2015, 'Behavioral economics as neoliberalism: Producing and governing homo economicus', *Contemporary Political Theory*, 14, pp. 137–58.

Mehta, J. 2013, 'The discourse of bounded rationality in academic and policy arenas: Pathologising the errant consumer', *Cambridge Journal of Economics*, 37(6), pp. 1243–61.

Metcalfe, J. and Mischel, W. 1999, 'A hot/cool-system analysis of delay of gratification: Dynamics of willpower', *Psychological review*, 106(1), p. 3–19.

Mullainathan, S. and Shafir, E. 2013, *Scarcity*, Henry Holt and Company, New York.

Murphy, K. 2006, 'Obesity and the economic man', presentation at the McGill Health Challenge Think Tank, Montreal, Canada, 25–7 October.

Nordgren, L.F., Van Harreveld, F. and Van Der Pligt, J. 2009, 'The restraint bias: How the illusion of self-restraint promotes impulsive behavior', *Psychological Science* 20(12), pp. 1523–8.

O'Donoghue, T. and Rabin, M. 2000, 'The economics of immediate gratification', *Journal of Behavioral Decision Making*, 13(2), pp. 233–50.

O'Donoghue, T. and Rabin, M. 2006, 'Optimal sin taxes', *Journal of Public Economics*, 90(10–11), pp. 1825–1949.

Otero, G. 2018, *The Neoliberal Diet*, University of Texas Press, Austin.

Pastore, C., Schurer, S., Tymula, A., Fuller, N. and Caterson, I. 2020, 'Economic preferences and obesity: Evidence from a clinical lab-in-field study', *IZA Discussion Paper Nr. 13915*, December, accessed 7 April 2022, <https://www.iza.org/publications/dp/13915/economic-preferences-and-obesity-evidence-from-a-clinical-lab-in-field-experiment>.

Pedwell, C. 2017, 'Habit and the politics of social change: A comparison of nudge theory and pragmatist philosophy', *Body and Society*, 23(4), pp. 59–94.
Petracca, E. 2017, 'A cognition paradigm clash: Simon, situated cognition and the interpretation of bounded rationality', *Journal of Economic Methodology*, 24(1), pp. 20–40.
Pfeffer, I. and Strobach, T. 2022, 'Physical activity automaticity, intention, and trait self-control as predictors of physical activity behaviour – A dual-process perspective', *Psychology, Health and Medicine*, 27(5), pp. 1021–34.
Philipson, T. and Posner, R. 2003, 'The long run growth of obesity as a function of technological change', *Perspectives in Biology and Medicine*, 46(3), pp. 87–108.
Philipson, T.J. and Posner, R.A. 2008, 'Is the obesity epidemic a public health problem? A review of Zoltan J. Acs and Alan Lyles's obesity, business and public policy', *Journal of Economic Literature*, 46(4), pp. 974–982.
Primrose, D. 2017, 'The subjectification of homo economicus in behavioural economics', *Journal of Australian Political Economy*, 80, pp. 88–128.
Primrose, D. 2022, 'Behavioural economics and neuroeconomics', in Stilwell, F., Primrose, D. and Thornton, T.B. (eds), *Handbook of Alternative Theories of Political Economy*, Edward Elgar, Cheltenham, pp. 390–410.
Rabin, M. 2002, 'A perspective on psychology and economics', *European Economic Review*, 46(4), pp. 657–85.
Read, D. and Van Leeuwen, B. 1998, 'Predicting hunger: The effects of appetite and delay on choice', *Organizational Behavior and Human Decision Processes*, 76(2), pp. 189–205.
Richards, T.J. and Hamilton, S.F. 2012, 'Obesity and hyperbolic discounting: An experimental analysis', *Journal of Agricultural and Resource Economics*, 37(2), pp. 181–98.
Roberto, C.A. and Kawachi, I. 2016, 'An introduction to behavioral economics and public health', in Roberto, C.A. and Kawachi, I. (eds), *Behavioral Economics and Public Health*, Oxford University Press, New York, pp. 1–26.
Ruhm, C.J. 2012, 'Understanding overeating and obesity', *Journal of Health Economics*, 31(6), pp. 781–96.
Santos, A.C. and Rodrigues, J. 2014, 'Neoliberalism in the laboratory? Experimental economics on markets and their limits', *New Political Economy*, 19(4), pp. 507–33.
Scharff, R.L. 2009, 'Obesity and hyperbolic discounting: Evidence and implications', *Journal of Consumer Policy*, 32, pp. 3–21.
Schorb, F. 2022, 'Fat as a neoliberal epidemic: Analyzing fat bodies through the lens of political epidemiology', *Fat Studies*, 11(1), pp. 70–82.
Sen, A. 1977, 'Rational fools: A critique of the behavioural foundations of economic theory', *Philosophy and Public Affairs*, 6(4), pp. 317–44.
Sent, E.-M. 2004, 'Behavioral economics: How psychology made its (limited) way back into economics', *History of Political Economy*, 36(4), pp. 735–60.
Shaikh, A. 2016, *Capitalism*, Oxford University Press, New York.
Simon, H.A. 1955, 'A behavioral model of rational choice', *Quarterly Journal of Economics*, 69(1), pp. 99–118.
Smith, M. and Toprakkiran, N. 2019, 'Behavioural insights, nudge and the choice environment in obesity policy', *Policy Studies*, 40(2), pp. 173–87.
Strauss, K. 2009, 'Cognition, context, and multimethod approaches to economic decision making', *Environment and Planning A*, 41(2), pp. 302–17.
Streeck, W. 2010, 'Does "behavioural economics" offer an alternative to the neoclassical paradigm?', *Socio-Economic Review*, 8(2), pp. 387–97.
Thaler, R. 1987, 'Anomalies: The January effect', *Journal of Economic Perspectives*, 1(1), pp. 197–201.
Thaler, R. 2000, 'From homo economicus to homo sapiens', *Journal of Economic Perspectives*, 14(1), pp. 133–41.
Thaler, R. 2015, *Misbehaving*, WW Norton & Company, New York.
Thaler, R. and Sunstein, C.R. 2008, *Nudge*, Yale University Press, New Haven.
Tversky, A. and Kahneman, D. 1973, 'Availability: A heuristic for judging frequency and probability', *Cognitive Psychology*, 5(2), pp. 207–32.
Tversky, A. and Kahneman, D. 1974, 'Judgement under uncertainty: Heuristics and biases', *Science*, 185 (4157), pp. 1124–31.

Tzotzes, S. and Milonakis, D. 2021, ‘Paradigm change or assimilation? The case of behavioral economics’, *Review of Radical Political Economics*, 53(1), pp. 173–92.
Veblen, T. 1898, ‘Why is economics not an evolutionary science?’, *The Quarterly Journal of Economics*, 12(4), pp. 373–97.
Wansink, B. 2004, ‘Environmental factors that increase the food intake and consumption volume of unknowing consumers’, *Annual Review of Nutrition*, 24, pp. 455–79.
Wansink, B. 2016, *Slim by Design*, Hay House, California.
Ward, A. and Mann, T. 2000, ‘Don’t mind if I do: Disinhibited eating under cognitive load’, *Journal of Personality and Social Psychology*, 78(4), pp. 753–63.
White, M.D. 2017, ‘“Preferences all the way down”: Questioning the neoclassical foundations of behavioural economics and libertarian paternalism’, *Oeconomica*, 7(3), pp. 353–73.
Whitehead, M., Jones, R., Lilley, R., Pykett, J. and Howell, R. 2017, *Neuroliberalism*, Routledge, London.
WHO. 2000, *Obesity: Preventing and Managing the Global Epidemic*, World Health Organization, Geneva.
WHO. 2021, ‘Obesity and overweight’, *fact sheet*, World Health Organization, 9 June, accessed 14 July 2022, <https://www.who.int/news-room/fact-sheets/detail/obesity-and-overweight>.
Winson, A. 2013, *The Industrial Diet*, University of British Columbia Press, Vancouver.
Zimmerman, F.J. and Shimoga, S.V. 2014, ‘The effects of food advertising and cognitive load on food choices’, *BMC Public Health*, 14(1), pp. 1–10.
Žižek, S. 2012 [1994], ‘The spectre of ideology’, in Žižek, S. (ed), *Mapping Ideology*, Verso, New York, pp. 1–33.

PART II

Contemporary political-economic dimensions of health

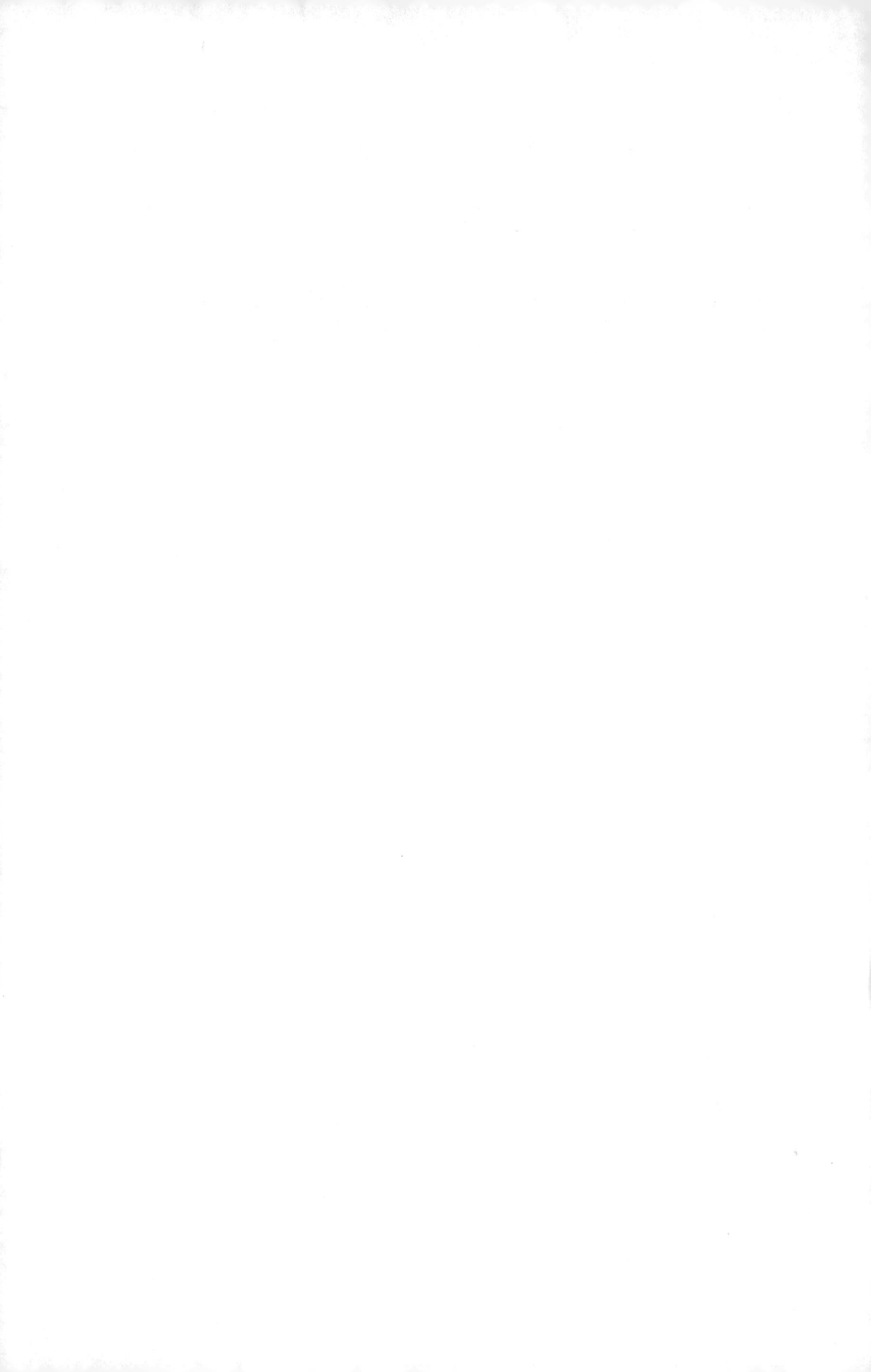

9

A CRITICAL POLITICAL ECONOMY OF HEALTH INEQUITIES

Arnel M. Borras

This chapter[1] is concerned with critical political economy and health inequities, emphasizing the co-constitutive character of class, gender, and racialized health inequities. The critical political economy approach incorporates the historical, economic, political, and cultural aspects of social life into its analysis of social and health inequities (Marx 1977 [1867]). It interrogates the links between health, illness, disease, and care; class, gender, and race relations; social structures and agency; and materials and ideas (Armstrong *et al.* 2001). Wealth and power inequalities between classes and groups figure prominently, in that they influence the production and distribution of societal resources through the political processes by which population health is transformed (Raphael 2015). Simultaneously, it also accounts for racism and sexism structured within and through economic and political systems that shape health inequities (Krieger *et al.* 1993; Syed 2016). In this respect, the approach is attentive to the roles played by the state, market, labor, and civil society in policy-making processes that shape the social determinants of health (Bryant 2016), and it scrutinizes the links between global neoliberal capitalism and health inequities (Navarro 2007). In all of these endeavors, the cornerstone of the critical political economy of health and healthcare remains social relations of power.

Some argue that critical political economy does not pay adequate attention to gender and race relations and that there is considerable overlap and tension with studies based on intersectionality. While space limitations here must restrict this discussion, Crenshaw (1989) coined the term *intersectionality* to examine the intersecting forms of oppression experienced by black women, non-white members of LGBT communities, and persons with disabilities, in reproducing the junctions of racism, sexism, ableism, and classism. Since then, others have described intersectionality as a normative and empirical research paradigm (Hankivsky *et al.* 2010), a method and disposition, a heuristic and an analytic tool (Carbado *et al.* 2013), a concept (Gopaldas 2013), and a theory (Bauer 2014). Collins (2015) has cautioned that understandings of intersectionality remain vague, and recently, Crenshaw has clarified that intersectionality is not identity politics but '*basically a lens, a prism* for seeing the way in which various forms of inequality often operate together' (Steinmetz 2020: n.p., emphasis added). These unresolved internal contestations suggest that intersectionality is not a fully developed theory.

On the contrary, Brown (2014: n.p.) asserts that '[a]lthough *Capital* is devoted to the critique of political economy', Marx's explanations of gender went beyond women in the factories to

DOI: 10.4324/9781003017110-11

include oppressive relations within the family. Anderson (2021: n.p.) advises that it is essential to understand Marx's 'generalizations about capitalist society and the very concrete ways in which he examined not only class but also gender, race, and colonialism, and what today would be called the intersectionality of all of these'. Similarly, Musto and Martinez (2022) have argued that Marx examined women and family, queer liberation, nationalism, colonialism, and ecology structured within and through existing economic and political relations, evident in his complete works, the *Marx-Engels-Gesamtausgabe*. They state that 'it is possible to read a very different Marx than the dogmatic, economistic, and Eurocentric theorist who has been criticized for so many years by those who have not read his work or have only done so superficially' (Musto and Martinez 2022: n.p.).

Compensating for the perceived limitations of critical political economy, I further draw on McNally's (2015: 131) explanations about the 'dialectics of unity and difference in the constitution of wage-labour', where he argues that 'the social relations of race, gender and sexuality, among others, were understood to be *internally constitutive* of class – rather than as radically external to it' (original emphasis). In other words, although class, race, and gender are analytically and conceptually distinct, in reality, they are internally related, co-constitutive, and irreducible to each other. Consequently, in this chapter, I use the terms *gendered capitalism, racialized capitalism, and racialized and gendered capitalism* to stress the co-constitutive character of the class, gender, and racial relations shaping health inequities.

Health inequities at a glance

The health gaps among classes and groups resulting from natural causes, for example genetic, are called *health inequalities.* In contrast, the preventable, systematic, and unfair health inequalities resulting from, for example, unsafe working and living conditions are called *health inequities* (Whitehead 1991).[2] Numerous studies have explained the causes and ways to address health inequities. For instance, *biological-genetic* theories hypothesize that biological-genetic differences underpin health gaps, whereas *behavioral-cultural* accounts emphasize lifestyle and behavioral factors such as smoking, diet, and exercise (Black *et al.* 1992). In contrast, *psycho-social* explanations focus on the psychological and mental impacts of social status, living, and working conditions, whereas the *materialist-structuralist* accounts prioritize social structures and socioeconomic factors, such as income and employment (Bartley 2016). *Life course* theory posits that life circumstances determine health outcomes from the uterus onward (Krieger 2001). The *macrosocial policies* approach to health accords particular emphasis to public policies (Mantoura and Morrison 2016), whereas *intersectionality* underscores the confluence of multiple forms of oppression (*e.g.* classism, racism, and sexism) (Hankivsky 2012). Finally, the *political economy* of health concentrates on examining the role of social structures of power and ideologies in engendering health inequities (Raphael 2015). Whereas the first two approaches presume health inequities originate at the individual, micro-level, the others posit explanations located at the societal macro-level.

Moreover, despite the articulation of many policy interventions and proposals designed to address health inequities within and between countries, their underlying social determinants persist (Raphael *et al.* 2020). Take, for example, the very blunt indicator of life expectancies (LE). While Japan's female and male LE at birth were 87 and 81 years in 2016, these were only 55 and 51 years in Lesotho. Canada's female and male LE were 85 and 80 years in 2016 (WHO 2019: 82–4); however, in Nunavut, the female and male LE at birth were only 74 and 69 years in 2013–2015 (Statistics Canada 2018: 1). Such marked discrepancies in LE correspond to the broader imbalances in political-economic conditions confronting each population. Similarly, we can consider prominent singular issues of morbidity and mortality, like the COVID-19 pandemic, where outcomes have varied wildly due, largely, to the prevailing social context. In my own region, Ontario, Canada, those most infected by the SARS-CoV-2 virus and its variants live in communities with a higher concentration of immigrants and visible minorities typified by poverty (Chung *et al.* 2020). If we wish to take seriously the relevance of such socio-material inequities and their impact on health outcomes, it will require new ways to interpret and explain the conditions under which people concretely live their lives. It is to this task, through a consideration of the multiple analytical lenses available to critical political economy, that this chapter now turns.

Class health inequities

Health inequities are rooted in social relations of production, a fact long recognized by Marx and Engels (Engels 1845; Marx 1977 [1867]). For example, in the Nineteenth Century, compared to the wealthy and capitalist class, the poor and working-class suffered higher morbidity and mortality due to toxic working conditions, subsistence wages, poverty, housing insecurity, and food deprivation. The capitalist economic system shapes these material and social conditions (Engels 1845) because, within capitalism, 'accumulation of wealth at one pole is at the same time accumulation of misery, agony of toil slavery, ignorance, brutality, mental degradation, at the opposite pole' (Marx 1977 [1867]: 451). Therein, women and children, immigrants, and enslaved people are further disadvantaged. In this sense, '[c]apital is reckless of the health or length of life of the laborer, unless under compulsion from society' (Marx 1977 [1867]: 181). Thus, contrary to Chadwick (1965 [1842]), who proposed solving social and health inequities through public policies within the capitalist system, Marx and Engels (1964 [1848]) recommended overthrowing capitalism and replacing it with communism or proletarian socialism.

In the Twentieth Century, Doyal and Pennell (1979) demonstrated that health inequalities within and between developed (UK) and underdeveloped countries are primarily produced not by biological differences, but rather by society's economic and social organization – the prevailing logic of which conforms to capitalism. Navarro (1986) also showed that capitalist labor processes in Western countries negatively impact workers' well-being by producing toxicity, accidents, stress, and fatigue, such that blue-collar workers are further disadvantaged than managers and professionals (Navarro 1991). On the contrary, some have divorced health inequities from the structure of capitalism, *per se*. For instance, Wilkinson (1989, 1992, 1997) has emphasized that joblessness and employment income variances result in low income and relative poverty, shaping mortality differences among social classes. Unfortunately, although Wilkinson proposed redistributive public policies to address health inequities, he neglected the structural importance of capitalist class relations in configuring such social determinants themselves.

More recently, the health effects of the advanced welfare state have been explored more thoroughly. For instance, with regard to infant mortality rates (IMR), Navarro and Shi (2001) find that when compared to Christian democratic countries, former fascist dictatorships, or liberal states (which record relatively high IMR), social democratic states exhibited the lowest mean IMR from 1960 to 1996. This, they posit, is a direct result of social relations, because redistributive public policies were weaker in the liberal welfare states due to the comparative powerlessness of social democratic parties and the working-class therein. In social democratic states, where the power of left-leaning parties and the working-class is more substantial and effective relative to the capitalist class (Navarro and Shi 2001), prevailing egalitarian ideologies bring about redistributive public policies (Navarro *et al.* 2003). Working-class power and socialist party representation are, thus, crucial to enhancing health equity.

More specific to the neoliberal era, Coburn (2004) provides a *class/welfare regime model* for explaining health inequalities. Coburn contends that economic globalization and neoliberalism, powered by capital, have defeated labor in the market and undermined extant welfare state systems. These conditions have weakened social cohesion and intensified social inequality, income inequality, poverty, and health inequality. As such, deregulation, privatization, liberalization, and austerity can all be understood as political tools used to undermine working-classes and weaken components of welfare state systems since the 1970s, and are primarily accountable for vast contemporary social and health inequities (Labonté and Stuckler 2016; Navarro and Muntaner 2004; Schrecker and Bambra 2015). Raphael (2015: S19) posits that 'the power and dominance of the business and corporate sector in the liberal welfare state translates into public policy that inequitably shapes the distribution of [the social determinants of health] in a whole range of public policy areas'. Such public policy areas might include, but are not limited to, employment, child development, and healthcare systems. Consequently, most people now experience greater social and material deprivation and psycho-social stress, resulting overall in less healthy coping behaviors and health inequalities (Bryant and Raphael 2020). Ultimately, neoliberal governments represent more than the political execution of a governing ideology; they are also an expression of the effects of class relations and class power, via electoral politics and public policy, on the exacerbation of health inequities.

Globally, the effects of neoliberal capitalism on wealth inequality – which, in turn, exacerbate class-based health inequities – are clear enough numerically. From 1980 to 2014, the global Gini coefficient skyrocketed from 0.657 (Bourguignon and Morrisson 2002: 732) to 0.922, with the wealthiest 10 percent gaining a global wealth share of 88.3 percent in 2014 (Davies *et al.* 2017: 731). In Canada, while the majority of the household incomes stagnated from 1990 to 2010, the household incomes of the wealthiest 0.01 percent increased by 145 percent (Peters 2012: 19). During this period, de-unionization and concessionary wages and benefits worsened, while contractual, temporary, and part-time employment practices became more widespread. Corporate downsizing and closures of many small- and medium-sized businesses resulted in unemployment, income losses, housing insecurity, and vast social inequalities (Banting and Myles 2013; Carroll and Sapinski 2018; Finkel 2018), along with their attendant health inequalities (Bryant and Raphael 2020). Moreover, neoliberalism continued to generate the so-called *precariat* – workers living in perennial states of material precariousness – many of whom live in poverty (Standing 2014). These precarious workers suffer from higher physio-pathological, behavioral, and psycho-social health risks than other classes (Muntaner *et al.* 2010). Moreover, as a gross indicator of health effects, between 1996–2001 and 2011–2016, the LE gap between Canadian women in the top and lowest income quintiles widened from 3.7 to 5.4 years, while growing from 6.7 to 7.7 years for men in the same categories (Bushnik *et al.* 2020: 8).

In Canada's largest urban area, Toronto, households above C$150,000 annual income recorded only 7 percent of COVID-19 cases during the early stages of the pandemic, despite constituting 21 percent of the population. In contrast, households below C$29,000 annual income recorded 27 percent of the COVID-19 cases, despite only comprising 14 percent of the population (City of Toronto 2020). As such, even in a metropolitan area in which public health infrastructure is relatively prolific, the capitalist economic system confers advantages to the capitalist class and the wealthy, while remaining disadvantageous to the working-class and poor. It is not surprising, then, that across a multitude of resource-poor settings worldwide, wealth accumulation and power concentration in the hands of the economic and political elite create penury for billions. This is the logical outcome of capitalism, where class relations remain a fundamental and prime mover of health inequities.

Class and gendered health inequities

Class relations never proceed in isolation and are always imbricated or entangled with other relations of exploitation or oppression. In this sense, gendered capitalism creates and maintains class and gendered health inequities. Doyal (1995) has argued convincingly that, due to poverty across developed and developing countries, women experience relatively higher rates of infectious diseases, malnutrition, depression, cancer, and less access to healthcare than men. Additionally, cancer primarily affects women more than men in middle- and low-income countries. In these countries, women with cervical or breast cancer have less survival expectancy than their counterparts in high-income countries, because of the differences in access to diagnosis, quality care, and affordability (Ginsburg *et al.* 2017). In Canada's workplaces, females generally experience higher rates of psychological and mental health issues, cardiovascular diseases, musculoskeletal problems, toxic chemical exposures, and cancers (Messing and de Grosbois 2001). Gendered health inequities have also been documented in occupational health and healthcare systems due to sexist practices and policies (Armstrong and Armstrong 2010; Morrow *et al.* 2008). Thus, although women have longer life expectancies, they exhibit higher morbidities than men (Scott-Samuel *et al.* 2009).

COVID-19 further revealed the inequities rendered by gendered capitalism. Here, for instance, the global loss in working hours due to employment termination, reduced working hours, or underemployment affected females more than males (ILO 2020a). The primary reasons for this are as follows: (1) fewer males (36.6 percent) than females (40 percent) were employed in significantly affected sectors; (2) out of 55 million domestic workers, 37 million females experienced higher working-hour losses; (3) almost 80 percent of females work in the healthcare and social work sector; and (4) the closures of childcare centers and schools increased unpaid domestic labor, 75 percent of which is shouldered by females (ILO 2020b). Worse still, lockdowns and subsequent job and income losses intensified violence against women. In Canada, gender-based violence figures surged: ranging from 20 percent to 400 percent in some areas (Patel 2020). These upsurges were facilitated by inevitable close contact with the abuser, disrupted social support, constrained legal aid, and reduced healthcare access (WHO 2020). While it should be noted that violence against women had already escalated with the shift to neoliberal policies (Morrow *et al.* 2004), the intensification of these dynamics under COVID-19 was adumbrated distinctly by gendered class relations.

Pre-existing class and gendered health inequities, as well as the uneven financial and health impacts of COVID-19, can be linked to the gendered inequity of wealth accumulation, which consistently works to the detriment of females. Currently, the total wealth of 2,153 billionaires – almost entirely males – is greater than the total wealth of 4.6 billion people. This wealth inequality is partly due to underpaid and unpaid labor provided by women and girls, amounting to US$10.8 trillion annually (Coffey *et al.* 2020: 8). Under such conditions of blatant inequality, class and gendered health inequities persist, because most women remain economically disadvantaged, culturally suppressed, and politically misrepresented (Borras 2021). In 2018, the World Economic Forum reported worldwide that gendered disparity for economic participation and opportunity exhibited a gap of 41.9 percent, while the figure for political empowerment was 77.1 percent (WEF 2018: vii). In the healthcare industry, females are in minority management and leadership positions despite comprising the majority of the workforce (OECD 2020) and, not surprisingly, females are paid less than males, with a gender pay gap of 28 percent across 104 countries (Boniol 2019). Undervalued by those who control economic, cultural, and political resources, women and girls are often unable to participate in societal activities, especially in decision-making processes in both private and public spheres. Gendered capitalism discriminates against females in the production of social life, adversely affecting their working, living, and health conditions. Accordingly, it is difficult to avoid the conclusion that class and gendered health inequities are fundamentally a question of the co-constitutive character of class and gender relations.

Class and racialized health inequities

Race and class, entangled with both the history of colonialism and capitalism, similarly have formative effects on health inequities. Structural racism, interlinked with settler colonialism and white supremacy, influences institutions, legal standards, public policies, and political systems that, in turn, shape health outcomes (NCCDH 2018). It produces and sustains racialized health inequities via state-sanctioned violence, land grabbing, hazardous environments, social inequities, inequitable distribution of social determinants of health, and psycho-social trauma (NCCDH 2018). None of this can be detached from capitalist political economy, currently in its neoliberal form, where racism and the legacy of colonialism continue to reproduce critical mechanisms of structural exploitation.

The co-constitutive effects of race and class can, for instance, be witnessed across the Anglo-American world. In the US, a country deeply submerged in neoliberal capitalism, whites are generally wealthier than blacks, Native Americans, and people of color. Indeed, whites in America exhibit lower unemployment, poverty, and health risks than any of the latter groups (Bailey *et al.* 2017). In New Zealand, Australia, and the Pacific, indigenous peoples have lower employment and income, shorter life expectancies, and higher IMR than non-indigenous (Anderson *et al.* 2006). In Canada, indigenous people suffer from higher poverty levels, inequitable healthcare access, and mental health problems (Nelson and Wilson 2017). Moreover, while the food insecurity level for the white Canadian population stood at 11.1 percent in 2017–18, levels of food insecurity for other racial groups ranged from 11.3 percent to 28.9 percent (Tarasuk and Mitchell 2020). Not surprisingly, for peoples who were marginally, moderately, or severely food-insecure, mortality rates were, respectively, 28 percent, 49 percent, and 160 percent higher than for food-secure persons (Gundersen *et al.* 2018). Poverty, here linked to structural racism via nutrition and caloric consumption, demonstrates one of many ways in which class and race combine to produce material-biological pathways to unequal health outcomes.

These effects can be further discerned among migrants, a highly racialized category deeply imbued in an international political economy of labor. For instance, migrant farmworkers experience significant financial and occupational health risks across the profit-driven capitalist food system, largely because they lack the social support and healthcare services provided to permanent residents and citizens. In Canada, temporary farmworkers regularly experience wage theft (MWAC 2020), and during the COVID-19 lockdowns, most were deprived of food, income, and information. Racism, surveillance, intimidation, and threats all compel these laborers to work overtime, even under exceptional (pandemic) circumstances. Most labor laws exempt employers of migrant labor from safeguards concerning overtime pay, minimum wage, or collective bargaining. Given of their temporary status, many racialized migrant workers also encounter difficulties in asserting their rights around fair employment practices, decent housing, and equitable healthcare services (MWAC 2020). During the early phase of the COVID-19 pandemic, although nearly 1,000 workers were infected with the SARS-CoV-2 virus in the Cargill meat facility in Alberta, Canada, governing authorities permitted this transnational corporation to reopen within just two weeks of the incident. Perhaps not surprisingly, the facility workforce primarily consists of temporary foreign workers: Chinese, Vietnamese, and Filipinos (Dryden and Rieger 2020). From sector to sector, the capitalist state, in sync with employers, prioritizes production and profit over health when it concerns racialized migrant workers. Again, as with gender, co-constitution is an unavoidable conclusion in relation to race and class relations inasmuch as health is concerned.

Class, race, and gendered health inequities

Bringing these axes into a singular analytical lens, class, race, and gender can be understood to form a mutually enforcing matrix of social relations that generate health inequities. For example, in Canada in 2019, unemployment for racialized citizens stood at 9.2 percent, whereas it remained at only 7.3 percent for the non-racialized population (Block *et al.* 2019). These categories could, however, be further disaggregated. In 2016, racialized women and men faced unemployment rates of 9.6 percent and 8.8 percent, respectively, whereas parallel non-racialized figures were 6.4 percent and 8.2 percent. Earning power by race is also revealing, where 'racialized men earned 78 cents for every dollar that non-racialized men earned' in 2015 – a gap that has remained unchanged since 2005. At the same time, accounting for gender, 'racialized women earned 59 cents for every dollar that non-racialized men earned, while non-racialized women earned 67 cents for every dollar that non-racialized men earned' (Block *et al.* 2019: 4–5). Where the social determinants literature links income level unmistakably to health outcomes, the Canadian labor market is actively shaping potential health inequities explicitly along racial and gender lines.

In the healthcare industry, Navarro (1976: 446) long ago demonstrated that the labor distribution in capitalist Western systems amounts to 'physicians being primarily upper-middle-class white males; nurses, lower-middle or working-class females; and auxiliary health workers, females of working-class backgrounds'. Again, however, it is important to note that, due to low pay, many racialized females in the industry work multiple jobs, exposing them to further health disadvantages. These mostly frontline healthcare workers experience heavy workloads, understaffing, casualization, contractualization, racism, sexism, violence, and abuses (Armstrong 2020; Armstrong *et al.* 2001; Daly *et al.* 2011; Syed 2016, 2020). Even in the health sector, which should be more sensitive to health inequities, gendered and racialized biases perpetuate these inequities in complex ways.

This set of effects was, not surprisingly, magnified under COVID-19. For instance, in the UK National Health Service, of the first ten physicians to die from COVID, 9 were from racialized backgrounds. Similarly, of the first 50 healthcare workers to die, 75 percent were from racialized communities (Nagpaul 2020). These health inequities can be linked to working arrangements in which many racialized workers are employed as medical staff or direct care providers, while a disproportionate number of non-racialized are non-medical staff and/or managers (GOV.UK 2020). In Canada, more than 9,650 long-term care workers were infected, which amounted in May 2020 to over 10 percent of the entire country's cases (Canadian Institute for Health Information 2020). One of the reasons that women remained so vulnerable to the disease was that they made up about 80 percent of the health sector's labor force and 90 percent of long-term care workers (Boniol 2019). Some argue that the state, in such cases, has 'sacrificed' the lives of healthcare workers, many of whom are racialized women (Brophy *et al.* 2021). The gendered and racialized elements of capitalism are not always obvious, but they often involve adverse effects on working people's life conditions and/or morbidity. More regrettably, they also – as in the case of COVID – can amplify the likelihood of death.

Conclusion: a way forward?

While Chadwick (1965 [1842]) suggested policy reforms to address social and health inequities within the capitalist system, Marx and Engels (1964 [1848]) recommended replacing capitalism with proletarian socialism or communism through class struggle. In light of this historical and conceptual backdrop, some have proposed stronger alliances among working-class and feminist organizations; occupational health scientists and feminists; and researchers and female workers (*e.g.* Messing and de Grosbois 2001). In an even more integrated manner, others examine the class, gender, and racial relations that underlie economic, cultural, and political structures which, in turn, shape health inequities (*e.g.* Borras 2021; Krieger *et al.* 1993; Morrow *et al.* 2008; Muntaner and Navarro 2004; Syed 2016, 2020). After all, as Navarro (2020: 1) has stated, 'the objective of any emancipatory project should be the elimination of any form of exploitation, whether of class, gender, race, nation, or the environment'. Doubtless, on some level, this will require the strengthening of labor, political, and social movements, in order to counter corporate power and compel the capitalist state to improve working and living conditions (Bryant and Raphael 2020).

On any road to potential change, we might draw on Wright (2019), who suggests that different struggles against social and health inequities have been informed by intermingling, but discrete, 'strategic logics': smashing, dismantling, taming, resisting, and escaping capitalism. Central to *smashing capitalism* is the idea that capitalism is irreformable, and its contradictory logic is manifest in the frequent economic crises prevailing in the capitalist system. Here, such crises are understood as potential 'ruptures', in the wake of which the possibilities for huge mobilizations to seize the state or systematically reconfigure social relations are understood as more likely. The goal is, ultimately, the end of capitalism and radical reconstitution of institutional structures, whereby some form of socialism would address social and health inequities. The historical track record, here, however, is not especially encouraging: in the Twentieth Century, 'revolutionary ruptures' failed to create an alternative world that brought about social and health equity, and often resulted in new forms of authoritarian political control.

For its part, *dismantling capitalism* does not perceive a radical rupture with capitalism, so much as a continuing transition to democratic socialism, more likely via state-led reforms that deliver gradual socialist alternatives within the capitalist economic system (Wright 2019). This strategic logic entails a secure democratic electoral politics and a socialist party that can win elections and capture state power over the long-term, continuously institutionalizing alternative economic structures that address social and health inequities. Such a reformist pathway to socialism continues to face relentless attacks from proponents of neoliberalism, because 'both smashing and dismantling capitalism [...] have revolutionary aspirations, even if they differ in their understanding of the necessary means for accomplishing their goals' (Wright 2019: 20).

Contrary to smashing and dismantling capitalism, *taming capitalism* does not attempt to replace capitalism with socialism (Wright 2019). This strategic logic guides social democratic parties and seeks to 'neutralize some of the harms of capitalism' via state redistributive policies and regulations, feasible through 'political will' and 'popular mobilization'. Exemplified by the post-World War Two era of capitalism – where states extended socialized insurance, progressive taxation, and workplace health and safety regulations – the logic here emphasizes state policy formulations to mitigate social and health inequities. Yet, this, too, can engender backlash, as the capitalist class and elected neoliberal governments have sought to 'claw back' those democratic gains since the 1980s.

Resisting capitalism means working outside the state (Wright 2019). This strategic logic informs many labor unions, grassroots organizations, and civil society groups in their response to social and health inequities. This might be exemplified by a workers' strike, which does not attempt to capture state power, but does challenge the economic and political elite through resistance beyond the state. While the primary struggle might involve general workers' actions against exploitation workplaces, such resistance is fueled by social identities, such as class, gender, and race relations – from the involvement of the women's movement in post-World War One strikes, to the intersectional nature of strikes by so-called support workers at the University of California.

Finally, *eroding capitalism* may emerge organically from the ongoing work of social movements (Wright 2019). This strategic logic integrates the bottom-up civil society-centric strategies of escaping and resisting capitalism and top-down state-centric strategies of dismantling and taming capitalism to respond to social and health inequities. Eroding capitalism is best exemplified by a combination of tactics emanating from the likes of Sanders, Corbyn, Syriza, and Podemos. It allows for the possibility of historical change – displacing capitalism from its dominance – without a singular agenda or directed program (Wright 2019). Here, where historical contingency remains central, a multi-pronged approach that struggles for a world beyond capitalism, with the reduction of class, gender, and racialized health inequities, still leaves open the possibility that socialistic practices remain a plausible – though not guaranteed – alternative.

Class, gender, and racialized health inequities are extensive. Indeed, the constellation of interrelated issues appears overwhelming, where a continuing ensemble of capitalism, sexism, colonialism, and racism set the scene. Imagining strategies to address this scene is no less difficult, and a way forward may mean any combination of smashing, dismantling, resisting, or eroding capitalism. One thing is certain: whatever form it takes, ignoring any one of the constituent parts of inequity is likely only to bring negative or disappointing returns. This chapter has contributed to current public and scholarly debates on preventing and reducing these health inequities by articulating the need for a *critical* political economy approach that accounts for the co-constitutive character of class, gender, and race. This offers the possibility for realistic and concrete assessments of the interwoven and complicated sources of health inequity, as well as opening up potential routes to address them.

Notes

1 This chapter builds on Borras (2021).
2 Some interchange between health inequalities and health inequities persists within existing scholarship, which serves to muddle both concepts (Borras 2021). For the purposes of this chapter, I maintain this distinction.

References

Anderson, I., Crengle, S., Kamaka, M.L., Chen, T.H., Palafox, N. and Jackson-Pulver, L. 2006, 'Indigenous health in Australia, New Zealand, and the Pacific', *The Lancet*, 367(9524), pp. 1775–85.

Anderson, K. 2021, 'Class, gender, race and colonialism: The "intersectionality" of Marx', *MR Online*, accessed 14 December 2022, <https://mronline.org/2021/02/08/theintersectionality-of-marx/>.

Armstrong, P. 2020, 'Viruses and care', *The Bullet*, accessed 14 December 2022, <https://socialistproject.ca/2020/04/viruses-and-care/>.

Armstrong, P., Armstrong, H. and Coburn, D. 2001, *Unhealthy Times: Political Economy Perspectives on Health and Care,* Oxford University Press, Toronto.Armstrong, P. and Armstrong, H. 2010, *Wasting Away: The Undermining of Canadian Health care*, Oxford University Press, Toronto.

Bailey, Z.D., Krieger, N., Agénor, M., Graves, J., Linos, N. and Bassett, M.T. 2017, 'Structural racism and health inequities in the USA: Evidence and interventions', *The Lancet,* 389(10077), pp. 1453–63.

Banting, K. and Myles, J. (eds) 2013, *Inequality and the Fading of Redistributive Politics*, UBC Press, Vancouver.

Bartley, M. 2016, *Health Inequality: An Introduction to Concepts, Theories and Methods*, John Wiley and Sons, Cambridge.

Bauer, G.R. 2014, 'Incorporating intersectionality theory into population health research methodology: Challenges and the potential to advance health equity', *Social Science and Medicine*, 110, pp. 10–7.

Black, D., Morris, J.N., Smith C. and Townsend, P. 1992, 'The black report', in Townsend, P. and Davidson, N. (eds), *Inequalities in Health: The Black Report and the Health Divide*, Penguin Books, London, pp. 33–213.

Block, S., Galabuzi, G.E. and Tranjan, R. 2019, *Canada's Colour Coded Income Inequality*, Canadian Centre for Policy Alternatives, Ottawa.

Boniol, M., McIsaac, M., Xu, L., Wuliji, T., Diallo, K. and Campbell, J. 2019, *Gender Equity in the Health Workforce: Analysis of 104 Countries*, No. WHO/HIS/HWF/Gender/WP1/ 2019.1, WHO, Geneva.

Borras, A.M. 2021, 'Toward an intersectional approach to health justice', *International Journal of Health Services*, 51(2), pp. 206–25.

Bourguignon, F. and Morrisson, C. 2002, 'Inequality among world citizens: 1820–1992', *American Economic Review*, 92(4), pp. 727–44.

Brophy, J.T., Keith, M.M., Hurley M. and McArthur, J.E. 2021, 'Sacrificed: Ontario healthcare workers in the time of COVID-19', *New Solutions*, 30(4), pp. 267–81.

Brown, H. 2014, 'Marx on gender and the family: A summary', *Monthly Review*, 66(2), pp. 48–57.

Bryant, T. 2016, *Health Policy in Canada*, 2nd edn, Canadian Scholars' Press Inc., Toronto.

Bryant, T. and Raphael, D. 2020, *The Politics of Health in the Canadian Welfare State*, Canadian Scholars, Toronto.

Bushnik, T., Tjepkema M. and Martel, L. 2020, 'Socioeconomic disparities in life and health expectancy among the household population in Canada', *Health Reports*, 31(1), pp. 3–14.

Canadian Institute for Health Information. 2020, *Pandemic Experience in the Long-Term Care Sector: How Does Canada Compare With Other Countries?*, CIHI, Ottawa.

Carbado, D.W., Crenshaw, K.W., Mays, V.M. and Tomlinson, B. 2013, 'Intersectionality: Mapping the movements of a theory', *Du Bois Review: Social Science Research on Race*, 10(2), pp. 303–12.

Carroll, W.K. and Sapinski, J.P. 2018, *Organizing the 1 Percent: How Corporate Power Works*, Fernwood Publishing, Nova Scotia.

Chadwick, E. 1965 [1842], *Report on the Sanitary Condition of the Labouring Population and on the Means of its Improvement*, Edinburgh University Press, Edinburgh.

Chung, H., Fung, K., Ferreira-Legere, L.E., Chen, B., Ishiguro, L., Kalappa, G., Gozdyra, P., Campbell, T., Paterson, J.M., Bronskill, S.E. and Kwong, J.C. 2020, *COVID-19 Laboratory Testing in Ontario: Patterns of Testing and Characteristics of Individuals Tested, as of April 30, 2020*, ICES, Toronto.

City of Toronto. 2020, *COVID-19: Status of Cases in Toronto – Ethno-Racial Group, Income, and Infection*, accessed 4 September 2020, <https://www.toronto.ca/home/covid-19/covid-19-latest-city-of-toronto-76.news/covid-19-status-of-cases-in-toronto/>.

Coburn, D. 2004, 'Beyond the income inequality hypothesis: Class, neo-liberalism, and health inequalities', *Social Science and Medicine*, 58(1), pp. 41–56.

Coffey, C., Revollo, P.E., Harvey, R., Lawson, M., Butt, A.P., Piaget, K., Sarosi, D. and Thekkudan, J. 2020, *Time to Care: Unpaid and Underpaid Care Work and the Global Inequality Crisis*, Oxfam International, Oxford.

Collins, P.H. 2015, 'Intersectionality's definitional dilemmas', *Annual Review of Sociology*, 41, pp. 1–20.

Crenshaw, K. 1989, 'Demarginalizing the intersection of race and sex: A black feminist critique of antidiscrimination doctrine, feminist theory and antiracist politics', *University of Chicago Legal Forum*, 1989(1), Article 8.

Daly, T., Banerjee, A., Armstrong, P., Armstrong, H. and Szebehely, M. 2011, 'Lifting the 'violence veil': Examining working conditions in long-term care facilities using iterative mixed methods', *Canadian Journal on Aging*, 30(2), pp. 271–84.

Davies, J.B., Lluberas, R. and Shorrocks, A.F. 2017, 'Estimating the level and distribution of global wealth, 2000–2014', *Review of Income and Wealth*, 63(4), pp. 731–59.

Doyal, L. 1995, *What Makes Women Sick: Gender and the Political Economy of Health*, Macmillan Press, London.

Doyal, L. and Pennell, I. 1979, *The Political Economy of Health*, Pluto Press, London.

Dryden, J. and Rieger, S. 2020, 'Inside the slaughterhouse', *Canadian Broadcasting Corporation,* 6 May, accessed 10 June 2020, https://newsinteractives.cbc.ca/longform/cargill-covid19-outbreak>.

Engels, F. 1845, *The Condition of the Working Class in England*, accessed 27 January 2017, <https://marxists.architexturez.net/archive/marx/works/download/pdf/condition-working-class-england.pdf>.
Finkel, A. 2018, *Compassion*, Macmillan International Higher Education, Basingstoke.
Ginsburg, O., Bray, F., Coleman, M.P., Vanderpuye, V., Eniu, A., Kotha, S.R., Sarker, M., Huong, T.T., Allemani, C., Dvaladze A., Gralow, J., Yeates, K., Taylor, C., Oomman, N., Krishnan, S., Sullivan, R., Kombe, D., Blas, M.M., Parham, G., Kassami, N. and Conteh, L. 2017, 'The global burden of women's cancers: A grand challenge in global health' *The Lancet,* 389(10071), pp. 847–60.
Gopaldas, A. 2013, 'Intersectionality 101', *Journal of Public Policy and Marketing*, 32(1), pp. 90–4.
GOV.UK. 2020, 'NHS workforce', accessed 18 May 2022, <https://www.ethnicity factsfigures.service.gov.uk/workforce-and-business/workforce-diversity/nhs-workforce/latest>.
Gundersen, C., Tarasuk, V., Cheng, J., De Oliveira, C. and Kurdyak, P. 2018, 'Food insecurity status and mortality among adults in Ontario, Canada', *PloS One*, 13(8), pp. 1–10.
Hankivsky, O. (ed.) 2012, *Health Inequities in Canada: Intersectional Frameworks and Practices*, UBC Press, Vancouver.
Hankivsky, O., Reid, C., Cormier, R., Varcoe, C., Clark, N., Benoit, C., and Brotman, S. 2010, 'Exploring the promises of intersectionality for advancing women's health research', *International Journal for Equity in Health*, 9(5), pp. 1–15.
International Labour Organization. 2020a, *ILO Monitor: COVID-19 and the World of Work, Third edition, Updated Estimates and Analysis 29 April 2020*, ILO, Geneva.
International Labour Organization. 2020b, *ILO Monitor: COVID-19 and the World of Work, Fifth edition, Updated Estimates and Analysis 30 June 2020*, ILO, Geneva.
Krieger, N. 2001, 'A glossary for social epidemiology', *Journal of Epidemiology and Community Health*, 55(10), pp. 693–700.
Krieger, N., Rowley, D.L., Herman, A.A., Avery, B. and Phillips, M.T. 1993, 'Racism, sexism, and social class: Implications for studies of health, disease, and well-being', *American Journal of Preventive Medicine*, 9(6), pp. 82–122.
Labonté, R. and Stuckler, D. 2016, 'The rise of neoliberalism: How bad economics imperils health and what to do about it', *Journal of Epidemiology and Community Health*, 70(3), pp. 312–8.
Mantoura, P. and Morrison, V. 2016, *Policy Approaches To Reducing Health Inequalities*, National Collaborating Centre for Healthy Public Policy, Quebec.
Marx, K. 1977 [1867], *Capital: A Critique of Political Economy*, Progress Publishers, Moscow.
Marx, K. and Engels, F. 1964 [1848], *The Communist Manifesto*, Simon and Schuster, New York.
McNally, D. 2015, 'The dialectics of unity and difference in the constitution of wage-labour: On internal relations and working-class formation', *Capital and Class*, 39(1), pp. 131–46.
Messing, K. and de Grosbois, S. 2001, 'Women workers confront one-eyed science: Building alliances to improve women's occupational health', *Women and Health*, 33(1–2), pp. 125–41.
Migrant Workers Alliance for Change. 2020, *Unheeded Warnings: COVID-19 and Migrant Workers in Canada*, Migrant Workers Alliance for Change, Toronto.
Morrow, M., Hankivsky, O. and Varcoe, C. 2004, 'Women and violence: The effects of dismantling the welfare state', *Critical Social Policy*, 24(3), pp. 358–84.
Morrow, M., Hankivsky, O. and Varcoe, C. (eds), 2008, *Women's Health in Canada: Critical Perspectives on Theory and Policy*, University of Toronto Press, Toronto.
Muntaner, C., Solar, O., Vanroelen, C., Martínez, J.M., Vergara, M., Santana, V., Castedo, A., Kim, I.H., Benach, J. and EMCONET Network. 2010, 'Unemployment, informal work, precarious employment, child labor, slavery, and health inequalities: Pathways and mechanisms', *International Journal of Health Services*, 40(2), pp. 281–95.
Musto, M. and Martinez, J. 2022, 'The unknown paths of the late Marx', translated by Flakin, N., *Left Voice Magazine*, accessed 14 December 2022, <https://www.leftvoice.org/the-unknown-paths-of-the-late-marx/>.
Nagpaul, C. 2020, 'The disproportionate impact of COVID-19 on ethnic minority healthcare workers', *Thebmjopinion*, accessed 14 December 2022, <https://blogs.bmj.com/bmj/2020/04/20/chaand-nagpaul-the-disproportionate-impact-of-covid-19-on-ethnic-minority-healthcare-workers/>.
National Collaborating Centre for Determinants of Health. 2018, *Let's Talk: Racism and Health Equity,* NCCDH, St. Francis Xavier University, Nova Scotia.
Navarro, V. 1976, 'Social class, political power and the state and their implications in medicine', *Social Science and Medicine*, 10(9–10), pp. 437–57.
Navarro, V. 1986, *Crisis, Health, and Medicine: A Social Critique*, Tavistock, New York.

Navarro, V. 1991, 'Race or class or race and class: Growing mortality differentials in the United States', *International Journal of Health Services*, 21(2), pp. 229–35.
Navarro, V. 2007, *Neoliberalism, Globalization and Inequalities*, Baywood Publishing Company, New York.
Navarro, V. 2020, 'What should be the objective of an emancipatory project?', *International Journal of Health Services*, 50(3), pp. 253–63.
Navarro, V., Borrell, C., Benach, J., Muntaner, C., Quiroga, A., Rodríguez-Sanz, M., Vergés, N., Gumá, J. and Pasarin, M.I. 2003, 'The importance of the political and the social in explaining mortality differentials among the countries of the OECD, 1950–1998', *International Journal of Health Services*, 33(3), pp. 419–94.
Navarro, V. and Muntaner, C. (eds) 2004, *Political and Economic Determinants of Population Health and Well-Being: Controversies and Developments*, Baywood Publishing Company, New York.
Navarro, V. and Shi, L. 2001, 'The political context of social inequalities and health', *International Journal of Health Services*, 31(1), pp. 1–21.
Nelson, S.E. and Wilson, K. 2017, 'The mental health of Indigenous peoples in Canada: Critical review of research', *Social Science and Medicine*, 176, pp. 93–112.
Organisation for Economic Co-operation and Development. 2020, *Women at the Core of the Fight Against the COVID-19 Crisis*, OECD, Paris.
Patel, R. 2020, 'Minister says COVID-19 is empowering domestic violence abusers as rates rise in parts of Canada', *CBC News*, 27 April, accessed 5 May 2020, <https://www.cbc.ca/news/politics/domestic-violence-rates-rising-due-to-covid19 1.5545851>.
Peters, J. (ed.) 2012, *Boom, Bust and Crisis: Labour, Corporate Power and Politics in Canada,* Fernwood Publishing, Nova Scotia.
Raphael, D. 2015, 'The political economy of health: A research agenda for addressing health inequalities in Canada', *Canadian Public Policy*, 41, pp. S17–S25.
Raphael, D., Bryant, T., Mikkonen, J. and Raphael, A. 2020, *Social Determinants of Health: The Canadian Facts*, Ontario Tech University Faculty of Health Sciences, Ontario.
Schrecker, T. and Bambra, C. 2015, *How Politics Makes Us Sick: Neoliberal Epidemics*, Palgrave Macmillan, London.
Scott-Samuel, A., Stanistreet, D. and Crawshaw, P. 2009, 'Hegemonic masculinity, structural violence and health inequalities', *Critical Public Health*, 19(3–4), pp. 287–92.
Standing, G. 2014, 'The precariat', *Contexts*, 13(4), pp. 10–2.Statistics Canada. 2018, 'Deaths and causes of deaths, 2015', *The Daily*, 23 February, accessed 10 October 2021, <https://www150.statcan.gc.ca/n1/en/daily quotidien/180223/dq180223c-eng.pdf?st=W7d6RKxu>.
Steinmetz, K. 2020, 'She coined the term "intersectionality" over 30 years ago. Here's what it means to her today', *Time Magazine*, 20 February, accessed 5 March 2020, <https://time.com/5786710/kimberle-crenshaw-intersectionality/>.
Syed, I.U. 2016, 'Labor exploitation and health inequities among market migrants: Political economy perspective', *Journal of International Migration and Integration*, 17(2), pp. 449–65.
Syed, I.U. 2020, 'Racism, racialization, and health equity in Canadian residential long-term care a case study in Toronto', *Social Science and Medicine*, 265, p. 113524.
Tarasuk, V. and Mitchell, A. 2020, *Household Food Insecurity in Canada, 2017–18*, research to identify policy options to reduce food insecurity (PROOF), Toronto.
Whitehead, M. 1991, 'The concepts and principles of equity and health', *Health Promotion International*, 6(3), pp. 217–28.
Wilkinson, R.G. 1989, 'Class mortality differentials, income distribution and trends in poverty 1921–1981', *Journal of Social Policy*, 18(3), pp. 307–35.
Wilkinson, R.G. 1992, 'Income distribution and life expectancy', *British Medical Journal*, 304, pp. 165–8,
Wilkinson, R.G. 1997, 'Socioeconomic determinants of health: Health inequalities – Relative or absolute material standards?', *British Medical Journal*, 314, p. 591.
World Economic Forum. 2018, *The Global Gender Gap Report 2018*, WEF, Geneva.
World Health Organization. 2019, *World Health Statistics Overview 2019: Monitoring Health for the SDGs, Sustainable Development Goals*, No. WHO/DAD/2019.1, WHO, Geneva.
World Health Organization. 2020, *COVID-19 and Violence Against Women: What the Health Sector/System Can Do*, No. WHO/SRH/20.04, WHO, Geneva.
Wright, E.O. 2019, *How to be an Anti-Capitalist in the 21st Century*, Verso, Brooklyn.

10

ISSUES OF SOCIAL REPRODUCTION AND THE POLITICAL ECONOMY OF HEALTH

Sarah Redikopp

Under the prevailing neoliberal paradigm of 'responsibilization' (Brown 2016), 'health' is predominantly rendered a matter of individual choice, where the impetus to achieve 'good health' is removed from the social, political, and historical contexts, which foster or foreclose health (Polzer and Power 2016). Conversely, this chapter aims to problematize the individualization of 'good health' and instead locate health outcomes, illness, disability, and death within historically specific and shifting material, political, and cultural frameworks. In this respect, 'health' is understood not simply as the absence of illness, but as 'the extent to which a person possesses the physical, social, and personal resources to identify and achieve personal aspirations, satisfy needs, and cope with the environment' (Raphael 2009: 2).

Specifically, I explore how *social reproduction*, as the quotidian renewal of life itself, is central to achieving and maintaining 'good health' on daily and generational scales. By engaging with feminist political economy (FPE) scholarship, I situate 'social reproduction' as the relational and caregiving labor that ensures the maintenance and re/production of healthy, viable laboring populations (Bezanson and Luxton 2006). In contexts of health and healthcare, the work of social reproduction figures in the social determinants of health (Armstrong 2009), as well as sites of formal and informal care provision: preparing food, cleaning homes and care facilities, changing bedding and bandages. It also underpins the comfort and affective support of those receiving care. Yet, despite its necessary function in these care milieus and the ongoing propagation of capitalism more broadly, social reproduction remains systemically devalued within extant economic discourse and institutions. Dismissed as 'women's work' – that is, unskilled work that is 'natural' to women – 'much of the work and many of the skills remain invisible both in terms of the acquired nature of women's capacities and in terms of their contributions to health' (Armstrong and Armstrong 2005: 175). In turn, the chapter reveals the ideological and material devaluation of care central to neoliberal projects of healthcare privatization, and demonstrates its profoundly gendered and racialized effects. Most pertinently, neoliberal cost-cutting measures have increasingly undermined crucial aspects of care: increasing labor demands on feminized and marginalized healthcare workers, while decreasing the time and resources available for safe and effective care provision (Bannerjee 2012; Spitzer 2004).

In seeking to render visible these contradictory configurations of social reproductive labor and care work, I locate my analysis within the specific parameters of the healthcare system of Ontario,

 DOI: 10.4324/9781003017110-12

Canada, as well as FPE traditions particular to Canada. Although Canada's publicly funded healthcare system is widely regarded as 'universal', in Ontario – Canada's most populous province – healthcare has been increasingly susceptible to neoliberal forms of restructuring and privatization, funding cuts, and the adoption of corporatized 'business management' strategies, which negatively impact those providing and receiving care. Locating my analysis in the Canadian context – where supposedly 'universal' healthcare is internationally renowned and ideologically cherished within the country itself – makes visible the often-insidious character of healthcare privatization in public services, and centralizes the devaluation of racialized and gendered social reproductive labor endemic to these privatization projects.

Social reproduction and feminist political economy in Canada

FPE in Canada has produced a range of scholarship attentive to the gendered dimensions of neoliberal capitalist systems of production. Emerging in the 1970s out of socialist feminist engagements with the economic value of women's domestic labor, Canadian FPE scholars highlighted the exclusion of women's work from 'malestream' political economy analyses (Smith 1989). Throughout the 1980s, Black, Indigenous, and women of color feminists systematically criticized FPE's failure to centralize processes of racialization and settler colonialism in critical engagements with women's work under capitalism (Brand 1999). Integrating these critical insights and attending to the gendered and racialized particularities of the reproduction of life under capitalism, feminist political economists have since produced scholarship that engages with myriad previously under-explored themes. This includes conceptualizing households and communities as economic units and sites of social provisioning (Bezanson and Luxton 2006; Braedley and Luxton 2010; Vosko 2006); situating gendered labor and care provision within transnational and racialized care contexts (Arat-Koc 2006; Bakan 1987; Lawson 2013); and particularizing the racialized and settler colonial foundations of neoliberal capitalism (Bakan and Dua 2014; Hall 2016). This literature has also explored the implications of neoliberal social policies for disabled Canadians (LeBlanc-Haley 2017) and analyzed how the systemic devaluation of social reproductive labor – disproportionately performed by working-class, racialized, and immigrant women in Canada – has 'enabled the specific forms that neoliberal capital accumulation has taken, and has mediated the social contradictions generated by neoliberal restructuring' (LeBaron 2010: 902).

Despite the scope of Canada's FPE scholarship, issues of social reproduction have been largely under-theorized in 'mainstream' political economy of health frameworks, which seek to situate dialectically health outcomes, health determinants, and healthcare systems within the prevailing capitalist mode of production (Coburn 2000; Panitch and Leys 2009). Despite this marginality, however, FPE analyses have formulated a range of influential contributions. These have highlighted the gendered nature of paid and unpaid healthcare work under capitalism (Anderson 2000; Razavi and Staab 2011); the gendered and racialized nature of social determinants of health (Armstrong 2009; de Leeuw and Greenwood 2011; Galabuzi 2009; Smylie 2009); and the impact of neoliberal restructuring on the provision of healthcare at various sites and levels of abstraction (Daly *et al.* 2015; Spitzer 2004; Syed 2020). This body of research has demonstrated how social reproduction occurs in the 'formal' provision of clinical healthcare services, including work performed by nurses, personal support workers, therapists, and home care workers. Yet, it also establishes the contribution of other necessary, albeit often ignored, forms of labor to social reproduction, such as that undertaken by ancillary workers and the menial, or 'dirty' work of care (Duffy 2005) (including cleaners, food service workers, laundry staff, and clerical workers), along with unpaid care performed disproportionately by women at home.[1] From here, we move to a more focused exploration of the conceptual parameters of social reproduction and its relevance for health and healthcare.

Conceptualizing social reproduction

In FPE traditions, social reproduction refers to the socially necessary paid and unpaid labor involved in reproducing and maintaining the laboring population on daily and generational scales (Bezanson and Luxton 2006). Rai *et al.* (2014: 87) offer a helpful conceptualization of social reproduction as including the following:

- Biological reproduction (including reproducing labor) and, concomitantly, the provision of sexual, emotional, and affective services required to maintain family and intimate relationships;
- Unpaid production in the home of both goods and services, incorporating different forms of care, as well as social provisioning and voluntary work directed at meeting needs within the community;
- Reproduction of culture and ideology, which stabilizes (and sometimes challenges) dominant social relations.

The work of social reproduction is therefore affective, material, and ideological, encapsulating 'the political imaginaries, public policies, and material practices necessary to sustain and reproduce individuals, families, and communities on a daily and generational basis' (Brodie 2010: 1561). At the level of the everyday, social reproduction appears as what could normatively be conceived of as 'women's work': preparing food, cleaning house, doing laundry, raising, socializing, and educating children, and supporting and caring for people who are disabled, sick, injured, and dying. While predominantly theorized as occurring in the private sphere, social reproduction goes beyond narrow conceptualizations of domestic labor undertaken in individual households to implicate various institutions in this socially necessary work, including the state, the market, and volunteer sectors.

Although social reproduction is carried out at various sites and levels of abstraction, Meg Luxton (2006: 38) suggests that in capitalist societies such as Canada, domestic work in the home tends to 'act as a residual subsistence labor, expanding or contracting as much as possible to offset the impact of market forces, state practices, or changing family circumstances'. While the household serves as a key site in necessary social provisioning, 'women's labor in their homes is not endlessly elastic. Without sufficient support, standards of living drop, the most vulnerable households typically collapse, and a crisis in social reproduction is produced' (Luxton 2006: 38, citing Elson 1998). As care work under capitalism, social reproduction is inherently in crisis insofar as the capitalist drive for profit conflicts with the reproduction of the working-class (Luxton 2006). That is, while capitalism relies on the reproduction of the worker, the conditions of reproduction (including temporal, affective, and material resources needed for care work) are simultaneously undermined by the perpetual imperative to augment profit. Largely, these contemporary crises in social reproduction have been mitigated by invoking racialized transnational workers to meet provisioning needs, as social reproduction is increasingly commodified (Arat-Koc 2006; Bakan 1987). This has been evidenced, for example, in the increased practice of families employing (racialized) private companions to provide additional, one-on-one support for long-term care residents (Daly 2015).

Importantly, the work of social reproduction is socially, historically, and geographically specific, shifting over time 'so as to be reconstituted in ways that are more compatible with the priority of capital's accumulation' (LeBaron 2010: 898). Thus, it is important to examine how social reproduction has been reconfigured through the contemporary entrenchment and deepening of neoliberal ideology. The latter promulgates the penetration of market rule into myriad socio-economic spheres through 'political-economic strategies such as the retrenchment and redesign of state supports, the privatization of state assets, and the mobilization of an ideal, self-interested, self-reliant individual citizen through public and social policy' (Leblanc-Haley 2017: 3).[2] Accordingly, while the state is traditionally understood as responsible for mitigating the contradictions that arise between production and reproduction (Vosko 2006), the state's role in direct social provisioning has atrophied, thereby intensifying reliance on both the private market and individual households for social provisioning (Brodie 2010). Specifically, the work of social reproduction has been redefined as a privatized responsibility, commodified through the market for those who can afford it, and done 'at home' in unpaid capacities for those who cannot (Fraser 2017). Simultaneously, the state has broadened its policy-making activities to support business interests and private profit making (Luxton 2010). This widespread erosion of the welfare state has been theorized by FPE scholars as a form of 'new enclosures' (Federici 2004) which, rather than signaling a *withering-away* of the state, reflects a reorganization and proliferation of state surveillance as available state-provided social supports are hollowed out and their eligibility criteria intensified (Brodie 2010).

As discussed in the next section, as institutions and practices of social reproduction, Canadian healthcare follows these trends: increased reliance on unpaid, informal caregivers and/or privatized reproductive work to meet provisioning needs as the state withdraws from its role in direct social provisioning, and business management strategies infiltrate practices of care (Armstrong and Armstrong 1996; Whiteside 2018).

Social reproduction and healthcare in Canada

Analytic specificity necessitates a brief outline of the evolution of social reproduction and healthcare in Canada.[3] Forged through several decades of activism and collectivized demands at the height of Canada's postwar Keynesian welfare state, in 1968 the *Medical Care Insurance Program* (more popularly known as Medicare) combined coverage for all 'medically necessary' hospital and allopathic doctors' services under a decentralized federal-provincial cost-sharing formula and fee-for-service model, providing public funds for private provision (Armstrong and Armstrong 1999).[4] Technological advancements made prior to World War II demanded larger hospitals with greater numbers of skilled workers, including nurses, and the implementation of Medicare programs expanded investment in hospital infrastructure and doctors' services (Armstrong and Armstrong 2005). Simultaneously, biomedical and allopathic illness models were entrenched in healthcare provision and funding models (Armstrong and Armstrong 1996).

These postwar shifts and funding developments affected social reproduction in several ways (Armstrong and Armstrong 2005). First, healthcare became more accessible through the expansion of healthcare services and lack of user fees (though Indigenous, racialized, and immigrant Canadians, and particularly women, did not benefit from these shifts to the same extent as their white counterparts and continue to experience systemic inequity and racialized violence in Canada's healthcare system).[5] Second, the increased provisioning of care work in the public sector reallocated the burden of social reproduction more equitably between the state, individual households, and the private sector, thus decreasing demands on women to provide unpaid care at home. Third, the expansion of women's employment as nurses in the public sector allowed these workers to leverage their organizing power for unionization, better wages, and improved working conditions (Armstrong and Armstrong 2005).

The professionalization of registered nursing in Canada recognized it as skilled labor, while informing the fracturing of care work into 'skilled' and 'unskilled' factions (Armstrong and Armstrong 2005). The 1970s saw a proliferation of nursing categories, including nursing aides, orderlies, therapists, and nursing assistants, along with established divisions between Registered Nurses and Registered Practical Nurses – no longer simply 'nurses', but specialized workers performing discrete tasks (Armstrong and Armstrong 1996: 111). As registered nursing was increasingly defined in clinical/professionalized terms, more of the 'dirty work' of care, such as cleaning, feeding, and comforting patients, was devolved to nursing assistants, personal support workers, general aides, clerks, cleaners, and laundry and dietary workers. These quickly trained, low-paid workers functioned as a cost-saving measure, who were – and remain – largely immigrant and racialized women. Although these 'unskilled' (non-clinical) care workers fared better in the public sector than in the private sector – with relatively better pay and working conditions (Armstrong and Armstrong 2005) – the ideological and material devaluation of this 'unskilled' and racialized caregiving labor has been central to contemporary neoliberal privatization projects in Ontario healthcare.

In 1977, the Canadian Federal Government implemented the *Federal-Provincial Fiscal Arrangements and Established Programs Act* (EPF), which instituted a block-funding policy devolving power of funding allocation to the provinces. This shift negated the capacity of the Federal Government to ensure national standards for healthcare delivery and raised concerns about inconsistent healthcare implementation among the provinces. The subsequent *MacDonald Report* (1985) – which Whiteside (2009: 90) identifies as symbolizing 'the onset of a shift towards neoliberalism in Canada' – initiated the onslaught of federal funding cuts to the provinces throughout the 1990s, culminating in the eventual consolidation of the Canada Assistance Plan (CAP), the social assistance and welfare fund, and the EPF into a new block fund called the *Canada Health and Social Transfer* (CHST) in 1995. The CHST dramatically reduced transfer payments to the provinces, while healthcare costs continued to rise (Whiteside 2009). While federal transfers initially covered 50 percent of healthcare expenses, federal funds today cover only 22 percent of provincial health services, with the remainder of funding responsibility left to individual provinces, leaving provincial healthcare systems vulnerable to privatization (Ontario Health Coalition 2020).

In keeping with neoliberalism's commitment to market principles and the unfettered liberation of capital and marketplace competition as fostering efficiency, rising healthcare costs in Canada have increasingly engendered funding cuts and the adoption of for-profit managerial strategies. This has manifested in establishment of public-private partnerships in healthcare infrastructure (Whiteside 2018); privatization or contracting out of ancillary services (Armstrong *et al.* 2008; Mehra 2018); staff reductions and increased reliance on part-time, temporary laborers (Armstrong *et al.* 2009; Spitzer 2004); and increased emphasis on outpatient surgeries, ambulatory and community-based treatments, and decentralization of care from hospitals to individual homes (Armstrong and Armstrong 1996). Simultaneously, with hospitals' and doctors' services increasingly defined in terms of acute care and facing reduced staffing levels, patients are sent home earlier and sicker, the quantity of hospital beds has decreased, eligibility criteria for state-provided home care services have tightened, and healthcare workers are expected to do more in less time (referred to as the '90-second minute') (Armstrong and Armstrong 1996: 129; Armstrong and Armstrong 2005).

As workers engaged in paid social reproduction, Canada's healthcare workforce is intensely gendered and particularly racialized. To illustrate, 90 percent of nurses, 90 percent of personal support workers (PSWs), and two thirds of hospital cleaners and ancillary staff are women, while immigrant women, making up 15 percent of the total workforce, constitute 23 percent of Canada's nurses and 29 percent of long-term care workers (Salami 2020). Moreover, healthcare labor in Canada is hierarchicalized in ways that reflect dominant racial and gendered configurations. Teaching, research, supervisory, administrative, and professionalized positions are largely occupied by white women, while licensed practitioners, aides, and PSWs – those responsible for the time-intensive, menial, and devalued emotional and physical care of patients – are disproportionately women of color (Duffy 2007; Glenn 1992; Lorber and Moore 2000: 41). These forms of occupational segregation reflect the valuation of care work more broadly, where 'menial' or 'unskilled' care tasks are increasingly positioned as 'outside' of healthcare, susceptible to privatization and contracting out, and increasingly undertaken by precarious racialized and immigrant women (Daly 2015).

Neoliberal measures operationalized in the name of 'cost-saving' and 'efficiency' rely on the widespread devaluation of social reproductive work, which has embodied effects for formal and informal care providers (Anderson 2000). In Canada, women are largely viewed as responsible for raising children and caring for families, including aging parents, and are more likely to parent alone than men. Simultaneously, women earn less, are more likely to work part-time or precariously, receive less workplace benefits, and are disproportionately employed in low-status and low-paying jobs – all of which contribute extensively to gendered health outcomes (Armstrong 2009). These burdens of social reproductive work are compounded by processes of racialization, informed by ongoing structures of settler colonialism and white supremacy. Most conspicuously, the systemic marginalization of Indigenous, racialized, and immigrant women in Canada informs their ghettoization in low-paying jobs with limited time to seek medical care – which, in turn, is seldom culturally appropriate and often discriminatory – thereby resulting in poorer health outcomes than middle-class white women (Anderson and Reimer-Kirkham 1998; Egan and Gardner 1999; Oxman-Martinez and Hanley 2011). In what follows, I undertake a brief consideration of how reconfigurations of social reproduction under neoliberal capitalism influence the day-to-day work of social provisioning in Canadian healthcare contexts.

Locating social reproduction: clinical healthcare workers

Neoliberal cost-saving measures shape social reproductive work in the formal healthcare system in numerous ways, impacting hospitals, long-term residential care facilities, and home care workers. Some impacts include the fragmentation of care work through the implementation of managerial strategies in care provision; increased healthcare worker precarity and reliance on part-time and temporary labor; high rates of workplace violence and decreased worker satisfaction; and decreased quality of care for patients and care recipients. For example, Armstrong and Armstrong (1996: 121–33) have explored the impact of Total Quality Management techniques, including time-budget measurements, on nursing labor as a new means of monitoring and controlling nurse activities, standardizing care, and cutting labor costs. Fragmented care work is increasingly transferred to the 'Lowest Paid Care Provider' (LCCP), understood as 'a person who has been given the minimum amount of training to acquire a particular technical skill' (Armstrong and Armstrong 1996: 129). The result of this fragmentation and devolution is a lack of continuity of care – nurses, like patients, are not seen as complex care providers, but as workers who must maintain regimes of efficiency embedded within a 'business paradigm' of healthcare services (Armstrong 2001).

In addition to the fragmentation of caregiving labor into discrete tasks monitored for time and efficiency, funding cuts result in reduced staff and labor costs, increased reliance on part-time and temporary workers, rushed patient care, and a lack of worker satisfaction (Armstrong *et al.*

2009). Denise Spitzer (2004: 496), in her analysis of the effects of healthcare reform measures on Canadian nursing staff, argues that

> [r]apid turnover [of staff] and increased patient load have reshaped nurses' duties within the institution, contracting the amount of time available for intimate patient interaction. Although caring work has often been cited as the source of the nursing profession's denigrated status vis-`a-vis other health professions, nurses unanimously reported this to be the most rewarding aspect of their work and the major attraction of the profession.

Spitzer also found that time-stressed nursing staff practiced 'avoidance patterns' with high-maintenance and/or time-intensive patients, especially those marked 'problematic' as racialized subjects, underscoring the racist effects of time-management strategies in nursing and healthcare work (Spitzer 2004: 491). In long-term care, which is largely privatized in Canada (Liu *et al.* 2020), residents receive insufficient social engagement, as well as physical neglect, largely due to chronic understaffing and budget cuts, while violence levels against staff have increased (Bannerjee *et al.* 2012). Families of these residents are increasingly hiring privatized companion workers to meet the needs of residents in long-term care, providing 'different combinations of social and emotional care as well as body work for residents, which involves toileting, washing the body and assisting with eating' (Daly 2015: 247). These workers, hired through agencies or independently, are under-protected by labor laws and regulations, rendering them particularly vulnerable as workers.

Decreased funding, chronic understaffing, and increased demands for complex care expose nurses, personal support workers, occupational therapists, nursing aides, and other 'formal' care providers to hazardous, unsafe, and unsatisfactory working conditions (Banerjee *et al.* 2012; Syed 2020). A 2009 comparative study of Canadian long-term care workers, including nurses and personal support workers, found alarming rates of missed breaks, starting shifts early and leaving late, while 40 percent of Canadian long-term care workers reported feeling inadequate in terms of the care they provided (Armstrong *et al.* 2009: 113). While it is beyond the scope of this chapter to locate the varying experiences of formal healthcare staff across Canada, it is notable that formalized work of social reproduction is increasingly devalued, hazardous, and poorly remunerated. Importantly, the effects of these healthcare transformations are not contained to the workplace, but have implications for the quality of provisioning work performed at home as well, affecting the overall health of individuals, families, and communities (Armstrong *et al.* 2009).

Ancillary workers and social reproduction: 'outside' healthcare?

Issues of social reproduction in the political economy of health show up not only in the provision of clinical care but also in ancillary and hospital-support facilities such as cleaning, food services, laundry, and maintenance. In Canada, ancillary services were first distinguished from 'direct healthcare services' by the 2002 *Romanow Report*. Subsequently, they have been conceptualized as 'outside' of healthcare (or outside the bounds of allopathic medicine) and, therefore, rendered susceptible to private contracting (Griffin-Cohen and Cohen 2006). Yet, as Armstrong *et al.* (2008) powerfully argue, ancillary services such as hospital cleaning, laundry, and food services are not 'outside' of healthcare, but are integral to the conditions of good health. The re-definition of cooking, cleaning, and laundry in healthcare contexts as ancillary services has been mobilized to justify the contracting out of this 'unskilled' work to large for-profit firms. The latter deliver these services primarily through low-paid, precarious, racialized, and immigrant women whose labor is intensely devalued and who undertake this work for low pay and limited-to-no benefits (Griffin-Cohen and Cohen 2006). Such cost-cutting measures have been directly linked to illness and death, underscoring the centrality of this labor to health. For example, Whiteside (2018: 19) cites the development of an 'antibacterial-resistance superbug', *c. difficile,* in a BC hospital in 2009 as having arisen from understaffing and improper training by a private contractor, which led to crucial errors in sanitization protocol. Ancillary work is deeply gendered, predominantly performed by women – especially racialized and immigrant women – and this association with 'women's work' informs its devaluation and invisibilization as unskilled labor, as well as the heightened hazards to which female workers are subjected (Armstrong *et al.* 2008: 5, 10).

Filling care gaps: social reproduction and informal care providers

While discussions of paid work tend to dominate most discussions of healthcare labor, unpaid caregivers play an increasingly necessary role in the provision of care labor. As states increasingly pull back from the provision of caregiving for sick citizens and aging populations, the onus of care predictably falls to middle-aged and older women, many of whom also support children and face transitioning from full- to part-time employment or leaving the paid workforce (Funk and Kobayashi 2011). According to the Canadian Institute of Health Information (CIHI), family members, friends, and community volunteers comprise the largest group of informal and unregulated care providers in Canada. In Ontario, 97 percent of adults receiving publicly funded home care have at least one additional unpaid caregiver, usually a family member, friend, or neighbor (CIHI 2020).

These burdens of unpaid care have detrimental effects on the health of care providers. For instance, one third of these caregivers reported feeling distressed, that they were unable to keep up with care demands, and experienced deleterious health effects such as chronic stress, anxiety, back pain, and other forms of injury. Such shifts are occurring as services and funding for home care workers have withered, home care is increasingly privatized, and patients are living longer with more complex conditions requiring more complex care (CIHI 2020). This 'closer to home' model of care, increasingly adopted as a form of cost-saving, has implications for both the caregiver and the care receiver, as 'increasingly sophisticated care tasks are being sent home to be done by relatives or friends' with little-to-no training (Armstrong and Armstrong 1996). Informal care providers are gradually more essential, both at home and in care facilities, as (female) family members are expected to provide emotional care within hospitals, as well as bathing, feeding, even monitoring IVs of sick children (Armstrong and Armstrong 1996: 138). These family members plug care gaps left by understaffed and overburdened workers, therefore complicating the boundaries between home and hospital, and paid and unpaid care. As Armstrong and Armstrong (1996) argue, at the root of neoliberal deinstitutionalization and 'home care' policies is the assumption that there will be a woman at home who is willing and able to provide care for sick or disabled family members, undergirding the reliance of neoliberal cost-saving measures on unpaid and undervalued social reproductive labor.

Conclusion

Attention to social reproduction in contexts of health and healthcare highlights the material, affective, and ideological aspects of care work under capitalism, the racialized and gendered dimensions of care work, and the ways in which social reproduction is reconfigured in accordance with the demands of capital. In Canada, the widespread erosion of state provisioning and increased privatization of social reproduction impact the working conditions, remuneration, and valuation of these necessary workers (Armstrong *et al.* 2008; Armstrong *et al.* 2019), while increasing reliance on the unpaid work of family members and loved ones in healthcare provision. These shifts disproportionately impact women, particularly racialized women, who are both disproportionately employed as healthcare workers and bear the burden of social reproduction and unpaid labor to 'pick up the slack' of the state (Anderson 2000).

As a site of feminist analysis, attention to social reproduction provides not only sites of critique but also pathways for enabling the re-imagining of the organization of care and care work under capitalism. Rebecca Hall (2016: 88) suggests that 'One of the great strengths of social-reproduction feminism is that it makes visible, denaturalizes and politicizes processes of care and unpaid labor'. Critical and feminist scholars within Canada and beyond are increasing calls for the fair valuation of social reproduction as necessary work central to health and healthcare under capitalism. Centering social reproduction in political economy of health analyses undergirds the necessity of devalued care labor to projects of healthcare profitization in Canada and beyond, as well as the intimate and embodied confluences of state, market, and capital in caregiving work.

Notes

1 Though these sites of social reproduction are not easily parsed into discrete categories, my identification of these three 'streams' of care is primarily heuristic and reflective of debates and sites of analysis in the field.
2 See also: Braedley and Luxton (2010); and Connell (2010).
3 For extended surveys of healthcare in Canada, see: Armstrong and Armstrong (1996, 1999); and Whiteside (2009).
4 Notably, 'medically necessary' excludes prescription drug services, optometry, prosthetic services, home care, residential care, chiropractors, naturopathic care, doula services, and dentistry not performed in-hospital. Instead, these services must be covered by individual insurance plans or paid for out-of-pocket.
5 See: Anderson and Reimer-Kirkham (1998); Kelm (1998); Egan and Gardner (1999); Tang and Browne (2008); and Boyer (2017).

References

Anderson, J.M. 2000, 'Gender, "race", poverty, health and discourses of health reform in the context of globalization: A postcolonial feminist perspective in policy research', *Nursing Inquiry*, 7(4), pp. 220–9.

Anderson, J. and Reimer-Kirkham, S. 1998, 'Constructing nation: The gendering and racializing of the Canadian healthcare system', in Strong-Boag, V. (ed), *Painting the Maple: Essays on Race, Gender, and the Construction of Canada*, University of British Columbia Press, Vancouver, pp. 249–68.

Arat-Koc, S. 2006, 'Whose social reproduction? Transnational motherhood and challenges to feminist political economy', in Bezanson, K. and Luxton, M. (eds), *Social Reproduction: Feminist Political Economy Challenges Neoliberalism*, McGill-Queens University Press, Montreal and Kingston, pp. 75–92.

Armstrong, P. 2000, 'Gender, health, and care', in Raphael, D., Bryant, T., Rioux, M. and Teeple, G. (eds), *Staying Alive: Critical Perspectives on Health, Illness, and Healthcare,* Canadian Scholars' Press and Women's Press, Toronto, pp. 287–305.

Armstrong, P. 2001, 'Evidence-based healthcare reform: Women's issues', in Armstrong, P., Armstrong, H. and Coburn, D. (eds), *Unhealthy Times: Political Economy Perspectives on Health and Care in Canada*, Oxford University Press, Toronto, pp. 121–45.

Armstrong, P. 2009, 'Public policy, gender, and health', in D. Raphael (ed), *Social Determinants of Health: Canadian Perspectives*, Canadian Scholar's Press, Toronto, pp. 350–62.

Armstrong, P. and Armstrong, H. 1996, *Wasting Away: The Undermining of Canadian Healthcare*, Oxford University Press, Toronto.

Armstrong, P. and Armstrong, H. 1999, 'Decentralised healthcare in Canada', *British Medical Journal*, 318(7192), pp. 1201–4.

Armstrong, P. and Armstrong, H. 2005, 'Public and private: Implications for care work', *The Sociological Review*, 53(2), pp. 167–87.

Armstrong, P., Armstrong, H. and Scott-Dixon, K. 2008, *Critical to Care: The Invisible Women in Health Services*, University of Toronto Press, Toronto.Armstrong, P., Banerjee, A., Szebehely, M., Armstrong, H., Daly, T. and Lafrance, S. 2009, *They Deserve Better: The Long-Term Care Experience in Canada and Scandinavia,* Canadian Centre for Policy Alternatives, Ottawa.

Bakan, A. 1987, 'The international market for female labour and individual deskilling: West Indian women workers in Toronto', *Canadian Journal of Latin American and Caribbean Studies*, 12(24), pp. 69–85.
Bakan, A.B. and Dua, E. (Eds.) 2014, *Theorizing Anti-Racism: Linkages in Marxism and Critical Race Theories*. University of Toronto Press, Toronto.
Banerjee, A., Daly, T., Armstrong, P., Szebehely, M., Armstrong, H. and Lafrance, S. 2012. 'Structural violence in long-term, residential care for older people: Comparing Canada and Scandinavia', *Social Science and Medicine*, 74(3), pp. 390–8.
Bezanson, K. 2006, 'The neo-liberal state and social reproduction: Gender and household insecurity in the late 1990s', in Bezanson, K. and Luxton. M. (eds), *Social Reproduction: Feminist Political Economy Challenges Neoliberalism*, McGill-Queen's University Press, Montreal and Kingston, pp. 173–214.
Boyer, Y. 2017, 'Healing racism in Canadian healthcare', *Canadian Medical Association Journal* 189(46), pp. E1408–9.
Braedley, S. and Luxton, M. 2010, 'Competing philosophies: Neoliberalism and challenges of everyday life', in Braedley, S. and Luxton, M. (eds), *Neoliberalism and Everyday Life*, McGill-Queen's University Press, Montreal and Kingston, pp. 3–21.
Brand, D. 1999, 'Black women and work: The impact of racially constructed gender roles on the sexual division of labour', in Dua, E. and Robertson, A. (eds), *Scratching the Surface: Canadian Anti-Racist Feminist Thought*, Women's Press, Toronto, pp. 83–96.
Brodie, J. 2010, 'Globalization, Canadian family policy, and the omissions of neoliberalism', *North Carolina Law Review*, 88(5), pp. 1559–91.
Brown, W. 2016, 'Sacrificial citizenship: Neoliberalism, human capital, and austerity politics', *Constellations,* 23(1), pp. 3–14.
Canadian Institute for Health Information. 2020, '1 in 3 unpaid caregivers in Canada are distressed', 6 August, accessed 14 July 2021, <https://www.cihi.ca/en/1-in-3-unpaid-caregivers-in-canada-are-distressed>.
Coburn, D. 2000, 'Health and healthcare: A political economy perspective', in Raphael, D., Bryant, T., Rioux, M. and Teeple. G. (eds), *Staying Alive: Critical Perspectives on Health, Illness, and Healthcare*, Canadian Scholars' Press and Women's Press, Toronto, pp. 59–85.
Connell, R. 2010, 'Understanding neoliberalism', in Braedley, S. and Luxton, M. (eds), *Neoliberalism and Everyday Life*, McGill-Queen's University Press, Montreal and Kingston, pp. 22–36.
Daly, T. 2015, 'Dancing the two-step in Ontario's long-term care sector: deterrence regulation = consolidation', *Studies in Political Economy*, 95(1), pp. 29–58.
Daly, T., Armstrong, P. and Lowndes, R. 2015, 'Liminality in Ontario's long-term care facilities: Private companions' care work in the space 'betwixt and between', *Competition and Change*, 19(3), pp. 246–63.
De Leeuw, S. and Greenwood, M. 2011, 'Beyond borders and boundaries: Addressing indigenous health inequities in Canada through theories of social determinants of health and intersectionality', in Hankivsky, O. (ed), *Health Inequities in Canada: Intersectional Frameworks and Practices*, University of British Columbia Press, Vancouver, pp. 53–71.
Duffy, M. 2005, 'Reproducing labour inequalities: Challenges for feminists conceptualizing care at the intersections of gender, race, and class', *Gender and Society*, 19(1), pp. 66–82.
Duffy, M. 2007, Doing the dirty work: Gender, race, and reproductive labor in historical perspective', *Gender and Society*, 21(3), pp. 313–36.
Egan, C. and Gardner, L. 1999, 'Racism, women's health, and reproductive freedom', in Dua, E. and Robertson, A. (eds), *Scratching the Surface: Canadian Antiracist Feminist Thought*, Women's Press, Toronto, pp. 295–308.
Elson, D. 1998, 'The economic, the political and the domestic: Businesses, states and households in the organization of production', *New Political Economy,* 3(2), pp. 189–208.
Federici, S. 2004, *Caliban and the Witch: Women, the Body, and Accumulation*, Autonomedia, Brooklyn.
Fraser, N. 2017, 'Crisis of care? On the social-reproductive contradictions of contemporary capitalism', in Bhattacharya, T. (eds), *Social Reproduction Theory: Remapping Class, Recentering Oppression*, Pluto Press, London, pp. 22–36.
Funk, L. and Kobayashi, K. 2011, '"Choice" in unpaid intimate labour: Adult children with aging parents', in Benoit, C. and Hallgrimsdóttir, H. (eds), *Valuing Care Work: Comparative Perspectives*, University of Toronto Press, Toronto, pp. 171–92.
Galabuzi, G.E. 2009, 'Social exclusion', in Raphael, D. (ed), *Social Determinants of Health: Canadian Perspectives*, Canadian Scholar's Press, Toronto, pp. 252–69.

Glenn, E.N. 1992, 'From servitude to service work: Historical continuities in the racial division of paid reproductive labor', *Signs: Journal of Women in Culture and Society*, 18(1), pp. 1–43.

Griffin-Cohen, M. and Cohen, M. 2006, 'Privatization: A strategy for eliminating pay equity in healthcare', in Bezanson, K. and Luxton, M. (eds), *Social Reproduction: Feminist Political Economy Challenges Neoliberalism*, McGill-Queens University Press, Montreal and Kingston, pp. 117–45.

Hall, R. 2016, 'Reproduction and resistance', *Historical Materialism*, 24(2), pp. 87–110.

Kelm, M. 1998, *Colonizing Bodies: Aboriginal Health and Healing in British Columbia, 1900-50*, University of British Columbia Press, Vancouver.

Lawson, E. 2013, 'The gendered working lives of seven Jamaican women in Canada: A story about "here" and "there" in a transnational economy', *Feminist Formations*, 25(1), pp. 138–56.

LeBaron, G. 2010, 'The political economy of the household: Neoliberal restructuring, enclosures, and daily life', *Review of International Political Economy*, 17(5), pp. 889–912.

LeBlanc-Haley, T. 2017, *Transinstitutionalization: A Feminist Political Economy Analysis of Ontario's Public Mental Healthcare System*, unpublished doctoral dissertation, York University, Toronto.

Liu, M., Maxwell, C.J., Armstrong, P., Schwandt, M., Moser, A., McGregor, M.J., Bronskill, S.E. and Dhalla, I.A. 2020, 'COVID-19 in long-term care homes in Ontario and British Columbia', *Canadian Medical Association Journal* 192(47), pp. E1540–E1546.

Lorber, J. and Moore, L.J. 2000, *Gender and the Social Construction of Illness*, Altamira Press, New York.

Luxton, M. 2006, 'Feminist political economy in Canada and the politics of social reproduction', in Bezanson, K. and Luxton, M. (eds), *Social Reproduction: Feminist Political Economy Challenges Neoliberalism*, McGill-Queens University Press, Montreal and Kingston, pp. 11–45.

Luxton, M. 2010, 'Doing neoliberalism: Perverse individualism in personal life', in Braedley, S. and Luxton, M. (eds), *Neoliberalism and Everyday Life*. McGill-Queen's University Press, Montreal, pp. 163–183.

Mehra, N. 2018, 'Three waves of healthcare corporatization in Ontario hospitals', in Brownlee, J. Hurl, C. and Walby, K. (eds), *Corporatizing Canada: Making Business Out of Public Service*, Between the Lines, Toronto, pp. 27–40.

Ontario Health Coalition. 2020, 'Health coalitions call for increased federal healthcare funding and accountability', 10 December, accessed 14 July 2021, <https://www.ontariohealthcoalition.ca/index.php/release-health-coalitions-call-for-increased-federal-health-care-funding-and-accountability/>.

Oxman-Martinez, J. and Hanley, J. 2011, 'An intersectional lens on various facets of violence: Access to health and social services for women with precarious immigration status', in Hankivsky, O. (ed), *Health Inequities in Canada: Intersectional Frameworks and Practices*, University of British Columbia, Vancouver, pp. 221–39.

Panitch, L. and Leys, C. 2009, 'Preface', in Panitch, L. and Leys, C. (eds), *Socialist Register: Morbid Symptoms – Health Under Capitalism*, Merlin Press, Pontypool, pp. 1–6.

Polzer, J. and Power, E. 2016, 'Introduction: The governance of health in neoliberal societies', in Power, E., Polzer, J., Cayen, L., Katzman, E., Laliberte-Rudman, D., Knabe, S. and Orchard, T. (eds), *Neoliberal Governance and Health: Duties, Risks, and Vulnerabilities*, McGill-Queens University Press, Montreal and Kingston, pp. 3–42

Rai, S., Hoskyns, C. and Thomas, D. 2014, 'Depletion: The cost of social reproduction', *International Feminist Journal of Politics*, 16(1), pp. 86–105.

Raphael, D. 2009, 'Social determinants of health: An overview of key issues and themes', in Raphael, D. (ed), *Social Determinants of Health: Canadian Perspectives*, Canadian Scholar's Press, Toronto, pp. 2–20.

Razavi, S. and Staab, S. 2011, 'Underpaid and overworked: A cross-national perspective on care workers', *International Labour Review*, 149(4), pp. 407–22.

Salami, B. 2020, 'Intersectionality, COVID-19, and healthcare workers', *IG in Conversation, University of Alberta*, accessed 14 July 2021, <https://www.ualberta.ca/intersections-gender/news-events/news2020/conversation-bukola-salami.html>.

Smith, D. 1989, 'Feminist reflections on political economy', *Studies in Political Economy*, 30, pp. 37–59.

Smylie, J. 2009, 'The health of aboriginal peoples', in Raphael, D. (ed), *Social Determinants of Health: Canadian Perspectives*, Canadian Scholar's Press, Toronto, pp. 280–305.

Spitzer, D. 2004, 'In visible bodies: Minority women, nurses, time, and the new economy of care', *Medical Anthropology Quarterly*, 18(4), pp. 490–508.

Syed, I. 2020, 'Racism, racialization, and health equity in Canadian residential long term care: A case study in Toronto', *Social Science and Medicine*, 265(3), p. 113524.

Tang, S. and Browne, A. 2008, '"Race" matters: racialization and egalitarian discourses involving Aboriginal people in the Canadian healthcare context', *Ethnicity and Health*, 13(2), pp. 109–27.

Vosko, L.F. 2006, 'Crisis tendencies in social reproduction: The case of Ontario's early years plan', in Bezanson, K. and Luxton, M. (eds), *Social Reproduction: Feminist Political Economy Challenges Neoliberalism*, McGill-Queens University Press, Montreal and Kingston, pp. 145–72.

Whiteside, H. 2009, 'Canada's healthcare "crisis": Accumulation by dispossession and the neoliberal fix', *Studies in Political Economy,* 84, pp. 79–100.

Whiteside, H. 2018, 'Health profit: Private finance and public hospitals', in Brownlee, J., Hurl, C. and Walby, K. (eds), *Corporatizing Canada: Making Business Out of Public Service*, Between the Lines, Toronto, pp. 15–26.

11
HEALTH AND THE CORPORATE AGRI-FOOD SYSTEM

Jennifer Lacy-Nichols and Gyorgy Scrinis

Transnational and national corporations now dominate virtually every sector of global and national food systems, including agricultural production, trade, food manufacturing, food retail and the fast-food sectors. The practices and products of these corporations have engendered substantial social, health, ecological and animal welfare impacts. The ultra-processed foods and beverages that they manufacture, distribute and heavily market are a substantial driver of poor-quality dietary patterns, and have been implicated in poor health outcomes. Over the past couple of decades, their products and practices have come under scrutiny by both governments and health-conscious consumers.

Yet, most corporations have been actively responding to these political and market challenges to their profits. This chapter identifies two forms of response instigated by Big Food corporations: the strategy of opposing public health policies, and the strategy of presenting themselves as 'part of the solution' to the health problems associated with poor diets. This two-pronged approach has served to protect Big Food's market and political influence, while undermining collaborative efforts to transform the industrial food system.

Corporate power in the food system

Within food systems scholarship, a key conceptual approach is the three-dimensional corporate power framework set out in Clapp and Fuchs' (2009) analysis of corporate power in the food system. This framework draws on Lukes' (1974) three faces of power. Each form of power exerts a different form of political influence. *Instrumental power*, the 'first face of power', exerts a direct influence on decision-making by means of lobbying and campaign contributions from interest groups, as well as efforts to increase access to decision-makers via the 'revolving door' between industry and politicians or the development of public-private partnerships (Fuchs 2007; Clapp and Fuchs 2009; Clapp and Scrinis 2017). Instrumental power draws attention to the ways in which decision outcomes are changed due to the influence of one actor over another, and highlights the relationships corporations have with other stakeholders involved in policymaking.

Structural power, the 'second face of power', influences the agenda-setting process that precedes decision-making, and can limit the range of choices available to policymakers. It can also

 DOI: 10.4324/9781003017110-13

involve the acquisition of decision-making power by corporations themselves via self-regulation (Clapp and Fuchs 2009). The exercise of structural power attempts to shape the circumstances in which decisions are made, to make some options more appealing than others or to limit the scope of debate to issues that are innocuous to the industry. For this reason, structural power is also known as 'non–decision-making' power that keeps unwanted issues off the political agenda (Bachrach and Baratz 1962).

Lastly, *discursive power*, the 'third face of power', influences the norms and ideas that underpin and precede agenda-setting and political decision-making. Discursive power uses media and public relations to shape public understanding of issues (and non-issues), as well as what solutions are most appropriate (Haugaard 2002; Clapp and Fuchs 2009). The exercise of power can also be more or less coercive or persuasive – the latter of which can be understood as a more hegemonic approach to retain power in the face of countervailing threats through incremental concessions (Lacy-Nichols and Williams 2021).

A range of factors and circumstances enable or constrain corporate power in the food system. A key strength of corporations is their market resources, including their revenue, market concentration, global supply chains, intellectual property, access to commercially sensitive information, marketing expertise, and their research and development capabilities (Lang and Heasman 2004; Clapp and Fuchs 2009; Carolan 2011). In addition to (and often due to) financial resources, large food companies and their trade associations are often politically well-connected (Miller and Harkins 2010; Nestle 2013; Williams 2015; Gómez 2018). Food companies also exist in different political and market contexts, and face differing regulatory threats and market opportunities due to the different foods (and non-foods) in their portfolios (Lang *et al.* 2006; Hawkes and Harris 2011; Access to Nutrition Index 2018).

These differences point to the need to recognize that, alongside common business interests and agendas, there are significant divergences within the food industry (Falkner 2008; Clapp and Fuchs 2009). Food companies differ in size, geographic scale, revenue and industry concentration (Heffernan *et al.* 1999; Lang and Heasman 2004; Carolan 2011). Depending on their location in the food supply chain, food companies exercise varying degrees of influence over other food companies, producers or eaters (Winson 2004; Burch and Lawrence 2009). The global, national and local food industries are vast and heterogeneous, including smallholder subsistence farmers, artisanal bakeries and local farmers markets, through to transnational agrochemical companies, ultra-processed food manufacturers and hypermarkets (Monteiro *et al.* 2021). These latter entities are wealthy, horizontally and vertically concentrated, and wield market and political influence on par with nation-states (IPES-Food 2017). These powerful food industry actors – Big Food – constitute the focus of this chapter.

Big Food strategy one: opposing public health policies

Policies designed to reduce the production and consumption of ultra-processed foods present a threat to the business status quo of Big Food. In the early-2000s, leading global investment firms raised concerns about the exposure of the packaged and fast-food industry to obesity-related litigation and regulation (Lang *et al.* 2006). Over the next decade, it became clear that businesses invested in sugary drinks and other ultra-processed foods faced considerable financial and regulatory risks.

A growing number of governments are developing policies and regulations to reduce the consumption of ultra-processed foods (though these often focus on specific products, such as sugary

Table 11.1 Big Food's oppositional political strategies

Oppositional strategy	*Examples*
Influence and distort science	Coca-Cola funded the Global Energy Balance Network to conduct and publish research showing that exercise, not dietary change, is the best solution to obesity (Gertner and Rifkin 2017).
Lobbying	In 2013, the American soft drink industry (Coca-Cola, PepsiCo and the American Beverage Association) spent $10.9 million dollars lobbying the US government (Nestle 2015).
Campaign financing	In 2012, the American soft drink industry (Coca-Cola, PepsiCo and the American Beverage Association) gave US$5.5 million in US campaign contributions (Nestle 2015).
Revolving door	PepsiCo hired Derek Yach, former director of non-communicable diseases at the WHO, to be Senior Vice President of Global Health Policy (Nestle 2015).
Astroturf	The American soft drink industry funded the 'Community Coalition Against Beverage Taxes' to oppose a sugary drink tax in Richmond, California (Mejia *et al.* 2014).
Criticize public health policies	The EU lobby group FoodDrinkTax portrayed a sugar tax as a 'nanny state' intervention that limits 'personal freedom' (Tselengidis and Östergren 2019).
Litigation	The American soft drink industry filed a lawsuit opposing the Philadelphia sugary drink tax (Huehnergarth 2015).
Fragment and discredit public health professionals	The Center for Consumer Freedom attacked public health organizations and nutritionists, including Michael Jacobson (of the Center for Science in the Public Interest) and Marion Nestle (Simon 2006).
Threaten job or investment losses	The EU Soft Drinks Association (UNESDA) argued that the UK sugary drink tax would lead to job losses (Tselengidis and Östergren 2019).

drinks, or on the nutrient profile of foods). The NOURISHING Framework (developed by the World Cancer Research Fund) sets out a comprehensive set of policy actions across three domains – food environment, food system and behaviour change – that collectively promote healthier eating (Hawkes *et al.* 2013). On the one hand, the existence of these policies speaks to the successful advocacy from public health organizations and researchers in support of them. However, many of the implemented policies focus on downstream, behaviour change strategies that influence awareness and acceptability, but do little to alter the availability or affordability of sugary drinks (or other ultra-processed foods). Indeed, a 2020 analysis of nutrition policies in high-income countries found the majority focused on behaviour change, with few economic tools, such as taxation, used (Lee *et al.* 2020). Moreover, many policies were voluntary.

As regulatory threats loomed large, Big Food has not been passive, pursuing a range of strategies to deny, resist and undermine public health research and policies that it perceives as threatening to business interests. Research analysing Big Food's oppositional responses to obesity documents a vast range of political strategies used to protect the industry's interests. A growing body of international and interdisciplinary literature investigates not only the market strategies food corporations use to promote unhealthy commodities, but also the political strategies they use to protect their business interests (Wiist 2010; Stuckler *et al.* 2012; Moodie *et al.* 2013;

Freudenberg 2014; Mialon *et al.* 2015; Kickbusch *et al.* 2016; Moodie 2016; Buse *et al.* 2017). Collectively, this body of scholarship illuminates Big Food's more overt and confrontational efforts to shape the political environment in its favour. In Table 11.1, we summarize the oppositional political tactics identified in the literature, utilizing illustrative examples from the soft drink industry.

A significant body of research analyses the breadth of oppositional strategies used by the packaged food and beverage industry to protect its business interests. One strategy is to attack, confuse or undermine the body of scientific evidence linking consumption of ultra-processed foods (or other unhealthy products) to obesity and other non-communicable diseases (Legg *et al.* 2021). This includes funding research that does not show a relationship between sugary drinks and obesity, and disseminating information about the importance of energy balance and exercise in addressing obesity. A second dimension of the packaged food and beverage industry's oppositional strategies focuses on policymaking, and works to block or undermine public health policies that it perceives as threatening to its business interests. The latter includes lobbying policymakers to influence the development of nutrition policies, using campaign donations to influence voting, exercising influence through the 'revolving door' between political office and corporate positions (Williams 2015), funding 'astroturf' groups to oppose policies,[1] criticizing public health policies and using litigation to oppose unwanted policies (Ulucanlar *et al.* 2016; Mialon *et al.* 2020). Lastly, a third dimension of the packaged food and beverage industry's oppositional strategy

Table 11.2 Big Food's corporate health promotion activities

Health promotion activity	*Examples*
Product reformulation	PepsiCo pledged to reduce added sugar in beverages by 25 per cent by 2020 (Yach *et al.* 2010).
Nutrition labelling	PepsiCo pledged to display calorie count and key nutrients (Yach *et al.* 2010)
Restrict marketing to children	The Australian Beverages Council, the Union of European Beverage Associations and the International Council of Beverage Associations developed pledges on marketing to children (Hawkes and Harris 2011).
Nutrition education	Coca-Cola sponsored *Energy Balance 101* in the US, which taught children that there are no 'good' or 'bad' foods (Powell and Gard 2014).
Promote physical activity	Coca-Cola sponsored physical activity programmes in Mexican schools (Gómez *et al.* 2011)
Public-private partnerships	Coca-Cola, PepsiCo and Cadbury-Schweppes partnered with the Clinton Foundation and the American Heart Association to develop the Alliance for a Healthier Generation (Mello *et al.* 2008).
Self-regulation	The Australian Food and Grocery Council (of which Coca-Cola is a member) developed a voluntary front-of-pack labelling code of practice (Carter *et al.* 2013).
Remove products from schools	The alliance for a healthier generation (including Coca-Cola, PepsiCo and Cadbury-Schweppes) voluntarily removed sugary soft drinks from American primary schools (Mello *et al.* 2008).

works to fragment and discredit its opposition within the public health nutrition community (Mialon *et al.* 2018).

Public health researchers draw parallels between Big Food's oppositional responses to obesity and the tobacco industry's efforts to deny evidence and oppose public health policies (Brownell and Warner 2009; Capewell and Lloyd-Williams 2018). Concern about the role of powerful commercial actors in causing public health problems and blocking effective responses to them has led some scholars to propose the concept of 'industrial epidemics' caused by the business practices of powerful corporations (Jahiel 2008). Building on epidemiological models, the concept frames the private sector as a vector that spreads disease in a manner akin to how mosquitos are a vector for the malaria virus. This has sparked calls for critical scrutiny and investigation of the 'commercial determinants of health' (Kickbusch *et al.* 2016) and the 'effect of corporate behaviour on health' (Stuckler *et al.* 2012; Moodie *et al.* 2013; Williams 2015; Moodie 2016). Much of this literature takes the position that the commercial interests of many private sector actors run counter to public health interests, a perspective epitomized in the title of Wiist's (2010) book, *The Bottom Line or Public Health.*

Big Food strategy two: be 'part of the solution'

In addition to its overtly oppositional strategies, Big Food is now pursuing a second, parallel strategy to present itself as 'part of the solution' to obesity. To illustrate, the Coca-Cola Company (2013) explicitly stated that while '[o]besity is today's most challenging health issue [...] We are committed to being part of the solution, working closely with partners from business, government and civil society'. The spectrum of industry strategies that fall under this 'part of the solution' umbrella is broad, and analyses of these strategies differ in what they include and exclude from this group. Deploying illustrative examples from the soft drink industry once again, Table 11.2 summaries key corporate activities, which broadly correspond to the five commitments that the International Food and Beverage Alliance (IFBA) made to the WHO in 2008: product reformulation; nutrition labelling and information; advertising to children; educational and physical activity programmes; and public-private partnerships (International Food and Beverage Alliance 2009). We also include two categories not part of the IFBA's commitment that are analysed in the literature: the development of self-regulation, and the voluntary removal of soft drinks from schools. These strategies are a form of *corporate health promotion* – where corporations undertake activities that public health actors have recommended. Importantly, these often fall short of public health goals.

Most evaluations of corporate health promotion focus on two metrics: the extent of its positive nutritional impact on population health, and/or the political benefits it offers the packaged food and beverage industry. Both lines of research offer important insights into the motivations for, and consequences of, corporate health promotion.

According to Big Food, its corporate health promotion interventions generate positive health outcomes and contribute towards the reduction of obesity and other dietary and nutritional health concerns (Nixon *et al.* 2015). Public health nutrition research of corporate health promotion offers a more complex narrative. While some public health researchers acknowledge that corporate health promotion is an improvement on the status quo, they conclude that the initiatives are weaker alternatives to proposed public health policies (Mello *et al.* 2008; Nestle, 2015). Most evaluations of corporate health promotion strategies focus on specific commitments or programmes, and compare them to evidence-based, public health nutrition policies, such as those proposed in the

NOURISHING Framework from the World Cancer Research Fund, or to the WHO's proposed fiscal policies to tackle non-communicable diseases (Hawkes *et al.* 2013; World Cancer Research Fund; 2015; World Health Organization 2016). Public health researchers have identified several limitations of Big Food's corporate health promotion strategies. These limitations include the following: weak targets and loopholes (for example, permissive interpretations of the terms 'children' and 'marketing') (Hawkes and Harris 2011); the use of industry-friendly nutrient profiling systems (Drewnowski 2017); the inconsistent implementation of initiatives (Scrinis 2016); and the question of whether physical activity promotion undermines the message of dietary change (Nestle 2015).

Partly because of the above limitations of corporate health promotion initiatives, public health nutrition researchers have expressed scepticism over whether corporate actions would match corporate rhetoric. The idea that corporate health promotion serves a business or political purpose is at the core of a growing body of scholarship that critically analyses the corporate health promotion strategies of Big Food. One political benefit of corporate health promotion is its potential to improve Big Food's public image. Sports sponsorship has been shown to create a positive brand image, and positions the industry as a community benefactor (Richards *et al.* 2015). Further, corporate health promotion can create a 'health halo' for a company, making its portfolio appear healthier (Nestle 2015). Voluntary initiatives to reformulate products and market 'healthier' alternatives also present public relations opportunities (Lacy-Nichols *et al.* 2020a).

Corporate health promotion can also help to foster relationships with key stakeholders (Panjwani and Caraher 2014; Jane and Gibson 2018). Corporate health promotion can facilitate public-private partnerships between the Big Food, governments and public health organizations. These partnerships can offer credibility and legitimize corporate participation in nutrition policy development (Ken 2014). These relationships affiliate powerful commercial actors with credible stakeholders, and offer opportunities to influence nutrition professionals. Similarly, corporate sponsorship of nutrition research and organizations can help to 'win friends' or 'silence critics' (Nestle 2015).

Corporate health promotion initiatives also directly or indirectly promote personal, not corporate, responsibility for obesity. Analysis of corporate school nutrition education programmes finds that, despite different curricula, they share the 'steady mantra of personal fault and responsibility' (Powell and Gard 2014). While product reformulation could be seen as an exception to this, initiatives that require consumers to 'choose' healthier alternatives similarly require consumers to exercise personal responsibility (Herrick 2009; Scrinis 2016). These initiatives situate responsibility with consumers and minimize the extent to which Big Food is held accountable for obesity. Corporate health promotion initiatives can also distract from, or minimize, the perceived health harms from individual foods and beverages. Big Food's voluntary front-of-pack labelling initiatives face criticism for highlighting the beneficial attributes of foods (such as the vitamin or fibre content), and obscuring the high levels of salt, sugar or fat (Bix *et al.* 2015; Scrinis 2016). Similarly, reformulated food products are marketed as 'low in' or 'reduced', which can mislead consumers about the overall healthfulness of the product (Monteiro and Cannon 2012; Scrinis and Monteiro 2018).

Corporate health promotion helps the industry to diffuse the threat of unwanted regulations. Several scholars have noted that Big Food develops self-regulation with the intention of pre-empting mandatory government policies (Brownell and Warner 2009; Sharma *et al.* 2010; Moodie *et al.* 2013; Lacy-Nichols *et al.* 2020b). Brownell and Koplan (2011) describe Big Food's launch of a voluntary labelling initiative during deliberations on a national labelling policy. They argue that the launch of a voluntary alternative was a deliberate strategy to co-opt the momentum for a national front-of-pack nutrition label and provide a weaker, industry-friendly alternative.

Product reformulation and portfolio diversification into 'healthier' products deserve particular scrutiny. On the one hand, it offers the direct benefit of expanding the company's market share and revenue which, in turn, have facilitated their expansion into the Global South (Scrinis 2016). Nutritional reformulation is profitable. However, this profit fundamentally strengthens the market position and financial resources of Big Food – resources that are easily transformed into political influence.

Financial resources underpin and enable many of Big Food's political strategies. We can observe that the ability of corporations to influence political decision-making via lobbying is facilitated by their financial reserves (Nestle 2015). Moreover, the contrast between the lobbying and campaign expenditures of the American soft drink industry, and those of public health advocates, highlights the resource disparities between these two groups and the advantages that the soft drink industry has in engaging in this political practice (Paarlberg *et al.* 2017). Political influence is likewise facilitated by market resources: larger corporations tend to generate greater tax revenue for governments and employ more voters/constituents, leading to a greater threat of relocation or job loss which, even if only implicit, can exert significant regulatory chill (Fuchs 2007; Milsom *et al.* 2021). Big Food's nutrition initiatives and self-regulation also require financial investments (such as in research and development, monitoring, auditing and reporting). The soft drink industry's financial resources facilitate widespread advertising campaigns and a vocal online and social media presence. Corporate relationships with, and ownership of, media outlets further enable Big Food to shape public understanding of the issue and to normalize industry-friendly solutions (McKee and Stuckler 2018). By highlighting the role of market resources in political strategies, this analysis accentuates the interconnections between a corporation's economic, political and social environments (Levy and Newell 2002; Levy and Egan 2003). The relationship between material resources and the exercise of power also underscores the distinct advantages held by the private sector in exerting political influence relative to less well-resourced public health organizations.

The debate over whether and, if so, how to engage with commercial actors continues

This chapter has identified some of the risks and opportunities of Big Food's corporate health promotion initiatives. These food companies dominate ultra-processed food markets, and so even incremental changes on their part can potentially have global implications for public health. Yet, there is a risk that support for incremental changes (such as those found in most corporate health promotion initiatives) will diminish pressure for the structural changes needed to create healthy, sustainable and equitable food systems.

This ambiguity and contestation over how to evaluate the food industry's corporate health promotion presents real risks to food system governance, sustainability, health and justice – issues encapsulated in the controversy surrounding the 2021 UN Food Systems Summit. The organizers of the Summit argued that it was inclusive and democratic (referring to it as a 'People's Summit') – indeed, hundreds of NGOs, research institutions, and other food and health organizations participated in the international forum. However, critics, including the UN Special Rapporteur on the Right to Food, argued that the inclusion of corporate actors in the design of the Summit (the World Economic Forum, in particular) led to the corporate capture of the Summit, along with the disempowerment of the small-scale producers it purported to support (Canfield *et al.* 2021; Nisbett *et al.* 2021).

These developments demonstrate how Big Food corporations are positioning themselves for a more direct role in governing food systems, and how this undermines moves by independent governments to challenge the role of these corporations in creating the very problems they now claim to be solving. It also demonstrates the difficulties in attempting to challenge the practices and products of Big Food corporations as long as they maintain their political-economic power.

Note

1 The term 'astroturf' refers to industry-funded organizations that pose as genuine community (grassroots) organizations to disguise the role of the private sector in generating support or opposition to an issue (Nestle 2015).

References

Access to Nutrition Foundation. 2018, *Access to Nutrition Index: Global Index 2018*, accessed 21 December 2022, <https://accesstonutrition.org/index/global-index-2018/>.

Bachrach, P. and Baratz, M.S. 1962, 'Two faces of power', *American Political Science Review*, 56(4), pp. 947–52.

Bix, L., Sundar, R.P., Bello, N.M., Peltier, C., Weatherspoon, L.J. and Becker, M.W. 2015, 'To see or not to see: Do front of pack nutrition labels affect attention to overall nutrition information?' *Plos One,* 10(10), p. e0139732.

Brownell, K.D. and Koplan, J.P. 2011, 'Front-of-package nutrition labeling: An abuse of trust by the food industry?', *New England Journal of Medicine,* 364(25), pp. 2373–5.

Brownell, K.D. and Warner, K.E. 2009, 'The perils of ignoring history: Big tobacco played dirty and millions died. How similar is big food?' *The Milbank Quarterly*, 87(1), pp. 259–94.

Burch, D. and Lawrence, G. 2009, 'Towards a third food regime: Behind the transformation', *Agriculture and Human Values*, 26, pp. 267–279.

Buse, K., Tanaka, S. and Hawkes, S. 2017, 'Healthy people and healthy profits? Elaborating a conceptual framework for governing the commercial determinants of non-communicable diseases and identifying options for reducing risk exposure', *Globalization and Health*, 13, article 34.

Canfield, M., Anderson, M.D. and Mcmichael, P. 2021, 'UN Food Systems Summit 2021: Dismantling democracy and resetting corporate control of food systems', *Frontiers in Sustainable Food Systems*, 5, p. 661552.

Capewell, S. and Lloyd-Williams, F. 2018, 'The role of the food industry in health: Lessons from tobacco?' *British Medical Bulletin,* 125(1), pp. 131–43.

Carolan, M. 2011. *The Real Cost of Cheap Food*, Earthscan, London.

Carter, O.B.J., Mills, B.W., Lloyd, E. and Phan, T. 2013, 'An independent audit of the Australian food industry's voluntary front-of-pack nutrition labelling scheme for energy-dense nutrition-poor foods', *European Journal of Clinical Nutrition*, 67(1), pp. 31–5.

Clapp, J. and Fuchs, D. 2009, *Corporate Power in Global Agrifood Governance*, MIT Press, Cambridge.

Clapp, J. and Scrinis, G. 2017, 'Big food, nutritionism, and corporate power', *Globalizations*, 14(4), pp. 1–18.

Drewnowski, A. 2017, 'Uses of nutrient profiling to address public health needs: From regulation to reformulation', *Proceedings of the Nutrition Society*, 76(3), pp. 220–9.

Falkner, R. 2008, *Business Power and Conflict in International Environmental Politics*, Palgrave Macmillan, Basingstoke.

Freudenberg, N. 2014, *Lethal But Legal: Corporations, Consumption, and Protecting Public Health*, Oxford University Press, New York.

Fuchs, D. 2007, *Business Power In Global Governance*, Lynne Rienner, Boulder, Colorado.

Gertner, D. and Rifkin, L. 2017, 'Coca-Cola and the fight against the global obesity epidemic', *Thunderbird International Business Review*, 60(2), pp. 161–73.

Gómez, E.J. 2018, 'The transnational and domestic contexts facilitating sugary beverage and fast food industry policy and research manipulation in Mexico, Brazil, and India', *Annual Meeting of the American Political Science Association*, Boston.

Gómez, L., Jacoby, E., Ibarra, L., Lucumi, D., Hernandez, A., Parra, D., Florindo, A. and Hallal, P. 2011, 'Sponsorship of physical activity programs by the sweetened beverages industry: Public health or public relations?' *Revista de Saude Publica*, 45(2), pp. 423–7.

Haugaard, M. 2002, *Power: A Reader*, Manchester University Press, Manchester.
Hawkes, C. and Harris, J.L. 2011, 'An analysis of the content of food industry pledges on marketing to children', *Public Health Nutrition*, 14(8), pp. 1403–14.
Hawkes, C., Jewell, J. and Allen, K. 2013, 'A food policy package for healthy diets and the prevention of obesity and diet-related non-communicable diseases: The nourishing framework', *Obesity Reviews*, 14(Suppl. 2), pp. 159–68.
Heffernan, W., Hendrickson, M. and Gronski, R. 1999, *Consolidation in the Food and Agriculture System: Report to the National Farmers Union*, Department of Rural Sociology, University of Missouri.
Herrick, C. 2009, 'Shifting blame/selling health: Corporate social responsibility in the age of obesity', *Sociology of Health and Illness*, 31(1), pp. 51–65.
Huehnergarth, N. 2015, 'Beverage industry sues to block philadelphia's soda tax', *Forbes*, accessed 20 August 2018, <https://www.forbes.com/sites/nancyhuehnergarth/2016/09/14/beverage-industry-sues-to-block-philadelphias-soft-drink-tax/#151ee5e41164>.
International Food and Beverage Alliance. 2009, *IFBA First Progress Report 2008*, accessed 19 December 2022, <https://ifballiance.org/publications/ifba-first-progress-report-2008/>.
IPES-Food. 2017, *Too Big to Feed: Exploring the Impacts of Mega-Mergers, Consolidation and Concentration of Power in the Agri-Food Sector*, accessed 28 August 2020, <http://www.ipes-food.org/_img/upload/files/concentration_fullreport.pdf>.
Jahiel, R.L. 2008, 'Corporation-induced diseases, upstream epidemiologic surveillance, and urban health', *Journal of Urban Health: Bulletin of the New York Academy of Medicine*, 85(4), pp. 517–31.
Jane, B. and gibson, K. 2018, 'Corporate sponsorship of physical activity promotion programmes: Part of the solution or part of the problem?' *Journal of Public Health*, 40(2), pp. 279–88.
Ken, I. 2014, 'A healthy bottom line: Obese children, a pacified public, and corporate legitimacy', *Social Currents*, 1(2), pp. 130–48.
Kickbusch, I., Allen, L. and Franz, C. 2016, 'The commercial determinants of health', *The Lancet Global Health*, 4(12), pp. E895–6.
Lacy-Nichols, J., Scrinis, G. and Carey, R. 2020a, 'The evolution of Coca-Cola Australia's soft drink reformulation strategy 2003–2017: A thematic analysis of corporate documents', *Food Policy*, 90, p. 101793.
Lacy-Nichols, J., Scrinis, G. and Carey, R. 2020b, 'The politics of voluntary self-regulation: Insights from the development and promotion of the australian beverages council's commitment', *Public Health Nutrition*, 23(3), pp. 564–75.
Lacy-Nichols, J. and Williams, O. 2021, '"Part of the solution:" Food corporation strategies for regulatory capture and legitimacy', *International Journal of Health Policy Management*, 10, pp. 845–56.
Lang, T. and Heasman, M. 2004, *Food Wars: The Global Battle for Minds, Mouths, and Markets*, Earthscan, London.
Lang, T., Rayner, G. and Kaelin, E. 2006, *The Food Industry, Diet, Physical Activity and Health: A Review of Reported Commitments and Practice of 25 of the World's Largest Food Companies*, Centre For Food Policy, City University London, London.
Lee, A.J., Cullerton, K. and Herron, L-M. 2020, 'Achieving food system transformation: Insights from a retrospective review of nutrition policy (in) action in high-income countries', *International Journal of Health Policy Management*, 10(12), pp. 766–83.
Legg, T., Hatchard, J. and Gilmore, A.B. 2021, 'The science for profit model: How and why corporations influence science and the use of science in policy and practice', *Plos One*, 16, p. e0253272.
Levy, D.L. and Egan, D. 2003, 'A neo-Gramscian approach to corporate political strategy: Conflict and accommodation in the climate change negotiations', *Journal of Management Studies*, 40(4), pp. 803–29.
Levy, D.L. and Newell, P.J. 2002, 'Business strategy and international environmental governance: Toward a neo-Gramscian synthesis', *Global Environmental Politics*, 2(4), pp. 84–101.
Lukes, S. 1974, *Power: A Radical View*, Macmillan, London.
Mckee, M. and Stuckler, D. 2018, 'Responding to the corporate and commercial determinants of health', *American Journal of Public Health*, 108(9), pp. E1–4.
Mejia, P., Nixon, L., Cheyne, A., Dorfman, L. and Quintero, F. 2014, 'Two communities, two debates: News coverage of soda tax proposals in Richmond and El Monte', in Dorfman, L. (ed), *Issue 21*. Berkeley Media Studies Group, Berkley, pp. 1–32.
Mello, M. M., Pomeranz, J. and Moran, P. 2008, 'The interplay of public health law and industry self-regulation: The case of sugar-sweetened beverage sales in schools', *American Journal of Public Health*, 98(4), pp. 595–604.

Mialon, M., Crosbie, E. and Sacks, G. 2020, 'Mapping of food industry strategies to influence public health policy, research and practice in South Africa', *International Journal of Public Health*, 65(7), pp. 1027–36.
Mialon, M., Julia, C. and Hercberg, S. 2018, 'The policy dystopia model adapted to the food industry: The example of the nutri-score saga in france', *World Nutrition*, 9(2), pp. 109–20.
Mialon, M., Swinburn, B. and Sacks, G. 2015, 'A proposed approach to systematically identify and monitor the corporate political activity of the food industry with respect to public health using publicly available information', *Obesity Reviews*, 16(7), pp. 519–30.
Miller, D. and Harkins, C. 2010, 'Corporate strategy, corporate capture: Food and alcohol industry lobbying and public health', *Critical Social Policy*, 30(4), pp. 564–89.
Milsom, P., Smith, R., Modisenyane, S.M. and Walls, H. 2021, 'Do international trade and investment agreements generate regulatory chill in public health policymaking? A case study of nutrition and alcohol policy in South Africa', *Globalization and Health*, 17, pp. 1–17.
Monteiro, C.A. and Cannon, G. 2012, 'The food system: Product reformulation will not improve public health', *World Nutrition*, 3(9), pp. 406–34.
Monteiro, C.A., Lawrence, M., Millett, C., Nestle, M., Popkin, B.M., Scrinis, G. and Swinburn, B. 2021, 'The need to reshape global food processing: A call to the united nations food systems summit', *BMJ Global Health*, 6, p. e006885.
Moodie, R. 2016, 'Corporations taking deadly aim', *American Journal of Public Health*, 106(5), pp. 781–2.
Moodie, R., Stuckler, D., Monteiro, C., Sheron, N., Neal, B., Thamarangsi, T., Lincoln, P. and Casswell, S. 2013, 'Profits and pandemics: Prevention of harmful effects of tobacco, alcohol, and ultra-processed food and drink industries', *The Lancet*, 381(9869), pp. 670–9.
Nestle, M. 2013, *Food Politics: How the Food Industry Influences Nutrition and Health*, University of California Press, Berkley.
Nestle, M. 2015, *Soda Politics: Taking on Big Soda (and Winning)*, Oxford University Press, New York.
Nisbett, N., Friel, S., Aryeetey, R., Da Silva Gomes, F., Harris, J., Backholer, K., Baker, P., Jernigan, V. B.B. and Phulkerd, S. 2021, 'Equity and expertise in the UN Food Systems Summit', *BMJ Global Health*, 6(7), p. e006569.
Nixon, L., Mejia, P., Cheyne, A., Wilking, C., Dorfman, L. and Daynard, R. 2015, '"We're part of the solution": Evolution of the food and beverage industry's framing of obesity concerns between 2000 and 2012', *American Journal of Public Health*, 105(11), pp. 2228–36.
Paarlberg, R., Mozaffarian, D. and Micha, R. 2017, 'Can US local soda taxes continue to spread?' *Food Policy*, 71, pp. 1–7.
Panjwani, C. and Caraher, M. 2014, 'The public health responsibility deal: Brokering a deal for public health, but on whose terms?' *Health Policy*, 114(2–3), pp. 163–73.
Powell, D. and Gard, M. 2014, 'The governmentality of childhood obesity: Coca-Cola, public health and primary schools', *Discourse: Studies in the Cultural Politics of Education*, 36(6), pp. 854–67.
Richards, Z., Thomas, S.L., Randle, M. and Pettigrew, S. 2015, 'Corporate social responsibility programs of big food in Australia: A content analysis of industry documents', *Australian and New Zealand Journal of Public Health*, 39(6), pp. 550–6.
Scrinis, G. 2016, 'Reformulation, fortification and functionalization: Big food corporations' nutritional engineering and marketing strategies', *Journal of Peasant Studies*, 43(1), pp. 17–37.
Scrinis, G. and Monteiro, C.A. 2018, 'Ultra-processed foods and the limits of product reformulation', *Public Health Nutrition*, 21(1), pp. 247–52.
Sharma, L.L., Teret, S.P. and Brownell, K.D. 2010, 'The food industry and self-regulation: Standards to promote success and to avoid public health failures', *American Journal of Public Health*, 100(2), pp. 240–6.
Simon, M. 2006, *Appetite For Profit: How the Food Industry Undermines Our Health and How to Fight Back*, Nation Books, New York.
Stuckler, D., Mckee, M., Ebrahim, S. and Basu, S. 2012, 'Manufacturing epidemics: The role of global producers in increased consumption of unhealthy commodities including processed foods, alcohol, and tobacco', *Plos Medicine*, 9(6), p. e1001235.
The Coca-Cola Company. 2013, 'Coca-Cola announces global commitments to help fight obesity', accessed 16 November 2016, <http://www.coca-colacompany.com/press-center/press-releases/coca-cola-announces-global-commitments-to-help-fight-obesity>.
Tselengidis, A. and Östergren, P.-O. 2019, 'Lobbying against sugar taxation in the european union: Analysing the lobbying arguments and tactics of stakeholders in the food and drink industries', *Scandinavian Journal of Public Health*, 47(5), pp. 565–75.

Ulucanlar, S, Fooks, G.J. and Gilmore, A.B. 2016, 'The policy dystopia model: an interpretive analysis of tobacco industry political activity', *Plos Medicine*, 13(9), p. e1002125.

Wiist, W.H. 2010, *The Bottom Line or Public Health: Tactics Corporations Use To Influence Health and Health Policy, and What We Can Do To Counter Them*, Oxford University Press, Oxford.

Williams, S.N. 2015, 'The incursion of "big food" in middle-income countries: A qualitative documentary case study analysis of the soft drinks industry in China and India', *Critical Public Health*, 25(4), pp. 455–73.

Winson, A. 2004, 'Bringing political economy into the debate on the obesity epidemic', *Agriculture and Human Values*, 21, pp. 299–312.

World Cancer Research Fund. 2015, *Curbing Global Sugar Consumption: Effective Food Policy Actions To Help Promote Healthy Diets and Tackle Obesity*, accessed 21 December 2022, <https://www.wcrf.org/policy/our-publications/curbing-global-sugar-consumption/>.

World Health Organization. 2016, *Fiscal Policies for Diet and the Prevention of Noncommunicable Diseases*, WHO, Geneva.

Yach, D., Khan, M., Bradley, D., Hargrove, R., Kehoe, S. and Mensah, G. 2010, 'The role and challenges of the food industry in addressing chronic disease', *Globalization and Health*, 6, article 10.

12

NEOLIBERALISM AND HEALTH IN GLOBAL CONTEXT

The role of international organizations

Timon Forster, Thomas H. Stubbs and Alexandros E. Kentikelenis

The global COVID-19 pandemic stretched health systems to their limits and threatened to unravel decades of socio-economic progress. As governments struggled to safeguard the well-being of their people, intergovernmental organizations (IGOs) stepped up their efforts to help mitigate the crisis (Hanrieder 2020; Kentikelenis *et al.* 2020; Stubbs *et al.* 2021). Yet, IGOs have long shaped country responses to socio-economic crises, exerting profound influence on global health via policy prescriptions attached to structural adjustment lending programs and through more subtle processes of policy norm diffusion (Chorev 2012; Hanrieder and Kreuder-Sonnen 2014; Kentikelenis and Stubbs 2023).

This chapter examines how IGOs act as 'agents of neoliberalism' (Babb and Kentikelenis 2018) in global health. We define neoliberalism as a set of policies promoting market-oriented solutions for a range of policy problems. Of course, not all IGOs are carriers and transmitters of neoliberal ideas about appropriate policy, but a subset of IGOs has been central in globalizing this paradigm. We focus on the role of three especially powerful such organizations: the World Health Organization (WHO), International Monetary Fund (IMF), and World Bank.

IGOs as carriers of neoliberal ideas

The global ascendancy of neoliberalism has its roots in the 1980s. Structural changes in the world economy, following the collapse of the Bretton Woods system and the 1970s oil crises, posed a range of economic challenges for developing countries. To adjust to the new global economic system, these countries – commonly facing high debt burdens and national or regional economic crises – turned to IGOs' policy advice to reform their economies. At the same time, IGOs – under the influence of their most powerful members, like the US – became increasingly committed to economic ideas about the merits of free markets in driving sustainable growth and development (Kentikelenis and Babb 2019). Consequently, IGOs acted as key agents in designing and overseeing market-oriented reforms of developing countries (Babb and Kentikelenis 2018; Forster *et al.* 2022; Kentikelenis and Stubbs 2023). Numerous countries restructured their domestic political economies according to neoliberal doctrine: privatizing state-owned enterprises, deregulating markets, and liberalizing trade (Harvey 2005). IGOs prompted this transition via two key channels of influence: normative pressures through IGOs' policy advice and technical assistance (Simmons *et al.*

DOI: 10.4324/9781003017110-14

2008), and coercive pressures through loans in exchange for policy reforms (Babb and Carruthers 2008). We discuss each of these channels in turn.

Policy norms

IGOs foster the adoption of neoliberal policies through normative processes – spreading policy norms by using their authority to define what policy ideas are 'appropriate' (Simmons *et al.* 2008: 31–40) as seemingly impartial actors (Heinzel *et al.* 2021). IGOs derive this authority from the knowledge and expertise their bureaucracies build through formal training and socialization. These organizations commonly recruit a narrow band of technocrats with degrees in orthodox economics and related social sciences from elite Anglo-Saxon universities (*e.g.* for the IMF, see: Weaver *et al.* 2022). In turn, these experts possess the credentials in neoclassical theories of trade, finance, and development to define contemporary issues, as well as to propose universally applicable neoliberal solutions to address them with professional legitimacy (Barnett and Finnemore 2004).

Neoliberal policy norms are diffused by IGOs through various means. For example, the process of normative emulation suggests that similar organizational structures and norms determine converging behavior (DiMaggio and Powell 1983). Or, more directly, IGOs engage in transnational policy training to disseminate norms to national officials, thereby increasing the number of domestic reformers who are sympathetic to their prescriptions for policy change (Broome and Seabrooke 2015).

Coercive pressures

In addition to normative processes, the diffusion of neoliberalism from IGOs to domestic policy is commonly achieved through the practice of conditional lending by international financial institutions (IFIs), a subset of IGOs. Among IFIs, the IMF and World Bank are the most influential (Babb and Kentikelenis 2018): granting loans to governments suffering from economic imbalances in exchange for a range of policy reforms, collectively known as 'conditionality' (*e.g.* Babb and Carruthers 2008; Kentikelenis and Stubbs 2023).

The IMF and World Bank, founded in 1944, are mandated to maintain global financial stability and finance development projects, respectively. Both organizations have been instrumental in promoting market-liberalizing reforms as part of their lending operations from as early as the 1980s (Babb and Kentikelenis 2018). Against a background of debt crises, their 'structural adjustment programs' – the vehicles through which conditionality is administered – achieved notoriety for coercing indebted developing countries to adopt four key neoliberal pillars: stabilization, liberalization, deregulation, and privatization of the economy (Babb and Kentikelenis 2018; Kentikelenis and Babb 2019). First, stabilization entails fiscal, monetary, and exchange rate policies aimed at resolving balance-of-payments issues and controlling inflation, including fiscal consolidation measures (or 'austerity'). Second, liberalization involves easing restrictions on flows of goods and capital to facilitate a higher degree of integration with the global economy and a more efficient allocation of capital. Third, deregulation encompasses measures enlarging the scope of free markets to limit state interference and corruption in economic processes, such as through reducing the number of procedures, time, and costs to register a company. Finally, privatization entails the commodification of state-owned enterprises and natural resources to private interests to promote the economic growth of industries hitherto sheltered from market forces.

Following extensive controversy over their handling of the Asian Financial Crisis during the late-1990s (Babb and Carruthers 2008), the IMF and World Bank claimed to have reformed the *modus operandi* of structural adjustment. According to them, revised programs incorporated 'flexible' policy design, 'streamlined' conditionality, adopted a 'pro-poor' orientation, and enabled borrowing-country 'ownership' (IMF 2009; World Bank 2009). Yet, at least for the IMF, studies find the advertised changes are not consistent with their actual lending practices (Kentikelenis *et al.* 2016; Mariotti *et al.* 2017; Forster *et al.* 2019). Instead, neoliberal-type conditionality has remained common in cross-country experiences of structural adjustment programs (Babb and Carruthers 2008; Kentikelenis *et al.* 2016; Labonté and Stuckler 2016; Kentikelenis and Stubbs 2023).

IGOs, neoliberalism, and global health

Since the 1980s, IGOs have encouraged and frequently compelled countries to adopt neoliberal policy reforms. These have had significant consequences on global health. From as early as 1987, in a landmark report on structural adjustment and child health, UNICEF acknowledged that the IMF and World Bank had engendered detrimental effects on health outcomes (Cornia *et al.* 1987). As the two most powerful IFIs (Babb and Kentikelenis 2018), the IMF and the World Bank warrant particular attention. In addition, we discuss the role of the WHO, as the IGO formally tasked with promoting human health and well-being.

Figure 12.1 depicts three main pathways through which neoliberalism affects health outcomes. First, direct effects originate from two nodes: IGOs deploy structural adjustment programs to impose conditions directly related to health systems, and draw on their expert authority to influence health policy discourse and reforms. Second, indirect effects on health systems stem from macroeconomic and institutional policies and norms. Third, the social determinants of health, such as

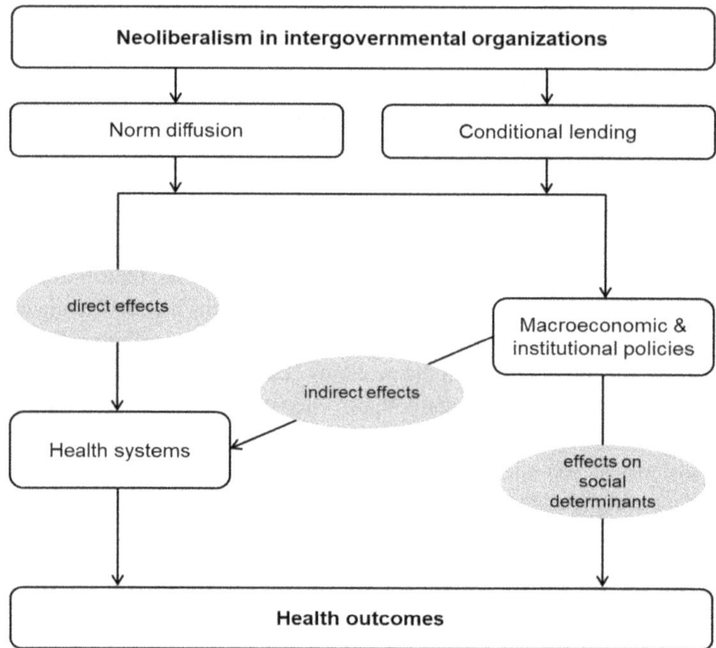

Figure 12.1 Impact of neoliberalism on health – overview of mechanisms.
Source: Authors, adapted from Kentikelenis (2017).

education and income, are impacted by a country's macroeconomic and institutional framework. We first provide evidence on the effects from norm diffusion, and then turn our attention to the relationship between structural adjustment and health.

Norm diffusion and health

IGOs utilize their 'expert' authority (Barnett and Finnemore 2004) to disseminate neoliberal policy ideas to affect global health. The normative nature of these processes in relation to health has received relatively little attention (for an exception, see: Murdie and Hicks 2013), partly because of empirical difficulties associated with identifying non-coercive diffusion of norms. For instance, policy reports might use deliberately vague language that invites ambiguity in the specificities of their proposals, and sometimes favor ideological principles over science (*e.g.* Navarro 2000). Still, the three pathways in Figure 12.1 have explanatory power. The framework can illuminate how neoliberal norms affect health. To demonstrate, we discuss how the WHO, World Bank, and IMF have consistently advocated for a wider role of the private sector in the provision of healthcare.

First, during the late-1990s, the WHO faced a crisis on three fronts: limited financial resources, alternative agencies competing in health governance, and uncertainty about its leadership. The WHO adopted a new agenda with various neoliberal features, responding selectively and strategically to these exogenous pressures (Chorev 2013). A 'neoliberal transformation was evident in every layer of operation' of the WHO (Chorev 2012: 187), and the organization supported market-oriented solutions and the involvement of the private sector. The *World Health Report 2000* on health systems (WHO 2000) – written by a team incorporating former World Bank economists to strengthen its legitimacy – was supposed to address concerns about privatization and market reforms in healthcare (Chorev 2012: 175–6). However, the report failed to achieve this target (Ollila and Koivusalo 2002). Instead, the recommendations were biased toward private health and encouraging competition, while voices criticizing the conventional wisdom at that time were absent (Navarro 2000). While the privatization of health services carries potential gains in terms of cost efficiency, it may reduce access for people who cannot afford to pay for private health services (Stuckler and Basu 2013).

Second, the World Bank, through a series of reports (Akin *et al.* 1987; World Bank 1993; The Human Development Network 1997) – most notably its annual *World Development Report* – promoted some distinctively neoliberal policy advice (Armada *et al.* 2001). The Bank sought to redefine the state's role in healthcare, and promoted private-sector provision (de Beyer *et al.* 2000) to, *inter alia*, increase competition in health service delivery (Ruger 2005). While the Bank has drawn attention to strengthening health systems in an updated *Health, Nutrition, and Population* strategy (World Bank 2007), earlier versions of this policy paper advocated expanding private-sector provision and exposing public providers to greater market competition (McCoy 2007).

Third, the IMF has regularly emphasized 'inefficiencies' in health systems (Coady *et al.* 2012). As a result, the Fund argues that pro-market measures – such as increased competition or greater reliance on private financing – can improve efficiency in both advanced (Cottarelli 2010) and emerging (Jenkner *et al.* 2012) economies. For example, the IMF continues to view many state-owned enterprises as a 'burden to taxpayers and the economy', and thus encourages market-oriented reform (IMF 2020b). Yet as discussed below, these reforms are likely to affect adversely the capacity and structure of health systems (see: Table 12.1).

In addition to direct effects on health systems, IGOs advocate broader policy norms that dictate best practices in global health governance. By drawing on their expert authority to define the issues at stake, IGOs control and guide debates. For instance, despite external, neoliberal pressures,

Table 12.1 Structural adjustment and health systems, direct and indirect effects

Health(-related) outcome	*Policy area*	*Mechanism*
Financing and provision of healthcare	Health spending	Austerity can require governments to reduce public health expenditure or replace public with private – often, aid – financing (Sridhar and Woods 2010; Stubbs *et al.* 2017). Priority spending floors stipulate minimum expenditures on health and education that, in theory, safeguard spending on health from austerity (Gupta *et al.* 2000). However, in practice, they are accorded secondary importance to economic targets (Ruckert and Labonté 2012; Kentikelenis *et al.* 2015; Kentikelenis *et al.* 2016). *Programs have catalytic effects on aid flows for general budget support and debt relief, but not for health aid* (Stubbs *et al.* 2016).
	Labor market	Wage bill ceilings lead to redundancies, hiring freezes, or wage cuts (Stuckler and Basu 2009; Kentikelenis *et al.* 2015; Stubbs *et al.* 2017), which lower health system access (Forster *et al.* 2020) and prompt medical 'brain drain' to advanced countries (Lefrançois 2010; Marphatia 2010).
	Trade and capital account liberalization	*Removal of tariffs and customs duties lowers trade tax revenues in the short-run. In low-income countries, revenue from domestic taxes tends to be insufficient to recover these losses* (Baunsgaard and Keen 2010)*, which can undermine the fiscal basis of health policy. Further, even if these policy reforms may be neutral with regard to tax revenue, IMF structural adjustment replaces trade taxes with regressive consumption taxes* (Reinsberg *et al.* 2020).
	Privatization	*Privatization of state-owned enterprises can raise funds for cash-strapped governments in the short-term. Yet, in the medium- and long-term, this can result in losses of reliable public revenue sources that could otherwise have been used to fund the health sector* (King *et al.* 2009).
Coverage and utilization of health services	User fees	The introduction of user fees for healthcare and co-payments for medicines or services (Sen and Koivusalo 1998; Kentikelenis *et al.* 2015) can restrict access for poorer households (McIntyre *et al.* 2006).
	Health system decentralization	Fiscal and operational decentralization of health systems to the subnational level (Kentikelenis *et al.* 2015; Stubbs *et al.* 2017) may generate savings in the short-run, but can lead to health system coordination and budget execution problems if local authorities lack technical capacities or divert funds to alternative uses (Djibuti *et al.* 2007).
	Privatization	*State-owned enterprises may provide health coverage to employees, which can be withdrawn once privatized* (Stuckler *et al.* 2009; Stuckler and Basu 2013).

Note: Mechanisms in normal font are direct effects on health systems, while those in italics capture indirect effects on health systems.

the WHO advocated for greater investment in health – as opposed to budget cuts – in a 2001 report (Commission on Macroeconomics and Health 2001). This was possible because the organization actively framed health issues in terms of economic growth, deviating from its earlier notion of social development (Chorev 2012: 165–72). According to this conceptualization, better health for the population increases productivity and, thus, stimulates growth. Not only did the WHO respond strategically in economic terms, economists wrote policy papers and applied their own analytical techniques to support this case. As noted earlier, the WHO overcame its internal financial crisis and regained its authority by appealing to, and diffusing, the dominant doctrine at the time (Horton 2002; Chorev 2013). In addition, the strategic response empowered the WHO to engage closely with other agencies, such as the Bill and Melinda Gates Foundation (Chorev 2012: 189). Nonetheless, its immediate success may prove costly in the long-run. While the selective correspondence to neoliberal demands secured financial survival for the institution, its adoption of economic methods and language may engender difficulties in expanding the concept of health to broader social domains at a later stage (Weaver 2010).

Today, the WHO and World Bank promote universal health coverage (WHO 2013; World Bank 2014), which requires strengthening health systems (WHO 2019). Undoubtedly, these organizations are subject to discourse and policy norms at a global level, such as the Sustainable Development Goals. Yet, they can respond selectively and strategically to external demands and, in doing so, promote their own policy norms. For example, the IMF emphasized the need to strengthen health systems, bolster social safety nets, and scale up public investment in response to the COVID-19 pandemic (IMF 2020a, b). Simultaneously, it emphasized that countries recovering from COVID-19 should prioritize 'unwinding the large public interventions in firms [privatize state-owned enterprises] and managing the associated fiscal risks' (IMF 2020a: 20–1). Further, the IMF and other IFIs have been slow to disburse the financing at their disposal after the outbreak, thereby casting doubt on the efficacy of the proposed changes (Stubbs *et al.* 2021). This illustrates how IGOs' discourse should not be taken at face-value (Mariotti *et al.* 2017; Forster *et al.* 2019).

Structural adjustment and health

In Table 12.1, we identify direct and indirect impacts that structural adjustment has had on two key aspects of health systems. First, conditions pertaining to health spending, labor market reforms, trade and capital account liberalization, and privatization impede – or sometimes strengthen – the capacity of states to finance and provide health services. In turn, sharp changes in public health spending patterns affect the volume and quality of services provided, such as the number of health facilities available (Stuckler and Basu 2009).

Second, deregulation, decentralization, and privatization affect the coverage and utilization of health services. For instance, structural adjustment has mandated the introduction of user fees for access to healthcare and co-payments for medicines or services (Sen and Koivusalo 1998), thereby giving rise to health inequalities (Forster *et al.* 2018).

Structural adjustment programs also have a noticeable impact on health outcomes by reshaping the social determinants of health (Labonté and Schrecker 2007) – that is, the conditions 'in which people are born, grow, live, work, and age' (Marmot and Bell 2012: S4). For instance, neoliberal policies are frequently undertaken with the promise of increasing economic growth. At the same time, in the short-run, structural adjustment programs lead to lower rates of economic growth (Dreher 2006), with ensuing declines in per capita incomes and higher involuntary unemployment. These undermine the social determinants of health in multiple ways, including through increasing poverty and inequality (Oberdabernig 2013; Forster *et al.* 2019; Lang 2021; Stubbs *et al.* 2022). These effects, in turn, cause a cascade of pernicious health effects (Pickett and Wilkinson 2015).

Moreover, the negative consequences of neoliberal policy reforms on health outcomes occur over time. In addition to short-run appearances, some of these effects only materialize during the medium- to long-term. In particular, neoliberal reforms hollow out state administrative capacities and finances (Reinsberg *et al.* 2018). This explains why governments have failed to respond adequately to the COVID-19 pandemic (Jones and Hameiri 2022). In addition, the effects of structural adjustment are unevenly distributed across the entire population. For example, since UNICEF first drew attention to the gendered impact of structural adjustment (Cornia *et al.* 1987), considerable attention has been devoted to identifying how these policies uniquely and disproportionately affect women. In particular, structural adjustment programs have been associated with increased maternal and infant mortality (Pandolfelli *et al.* 2013; Thomson *et al.* 2017; Forster *et al.* 2020).

Conclusion

Moving beyond the mainstream literature on the social, political, commercial, and financial determinants of health, this chapter highlighted the international-bureaucratic determinants of health. While these factors interact with other determinants, a comprehensive understanding depends on grasping them as a unique set of factors in global policy-making because they offer a crucial, often neglected piece of the puzzle of 'upstream' determinants of health.

Intergovernmental organizations embody neoliberalism when they promote market-based solutions through both coercive and normative processes. These processes affect population health through a number of pathways. Before discussing their implications, however, two limitations should be noted. First, these pathways are relevant to countries' experiences with structural adjustment and norm diffusion, but they are not all operative at all times. Likewise, not all countries rely on IGO advice to the same extent. Thus, some states find the norms and ideas IGOs disseminate unappealing, or are able to resist external pressures for adoption. Second, the lending activities of other IFIs – such as the African Development Bank – have also been shown to affect health (Coburn *et al.* 2015a, b). However, in-depth assessments of their operations remain scarce. Similarly, other IGOs also engage in norm making and diffusion. Increasingly, actors such as consultants, private foundations, and transnational corporations must be considered, too – on their own merit, as well as their activities within IGOs (*e.g.* Eckl and Hanrieder 2023).

With these caveats in mind, we discussed examples of the most important evidence of how conditionality affects health systems and other upstream determinants of health. The World Bank and the IMF are the most relevant institutions in this respect. In the short-run, the pathways examined link structural adjustment to possibly adverse effects on health, due to both individual-level factors (such as unemployment, economic hardship, psycho-social distress) and institutional factors (such as availability and quality of healthcare services, health system operating principles). Nevertheless, individuals' socio-economic status is a key mediating factor, and the impact of structural adjustment policies varies by class, gender, and race. Equally importantly, the medium- and long-term effects of structural adjustment programs are more difficult to accurately estimate, and have received little attention in the literature. Neoliberal policies like trade liberalization may eventually create new employment opportunities and boost economic performance and tax revenues, but other structural adjustment reforms – like mass privatization – may contribute to long-term unemployment resulting in ill-health (Stuckler and Basu 2013). The underfunding, privatization, or decentralization of health systems may weaken capacity, which requires prolonged investment to be overcome.

IGOs are also empowered by the global trend toward technical rationality, and utilize the ideological power this has to dominate global health debates. The empirical evidence presented here supports the argument that the IGOs diffuse neoliberal policies through their research. IGOs encourage an increased role of the private sector in healthcare provision, and – to a lesser extent – favor the introduction of market mechanisms. Further, framing international health discussions, along with emphasizing the importance of measurement and data collection, reinforces IGOs' authority and offers an opportunity to promote neoliberal solutions. Moreover, we indicated how these IGOs – emanating from their knowledge – could easily extend their influence to other societal issues, such as education. This indirectly affects population health through undermining their broader social determinants.

In sum, the evidence regarding the impact of the reforms mandated and ideas advocated by IGOs to reconfigure global health – promoting market-based solutions over government 'intervention' in various forms – should raise alarm. Middle-income countries, in particular, are projected to face budget cuts in the coming years, thereby potentially compounding the adverse effects of the COVID-19 pandemic (Kentikelenis and Stubbs 2021; Ray *et al.* 2022). However, despite neoliberal dominance on health and its broader social determinants, there are also exceptions. Some policies – like the reliance on user fees – can be easily reversed, especially when governments cooperate with domestic and international partners to design alternative policy arrangements. For instance, user fee removal in Uganda quickly translated into increases in health service utilization, especially by the poor (Yates 2009). Similarly, collaborations with international donors, national-level planning, and appropriate tailoring to health needs have allowed some low-income countries to attenuate detrimental effects of structural adjustment on their health systems, while working to improve coverage (Meessen *et al.* 2006). Thus, options remain for sheltering and strengthening health policy. In addition, many UN Sustainable Development Goals for 2030 relate to health, which reflects member-states' acknowledgement of its global importance. Finally, the IGOs we discussed have sometimes reversed their neoliberal stances, or become more nuanced in advocating their policies, which puts these extant norms under more scrutiny. As the number of relevant actors in global health debates has increased substantially in recent decades – now including nation-states, inter- and non-governmental organizations, civil society groups, multinational corporations, and others – it is as important as ever to evaluate the impact of policy ideas put forward. Thus, researchers need to transcend exclusively mainstream economic evaluations of health systems and, instead, consider the social determinants of health.

References

Akin, J.S., Birdsall, N. and De Ferranti, D.M. 1987, *Financing Health Services in Developing Countries: An Agenda for Reform*, World Bank, Washington, DC.

Armada, F., Muntaner, C. and Navarro, V. 2001, 'Health and social security reforms in Latin America: The convergence of the world health organization, the world bank, and transnational corporations', *International Journal of Health Services*, 31(4), pp. 729–68.

Babb, S.L. and Carruthers, B.G. 2008, 'Conditionality: Forms, function, and history', *Annual Review of Law and Social Science*, 4(1), pp. 13–29.

Babb, S.L. and Kentikelenis, A.E. 2018, 'International financial institutions as agents of neoliberalism', in Cahill, D., Cooper, M., Konings, M. and Primrose, D. (eds), *The SAGE Handbook of Neoliberalism*, SAGE Publications, Thousand Oaks, pp. 16–27.

Barnett, M.N. and Finnemore, M. 2004, *Rules for the World: International Organizations in Global Politics*, Cornell University Press, Ithaca, NY.

Baunsgaard, T. and Keen, M. 2010, 'Tax revenue and (or?) trade liberalization', *Journal of Public Economics*, 94(9–10), pp. 563–77.

Broome, A. and Seabrooke, L. 2015, 'Shaping policy curves: Cognitive authority in transnational capacity building', *Public Administration*, 93(4), pp. 956–72.
Chorev, N. 2012, *The World Health Organization Between North and South*, Cornell University Press, Ithaca, NY.
Chorev, N. 2013, 'Restructuring neoliberalism at the world health organization', *Review of International Political Economy*, 20(4), pp. 627–66.
Coady, D., Clements, B.J. and Gupta, S. 2012, *The Economics of Public Health Care Reform in Advanced and Emerging Economies*, International Monetary Fund, Washington, DC.
Coburn, C., Restivo, M. and Shandra, J.M. 2015a, 'The African development bank and infant mortality: A cross-national analysis of structural adjustment and investment lending from 1990 to 2006', *International Journal of Comparative Sociology*, 56(3–4), pp. 275–96.
Coburn, C., Restivo, M. and Shandra, J.M. 2015b, 'The African development bank and women's health: A cross-national analysis of structural adjustment and maternal mortality', *Social Science Research*, 51, pp. 307–21.
Commission on Macroeconomics and Health. 2001, *Macroeconomics and Health: Investing in Health for Economic Development*, World Health Organization, Geneva.
Cornia, G.A., Jolly, R. and Stewart, F. 1987, *Adjustment With A Human Face, Vol. 1: Protecting the Vulnerable and Promoting Growth*, Oxford University Press, Oxford.
Cottarelli, C. 2010, 'Macro-fiscal implications of health care reform in advanced and emerging economies', policy paper 28, *International Monetary Fund*, accessed 17 January 2023, <https://www.imf.org/en/Publications/Policy-Papers/Issues/2016/12/31/Macro-Fiscal-Implications-of-Health-Care-Reform-in-Advanced-and-Emerging-Economies-Case-PP4522>.
de Beyer, J.A., Preker, A.S. and Feachem, R.G.A. 2000, 'The role of the World Bank in international health: Renewed commitment and partnership', *Social Science and Medicine*, 50(2), pp. 169–76.
DiMaggio, P. and Powell, W.W. 1983, 'The iron cage revisited: Collective rationality and institutional isomorphism in organizational fields', *American Sociological Review*, 48(2), pp. 147–60.
Djibuti, M., Rukhadze, N., Hotchkiss, D.R., Eisele, T.P. and Silvestre, E.A. 2007, 'Health systems barriers to effective use of infectious disease surveillance data in the context of decentralization in Georgia: A qualitative study', *Health Policy*, 83(2–3), pp. 323–31.
Dreher, A. 2006, 'IMF and economic growth: The effects of programs, loans, and compliance with conditionality', *World Development*, 34(5), pp. 769–88.
Eckl, J. and Hanrieder, T. 2023, 'The political economy of consulting firms in reform processes: The case of the World Health Organization', *Review of International Political Economy*, open access.
Forster, T., Kentikelenis, A.E. and Bambra, C. 2018, *Health Inequalities in Europe: Setting the Stage for Progressive Policy Action*, Foundation for European Progressive Studies and Think-tank for Action on Social Change, Dublin.
Forster, T., Kentikelenis, A.E., Reinsberg, B., Stubbs, T.H. and King, L.P. 2019, 'How structural adjustment programs affect inequality: A disaggregated analysis of IMF conditionality, 1980–2014', *Social Science Research*, 80(May), pp. 83–111.
Forster, T., Kentikelenis, A.E., Stubbs, T.H. and King, L.P. 2020, 'Globalization and health equity: The impact of structural adjustment programs on developing countries', *Social Science and Medicine*, 267, p. 112496.
Forster, T., Stubbs, T.H. and Kentikelenis, A.E. 2022, 'The politics of the International Monetary Fund', in Deciancio, M., Nemiña, P. and Deciancio, M. (eds), *Handbook on the Politics of International Development*, Edward Elgar Publishing, Cheltenham, pp. 376–91.
Gupta, S., Dicks-Mireaux, L., Khemani, R., McDonald, C. and Verhoeven, M. 2000, 'Social issues in IMF-supported programs', IMF Occasional Paper 191, accessed 17 January 2023, <https://www.imf.org/en/Publications/Occasional-Papers/Issues/2016/12/30/Social-Issues-in-IMF-Supported-Programs-3378>.
Hanrieder, T. 2020, 'Priorities, partners, politics: The WHO's mandate beyond the crisis', *Global Governance*, 26(4), pp. 534–43.
Hanrieder, T. and Kreuder-Sonnen, C. 2014, 'WHO decides on the exception? Securitization and emergency governance in global health', *Security Dialogue*, 45(4), pp. 331–48.
Harvey, D. 2005, *A Brief History of Neoliberalism*, Oxford University Press, Oxford.
Heinzel, M., Richter, J., Busch, P.O., Feil, H., Herold, J. and Liese, A. 2021, 'Birds of a feather? The determinants of impartiality perceptions of the IMF and the World Bank', *Review of International Political Economy*, 28(5), pp. 1249–73.

Horton, R. 2002, 'WHO: The casualties and compromises of renewal', *The Lancet*, 359(9317), pp. 1605–11.

IMF. 2009, *Creating Policy Space: Responsive Design and Streamlined Conditionality in Recent Low-Income Country Programs*, International Monetary Fund, Washington, DC.

IMF. 2020a, 'Fiscal monitor: Policies for the recovery', accessed 9 January 2023, <https://www.imf.org/en/Publications/FM/Issues/2020/09/30/october-2020-fiscal-monitor>.

IMF. 2020b, 'Fiscal monitor – April 2020', accessed 9 January 2023, <https://www.imf.org/en/Publications/FM/Issues/2020/04/06/fiscal-monitor-april-2020>.

Jenkner, E., Shang, B. and Clements, B.J. 2012, 'Health reform lessons from experiences of emerging economies', in Coady, D., Clements, B.J. and Gupta, S. (eds), *The Economics of Public Health Care Reform in Advanced and Emerging Economies*, International Monetary Fund, Washington, DC, pp. 125–32.

Jones, L. and Hameiri, S. 2022, 'COVID-19 and the failure of the neoliberal regulatory state', *Review of International Political Economy*, 29(4), pp. 1027–52.

Kentikelenis, A.E. 2017, 'Structural adjustment and health: A conceptual framework and evidence on pathways', *Social Science and Medicine*, 187, 296–305.

Kentikelenis, A.E. and Babb, S.L. 2019, 'The making of neoliberal globalization: Norm substitution and the politics of clandestine institutional change', *American Journal of Sociology*, 124(6), pp. 1720–62.

Kentikelenis, A.E., Gabor, D., Ortiz, I., Stubbs, T.H., McKee, M. and Stuckler, D. 2020, 'Softening the blow of the pandemic: Will the International Monetary Fund and World Bank make things worse?', *The Lancet Global Health*, 8(6), pp. E758–9.

Kentikelenis, A.E., King, L., McKee, M. and Stuckler, D. 2015, 'The international monetary fund and the Ebola outbreak', *The Lancet Global Health*, 3(2), pp. E69–70.

Kentikelenis, A.E., Stubbs, T.H. and King, L.P. 2016, 'IMF conditionality and development policy space, 1985–2014', *Review of International Political Economy*, 23(4), pp. 543–82.

Kentikelenis, A.E. and Stubbs, T.H. 2021, 'Austerity redux: The post-pandemic wave of budget cuts and the future of global public health', *Global Policy*, 13(1), pp. 5–17.

Kentikelenis, A.E. and Stubbs, T.H. 2023, *A Thousand Cuts: Social Protection in the Age of Austerity*, Oxford University Press, Oxford.

King, L.P., Hamm, P. and Stuckler, D. 2009, 'Rapid large-scale privatization and death rates in ex-communist countries: An analysis of stress-related and health system mechanisms', *International Journal of Health Services*, 39(3), pp. 461–89.

Labonté, R. and Schrecker, T. 2007, 'Globalization and social determinants of health: The role of the global marketplace (Part 2 of 3)', *Globalization and Health*, 3(1), p. 1–17.

Labonté, R. and Stuckler, D. 2016, 'The rise of neoliberalism: How bad economics imperils health and what to do about it', *Journal of Epidemiology and Community Health*, 70(3), pp. 312–18.

Lang, V.F. 2021, 'The economics of the democratic deficit: Ihe effect of IMF programs on inequality', *The Review of International Organizations*, 16(July), pp. 599–623.

Lefrançois, F. 2010, *The IMF, the Global Crisis and Human Resources for Health: Still Constraining Policy Space*, UK Consortium on AIDS & International Development and Action for Global Health UK, London.

Mariotti, C., Galasso, N. and Daar, N. 2017, 'Great expectations: Is the IMF turning words into action on inequality?', Oxfam briefing paper, accessed 21 December 2022, <https://policy-practice.oxfam.org/resources/great-expectations-is-the-imf-turning-words-into-action-on-inequality-620349/>.

Marmot, M. and Bell, R. 2012, 'Fair society, healthy lives', *Public Health*, 126, pp. S4–10.

Marphatia, A.A. 2010, 'The adverse effects of international monetary fund programs on the health and education workforce', *International Journal of Health Services*, 40(1), pp. 165–78.

McCoy, D. 2007, 'The world bank's new health strategy: Reason for alarm?', *The Lancet*, 369(9572), pp. 1499–501.

McIntyre, D., Thiede, M., Dahlgren, G. and Whitehead, M. 2006, 'What are the economic consequences for households of illness and of paying for health care in low- and middle-income country contexts?', *Social Science and Medicine*, 62(4), pp. 858–65.

Meessen, B., Van Damme, W., Tashobya, C.K. and Tibouti, A. 2006, 'Poverty and user fees for public health care in low-income countries: Lessons from Uganda and Cambodia', *The Lancet*, 368(9554), pp. 2253–7.

Murdie, A. and Hicks, A. 2013, 'Can international nongovernmental organizations boost government services? The case of health', *International Organization*, 67(3), pp. 541–73.

Navarro, V. 2000, 'Assessment of the World Health Report 2000', *The Lancet*, 356(9241), pp. 1598–601.

Oberdabernig, D.A. 2013, 'Revisiting the effects of IMF programs on poverty and inequality', *World Development*, 46, pp. 113–42.

Ollila, E. and Koivusalo, M. 2002, 'The world health report 2000: World health organization health policy steering off course – Changed values, poor evidence, and lack of accountability', *International Journal of Health Services*, 32(3), pp. 503–14.

Pandolfelli, L.E., Shandra, J.M. and Tyagi, J. 2013, 'The international monetary fund, structural adjustment, and women's health: A cross-national analysis of maternal mortality in Sub-Saharan Africa', *The Sociological Quarterly*, 55(1), pp. 119–42.

Pickett, K.E. and Wilkinson, R.G. 2015, 'Income inequality and health: A causal review', *Social Science and Medicine*, 128, pp. 316–26.

Ray, R., Gallagher, K.P. and Kring, W. 2022, "'Keep the receipts:" The political economy of IMF Austerity during and after the crisis years of 2009 and 2020', *Journal of Globalization and Development*, 13(1), pp. 31–59.

Reinsberg, B., Kentikelenis, A.E., Stubbs, T.H. and King, L. 2018, 'The world system and the hollowing-out of state capacity: How structural adjustment programs impact bureaucratic quality in developing countries', *American Journal of Sociology*, 143(3), pp. 1222–57.

Reinsberg, B., Stubbs, T.H. and Kentikelenis, A.E. 2020, 'Taxing the people, not trade: The international monetary fund and the structure of taxation in developing countries', *Studies in Comparative International Development*, 55(3), pp. 278–04.

Ruckert, A. and Labonté, R. 2012, 'The financial crisis and global health: The international monetary fund's (IMF) policy response', *Health Promotion International*, 28(3), pp. 357–66.

Ruger, J.P. 2005, 'The changing role of the world bank in global health', *American Journal of Public Health*, 95(1), pp. 60–70.

Sen, K. and Koivusalo, M. 1998, 'Health care reforms and developing countries: A critical overview', *The International Journal of Health Planning and Management*, 13(3), pp. 199–215.

Simmons, B.A., Dobbin, F. and Garrett, G. 2008, 'Introduction: The diffusion of liberalization', in Simmons, B.A., Dobbin, F. and Garrett, G. (eds), *The Global Diffusion of Markets and Democracy*, Cambridge University Press, Cambridge, pp. 1–63.

Sridhar, D. and Woods, N. 2010, 'Are there simple conclusions on how to channel health funding?', *The Lancet*, 375(9723), pp. 1326–8.

Stubbs, T.H., Kentikelenis, A.E., Stuckler, D., McKee, M. and King, L. 2017, 'The impact of IMF conditionality on government health expenditure: A cross-national analysis of 16 West African Nations', *Social Science and Medicine*, 174, pp. 220–7.

Stubbs, T.H., Kentikelenis, A.E. and King, L. 2016, 'Catalyzing aid? The IMF and donor behavior in aid allocation', *World Development*, 78, pp. 511–28.

Stubbs, T.H., Kentikelenis, A.E., Ray, R. and Gallagher, K.P. 2022, 'Poverty, inequality, and the International Monetary Fund: How austerity hurts the poor and widens inequality', *Journal of Globalization and Development*, 13(1), pp. 61–89.

Stubbs, T.H., Kring, W., Laskaridis, C., Kentikelenis, A.E. and Gallagher, K.P. 2021, 'Whatever it takes? The global financial safety net, Covid-19, and developing countries', *World Development*, 137, p. 105171.

Stuckler, D. and Basu, S. 2009, 'The international monetary fund's effects on global health: Before and after the 2008 financial crisis', *International Journal of Health Services*, 39(4), pp. 771–81.

Stuckler, D. and Basu, S. 2013, *The Body Economic: Why Austerity Kills*, Basic Books, New York.

Stuckler, D., King, L. and McKee, M. 2009, 'Mass privatisation and the post-communist mortality crisis: A cross-national analysis', *The Lancet*, 373(9661), pp. 399–407.

The Human Development Network. 1997, *Health, Nutrition, and Population Sector Strategy*, World Bank, accessed 7 April 2022, <http://documents.worldbank.org/curated/en/997651468779988699/Health-nutrition-population-sector-strategy>.

Thomson, M., Kentikelenis, A.E. and Stubbs, T.H. 2017, 'Structural adjustment programmes adversely affect vulnerable populations: A systematic-narrative review of their effect on child and maternal health', *Public Health Reviews*, 38(1), pp. 1–18.

Weaver, C. 2010, 'The strategic social construction of the world bank's gender and development policy norm', in Park, S. and Vetterlein, A. (eds), *Owning Development: Creating Policy Norms in the IMF and the World Bank*, Cambridge University Press, Cambridge, pp. 70–90.

'Weaver, C., Heinzel, M., Jorgensen, S., and Flores, J. 2022, 'Bureaucratic representation in the IMF and the World Bank', *Global Perspectives*, 3(1): 39684.

WHO. 2000, *The World Health Report 2000: Health Systems – Improving Performance*, World Health Organization, Geneva.

WHO. 2013, 'Launch of the world health report 2013: Research for universal health coverage', Accessed 2 February 2021, <https://www.who.int/director-general/speeches/detail/launch-of-the-world-health-report-2013-research-for-universal-health-coverage>.

WHO. 2019, 'Universal health coverage (UHC)', accessed 4 November 2020, <https://www.who.int/en/news-room/fact-sheets/detail/universal-health-coverage-(uhc)>.

World Bank. 1993, *World Development Report: Investing in Health. 1993*, The International Bank for Reconstruction and Development, Washington, DC.

World Bank. 2007, *Healthy Development: The World Bank Strategy for Health, Nutrition, and Population Results*, World Bank Group, Washington, DC.

World Bank. 2009, 'Development policy lending retrospective: Flexibility, customization, and results', accessed 19 September 2022, <http://documents.worldbank.org/curated/en/904211468327394724/2009-development-policy-lending-retrospective-flexibility-customization-and-results>.

World Bank. 2014, 'Speech by world bank group president Jim Yong Kim on universal health coverage in emerging economies', accessed 12 November 2016, <http://www.worldbank.org/en/news/speech/2014/01/14/speech-world-bank-group-president-jim-yong-kim-health-emerging-economies>.

Yates, R. 2009, 'Universal health care and the removal of user fees', *The Lancet*, 373(9680), pp. 2078–81.

13
NEOLIBERALISM AND MENTAL HEALTH

Jana Fey

The functioning of the human mind has long been a puzzle to solve for scientists. This is not only because of the huge potential that lies in uncovering truths about why people behave, think, or feel certain ways, but also because of how our realities are constructed. Holding the key to developing and maintaining healthy minds would be a key asset for producing societies that remain peaceful and economically productive. An attempt to define the relationship between the global economy and mental well-being has given rise to important critical interventions in recent years. While some have called into question the psychiatric hold on 'mental health' as a scientific concept (*e.g.* Davies 2016; Cohen 2018), others have provided close readings of neoliberal governance as a determinant of mental well-being (Ramon 2008; Collin 2015; Brijnath and Antoniades 2016). Nevertheless, there is scope for developing a more sustained critical engagement with mental health by scholars of global health economics. In order to expand the critiques of neoliberal systems (Teghtsoonian 2009; Esposito and Perez 2014) to the realm of mental health, an interdisciplinary approach that considers the varying social and cultural determinants of mental well-being can be a useful tool in making sense of the increase in diagnosable mental disorders globally. Simultaneously, mental health problems have been framed as a global economic burden, where the combined result of 'diminished productivity at work, reduced rates of labor participation, foregone tax receipts, and increased welfare payments' costs governments '10 billion days of lost work annually – the equivalent of US$1 trillion per year' – according to the most recent report on mental health by the World Bank Group (WBG 2016: 5).

This development also needs to be contextualized in a broader colonial history of the deployment of psychiatric knowledge and public health interventions for the purpose of establishing political hierarchies (Bashford 2004; Foucault 2006; Fanon 2008; Mills 2014; Fernando 2017). The option to diagnose people with mental disorders is a powerful tool of governance provided and facilitated by Western-dominated psychiatric systems, which also continue to promote racist understandings of what it means to be mentally healthy. This is because the psy (psychology and psychiatry) disciplines continue 'to reflect the culture and sociopolitical contexts in Euro-America at the time they developed' (Fernando 2017: 33; see also: Davar 2014; Mills 2014). The powerful dynamic of psychiatry and capitalist power in modernity has given rise to a symbiotic relationship between mental health and neoliberalism, where governing the political economy both necessitates and influences the maintenance of mental well-being in populations. Two of the most distinct ways

DOI: 10.4324/9781003017110-15

in which we see this are through the advent of consumption perceived as achievement (Brooks and Wee 2016) and the individualization of mental distress through psychopharmaceutical interventions (Esposito and Perez 2014; Davies 2017). Within this context arises a concern about the role that the state plays in facilitating the relationship between neoliberalism and mental health/mental distress, and how Western nations are drawing on psychiatric understandings to maintain global (economic) hierarchies.

This chapter sketches the relationship between mental health and neoliberalism by showing how it can be examined drawing on a variety of conceptual approaches. To do so, I refer to literature from across the Social Sciences (Rizq 2012, 2014a, 2014b; Esposito and Perez 2014; Collin 2015; Mills 2018; Tseris 2018), which has successfully mapped the conjuncture between an increase in diagnosable mental illnesses globally and the expansion of neoliberal modes of governance.

Before I discuss said literature further, I set out the parameters of terminology within which this chapter operates with regard to mental health. With much mental health discourse dominated by bio-medical understandings of distress, it is important to note that talking about mental illness and mental disorder is not the same as talking about mental distress. Taking my cue from an extensive and growing body of mental health service-user and survivor literature (Faulkner 2017; Cosgrove and Karter 2018; Voronka 2019), I approach this chapter with an attention to discourse. While *mental distress* captures a broad spectrum of (often-negative) emotions and experiences, the terms *mental illness* and *mental disorder* have typically been framed specifically within a bio-medical and psychiatric framework. This leaves little scope for comprehending mental health along a socially constructed spectrum of well-being. Therefore, the language of mental distress in this chapter is preferred when describing mental suffering in an attempt to escape the psychiatric gaze, while the terms mental illness and mental disorder are reserved for frameworks applied by governing institutions. To be clear, how one talks about mental health is immanently political. Consequently, beginning with a reflection on our own embeddedness within the current pharmaceutical and bio-medical economy is an important step in understanding the systemic breaking points that prompt our attention to mental distress in the first place (Trivelli 2014). At this stage, our own experience of mental well-being is deeply entwined with neoliberal governance, such that attention to our own subjectivity when working on mental well-being can aid us in developing empathy toward the lives and minds of others who are adversely affected by contemporary socio-economic structures.

Neoliberal personhood and the politics of mental well-being

Research on neoliberalism and mental health has covered a range of themes, such as the governance of healthcare institutions under neoliberal conditions (Rizq 2012, 2014a, b), the impact of neoliberalism in the form of austerity in causing mental distress (Mills 2018), and the production of neoliberal patients (Brijnath and Antoniades 2016) as an outcome of neoliberal governmentality. What these approaches share is a commitment to exposing the potential harms that psychiatric labels, as well as free-market–based models of healthcare, can cause if left unchecked. The advent of neoliberal policies in healthcare systems around the world has – to varying degrees – led to the treatment of patients as customers or consumers (Timimi 2011). Additional consequences have been the preferred use of pharmacological interventions as opposed to holistic healing practices (Esposito and Perez 2014) and the 'fetishization' of bureaucracy as a management approach (Rizq 2014b). Neoliberalism in the context of public health is conceptualized as a set of policy prescriptions that share a commitment to a liberalized market, individualization, and privatization. This chapter now traces some of the effects of neoliberal reforms and policies on mental health(care).

The British National Health Services (NHS) was confronted with a range of neoliberal policy reforms starting in the 1980s, and its current system serves as an example of a public healthcare approach that draws on management strategies usually found in private enterprise. The work by Rizq (2012, 2014a, b) on the state of therapeutic care in primary mental health services in the last ten years poignantly outlines the challenges brought on by an increase in self-management strategies for patients. Writing from a practitioner's perspective, and while working as a psychotherapist for the NHS in England, Rizq (2014a: 211) describes and criticizes the rise of an 'audit culture' for patients and mental health workers alike, which has seen the introduction of performance indicators as the primary determining factor in the allocation of funding for NHS Trusts. With the additional implementation of the indicator-based Improving Access to Psychological Therapies (IAPT) scheme in 2007, there is now a need for more 'accurate' psychiatric diagnoses from psychiatrists and psychotherapists in order to secure access to further mental health services for their patients. While IAPT was framed as a promising scheme that would replace outdated structures of psychiatric and psychological care in the NHS, it relies on the need for an exact psychiatric classification for patients while limiting the scope of help that can be accessed. For example, patients diagnosed with mental illnesses must have a proven record of improvement before further funding can be allocated to the relevant NHS authority. This has given rise to a management approach, which is more concerned with demonstrable (that is, measurable) outcomes than the very complex experiences and recovery journeys of people with mental distress.

This development can be understood as part of the ongoing neoliberal reforms within the NHS since the 1980s, which have served to undermine the potential success of mental healthcare services for a variety of reasons (Rizq 2014b). Most pertinently, there is an emphasis on scores and quality assurances that have constructed the patient as a service-user and/or customer who can (and should) be responsible for her own care. However, this shift from patient to purchaser not only means responsibility for care is shifted from the state to the individual, but also ensures the treatment of illness and suffering is converted into a satisfying and rewarding customer activity (Rizq 2014a: 213).

Clearly, the notion of the patient as a responsible and rational consumer is concurrent with a neoliberal approach, suggesting that well-being is an activity which one can choose to participate in and that its success is dependent on individual agency and initiative.

What is more, since public service and mental healthcare provision are increasingly driven by the private sector logic that prioritizes customer demand, mental health practitioners are now 'subject to intensified surveillance of their work' (Rizq 2012: 10). Self-management practices are rolled out to therapeutic and mental health services staff who are, in turn, held responsible for their performance in improving a patient's well-being, as well as the individual patient (Brijnath and Antoniades 2016). The responsibility for recovery is shifted to the level of the individual at all stages of care. This also leads to a complication of the therapeutic relationship between patient and psychiatric professional in an already wrought and unbalanced context of power and knowledge (Foucault 2006). An emphasis on performance indicators and the pressure of meeting numeric targets can, thus, hinder the provision of mental healthcare where the desire to manage and survey is artificially elevated over the need to care.

In addition, the question that Rizq (2014a: 212) comes to ask is: why 'despite the evident failings of neoliberal policies in the banking system and financial markets, do neoliberal philosophies continue to inform and inflect our public sector services'? One answer to such an important question is that neoliberalism has so deeply embedded itself within our psychologies that rethinking political-economic structures on a grand scale becomes increasingly difficult, precisely because it asks us to assess our own basic assumptions about what we value as a collective.

For example, the production of personhood within neoliberalism emphasizes the need for personal qualities and skills such as entrepreneurship, thriving under pressure, and equating achievement with the ability to consume. In this manner, the perception of ourselves through free-market logics becomes an important determinant of our mental well-being. It is those that thrive 'under competitive conditions' and 'are comfortable displaying these qualities in the context of public scrutiny' who are perceived as achievers (Brooks and Wee 2016: 218). It then comes as little surprise that mental health is dependent not only on the care and welfare that is made available by the state, but also on the type of personhood that is placed as ideal in society. Thus, the reach of neoliberalism extends beyond the boundaries of states, even if it is intimately bound up in public governance, economic policy, and welfare provision. This means that even a 'big' state could be compatible with neoliberalism as the dominant system structuring our realities. It is through the setting of acceptable boundaries of personhood that neoliberalism permeates to our well-being. Critically, unproductivity tends to be less tolerated under neoliberal structures:

> Accordingly, encouraging people to adjust their attitudes, habits, and behaviors to fit market demands is typically associated with functional/rational behavior. Not accepting or failing to become fully integrated into this market reality is, at best, regarded as a type of irrational/unproductive idealism, or, even more typically, associated with personal deviance and/or pathology.
> (Esposito and Perez 2014: 416)

This suggests that welfare claimants or people with disabilities and chronic illnesses fall out of the acceptable boundaries of neoliberal personhood. The association of unproductivity with pathology reminds us of Foucault's (2006: 166) work on psychiatric power in society, in which he draws attention to the disciplining power of psychiatry as 'the agent of reality itself' in its attempt to classify unusual behaviors in a scientific framework. At stake are the boundaries of what can be seen as 'rational' in modern society, a net that is cast rather tightly by neoliberal logics. As long as definitions of 'success' and 'achievement' are equated with material wealth and market productivity, the field of psychiatry offers limited solutions to these problems – be it through psychopharmaceutical intervention or diagnostic frameworks.

Indeed, the increased use of antidepressants and other psychopharmaceuticals for the treatment of diagnosed mental disorders has come under significant academic scrutiny (Timimi 2011; Esposito and Perez 2014) as part of the wider pharmaceuticalization of society (Abraham 2010; Tognetti Bordogna 2014). The concept of 'pharmaceuticalization' refers to a rise in chemical solutions offered for a growing list of issues in everyday life, including those that were not traditionally captured by a medical framework. Pharmaceuticalization has become an object of inquiry for scholars of global public health because of the vested financial interests of the pharmaceutical industry (Whitaker 2011) and its ready acceptance as an aspect of humanitarian intervention (Mills 2016). In the arena of communicable diseases, pharmaceuticalization is revealed to constitute an attempt by governments to 'secure populations pharmaceutically' in the face of 'new fears about our collective vulnerability to underlying microbiological processes', including the threats posed by future pandemics or bioterrorism (Elbe 2014: 924–36). For the treatment of mental distress, the evidence-base for pharmaceutical interventions – particularly for depression – is strikingly thin (Schultz 2015). This means that pharmaceutical intervention – for both communicable and non-communicable diseases – is embedded within the broader political economy of international security, development, and a political desire to secure human well-being.

Making sense of neoliberalism and mental well-being, thus, requires a wide lens that captures the complexity of competing economic interests involved in dealing with mental health.

We cannot dismiss the potential profitability of an ever-expanding – and, therefore, in need of intervention – set of mental disorders co-existing in a global capitalist economy that is based on unsustainable expectations of economic growth. The continuous increase in the prescription of drugs such as Abilify and Sertraline/Zoloft (Flore 2020) for a variety of mental disorders, including psychosis and generalized anxiety disorder, highlights how the chemical compounds of our bodies are posited as 'faults' to be fixed by pharmaceutical intervention.

Crucially, the use of medications for mental diseases not only validates a bio-medical understanding of illness, but also promotes the idea that there is a possible cure for mental disorders. Considering the complexity of mental distress, the ease with which psychopharmaceutical intervention has been normalized in society has given rise to a considerable body of literature investigating the meaning and processes of pharmaceuticalization over recent decades (Abraham 2010; Bell and Figert 2012; Tognetti Bordogna 2014). These contributions have been crucial in mapping theoretical debates about pharmaceuticalization, and reminding us of 'the symbolic and the real value of medication' as an answer to the pathologization of social life (Tognetti Bordogna 2014: 119–20). In the end, the status quo of psychopharmaceutical interventionism in Western societies has had a significant impact on those who refuse to engage in chemical treatments, and who live outside the sphere of 'acceptable' productivity. These people are often met with hostility and faced with paradoxical decisions: not doing anything can be taken as a sign of deviance, whereas choosing to rely on existing welfare systems brings about new forms of stigmatization and discrimination.

Austerity and the psychopolitics of welfare

The aftermath of the 2007–08 Global Financial Crisis has been marked by an increase in austerity-driven politics in Western liberal democracies. Austerity policies are designed to be temporary welfare reforms that mitigate the effects of the crisis. However, austerity as governance has since become the status quo of neoliberal modernity; it is difficult to think of these reforms as anything but a fundamental change in the role of the state from a welfare provider to a welfare denier. At the same time, an increase in suicides has been linked to the advent of austerity. These 'austerity suicides' should be contextualized

> [w]ithin an affective economy of the anxiety caused by punitive welfare retrenchment, the stigmatisation of being a recipient of benefits, and the internalisation of market logics that assigns value through 'productivity' and conceptualises welfare entitlement as economic 'burden'.
>
> (Mills 2018: 302)

In other words, the link between neoliberalism and mental health can be found in reforms that negatively affect the well-being of populations, with suicides as a potential consequence. To be clear, suicides have been identified as one outcome of austerity measures. However, death in relation to welfare reforms can also occur through the denial of essential benefits that force people to work although they are not able to. The key to understanding the link between suicides, mental health, and austerity is to pay attention to the discourse with which these suicides are discussed in the media. For example, even when families are quoted as suggesting that welfare cuts were the reason for a person's suicide or suicide notes naming the British government are found, 'newspaper coverage tends to report individual cases of suicide without making links to the wider pattern of such deaths' (Mills 2018: 304). The tragedy of mental well-being is framed within the context of psychiatric diagnosis, not the wider structural violence or shame that individuals may have experienced. In other words, research has shown that mental distress in an austere economic climate, in conjunction with internalized ideas of achievement, can have a profound impact on the recovery journeys of people.

Therefore, how we choose to talk and know about mental health matters, particularly when faced with a system that normalizes the experience of mental distress, while simultaneously demanding that individuals continue to be productive. However, the experience of mental distress under neoliberalism is linked to a multitude of factors, and not all can be explained by neoliberalism alone; yet, the socially engrained assumptions about acceptable personhood are striking examples of the neoliberal reach. Moreover, the reporting of suicides as an outcome of psychiatric disease, and not of state policies, is aligned with guidance by the World Health Organization, which posits that 'reporting suicidal behavior as an understandable response to social or cultural changes or degradation should be resisted' (WHO 2000, quoted in Mills 2018: 312). This suggests that mental health policy at the global level of governance is an important factor in determining the vocabulary with which mental distress is to be discussed. Nevertheless, there is a risk in depoliticizing the mental distress that emerges under neoliberal structures, because this provides a very narrow framework within which it can be addressed.

As such, another neoliberal approach to mitigate the effects of waning welfare provision is the rise of self-management as a healthcare strategy. Akin to the above discussion on mental health services and professionals by Rizq (2014a, b), Brijnath and Antoniades (2016) have sought to understand how self-management solutions in mental healthcare settings bring about a process of neoliberal subjectification in patients. Their findings show that study participants internalized neoliberal values through unsatisfying encounters with Australian healthcare services, which clearly directed patients toward absolving the state from its responsibilities. They 'neither talked about their right to state services nor about familial, social nor work reforms' and, instead, 'perceived that change needed to occur only within them for their depression to improve' (Brijnath and Antoniades 2016: 6). Even though all 58 of the study's interviewees initially sought help for depression from a GP, a psychiatrist, or social worker, the majority found it too difficult to navigate the healthcare system. Patients were told that the responsibility for finding adequate care (including the changing of providers) was theirs, but there was a consensus among the interviewees that it was nearly impossible to find affordable mental healthcare, particularly regular access to talking therapy.

Consequently, self-medication and self-care become preferred methods by individuals in neoliberal societies (see also: Trivelli 2014), and care proceeds without the involvement of healthcare professionals. Brijnath and Antoniades (2016) conclude that the participants were trained in self-management techniques by healthcare professionals that instructed patients to seek their own therapist, make appointments, manage their finances, and follow certain drug regimes. These neoliberal notions of responsibility and risk lead to a subjectification of the individual who, through the passing of responsibility from the provider to patient, undertakes the labor to manage herself and no longer expects the state to perform this task. Consequently, the figure of the neoliberal patient emerges successfully and clearly as an entity, which has internalized a responsibility for self-management.

At all levels – whether it be service provision at the structural level, the management of patients, or the psyche of individuals – a strong correlation between neoliberal logics and mental well-being can be observed. While there are some contestations in the literature about how research can be more inclusive of those who identify as mental health service-users or psychiatric system survivors (*e.g.* Cosgrove and Karter 2018), a broad consensus about the negative effects of neoliberalism has emerged. In particular, the slow erosion of comprehensive welfare provision (including austerity), the privatization of healthcare, and the advent of measurement-driven frameworks of the very definition of success are core aspects of neoliberal governance, which stand out in relation to the poor mental health of populations. In addition to the above examples, a growing body of literature draws attention to the harmful effects of racism and persistence of colonialism (Davar 2014; Mills 2014) on the mental well-being of people in non-Western countries. It is, thus, important to contextualize critiques of neoliberalism and its impact on mental health within an intersectional endeavor that equally prioritizes the rights and struggles of other social justice movements, such as Black Lives Matter, the Disability Rights Movement, and Mad Pride.

The pitfalls of governing mental well-being through public health campaigns

The global increase in diagnosable mental illnesses has been met with a variety of attempts to govern their economic impact, including the emergence of anti-stigma and mental health awareness programs. These campaigns constitute an interesting example of neoliberal governance, because they appear to work in favor of those with mental distress. However, a variety of criticisms (Jacob and Skinner 2015; Grey 2016; Tyler and Slater 2018) have emerged in recent years, directing us to question the legitimacy with which these programs can address mental health problems.

For example, Jacob and Skinner (2015) provide a critical reading of the 2010 Canadian *Defeat Denial* campaign, in which they examined how the mental health awareness intervention conveyed its message about mental illness to the public. The specific focus of the program was to provide an explanation of the nature of mental illness to the public, assuming that this would serve to 'correct' any misunderstandings. The authors (Jacob and Skinner 2015: 6) found that the language used by the campaign framed mental illness as a 'disruption in the brain circuitry', deeming the brain to be the source and site of mental illness. This powerful invocation of an imagery of mental illness as a 'flawed' brain was demonstrated to then reaffirm bio-medical hegemony in public discourse on mental health. The paradox of this is that the negative label attached to mental illness, and which anti-stigma campaigns seek to address, is rearticulated through this bio-medical framing of distress. In this case, the focus on individual brain anatomy has a profound impact on societal attitudes toward those diagnosed with a mental disorder, and wider implications for how we rationalize our own existence.

If mental distress is understood within the bio-medical framework of psychiatry, then obvious solutions are also aimed at the level of individual biology. This is where social determinants of mental distress, such as those introduced in the section above, are willfully excluded in favor of psychiatric explanations. A cycle develops where neoliberal modes of governance are continuously excused as potential causes or sources of perpetuation for mental distress, and psychiatric knowledge is prioritized as an explanatory framework which, in turn, prompts solutions that are pharmaceutical (Esposito and Perez 2014) and/or aimed at changing individual behavior (Tomlinson and Kelly 2013). Further, individualization through pathologization is aided by the normalized use of psychopharmaceuticals as a principal mode of intervention, because this frames the microbiological makeup of our brains and bodies as principal sites of ills. In this manner, individuals become burdened with the experience of mental distress, as well as the responsibility to recover or cope with the situation.

Moreover, public health interventions aimed at improving mental well-being often attempt to evoke empathy in the public as part of their messaging, but there is a problem when benevolence reaffirms problematic labels around mental illness. This point is made by Grey (2016), whose research in Australia encompassed the collection of a variety of texts, such as posters or advertisements on billboards, which he encountered in his everyday life, and which portray people with mental illnesses in a positive light. Grey argues that these texts constitute a form of 'benevolent othering' (2016: 241). In 2008, *Mind Australia*, a government-funded mental health organization, ran a poster campaign with the aim of challenging the stigma around mental illness. Simultaneously, it encouraged people to donate to *Mind* by directly speaking to the person viewing the poster – which read: 'Show that you care' – while depicting people covering their faces with their hands, hunched over on the floor, and 'crumpled' (Grey 2016: 242). These campaign posters, thus, offer a visual representation of people with mental illnesses as unable to cope or desperate. In order 'to be able to position itself as benevolent, *Mind* requires a needy other, one to whom benevolence can be given – people that *Mind* can help "recover"' (Grey 2016: 244).

In other words, the visual representation of people suffering from mental distress as part of public health promotion matters, insofar as it constructs identities through which those diagnosed with a mental illness can be portrayed as helpless and in need of aid, while service providers and donors are rendered as giving or benevolent. Hence, Grey's (2016) concept of benevolent othering can be a useful tool in approaching a critique of anti-stigma campaigns, because it helps conceptualize how those diagnosed with a mental illness and their experiences of distress are framed in particular ways, which then serve to construct a narrative about the nature of mental illness. The knowledge about personhood and disease that is produced in this manner associates mental distress with an abnormal and debilitating state of being. This is not to say that mental distress is not a debilitating condition, but rather to question whether distress could not be conceptualized as a rational response to adverse (austerity-driven) circumstances. Asking such questions about the purpose and effect of anti-stigma campaigns is important when assessing the political economy of mental healthcare, because it prompts deeper reflection on the political strategies that become available to policymakers and mental health advocates.

Finally, critical accounts of the concept of stigma, as deployed in mental health anti-stigma campaigns, reveal their association with social constructions of public attitudes and shame in relation to help-seeking (Tyler and Slater 2018). While anti-stigma campaigns tend to emphasize the need for people to become resilient, to practice self-care, and to seek conversations about their mental distress, this once again leverages responsibility at the level of the individual. Reminding us of self-management approaches (Rizq 2014a; Brijnath and Antoniades 2016), public health campaigning can be complicit in furthering neoliberal agendas that individualize responsibility. Despite evidence that stigma can be used as a tool of technology and that structural forms of stigma persist in excluding and labeling those deemed as undesirable (Tyler 2020), the apparent benevolence of anti-stigma campaigns makes them appear as bottom-up movements. Even if talking about mental distress can lessen some social stigma

> [a]nti-stigma initiatives which want to remove barriers to help-seeking, but that do not simultaneously address *either* the erosion of public service provision *or* the deeper social causes of increased levels of mental distress, will be limited in their impact.
>
> (Tyler and Slater 2018: 726, original emphases)

Ultimately, critical research on anti-stigma campaigns and wellness advocacy allows us to see how interdisciplinary approaches to the study of mental health and neoliberalism can successfully divert our gaze from ostensibly unassuming public health interventions. In this manner, something that initially appears as unquestionably good – raising awareness about mental illness and the alleviation of stigma – is revealed as a potentially dangerous tool for normalizing mental distress under neoliberal structures.

Conclusion: resisting the pathologization of mental distress

The key takeaway from this chapter is that neoliberal problems have generated, unfortunately, neoliberal solutions. As such, if the experience of mental distress under austerity politics is understood to be the symptom of a mental illness, then we risk omitting the structural effects and harms of neoliberalism. Where mental well-being has become a core aspect of governance for the state, research has shown that interventions are usually designed to change 'behaviors, rather than institutions, distributions and regulations' (Tomlinson and Kelly 2013: 151). This individualized approach, reminiscent of behavioral economics, is not only a sign of neoliberal logic, but it also perpetuates the bias of psychiatric knowledge to seek out solutions in a person's biology. The consequence of this is that structural concerns are willfully dismissed as drivers of mental distress, and social determinants are less likely to become the object of intervention. Where the individual body is both the facilitator of economic labor and the potential 'at-risk' site of (mental) disease, we can also spot the limitations of a neoliberal approach to political economy. It appears that an ever-present structural demand for economic growth and the erosion of welfare systems are unsustainable, given the rise in reported mental distress worldwide. However, through the creation of a mental wellness and awareness-driven industry, neoliberalism has become adaptable as a system that is far more than

> [s]imply a market economy, neoliberalism demands a *market society*, where definitions of normal, sane, and illness are determined primarily by market considerations that are conceived by large segments of the population as akin to natural law.
>
> (Esposito and Perez 2014: 432–3, original emphases)

It is through the normalization of expectations and measures of success that we can witness how neoliberalism and our mental well-being are intimately linked. This is why scholars concerned with mental health survivor-driven research (Cohen *et al.* 2018; see also: Cosgrove and Karter 2018) have argued that 'nothing short of an intellectual-insurgency needs to be deployed, spearheaded by a massive dosage of critical thinking' (Cohen *et al.* 2018: 192). The space that needs to be carved for counter-hegemonic thinking in relation to mental health also draws us to a radical rethinking of economic structures. Taking a critical political economy approach can, thus, address issues of neoliberal healthcare, especially if it remains skeptical about a bio-medical model that uses mental illness as an explanation for social ills or unwanted behaviors and, instead, focuses on the strengthening of social welfare structures.

What type of economic reforms can we imagine that would counter the ease with which mental distress becomes pathologized? As a first step, we need to consider how neoliberal logic determines not only our economic systems, but also our everyday encounters with ourselves and our own psyches. This means heeding the warning of scholars (Foucault 2006; Fanon 2008) who have shown how socio-political interests reflect on the development of scientific knowledge and the parameters with which normality is established in contemporary societies. While the boundaries of rationality and a 'healthy mind' might shift over time, their movement is deeply entwined with the needs of the global political economy. Attending to these definitions with a historicizing and interdisciplinary approach reveals the complexity of the systems of knowledge that are at stake. Future work might consider how the demands of an economic system based on growth and individual accomplishments can be balanced with the need to foster empathy and compassion for all (and beyond) humans, including ourselves.

References

Abraham, J. 2010, 'Pharmaceuticalization of society in context: Theoretical, empirical and health dimensions', *Sociology*, 44(4), pp. 603–22.

Bashford, A. 2004, *Imperial Hygiene: A Critical History of Colonialism, Nationalism and Public Health*, Palgrave Macmillan, London.

Bell, S.E. and Figert, A.E. 2012, 'Medicalization and pharmaceuticalization at the intersections: Looking backward, sideways and forward', *Social Science and Medicine*, 75(5), pp. 775–83.

Brijnath, B. and Antoniades, J. 2016, '"I am running my depression:" Self-management of depression in neoliberal Australia', *Social Science and Medicine*, 152, pp. 1–8.

Brooks, A. and Wee, L. 2016, 'The cultural production of consumption as achievement', *Cultural Politics*, 12(2), pp. 217–32.

Cohen, B.M.Z. (ed.) 2018, *Routledge International Handbook of Critical Mental Health*, Routledge, Abingdon.

Cohen, D., Gomory, T. and Kirk, S.A. 2018, 'The attributes of mad science', in Cohen, B. (ed), *Routledge International Handbook of Critical Mental Health*, Routledge, Abingdon, pp. 186–94.

Collin, J. 2015, 'Universal cures for idiosyncratic illnesses: A genealogy of therapeutic reasoning in the mental health field', *Health: An Interdisciplinary Journal for the Social Study of Health, Illness and Medicine*, 19(3), pp. 245–62.

Cosgrove, L. and Karter, J.M. 2018, 'The poison in the cure: Neoliberalism and contemporary movements in mental health', *Theory and Psychology*, 28(5), pp. 669–83.

Davar, B. 2014, 'Globalizing psychiatry and the case of "vanishing" alternatives in a neo-colonial state', *Disability and the Global South*, 1(2), pp. 266–84.

Davies, J. 2017, *The Sedated Society: The Causes and Harms of our Psychiatric Drug Epidemic*, Palgrave Macmillan, Basingstoke.

Davies, W. 2016, 'Externalist psychiatry,' *Analysis*, 76(3), pp. 290–296.

Elbe, S. 2014, 'The pharmaceuticalisation of security: Molecular biomedicine, antiviral stockpiles, and global health security', *Review of International Studies*, 40(5), pp. 919–38.

Esposito, L. and Perez, F.M. 2014, 'Neoliberalism and the commodification of mental health', *Humanity and Society*, 38(4), pp. 313–42.

Fanon, F. 2008 [1952], *Black Skin, White Masks*, Grove Press, New York.

Faulkner, A. 2017, 'Survivor research and mad studies: The role and value of experiential knowledge in mental health research', *Disability and Society*, 32(4), pp. 500–20.

Fernando, S. 2017, *Institutional Racism in Psychiatry and Clinical Psychology: Race Matters in Mental Health*, Palgrave Macmillan, London.

Flore, J. 2020, 'Ingestible sensors, data, and pharmaceuticals: Subjectivity in the era of digital mental health', *New Media and Society*, 23(7), pp. 2034–51.

Foucault, M. 2006, *Psychiatric Power, Lectures at the Collège de France, 1973–43*, translation by Graham Burchell, Palgrave Macmillan, Basingstoke.

Grey, F. 2016, 'Benevolent othering: Speaking positively about mental health service users', *Philosophy, Psychiatry, and Psychology*, 23(3–4), pp. 241–51.

Jacob, J.D. and Skinner, E. 2015, 'Exposing the expert discourse in psychiatry: A critical analysis of an anti-stigma/mental illness awareness campaign', *Aporia*, 7(1), pp. 5–16.

Mills, C. 2014, *Decolonizing Global Mental Health: The Psychiatrization of the Majority World*, Routledge, Abingdon.

Mills, C. 2016, 'Mental health and the mindset of development', in Grugel, J. and Hammett, D. (eds), *The Palgrave Handbook of International Development*, Palgrave Macmillan, London, pp. 535–54.

Mills, C. 2018, '"Dead people don't claim": A psychopolitical autopsy of UK austerity suicides', *Critical Social Policy*, 38(2), pp. 302–22.

Ramon, S. 2008, 'Neoliberalism and its implications for mental health in the UK', *International Journal of Law and Psychiatry*, 31(2), pp. 116–35.

Rizq, R. 2012, 'The perversion of care: Psychological therapies in time of IAPT', *Psychodynamic Practice*, 18(1), pp. 7–24.

Rizq, R. 2014a, 'Perversion, neoliberalism and therapy: The adult culture in mental health services', *Psychoanalysis, Culture and Society*, 19(2), pp. 209–18.

Rizq, R. 2014b, 'Perverting the course of therapy: The fetishisation of governance in public sector mental health services', *Psychoanalytic Psychotherapy*, 28(3), pp. 249–66.

Schultz, W. 2015, 'The chemical imbalance hypothesis: An evaluation of the evidence', *Ethical Human Psychology and Psychiatry*, 17(1), pp. 60–75.

Teghtsoonian, K. 2009, 'Depression and mental health in neoliberal times: A critical analysis of policy discourse', *Social Science and Medicine*, 69(1), pp. 28–35.

Timimi, S. 2011, 'Globalising mental health: A neo-liberal project', *Ethnicity and Inequalities in Health and Social Care*, 4(30), pp. 155–60.

Tognetti Bordogna, M. 2014, 'From medicalization to pharmaceuticalization: A sociological overview – New scenarios for the sociology of health', *Social Change Review*, 14(2), pp. 119–40.

Tomlinson, M.W. and Kelly, G.P. 2013, 'Is everybody happy? Politics and measurement of national well-being', *Policy and Politics*, 41(2), pp. 139–57.

Trivelli, E. 2014, 'Depression, performativity and the conflicted body: An auto-ethnography of self-medication', *Subjectivity*,7, pp. 151–70.

Tseris, E. 2018, 'Biomedicine, neoliberalism and the pharmaceuticalisation of society', in Cohen, B. (ed), *Routledge International Handbook of Critical Mental Health*, Routledge, Abingdon, pp. 169–76.

Tyler, I. 2020, *Stigma: The Machinery of Inequality*, Zed Books, London.

Tyler, I. and Slater, T. 2018, 'Rethinking the sociology of stigma', *The Sociological Review Monographs*, 66(4), pp. 721–43.Voronka, J. 2019, 'The mental health peer worker as informant: Performing authenticity and the paradoxes of passing', *Disability and Society*, 34(4), pp. 564–82.

Whitaker, R. 2011, *Anatomy of an Epidemic: Magic Bullets, Psychiatric Drugs, and the Astonishing Rise of Mental Illness in America*, Random House, New York.

World Bank Group. 2016, *Out of the Shadows: Making Mental Health a Global Development Priority*, accessed 29 July 2021 <http://documents1.worldbank.org/curated/en/270131468187759113/pdf/105052-WP-PUBLIC-wb-background-paper.pdf>.

14

OCCUPATIONAL HEALTH AND SAFETY IN THE GLOBAL GARMENT INDUSTRY

Patrick Neveling

Capacious and critical academic writing about occupational health and safety (OH&S) in the global textile and garment (TG) industry builds on a historical-realist perspective (Smith 2014). First, a historical evaluation of this industry is important as a means to identify continuities and changes in OH&S, particularly as production sites have moved around the globe since the onset of the Industrial Revolution. Accordingly, researchers can link historical and contemporary developments in TG manufacturing – from fin de siècle New York to the bonded warehouses and export processing zones of Twenty-First Century Bangladesh – via the red threads of sweatshop manufacturing, races to the bottom in labor standards and rights, government support for webs of subcontracting located in the shadow economy, and deadly industrial disasters (Bair *et al.* 2017). Second, a realist perspective (Porter 1993) directs critical attention to actually existing workplace conditions. It transcends pro-capitalist developmentalist narratives portraying particular stages of capitalist exploitation in the industry as 'transitional' and, thus, soon to be replaced with decent work and wages. Such fictions have been amplified by many commentaries within the social sciences, as they locate the crucibles of health and safety at the scale of the individual worker and/or the individual factory (see: Barab 2006). In this, they either echo corporate management claims about workers making poor lifestyle choices that affect their workplace performance and safety. In a similar vein, they reaffirm claims from TG sector umbrella organizations that OH&S problems have arisen from the actions of a few 'bad (corporate) apples', running counter to an otherwise diligently managed industry with ample scrutiny of its supply chains.

This chapter builds on such historical and realist insights to remind readers that abuse and extreme exploitation of workers have underpinned global TG production since British machine-made products flooded Asian markets in the 1800s, thereby destroying Indian, Chinese, and Japanese garment industries (Wolf 1997 [1982]: 251). One thrust of this approach is to invert mainstream structural-functionalist and symbolic-interactionist sociology of health paradigms centered on individuals and their well-being. According to the former, societies positively sanction ill-health individuals as long as they accept a 'sick role' that obliges them to follow expert advice for recovery (Parsons 1951; *cf.* Doyal and Pennell 1979). Shifting the analysis of health in general, and OH&S in particular, from the individual scale to that of an industrial sector firmly embedded in the capitalist world system, the chapter reviews the TG industry's sickening impact on hundreds of millions of workers over two centuries. Factory owners and corporations in this industry have

DOI: 10.4324/9781003017110-16

repeatedly refused to accept recommendations from commissions of public enquiry, labor rights groups, United Nations agencies, academics, and many others on how to improve OH&S (War on Want 1985 [1984]; Boris 2003; Prentice and de Neve 2017). As such, the TG industry analyzed in this chapter stands as emblematic of the overall social and planetary destruction by capitalist industrial manufacturing.

The following *longue durée* analysis of (the lack of) OH&S in the TG industry revisits key academic publications on its global historical development since around 1800, before identifying opportunities for future research on the spatio-temporal configurations erected to secure capital accumulation and worker exploitation in the sector. The emphasis throughout the chapter is on linking topical literature on TG sector health and safety (avoidance) strategies with a critical political-economic analysis of capitalism.

The rise of textile and garment sweatshops after the Industrial Revolution

Humans have made textiles and clothing for thousands of years. From protection to decoration and, later, fashion, textiles and clothing have always been central to everyday life, rituals, myths, religious beliefs, and social order (Riello and Parthasarathi 2009: 1–2). The Old Testament begins with a story about human desire and covering body parts with plant products. Buddhist and Hindu monks made robes from discarded fabric in early practices of TG recycling. As empires rose and fell, spinning, weaving, dyeing, and other production techniques spread around the globe. In the 1500s, cotton textiles became 'the first global commodity'. The Indian subcontinent initially dominated all production steps, from cotton and hemp agriculture to spinning, weaving, finishing, and global export. As Eric Hobsbawm (1999 [1968]) emphasized, the Eighteenth Century British imperial expansion targeted global domination in textile spinning and garment manufacturing and, thus, laid the grounds for the Industrial Revolution in England.

Textile and garment workers in the British Empire

The rapid ascent of the British TG industry during the late-Eighteenth and Nineteenth Centuries was, in large part, buttressed by the rapid expansion of British imperialism during this period and marked by various forms of political-economic violence at home and across the Empire. With the violent destruction of burgeoning global competition, imposition of import restrictions on Indian textiles to Britain, and enforced opening of South Asian and other markets for British produce, the British Empire laid the foundations for capitalist anti-markets as vehicles of economic policy in subsequent centuries. These processes also engendered the systematic super-exploitation of workers along the global supply chains for textiles and garments – from cotton harvesting, cleaning, transport, shipping, spinning, and weaving, to packaging and transport. Along these segments of the supply chains, uprisings were brutally quashed in the Peterloo Massacre in Manchester in 1819 and in the violent response to the Indian Mutiny in 1857, for example. Simultaneously, the British ruling classes developed elaborate ideologies to misrepresent working-class populations across the Empire as undeserving, ungrateful, lazy, deceitful and, ultimately, responsible for their own poverty (Wolf 1997 [1982]: 251). Within Britain itself, building on long-standing efforts to tarnish the discontented working-classes in Britain as the 'undeserving poor', the 1834 *Poor Law Amendment Act* codified Thomas Malthus' presumption that the poor would reproduce exponentially faster than agricultural and other resources could replenish themselves. With vagrancy now a public offense, the rural and urban poor were forced into workhouses planned and designed in the panopticon style of Jeremy Bentham, and purposed to supplement the reserve army of labor for capital (Hobsbawm and Rudé 1969).

William Blake's (1808) famous poetic reflections on the 'dark satanic mills' of the Industrial Revolution may have been aimed at the Albion flour mills of the last decade of the Eighteenth Century. Contemporaneous handloom weavers-turned-luddites, however, developed similar feelings about the steam-powered cotton spinning mills springing up across Britain and soon after in India, the United States of America, and across the globe in later waves of industrialization. In the revolutionary decades of the 1800s and 1900s, workers in the globalizing TG industry spearheaded organized strike actions. Perhaps most prominently, the origins of what has come to be known as 'International (Working) Women's Day' can be traced back to a mass walkout of female garment workers in New York in March of 1857, as well as the strike of female textile workers in Petrograd during February and March of 1917, which helped precipitate the Russian Revolution. In memory of the latter, Clara Zetkin established 8 March as a Communist holiday in 1922. Although a subsequent United Nations declaration on International Women's Day ignored the impact of socialism, it acknowledged the key role of garment workers during the late-Nineteenth and early-Twentieth Centuries in the fight for women's rights (Kaplan 1985).

Such industrial actions were a response, at least in part, to the poor working conditions prevailing within the TG industry. Reflecting on these circumstances, for instance, an International Labour Office (ILO 1983: 17–24) handbook, *Accident Prevention: A Workers' Education Manual*, includes a chapter on 'the origins of accident prevention' that sheds light on the feeble OH&S conditions prevailing within the TG industry as a pioneering sector in industrial capitalism. It details how, as the sector took off in the late-1700s, demand for cheap labor targeted pauper children, who had to work 14 to 15 hours per day in crowded factories filled with dirt, pollution from fibers, and constant noise from ever-accelerating machinery. Analogously, Jamie Bronstein's (2008: 14–5) monograph on workplace accidents in Nineteenth Century Britain describes how different work tasks exposed workers to accidents – from sweeping floors and being caught in the 'giant metal jaws of spinning mules', to clothing or hair caught in unguarded belts that transmitted power from steam or water. Indeed, the British Parliament received reports of accident-to-worker ratios of 1:176 for the cotton industry and 1:230 for the wool industry as late as 1870, despite repeated Royal Commissions reporting on the lack of OH&S across the sector since 1833.

Writing in 1844 about *The Condition of the English Working Class* based on two years of research in Manchester, Friedrich Engels (2009 [1892]) observed that there were so many cripples among the inhabitants of Manchester that it was 'like living in the midst of an army just returned from a campaign'. The *Factory Act of 1844* codified safeguards for machines and protection of workers, as well as inspections and accident reporting, in British law. The above-mentioned ILO handbook published in 1983 declares this a victory of public policy and political pressure groups campaigning against the refusal of mill owners to take responsibility for health and safety provisions, especially for young workers (International Labour Office 1983: 18). Yet, this depiction ignores the broader role of workers' uprisings and other revolutionary movements in the Nineteenth Century in pressing the British Parliament and capitalists to grant such concessions (Moos 2021).

Continental European and North American working conditions

The ILO handbook (1983: 20–2) dates early recommendations for medical and safety inspections in some German kingdoms to the 1830s, with binding legislation arising in Prussia, Saxony, and Bavaria from around 1872. The same sequence is evident in France for 1841 and 1893, while binding legislation for Denmark and Switzerland dates back to 1873 and 1877, respectively. The Kingdom of Belgium was an outlier, with an 1810 Napoleonic-era Imperial Decree protecting against dangerous and unhealthy undertakings. In the US, federal states had the power to legislate.

Massachusetts, in the northeastern heartlands of the TG industry, led the way with an Act on the prevention of accidents in factories in 1877, and a requirement for reporting accidents in 1886. New York, Rhode Island, and other federal states with significant industrial activity, foremost in textiles and garments, followed prior to the fin de siècle era. Along with health and safety regulations, private-sector insurance companies mushroomed and offered tailored cover for TG employers' legal liabilities. Soon, insurance companies sent out their own inspectors to workplaces. In the first half of the Twentieth Century, voluntary manufacturers' associations formed at the national scale in Europe and North America, Asia (Japanese Industrial Welfare Society 1928; Safety First Association of India 1931), and Latin America (Cuban National Safety Council 1936).

In this context, the term 'sweatshop' emerged in public policy debates and parliamentary inquiries on OH&S that supported the demand for binding legislation. TG work by women and immigrants was termed 'sweated' from the 1830s, when a mass market for ready-made garments (RMG) took shape. Investigations by the US House of Representatives and the British House of Lords into the 'sweating system' accorded the term 'sweatshop' common, transatlantic usage (Bender and Greenwald 2003: 4–6). Despite these transatlantic origins, New York's Lower East Side is today framed as the birthplace of what Alessandra Mezzadri (2017) has poignantly identified as a 'sweatshop regime', marked by super-exploitative and abusive labor relations that also include modern slavery (Bair *et al.* 2017). Mid-to-late-Nineteenth Century New York was an ideal location for the most violent ignorance of OH&S, as the low capital-to-labor ratio of its RMG sector could feed on immigrants vulnerable to the rags-to-riches stories pervading depictions of the American Dream (Soyer 1999).

Early US industrialization in the textile sector had been closely linked to UK developments, first via technology transfers and then by immigration of skilled workers – mostly handloom weavers – eager to escape power-loom industrialization once Britain allowed the emigration of skilled workers in 1824 (Van Vugt 1999: 64–6). The cradle of RMG production in Britain was military uniforms. Army bureaucracies standardized sizes and, hence, paved the way for mass production of standardized garments. Early industrialization of textile manufacturing depended on the invention of spinning jennies and steam-powered weaving tables. RMG industrialization hinged on another ground-breaking technology: the rise of Singer sewing machines suitable for industrial production in the 1860s. Importantly, the sector has not subsequently seen more recent major technological innovations after spinning jennies, power looms, and industrial sewing machines consolidated RMG manufacturing. This is one reason why capitalist competition in the TG sector is manifest foremost in the search for ever-cheaper labor – mostly from female workers controlled by a few male workers at higher wage rates – and not by the increased capitalization for technological innovation that is characteristic of some other industrial sectors (Godley 1997). The *absence of investment in technological innovation* is, thus, the first constant spatio-temporal feature determining OH&S in the TG sector.

Consolidating the sweatshops in praxis and ideology

Early US RMG mass production set the stage for three additional spatio-temporal features that have kept the contemporary TG industry trapped in the sweatshop phase of unhealthy and unsafe working conditions, both globally and in the *longue durée*. New York's rise to the world's RMG capital was initially driven by the demand for cheap clothing for enslaved workers on plantations in the southern states. In the late-1800s, cotton production helped turn the US into the world's largest exporter of cotton textiles. After the US Civil War, industrial production expanded into mass consumer markets, consolidating the happy-consumer image of US workers content with capitalist exploitation. Until this day, the *undervalued and unsafe labor of millions of exploited workers* constitutes the sector's second spatio-temporal feature. This secures a steady flow of surplus cheap textiles and garments for the world's consumer markets, thereby keeping consumers' costs of living down and, accordingly, allowing for wage cuts across other sectors.

The third spatio-temporal feature is the *division of labor* that emerged in New York's Lower East Side. Well into the 1920s, mass production stayed close to the display rooms of so-called jobbers, who subcontracted bulk orders to contractors, and then hired laborers – mostly female immigrants from southern and eastern Europe – on a piece-rate basis. Bair *et al.* (2017: 32) state that 'contracting was the core organizing principle of the apparel industry' by the 1880s, with the majority of cloak-houses and, later, warehouses preferring an 'outside system' where jobbers had contractors competing for orders, all to the detriment of workers' wages and safety. Output more than doubled from US$32 million in 1883 to US$68 million in 1885. Average weekly wages fell from US$15 to US$6 during the same short period. The three-tier structure with the contractors between jobbers and workers made direct complaints impossible. Workers organized and formed the International Ladies Garment Workers Union (ILGWU), a key trade union that would exert global influence for more than 100 years.

As the sector expanded, high rises not built for large-scale industrial manufacturing turned into shop floors. New York's largest garment manufacturer, the Triangle Shirtwaist Company (TSC), ran a factory on the three upper floors of the ten-story Asch building in Manhattan. TSC female workers organized in the ILGWU and demanded safer working conditions and better wages in a mass walkout in 1909, supported by the wealthy members of the Women's Trade Union League. The dispute dragged on for years. In 1911, a fire broke out in the Asch building, leading to 146 of 500 workers losing their lives – many of whom jumped out of windows when fire ladders could not reach the upper floors. Other victims were buried under collapsing fire escapes unfit for the use of the building as a factory. The disaster consolidated the organizational power of the ILGWU and its support by some wealthy New Yorkers. Yet, it took until 1933 for the New Deal-era *National Industry Recovery Act* (*NIRA*) to sink the 'outside system' and establish a firm link between (sub-) contracting and unionization via the so-called jobbers' agreement, which successfully reduced wage-driven competition between contractors into the 1980s and across the US (Bair *et al.* 2017: 41).

While workers fought against sweatshop wages and working conditions, *racialized capitalism* arose as the fourth spatio-temporal feature in a globalizing TG industry. The racialization of capitalist exploitation in the sector was facilitated by the entry of social Darwinism into the discipline of economics (see: Halliday 1971: 396–7; Hofstadter 2016 [1944]: 143–56). In the US, this facilitated an ideology that blamed the 'race' of workers themselves for the working conditions they endured and, thereby, sought to disguise capitalist exploitation as the guarantor of sweatshops. Such prescriptions claimed that the workforce, primarily comprising Jewish immigrants, were at fault for the ills of the sector. Sweatshops were driving 'American' factories out of the business. Conversely, inspectors fashioned themselves as 'protectors of civilization' against the Jewish workers' 'low racial status', which was held to confer on them a preference for individualistic, piece-rate work, and acceptance of unsafe working conditions that were spreading 'contagious diseases' (Bender 2003: 23–5). Immigrant workers, instead, forcefully resisted such racialized explanations for the sweatshop. When they had the opportunity to testify before public enquiries, they pointed to the responsibility of contractors and jobbers for factories without sufficient light and ventilation. Moreover, such enquiries revealed that competition between businesses and associated efforts to bolster profits via increased labor exploitation often manifest in employers paying immigrant workers wages so low that, in order to subsist, workers had to take work home to be completed by other household members (Bender 2003: 27–8).

Sweatshops and the rise of neoliberal globalization

Government legislation for health and safety, the entry of insurance companies and their investigators, and the rise of trade unions all helped improve OH&S for TG workers in the heartlands of the capitalist world system before the Second World War. The rise of socialist and anarchist movements, in conjunction with trade unions, gave workers a voice and means to collectively bargain for higher wages and safer workplaces. Capitalists' fear of successful working-class uprisings akin to the Russian Revolution, alongside the rapid economic development of the Soviet Union in the 1930s, buttressed these push factors and helped workers win social welfare and social policy concessions as a means to quell potential industrial unrest. This trend continued after the Second World War, leading many scholars to characterize the immediate post-War period as marked by a tripartite industrial entente. This structure lasted until the 1970s, when large-scale relocations from the industrial heartlands of capitalism to countries in the Global South globalized sweatshops and, thus, created a new international division of labor (Froebel *et al.* 1981; Rosen 2002).

Pertinently, the concessions won in the inter-War period did not apply to all workers in the Global North, nor were they immune to capital's drive to sustain the sweatshop-driven 'sick role' of the TG sector via unsafe and unhealthy working conditions. Of the labor unrests discussed so far, only the female textile workers of Petrograd engendered a structural expropriation of capitalists. All other successes manifest in Polanyian 'double-movements' (Silver 2003) – incremental and *post facto* reforms designed to protect society against the excesses of the capitalist market – that were, from the 1970s onward, largely unable to withstand the neoliberal '*counter* double-movement' promulgated by capital against such measures (Blyth 2003: 5). In the context of the crisis of post-War capitalism during the 1970s, TG employers in the US sought to circumvent the rising bargaining power of workers and national legislation codifying OH&S. In particular, they relocated their factories to southern states with laxer legislation and lower unionization rates, or employed new immigrants from Puerto Rico and other US colonies to break unionization in the north of the country. Detailed case-studies of northeastern manufacturing cities highlight further that employers used periods of low economic growth in the 1920s and 1950, and again in the 1970s, to push for rollbacks of (female) workers' rights and OH&S (Koistinen 2013). TG manufacturers in the Federal Republic of Germany (FRG) employed similar counter-movement tactics, with abysmal treatment of the so-called *Gastarbeiter* from southern Europe, hired since the 1950s to top up the national workforce after millions were killed under Nazi rule (Herbert 1990).

The rise of SEZs as new sweatshop locations

The four spatio-temporal features of exploitation and capitalist accumulation in the TG sector detailed above continued to dominate as the sector globalized from the 1930s onward. From the late-1940s, this dominance increasingly benefitted from the rise of export processing zones (EPZs) and special economic zones (SEZs) as the new locations for competition among countries over foreign investment and export-oriented industrialization in the era of decolonization and the Cold War (Neveling 2017). Rather than investing in technology to maintain or increase profit margins and secure OH&S, employers in the sector preferred mass layoffs and relocations to low-wage, low-unionization regions and postcolonial countries. The sector's racialized capitalism targeted new immigrant populations in Western nations after 1945, and projected this ideological configuration onto workers in postcolonial nations. Workers in former colonies were represented as inherently less productive, while Orientalist and sexist discourse claimed that women in Malaysia, Mauritius, Mexico, and elsewhere across the globe were ideal workers for RMG factories because of their 'nimble fingers'. Simultaneously, right-wing national governments declared that these female workers were undeserving of minimum wages because they were only supplementing household income from male breadwinners (Safa 1995; Neveling 2021).

In terms of production technologies, the globalization of the sector relied on Nineteenth Century innovations. Singer and other industrial sewing machines had facilitated mass production of RMG in countries like Mexico from the 1860s (de la Cruz-Fernández 2015). In the 1930s, the growing number of department stores drove the mass consumer revolution in leading capitalist countries. These stores were the first large-scale buyers on international markets and transnationalized New York's subcontracting system. Jobbers now sourced internationally: subcontracting embroidery and sewing work to Western colonies and newly independent nations that, from the 1960s, became mass suppliers for Western markets with millions of workers in SEZ factories.

Puerto Rico, a US colony, was one of the early locations for the globalization of the TG sector (Neveling 2015a). Ailing from centuries of Spanish rule and an onslaught of US agricultural trusts that rapidly dispossessed small cane planters into a landless urban proletariat, needlework industries producing for mainland department stores became the island's largest employer by the 1930s. The implementation of New Deal legislation and welfare in Puerto Rico (which included the *NIRA*) curbed mass strikes of female workers in urban sweatshops, but did little to ease the pressure on rural households embroidering textiles and garments at home for subcontractors. Local government legislation, backed by the US Treasury and supported by a Boston-based consulting corporation, established the world's first SEZ-style export-oriented development regime from 1947. Several new government agencies and a development bank lured mainland manufacturers and, later, international investors from Europe and Asia to Puerto Rico in the 1950s and 1960s. They advertised tax and customs holidays, low-wage labor without widespread unionization, government-funded factory buildings, government-backed guarantees on profits, and other investment incentives.

Government agencies and contractors supported investors with marketing campaigns and business planning (Neveling 2015a). Workers' rights protests were brutally quashed by local police forces, and OH&S ranked at the bottom of the industrialization agenda. A ten-year anniversary publication claimed that Puerto Rico's export-oriented industrialization program (called 'Operation Bootstrap') factories 'conform to modern codes of health, sanitation, and safety–all carefully enforced by the Department of Labor and Health' (Stead 1958: 92). Yet, that Department was anything but efficient, such that much of the historical reporting on accidents in the many new TG factories focused on monetary damage rather than workers' injuries. Concerns about health and safety in Puerto Rico's pioneering SEZ-style development program focused on healthy and safe profits for capital, rather than OH&S for workers (Neveling 2017: 131–2).

From Puerto Rico, the SEZ model – and, with it, TG industry sweatshops – spread persistently across an increasing number of postcolonial nations. Support for export-oriented and manufacturing-industrialization-driven economic development came from US departments and government institutions, along with new United Nations' (UN) commissions on economic development, UN technical assistance programs, the International Bank for Reconstruction and Development (IBRD), and other World Bank branches. US officials organized tours for Puerto Rican officials across the Caribbean and Latin American nations. The consulting corporation that designed much of the Puerto Rican scheme won grants to replicate this in Jamaica, Egypt, Honduras, and elsewhere. As the Cold War progressed, financial support for industrial infrastructure and preferential quotas for exports to Western markets became central means for supporting pro-capitalist dictatorships that showed little concern for OH&S. With EPZ policies in place in Taiwan in 1965, in Indonesia and South Korea in 1970, and in Bangladesh and Chile in 1973, among several other nations, TG sweatshops designed by Western and local planning agencies spread across the globe (Neveling 2015a).

Crucially, pro-zone policies became central to the agenda of international organizations as well. Around two dozen countries had SEZ-style development policies up and running, or in preparation, when the non-alignment movement's pressure for changing international terms of trade bore some fruit in the mid-1960s, when the United Nations Conference on Trade and Development (UNCTAD) and the United Nations Industrial Development Organization (UNIDO) began work in 1964 and 1966, respectively. With an approach based, to some extent, on surveys of existing policies, UNIDO became the powerhouse of SEZ promotion in the 1970s, despite the fact that the zones continued to give special rights to foreign investors and little oversight for national governments and, thus, were antagonistic to the New International Economic Order policies of many developing nations at the time. The debt crises of the 1980s put both socialist-bloc nations and non-aligned nations at the mercy of World Bank and International Monetary Fund structural adjustment programs, most of which came with requirements and regular monitoring to instigate SEZs. The number of zones rose above 1,000 in the 1990s, when governments in postsocialist nations in both Europe and Asia embraced neoliberalism (Neveling 2015a).

UNIDO had supported China with training and workshops since its economic liberalization, marked by the introduction of SEZs in 1979. With an increasing number of bilateral trade agreements, Chinese TG production increased rapidly in the 1990s, and grew exponentially when the country became a full member of the World Trade Organization in 2001. Among other Twenty-First Century WTO entrants, Nepal (2004), Cambodia (2004), and Vietnam (2007) experienced veritable TG booms, again coupled with the rapid expansion of SEZs and also economic corridors that link production sites across mainland Southeast Asia, for example (Arnold 2012; Shakya 2018). Subsequently, SEZs with similarly low wages and lax labor rights provision and policing facilitated the expansion of TG manufacturing for international markets in India (Mezzadri 2017), Bangladesh (Ashraf and Prentice 2019), and Thailand and Myanmar, fueled by huge numbers of regional migrant workers (Campbell 2018). Despite this internationalization trend, some Western countries – notably the US, Italy, Spain, and the Federal Republic of Germany – maintain positions as leading producers and exporters of textiles and garments, primarily because of an emphasis on high-tech products and *haut de gamme* fashion products.

Occupational health and safety in global SEZ sweatshops

The fact that the *ILO Handbook for Workers Education to Prevent Accidents* was published in 1983 indicates that attention to OH&S remained miniscule as the TG industry went global from the 1960s. In the US, advances from the jobbers' agreement of the 1930s were sustained into the 1980s, while the numbers of workers in the sector steadily declined. In Western Europe, TG manufacturing declined from the 1950s, first through competition from southern Europe, and then from Southeast Asia. Manufacturers in the Federal Republic of Germany, for example, followed this trend and moved production to Italy, then Poland and Hungary in the 1960s, before moving to Hong Kong, Mauritius, and Taiwan in the 1970s (Froebel *et al.* 1981). Again, such moves were motivated by the lure of longer working hours and limited government protections for workers.

Western governments, consultants, and international development organizations paid little attention to health and safety standards in what came to be known as 'newly industrializing countries' (NICs). As late as the 1970s, reports that carried 'health' and/or 'safety' in their titles commonly devoted limited attention to reporting on industrial accidents, and showed little interest in monitoring oversight bodies. If anything, that trend toward ignoring workers' health and safety rights violations was exacerbated by the structural adjustment programs of the 1980s and 1990s. Fiscal policies, deregulation of protectionist measures, and implementation of investment incentives by indebted governments were meticulously monitored in bi-annual reports over hundreds of pages, while the same huge bureaucratic apparatus had no interest in monitoring workers' rights provisions (Neveling 2017: 137). In sum, the credo that emerged in the late-1930s Puerto Rican TG manufacturing – health and safety for capital and investors, rather than for factory workers – went global in the following decades.

When UNIDO, other international organizations, corporate think-tanks, and industrial sector interest groups produced their first overviews of the global spread and operations of SEZs in the 1970s, OH&S was of little concern. Checklists produced by the government-funded German Institute for Economic Research for TG companies, for instance, emphasized low-wage costs, longer working hours, 'freedom to hire and fire', the absence of 'militant or communist influenced trade unions', and other anti-workers' rights variables as positive items to observe before determining new manufacturing locations (Froebel *et al.* 1981: 147). Even publications highly critical of global manufacturing – like the excellent working paper series by the UN's Centre on Transnational Corporations and the ILO's Multinational Enterprise Programme in the 1980s, or the seminal *No Logo* (Klein 2000) of the late-1990s and 2000s global anti-sweatshop campaign – lack comprehensive reviews of OH&S in the global TG sector. The shortcomings of those decades, thus, must be pieced together from a range of exemplary sources.

An SEZ-style scheme for Mexico, developed since around 1960, went live in 1965 as the Border Industrialization Programme (BIP), and gave rise to the widely criticized maquila factories where young women – many of them migrants from rural Mexico and other Latin American nations – toil for long hours under terrible sweatshop conditions while suffering sexist abusive from foremen and factory managers. Health hazards in maquilas in Nogales and elsewhere were representative of global conditions in the sector in the 1980s (Neveling 2017), making it worth reproducing a summary study in detail:

> Hazards of the workplace include exposure to toxics as well as mutagenic and carcinogenic chemicals, the operation of dangerous and antiquated machinery that lacks safeguards to prevent injury, lack of protective equipment and clothing, stress or disease caused by long hours and repetitive motion, and a denial of information on chemicals in the workplace. Community-level risks include chemical exposure due to improper disposal of industry chemicals, lack of hygienic water delivery, storage and drainage in squatter communities, housing vulnerability to flood damage, and transportation accidents in an overcrowded city.
>
> (Cravey 1998: 96)

Further reports from independent researchers and local workers' rights groups in the 1980s (cited in Cravey 1998: 96–7) amplify that industrial pollution goes beyond the workplace to impact entire communities of workers. The continuity of such environmental and workplace pollution into the present is evident in recent reporting (Grassi 2020) on Nogales, Mexico's 'Blue-Jeans capital', where around 300 factories and 25 laundries pollute rivers and drinking water, migrant TG workers live in extreme poverty in unsafe squatter settlements without running water, and factory workers report frequent sexual harassment, workplace abuse, exposure to toxic chemicals and fumes, and long working hours. Without government support, a local worker movement had to fight corporations for many years to win basic fire safety and other life-saving industrial protection.

Industrial hazards are well known in Nogales and all other TG factory production sites – not only to workers, but also to factory managers, owners, and most brands that subcontract production to SEZs, bonded warehouses, and other 'special' zone locations. Production techniques such as the sandblasting of denim jeans, for instance, are widely known to cause silicosis among workers, a long-term and often deadly lung disease (Hobson 2013). Yet, much like the garment stores of New York's Lower East Side around the time of the Triangle Shirtwaist Factory Fire, Twenty-First Century high-street retailers and fashion brands seek to outsource responsibility for OH&S while simultaneously subcontracting production. The rapidly expanding TG sector in Bangladesh had seen numerous accidents, and many of them deadly, before the Rana Plaza building collapse killed more than 1,000 mostly female garment workers on 24 April 2013. As in 1911 New York, the building was not constructed for industrial manufacturing. In the days before the disaster, workers from businesses on other floors of the building had been warned to stay home because cracks had appeared in the walls and ceilings of the building (Siddiqi 2015). After the disaster, pictures of garments among the rubble bearing the logos of brands and retailers made international news headlines. As global pressure on high-street retailers mounted, international workers' rights groups and Bangladeshi trade unions finally won the *Bangladesh Accord on Fire and Building Safety*, ratified in 2013 (Siddiqi 2015). This was after concerns over lacks of OH&S had been raised for decades, even by otherwise-supportive authors of the country's EPZ regime (*e.g.* Dowla 1997).

Critical scholars highlight the dangers of normalizing effects that arose from compensation payments that allegedly indemnified grieving families after the deadly Tazreen Fashions factory fire in Dhaka in 2012, and also the Rana Plaza factory collapse (Sumon *et al.* 2017). 2017 saw another garment factory fire in Bangladesh. For the period from 1 January 2021 to 13 June 2022 alone, the international workers' rights activist group, *Clean Clothes Campaign*, has listed 56 incidents internationally, with 131 workers dead and 279 injured in TG factories in Pakistan, India, Egypt, Morocco, China, and Cambodia. Adding to the list of obvious industrial hazards from lack of adequate OH&S measures are factory fires in Argentina, Chile, Turkey, and Peru that, fortunately, did not cost any lives.[1]

During the peak lockdowns of the global COVID-19 pandemic, many workers in TG factories had to show up for work, as production was hastily switched to incorporate protective equipment against the virus. Rural migrant workers in Bangladesh, India, and elsewhere received no compensations for temporary layoffs and were sent back-and-forth between their workplaces and hometowns like expendable pawns on a chessboard (Carswell *et al.* 2020; Siddiqi 2021). Millions of new forced migrants from regions marked by escalating wars are now vulnerable to super-exploitative factory regimes with hardly any oversight, as neoliberal development economists – like former Oxford Professor, Paul Collier, and ex-World Bank consultant, Lotta Moberg – promote construction of SEZs next to refugee camps so that capital may draw from an expanded reserve army of laborers in dire straits (Neveling 2015b). The death of Syrian migrants in a recent garment factory incident in Istanbul (see: Footnote 1) may, thus, be a first sign of an even more dangerous future for garment workers.

Stitching it up

This short overview of past and present developments in OH&S in the global TG sector has uncovered the long history of an industrial sector deliberately opting for the 'sick role'. The spatio-temporal features of the sector that have undergirded its accumulation of capital and exploitation of labor – lack of investment in technological innovation, undervalued and unsafe labor, opaque subcontracting networks, and racialized exploitation – have been surprisingly stable for more than a century. Innovation has been focused on globalizing the TG commodity chain so that capital investment in technology could remain low, while racist stereotyping of 'undeserving workers' has supported the poor provision of OH&S across the historical evolution of production hotspots. Dynamic webs of subcontracting have been maintained since the sector was at the center of Britain's pioneering industrialization drive at the turn of the Nineteenth Century. Retailers, contractors, and subcontractors have shown an impressive versatility in labor exploitation via global labor arbitrage – allowing them to tap into the lowest-paid pools of capitalism's industrial reserve army via, alternatively, incorporating incoming impoverished migrants in existing production sites, or relocating to regions with lower wages, lax government oversight, and minimal OH&S regulations. The latter strategy has supported capital's ability to avoid collective bargaining and unionization, which is particularly important for this chapter's topic, as successful struggles for workers' rights and support from progressive consumer publics have proven to be the only means to improve OH&S in the sector over more than 200 years. In the same period, capital has enjoyed healthy and safe profits from TG manufacturing, while showing little interest in improving OH&S on the global scale of the sector's activities.

Note

1 For more information, see: <https://cleanclothes.org/campaigns/protect-progress/deaths-and-injuries-in-the-global-garment-industry> (accessed 2 August, 2022).

References

Arnold, D. 2012, 'Spatial practices and border SEZs in Mekong Southeast Asia', *Geography Compass*, 6(12), pp. 740–51.

Ashraf, H. and Prentice, R. 2019, 'Beyond factory safety: Labor unions, militant protest, and the accelerated ambitions of Bangladesh's export garment industry', *Dialectical Anthropology*, 43(1), pp. 93–107.

Bair, J., Anner, M. and Blasi, J. 2017, 'Sweatshops and the search for solutions, yesterday and today', in Prentice, R. and de Neve, G. (eds), *Unmaking the Global Sweatshop: Health and Safety of the World's Garment Workers*, University of Pennsylvania Press, Philadelphia, pp. 29–56.

Barab, J. 2006, 'Acts of God, acts of man: The invisibility of workplace death', in Mogensen, V. (ed), *Worker Safety Under Siege: Labor, Capital, and the Politics of Workplace Safety in a Deregulated World*, Routledge, London, pp. 3–16.

Bender, D.E. 2003, '"A foreign method of working" –Racial degeneration, gender disorder and the sweatshop danger in America', in Bender, D.E. and Greenwald, R.A. (eds), *Sweatshop USA: The American Sweatshop in Historical and Global Perspective*, Routledge, New York, pp. 19–36.

Bender, D.E. and Greenwald, R.A. 2003, 'Introduction – Sweatshop USA: The American sweatshop in global and historical perspective', in Bender, D.E. and Greenwald, R.A. (eds), *Sweatshop USA: The American Sweatshop in Historical and Global Perspective*, Routledge, New York, pp. 1–18.

Blake, W. 1808, 'And did those feet in ancient time', *Poetry Foundation*, accessed 1 November 2022, <https://www.poetryfoundation.org/poems/54684/jerusalem-and-did-those-feet-in-ancient-time>.

Blyth, M. 2003, *Great Transformations: Economic Ideas and Institutional Change in the Twentieth Century*, Cambridge University Press, Cambridge.

Boris, E. 2003, 'Consumers of the world unite!: Campaigns against sweating, past and present', in Bender, D.E. and Greenwald, R.A. (eds) *Sweatshop USA: The American Sweatshop in Historical and Global Perspective*, Routledge, New York, pp. 203–24.

Bronstein, J.L. 2008, *Caught in the Machinery: Workplace Accidents and Injured Workers in Nineteenth-Century Britain,* Stanford University Press, Stanford.

Campbell, S. 2018, *Border Capitalism, Disrupted: Precarity and Struggle in a Southeast Asian Industrial Zone*, Cornell University Press, Ithaca.

Carswell, G., Neve, G.D. and Yuvaraj, S. 2020, 'Fifty days of lockdown in India: A view from two villages in Tamil Nadu', *Economic and Political Weekly*, 55(25), pp. 2–10. epw.in/sites/default/files/engage_pdf/2020/06/19/157090.pdf.

Cravey, A.J. 1998, *Women and Work in Mexico's Maquiladoras*, Rowman and Littlefield, Lanham.

de la Cruz-Fernández, P.A. 2015, 'Multinationals and gender: Singer sewing machine and marketing in Mexico, 1890–1930', *Business History Review*, 89(3), pp. 531–49.
Dowla, A. 1997, 'Export processing zones in Bangladesh: The economic impact', *Asian Survey*, 37(6), pp. 561–74.
Doyal, L. and Pennell, I. 1979, *The Political Economy of Health,* Pluto Press, London.
Engels, F. 2009 [1892], *The Condition of the Working Class in England*, Penguin, London.
Froebel, F., Heinrichs, J. and Kreye, O. 1981, *The New International Division of Labour: Structural Unemployment in Industrialised Countries and Industrialisation in Developing Countries*, Cambridge University Press, Cambridge.
Godley, A. 1997, 'The development of the clothing industry: Technology and fashion', *Textile History*, 28(1), pp. 3–10.
Grassi, L. 2020, 'Textile industries and pollution in Tehuacan, Mexico', *Environmental Justice Atlas*, accessed 2 August 2020, <http://www.cevreadaleti.org/conflict/textile-industries-in-tehuacan-mexico-have-contaminated-underground-water-used-to-be-bottled-for-sales>.
Halliday, R.J. 1971, 'Social Darwinism: A definition', *Victorian Studies*, 14(4), pp. 389–405.
Herbert, U. 1990, *History of Foreign Labour in Germany: 1880–1980*, University of Michigan Press, Ann Arbor,
Hobsbawm, E.J. 1999 [1968], *Industry and Empire: From 1750 to the Present Day*, The New Press, New York.
Hobsbawm, E.J. and Rudé, G.F.E. 1969, *Captain Swing*, Lawrence and Wishart, London.
Hobson, J. 2013, 'To die for? The health and safety of fast fashion', *Occupational Medicine*, 63(5), pp. 317–9.
Hofstadter, R. 2016 [1944], *Social Darwinism in American Thought: 1850–1915*, University of Pennsylvania Press, Philadelphia.
International Labour Office. 1983, *Accident Prevention: A Workers' Education Manual*, Report, International Labour Office, Geneva.
Kaplan, T. 1985, 'On the socialist origins of international women's day', *Feminist Studies*, 11(1), pp. 163–171.
Klein, N. 2000, *No logo: No Space, No Choice, No Jobs, Taking Aim at the Brand Bullies*, Flamingo, London.
Koistinen, D. 2013, *Confronting Decline: The Political Economy of Deindustrialization in Twentieth-Century New England*, University Press of Florida, Gainesville.
Mezzadri, A. 2017, *The Sweatshop Regime: Labouring Bodies, Exploitation, and Garments Made in India*, Cambridge University Press, New York.
Moos, K.A. 2021, 'The political economy of state regulation: The case of the British factory acts', *Cambridge Journal of Economics*, 45(1), pp. 61–84.
Neveling, P. 2015a, 'Export processing zones, special economic zones and the long march of capitalist development policies during the Cold War', in James, L. and Leake, E. (eds), *Negotiating Independence: New Directions in the Histories of the Cold War and Decolonisation*, Bloomsbury, London, pp. 63–84.
Neveling, P. 2015b, 'Free trade zones, export processing zones, special economic zones and global imperial formations, 200 BCE to 2015 CE', in Ness, I. and Cope, Z. (eds), *The Palgrave Encyclopaedia of Imperialism and Anti-Imperialism*, Palgrave Macmillan, Basingstoke, pp. 1007–16.
Neveling, P. 2017, 'Capital over labor: Health and safety in export processing zones garment production since 1947', in Prentice, R. and de Neve, G. (eds), *After Rana Plaza: Rethinking the Health and Safety of Global Garment Workers*, University of Pennsylvania Press, Philadelphia, pp. 123–46.
Neveling, P. 2021, 'The anthropology of special economic zones (free ports, export processing zones, tax havens)', in Aldenderfer, M. (ed), *Oxford Research Encyclopaedia: An*thropology, Oxford University Press, accessed 4 November 2022, < https://oxfordre.com/anthropology>.
Parsons, T. 1951, *The Social System*, The Free Press, Glencoe.
Porter, S. 1993, 'Critical realist ethnography: The case of racism and professionalism in a medical setting', *Sociology*, 27(4), pp. 591–609.
Prentice, R. and de Neve, G. 2017, *Unmaking the Global Sweatshop: Health and Safety of the World's Garment Workers*, University of Pennsylvania Press, Philadelphia.
Riello, G. and Parthasarathi, P. 2009, *The Spinning World: A Global History of Cotton Textiles, 1200–1850*, Oxford University Press, Oxford.
Rosen, E.I. 2002, *Making Sweatshops: The Globalization of the U.S. Apparel Industry*, University of California Press, Berkely.
Safa, H.I. 1995, *The Myth of the Male Breadwinner: Women and Industrialization in the Caribbean*, Westview Press, Boulder.

Shakya, M. 2018, *Death of an Industry: The Cultural Politics of Garment Manufacturing During the Maoist Revolution in Nepal*, Cambridge University Press, New Delhi.
Siddiqi, D.M. 2015, 'Starving for justice: Bangladeshi Garment Workers in a "Post-Rana Plaza" World', *International Labor and Working-Class History*, 87(Spring), pp. 165–73.
Siddiqi, D.M. 2021, 'Re-scripting empowerment? Post-COVID lessons from Bangladeshi garment workers', *Kohl: A Journal for Body and Gender Research*, 7(2), pp. 2–20.
Silver, B.J. 2003, *Forces of Labor: Workers' Movements and Globalization Since 1870*, Cambridge University Press, Cambridge.
Smith, G. 2014, *Intellectuals and (Counter-) Politics: Essays in Historical Realism*, Berghahn Books, New York.
Soyer, D. 1999, 'Garment sweatshops, then and now', *New Labor Forum*, 4, pp. 35–46.
Stead, W.H. 1958, *Fomento: The Economic Development of Puerto Rico*, National Planning Association, Washington, DC.
Sumon, M.H., Shifa, N. and Gulrukh, S. 2017, 'Discourses of compensation and the normalization of negligence: The experience of the Tazreen Factory fire', in Prentice, R. and de Neve, G. (eds), *After Rana Plaza: Rethinking the Health and Safety of Global Garment Workers*, University of Pennsylvania Press, Philadelphia, pp. 147–72.
Van Vugt, W.E. 1999, *Britain to America: Mid-Nineteenth-Century Immigrants to the United States*, University of Illinois Press, Urbana.
War on Want. 1985 [1984], *Women Working Worldwide: The International Division of Labour in the Electronics, Clothing and Textiles Industries*, War on Want, London.
Wolf, E.R. 1997 [1982], *Europe and the People Without History*, University of California Press, Berkeley.

15

POLITICAL ECONOMY AND SOCIAL EPIDEMIOLOGY IN THE CONTEXT OF THE HIV EPIDEMIC IN SUB-SAHARAN AFRICA

Kevin Deane

The discipline of epidemiology has been catapulted into the limelight due to the ongoing global COVID-19 pandemic, with the public across the world gaining greater competency in core epidemiological concepts, such as 'R' (the effective reproduction number). Epidemiological data during the pandemic has been vital in tracking its progression and in shaping the response. Data describing the distribution of the disease across the population and identifying risk factors has, for example, informed prevention policies such as shielding and the timing of lockdowns and associated control measures, as well as the population sub-groups to be prioritized in the vaccine rollout in the Global North. It may, therefore, seem a peculiar moment for a chapter that seeks to provide a critical perspective on some aspects of epidemiology. Further, as a key source of information regarding population health, political economists are often reliant on epidemiological data when engaging with different health issues. However, given this reliance, it is of vital importance for political economists to understand the limitations of the epidemiological approach, as well as more problematic tendencies within the discipline that (intentionally or unintentionally) have implications for how the drivers of poor health are understood. A critical understanding of these issues should also inform the development of a political economy research agenda and the construction of alternative narratives concerning health.

This issue has become more pertinent given the rise of social epidemiology as a sub-discipline of epidemiology. Social epidemiology has, at heart, a progressive agenda: acknowledging that population health stems from interactions between biological and social processes, and emphasizing focus on the social determinants of health and the social gradient (*i.e.* that most health outcomes are negatively correlated with increasing wealth) that is observed with respect to most health conditions across the globe.[1] The social determinants of health approach to understanding the drivers of health inequities[2] rose to prominence in the early-2000s (Marmot 2005). Subsequently, the WHO Commission on Social Determinants of Health produced an influential report in 2008 that collated a growing body of evidence on the social drivers of poor health and health inequities, and called for a new global health agenda to 'close the gap' (CSDH 2008). The report provided three overarching recommendations:

DOI: 10.4324/9781003017110-17

1 Improve daily living conditions
2 Tackle the inequitable distribution of power, money and resources
3 Measure and understand the problem and assess the impact of action (CSDH 2008).

The implicit recognition embedded in the report was that existing approaches focusing on individual health behaviours were poorly placed to explain observed health disparities. This opened up a space for theoretical approaches that engage with social structures, power and concerns regarding the distribution of wealth to come to the fore. Political economists have the theoretical tools to engage with these concerns, and so were (and are) well placed to respond to this agenda.

However, to a large extent, work on the social determinants of health has come to be dominated by social epidemiologists, such as in the literature on the structural drivers of HIV in sub-Saharan Africa. Rather than according space for the deployment of a wide range of theoretical and empirical approaches deriving from the social and political sciences, standard techniques from epidemiology have been applied to this issue, thereby constituting a form of scientific imperialism in which quantitative, positivist methods continue to colonize the social sciences. The concrete ways in which social epidemiology has applied and adapted traditional epidemiological methods to study the social aspects of health have resulted in analyses that, despite focusing on social determinants, continue to perpetuate epistemological and policy attention on individual behaviour (McMichael 1999; O'Laughlin 2015). This emphasizes more than ever the need for critical engagement in health issues by political economists.

This chapter provides some critical reflections on epidemiology and social epidemiology, using the case-study of migration, population mobility and HIV in sub-Saharan Africa as an illustration of how these issues play out with regard to concrete health issues. However, to clarify, it is not the contention of this chapter that the baby should be thrown out with the bathwater. Rather, it demonstrates that the application of epidemiological methods and statistical techniques to social and systemic drivers of health, and the resulting evidence produced, must be treated with caution. The structure of this chapter is as follows. First, a brief overview of epidemiology and social epidemiology is presented. The following section offers some critical perspectives on social epidemiology. The case-study of migration, mobility and HIV is then articulated in the next section to illustrate some of the limitations of social epidemiology, with an alternative political economy narrative discussed in the subsequent section that highlights core tools, concepts and categories at the disposal of political economists. The chapter concludes by reflecting on the policy implications of the preceding analysis, followed by some closing remarks.

From epidemiology to social epidemiology

Whilst numerous definitions of epidemiology have been forwarded in recent decades (Frérot *et al.* 2018), one recent authoritative definition is that it is 'the study of the distribution and determinants of health-related states and events (including disease) and the application of this study to the control of disease and other health problems' (Last 2001). This definition captures the main themes that reoccur in the literature. The history of epidemiology can be traced far back as the Fifth Century (Bracken 2003), though the establishment of 'modern epidemiology' gathered pace after the Second World War (Camargo Jr. *et al.* 2013). By the 1980s, the discipline had crystallized around a core set of statistical techniques. The discipline is characterized by a range of different approaches and sub-disciplines, which can be disease-specific, such as the SIR model used in infectious disease epidemiology (Avery *et al.* 2020). However, the dominant approach is risk-factor epidemiology, a method that seeks, through descriptive statistics and multiple regression techniques, to establish statistically significant independent risk factors for a disease or health condition. These methods have much in common with statistical techniques used in economics and should be familiar to political economists.

Traditionally, risk-factor epidemiology was largely concerned with patterns of exposure and causes of disease, and was rooted in a primarily biomedical approach that focused on the proximal causes of disease. However, the early-1990s saw the emergence of social epidemiology as a sub-discipline, as it was increasingly recognized that health outcomes were shaped by social, contextual and structural factors. Accordingly, social epidemiology incorporates the distal determinants of health (often referred to as the 'causes of the causes') into the analysis. Social epidemiology incorporates the distal determinants of health, with an emphasis on the pathways that link social factors with behaviours and biological processes (Galea and Link 2013). It has also been recognized that rather than constituting a linear process, the social determinants must be conceptualized as a web of causality operating at different levels that involves interactions between different social factors and feedback loops (Krieger 1994; McMichael 1999). However, whilst there have been considerable methodological advances and debates within the discipline, as well as increasing dialogue with the social sciences (Galea and Link 2013), the application of the standard 'risk-factor' approach continues to dominate social epidemiology (Kaplan 2004; Camargo Jr. *et al.* 2013), with social variables seamlessly incorporated into standard regression models. In this sense, traditional risk-factor epidemiology has been able to maintain its place as the core methodological approach, despite increasing polarization within the broader epidemiological discipline about the role of social factors and whether these should be within the scope of epidemiological inquiry (Galea and Link 2013; Wemrell *et al.* 2016).

Some critical reflections on social epidemiology

The critical analysis of social epidemiology presented here reflects observations that social epidemiologists themselves have made about traditional risk-factor epidemiology, though given the application of this method in social epidemiology, these points remain relevant to the present discussion. Critical reflections also arise from engagement with the social sciences and debates within the social epidemiology regarding the direction of future travel. Some will be immediately recognizable to political economists, as there are often parallels with critical engagements with mainstream economics regarding the use of statistical methods such as multiple regression, and the extent to which they are appropriate to apply to social issues.

Firstly, there is an inherent (yet, perhaps unintended with respect to social epidemiology) methodological individualism. Whilst social epidemiology attempts to address the social/structural determinants of health, the data used in risk-factor approaches is primarily collected from individuals (Kaplan 2004), often originating from cross-sectional demographic surveys that gather data on a range of demographic, social and behavioural variables. As a result, social epidemiology still studies individuals (as opposed to structures), with Kaplan (2004: 130) noting that 'this focus on individuals is found even when studying factors such as social networks and social support, where the concepts refer to exchanges between individual persons and participation in groups'. This methodological individualism also shapes the nature of the social epidemiological analyses that attempt to engage with the structural and social drivers of disease by mapping linear pathways from the more distal determinants of disease to the proximal causes. However, this insistence on being able to map and quantify these relationships limits the extent to which structures are incorporated into the analysis, and result in policy prescriptions that target individuals. This has become known as the 'prison of the proximate' (McMichael 1999; O'Laughlin 2015), in which social epidemiology that attempts to engage with structures is unable to escape the clutches of methodological individualism.

Secondly, there is an underlying positivism, reflected in the statistical methods used, that assumes the existence of quantifiable causal relationships between different variables. Whilst the social sciences and, indeed, many from within social epidemiology emphasize the messiness of the real-world and non-linear processes of uncertain social and structural change, social epidemiology seeks to impose a positivist framework on these issues. Further, and by implication, the solution to challenges within social epidemiology is primarily reduced to calls for more (and better) data and more complex modelling. This is reminiscent of the response by mainstream economists to failures to predict the Global Financial Crisis, with calls for improved modelling presented as the solution to methodological shortcomings of existing models (Colander *et al.* 2008), rather than reflecting deeper epistemological and ontological issues embedded within the models (Lawson 2009).

The application of risk-factor epidemiology and other statistical modelling also requires the conversion of complex social phenomena into variables that can be incorporated into statistical analyses. In many cases, this process entails a necessary reductionism that strips away the social content of core categories and concepts. For example, income is often used as a key measure of 'Socioeconomic Status' (SES) or 'Socioeconomic Position' (SEP). However, viewed from a political economy perspective, these types of income measures act as an imperfect proxy for class, a category of analysis that is not so easily reducible to a variable given that it is a relational concept. In the process of creating these variables, SES or SEP appears as sanitized, de-politicized representations of class, stripped of much of its social content. It has also been highlighted that the inclusion of variables that represent the social world can lead to an essentialism that can shape the research and policy agenda. For instance, the use of variables that capture 'race' or 'ethnicity' can obscure the fact that race itself is a social construct, which has implications for how study results are framed and interpreted. As Kaplan (2004 132) notes:

> While most social epidemiologists would acknowledge that race and ethnicity are mainly social constructions, many studies discuss 'race' or 'ethnicity effects when what they are really observing are the social, environmental, economic, and historical facts that lie underneath those terms.

Relatedly, the notion of what constitutes a 'risk factor', as used in social epidemiology, is to some extent conceptually muddled. On the one hand, a risk factor can reflect the underlying biological processes of specific diseases and/or factors that may increase exposure, and on the other, contextual/socio-economics/background/demographic risk factors are used to describe/identify/predict who may be at higher risk of contraction (Stampfer *et al.* 2004; Magadi and Desta 2011). In relation to HIV, for instance, a risk factor related to biological processes is having unprotected sex, as this has the potential to increase exposure to the virus and, thus, risk of infection. Conversely, other risk factors, such as age, gender and poverty/wealth, do not necessarily increase exposure to the virus, but operate in a range of ways that can enhance the likelihood of infection indirectly. For example, being poor may increase the need for a woman to engage in survival or transactional sex, but being poor in itself does not lead to increased exposure. However, these risk factors, which reflect differences in 'predictive' and 'explanatory' studies, are often conflated (Schooling and

Jones 2018). Despite these conceptual distinctions, different types of risk factors are not treated differently within statistical analyses, and are presented and described in similar ways.

This also has implications for the thorny problem of causality and correlation, an issue frequently encountered within mainstream econometric work. The risk-factor approach has been labelled as 'black-box epidemiology', with critics pointing out that statistically significant risk factors are, by sleight of hand, ascribed a degree of causality, but do not shed light on underlying causal processes (Skrabanek 1994). As a result, some studies report a seemingly unrelated set of statistically significant risk factors, which often do not advance our understanding of the problem. This lack of explanatory power can also be clarified through another criticism levelled at social epidemiology: its limited engagement with social theory (Camargo Jr. *et al.* 2013; Wemrell *et al.* 2016). When such theory is considered, there is a tendency to engage with a narrow set of behavioural models that are easily accommodated into the standard quantitative approach, with social theories emphasizing the importance of structures more difficult to embed in logistic regression models.

The case of migration, population mobility and HIV

The literature on the role of migration and population mobility in the HIV epidemic in sub-Saharan Africa is a good case-study through which to illustrate concretely these critical reflections. Migration and population mobility, more generally, are intimately intertwined with the spread and transmission of infectious diseases, most recently illustrated by the COVID pandemic. The HIV epidemic in sub-Saharan Africa has attracted (and continues to attract) a great deal of scholarship on the relationship between migration and population mobility and HIV transmission. Initially, the literature focused on routes of transmission and the role that certain forms of mobility, such as circular and seasonal migration, played in linking geographically separate epidemics and transmitting the virus from places of high prevalence to areas where it was not present (Deane *et al.* 2010; Deane *et al.* 2013). However, a second, now dominant, strand of literature that primarily draws on the risk-factor epidemiological approach seeks to link migration with higher rates of HIV and related risk behaviours summarized in Table 15.1. Whilst early studies on migration focused on specific mobile groups such as mineworkers and truck drivers (Carswell *et al.* 1989; Ramjee and Gouws 2002; Lurie *et al.* 2003; Zuma *et al.* 2003; Zuma *et al.* 2005), the narrative developed from these groups has been applied to migration and mobility more generally. Statistical analyses typically use cross-sectional survey data gathered in specific study sites or from nationally representative surveys, such as the Demographic Health Surveys (DHS). Surveys include a question on mobility (for example, 'have you spent more than one week away from the household in the last year?'), which enables the sample to be divided into different mobility categories. These can, in turn, be subjected to statistical tests to establish whether mobility is a 'risk factor' or not, and/or whether there are statistically significant differences in HIV prevalence and self-reported risk behaviours between different mobile and non-mobile groups.

A critical assessment of this approach illustrates the reflections outlined in the previous section. Firstly, whilst migration and mobility can be theorized as dynamic, historical socio-economic processes – including 'urbanization, seasonal and circulatory migration, rural to rural migration, commuting, internal displacement and international forced migration' (Deane *et al.* 2010) – there is an embedded methodological individualism. Data is gathered from individuals, and migration and mobility are, thus, reduced to individual behaviours, *i.e.* whether an individual has migrated or not. This deflects attention from considering migration as a structural driver of HIV, instead treating migration and mobility as analogous to individual characteristics.

Table 15.1 Examples of definitions of migration and mobility used in epidemiological studies

Study	*Categories of mobility*	*Definitions of mobility*
Lagarde *et al.* 2003	Short-term mobility	Been away for at least one day and one night in the last 4 weeks
	Long-term mobility	Been away for at least one month in the last 12 months
Lydie *et al.* 2004	No absence	No overnight trips in last 12 months
	Absence ≤ 31 days	Between 1 and 31 nights away in last 12 months
	Absence ≥ 31 days	More than 31 nights away in last 12 months
Kishamawe *et al.* 2006	Resident	Did not sleep or live elsewhere at the time of the demographic rounds
	Short-term mobile	Slept outside the household at least once the night before one of the five demographic rounds
	Long-term mobile	Lived elsewhere at least once the night before one of the five demographic rounds
Vissers *et al.* 2008	Non-mobile	Slept outside the household at most ten times in the last year
	Mobile	Slept outside the household more than ten times in the last year
Khan *et al.* 2008	Non-mobile	Lived in study town for more than 12 months
	Traveller	Lived outside but travelled to study town
	Migrant	Moved to the current town of residence within the last 12 months
Palk and Blower 2015		No overnight trips in the preceding year
		one to four overnight trips in the preceding year
	Frequent travellers	five or more trips in the preceding year
McGrath *et al.* 2015		Migrated at least once in past two years
	External migration event	Migration of an individual or household within the demographic surveillance area (DSA) to a household outside the DSA
		Spent <ten nights away from DSA household in past six months
Olawore *et al.* 2018	Permanent resident	No migration history
	Recent in-migrant	≤two years in community
	Non-recent in-migrant	>two years in community

There is also a challenge concerning how to define migration and turn it into a variable suitable for incorporation into statistical analysis. Table 15.1 illustrates the wide range of different definitions that have been used in the literature, with mobility and migration in general related to the length of time spent away from the household. These definitions are easily translatable into survey questions, and enable different mobility/migration categories to be constructed and compared to a 'non-mobile' category within the sample. However, these definitions are abstract and lack any social content. They conflate many forms of mobility that are likely to be qualitatively different (Deane *et al.* 2010). For example, being away from the household for a certain length of time may arise from economic reasons, such as formal employment or informal sector trading, or, in contrast, to care for sick relatives. Further, the distinction between different forms of mobility – including that between international and internal migration – disappears, with the primary focus on 'being away' for different periods deemed to be the primary marker of risk. This stripping of social content has parallels with the issue of race as a variable discussed above. Studies that present migrants as either engaging in higher levels of risky sexual behaviours than non-migrants or having higher HIV prevalence or incidence may inadvertently feed into xenophobic and stigmatizing narratives around migrants as risk takers and spreaders of disease – as those observed in South Africa (Petros *et al.* 2006).

This example also illustrates concerns related to what a risk factor is. It is questionable to what extent migration and mobility are risk factors in the traditional sense. Unlike having unprotected sex, moving in itself does not increase exposure to the virus (Colebunders and Kenyon 2015). Accordingly, it is problematic, if not entirely incorrect, to label migration and the various forms of mobility defined in Table 15.1 as a risk factor, though this is what much of the literature implies. Further, when migration or mobility is established as a risk factor, it implies that it acts as a risk factor in the same way across the sample, despite the many different reasons for, and experiences of engaging in, migration and mobility.

The result is an expanding literature that reports results that are often inconclusive and contradictory, leading to few firm conclusions (when viewed as a whole) regarding to what extent mobility is a risk factor for HIV and for whom. For instance, some studies have demonstrated statistically significant relationships (between mobility and HIV and/or risk behaviours) for men and not women, whereas others have found significant results for women but not men, and in relation to different lengths of being away (Deane *et al.* 2010; Colebunders and Kenyon 2015). Many studies also contain large numbers of results that are not statistically significant alongside one or two that are bringing into question their concluding statements and key findings. This leads to a confusing evidence base from which few consistent conclusions can be made, due to studies being conducted across different times and study sites regarding whether mobility increases HIV transmission.

A political economy perspective on migration, population mobility and HIV

Reflecting back on the core components of the research agenda forwarded to address the social determinants of health and the critical reflections on the risk-factor approach outlined in the previous section, political economists have a range of categories and concepts that are well placed to provide an alternative narrative regarding migration and HIV. However, as there has been relatively little work from the social sciences that explicitly adopt a political economy approach, this section attempts to summarize some of the main themes identified, drawing on the political economy research of O'Laughlin (2013) and Hickel (2012), as well as other critical social science literature that sheds light on the broader historical processes involved. It draws on the case-study of mineworkers in South Africa, the most prominent case presented in relation to migration and HIV within the literature.

At an early stage of the HIV epidemic, miners working in the gold and diamond mines of South Africa were identified as a population sub-group at high risk (Lurie *et al.* 2003; Zuma *et al.* 2005; Avery *et al.* 2020). As Msimang (2003) describes vividly in their description of a recipe for AIDS, male migrant flows were accompanied by female migrants attracted to the relative wealth at the mines:

> Steal some land and subjugate its people. Take some men from rural areas and put them in hostels far away from home, in different countries if need be. Build excellent roads. Ensure

> that the communities surrounding the men are impoverished so that a ring of sex workers develops around each mining town. Add HIV. Now take some miners and send them home for holidays to their rural, uninfected wives. Add a few girlfriends in communities along the road home. Add liberal amounts of patriarchy, both home-grown and of the colonial variety. Ensure that women have no right to determine the conditions under which sex will take place. Make sure that they have no access to credit, education, or any of the measures that would give them options to leave unhappy unions, or dream of lives in which men are not the center of their activities. Shake well and watch an epidemic explode.

This recipe highlights the central role of a historical political-economic perspective, in which poor health and development of the HIV epidemic in Southern Africa are located within the dynamics of contemporary capitalism since the colonial period. With respect to labour migration and the mines in Southern Africa, colonial administrations created a 'regional system of spatial and social divisions, cutting across what are now national boundaries, controlling both the flow of labour and the conditions of work' (O'Laughlin 2013). Patterns of forced male labour migration, in which young men were recruited for work on mines and plantations, were reinforced in post-colonial states. This was especially the case in countries of Southern Africa with large settler communities and apartheid regimes.

The beneficiaries of inflows of male labour from across Southern Africa to the gold mines in South Africa were (and often continue to be) international capital, reliant on sustained flows of cheap labour. Up until the mid-1990s, labour laws often prevented black workers from resettling, embedding the separation of male labour from rural households. Mine-owners did not provide family housing, and contracts were often temporary, requiring annual trips home whilst they were renewed. Male labour migration was also accompanied by female migration to the mines, with women moving to take advantage of economic opportunities to provide food and cleaning services to men, and to engage in sex work or transactional sex (Crush *et al.* 2005). This gendered migration is reflective of broader gendered inequalities, with women's access to land, other productive assets, formal employment and other income-generating activities limited.

Whilst this form of labour migration is slowly being eroded, new forms of migration have emerged due to neoliberalism and the structural adjustment programs of the 1990s. Increasing poverty during this period, the loss of manufacturing jobs and increased casualization of the workforce have since contributed to increased migratory flows as households diversify livelihood activities and attempt to maintain access to land in rural areas (Hickel 2012). There are also lingering aspects of the colonial era, with rural labour important in maintaining urban, casual labour that, in turn, underpins the profitability of capital. This narrative emphasizes the extent to which the penetration of capitalist relations, building on extractive and exploitative practices of the colonial era, combined with neoliberal economic reforms enforced on the continent to create a 'fertile environment' (Stillwaggon 2002) for the virus to be rapidly transmitted. Accordingly, this has led some to dub HIV a 'neoliberal plague' (Hickel 2012). This political economy analysis provides theoretical depth to our understanding of the way in which the inequitable distribution of power, money and resources has intensified the spread of HIV.

A second theme that is prominent in the literature on mineworkers draws attention to the material conditions of work, drawing on the political economy of Marx. In *Capital Volume One*, Marx (1976 [1867]) discusses in great detail how the labour process, working conditions in the industrial sector, class struggles over the length of the working day and employment practices during the early stages of industrial capitalism ultimately shortened the lives of workers. In relation to the cases of mineworkers in Southern Africa, there has been a focus on the role of poor working conditions in explaining high rates of 'risky' sexual behaviour and HIV prevalence. For example, as Hickel (2012) notes, mineworkers 'work six days a week with a 42 per cent injury rate and are often supplied with alcohol and prostitutes to prevent worker militancy and to alleviate the depression caused by loneliness, the daily threat of death and squalid working and living conditions'. Similarly, Campbell (1997) observes that many mineworkers 'said that they were expected to engage in physically taxing and dangerous work for up to eight hours with infrequent breaks, sometimes with minimal access to food or water, under conditions of tremendous heat, in air that was frequently stale and dusty, and sometimes with unpleasantly noisy machinery'. These accounts emphasize that the work is inherently risky and demanding, with injuries and deaths in the mines common. In turn, this fosters fatalistic attitudes and the development of dangerous forms of masculinities, and facilitates risk-taking (Campbell 1997) which, in turn, enhances the likelihood of HIV transmission amongst the workforce. These identities and attitudes are embedded in, and arise from, the material conditions of work. This alternative assessment draws attention away from the 'being-away' narrative embedded in the epidemiological approach.

The response from the mining sector illustrates the tensions in capital-labour relations in capitalist enterprises and the primacy of accumulation. Instead of focusing on the material living and working conditions of workers, the mining sector has explicitly promoted the implementation of workplace programs that prioritize biomedical and behavioural responses, such as education programs, the provision of treatment in some cases and condom promotion (Deane *et al.* 2019). As with many other health conditions related to the workplace, this does not address the underlying issues and locates the 'problem' solely in the behaviours of the miners. This response is often stimulated when profitability is threatened, for instance, when employers are faced with rising costs associated with reproducing the workforce, or to foster a positive external image for corporate social responsibility purposes. Further, many firms have attempted to 'shift the burden' of HIV onto households and the state through reducing employment benefits and health insurance schemes, firing HIV-positive workers, casualizing employment and engaging in pre-employment screening for HIV (Rosen and Simon 2003; Sprague *et al.* 2011). In times of crises, the response of capital is to maintain profitability through externalizing costs, whilst relying on the state to step in to secure social reproduction of the workforce.

Implications for HIV policy

The two approaches to understanding the issue of migration and HIV discussed above have very different implications for health policy. There are acknowledged limits regarding the extent to which social epidemiology, in its risk-factor form, can contribute to policy formation. Nevertheless, the findings are primarily used to emphasize that mobile individuals should be prioritized or targeted with the standard package of interventions, such as information/education campaigns and condom promotion, that reinforce the 'biomedical and behavioural paradigm' (Campbell and Williams 1999) and individualistic responses. Other policy suggestions, such as 'encouraging partners to move together', are formulated in a social vacuum and do not account for the varied forms of migration and mobility occurring across the continent.

In contrast, political economy and social science approaches applied to the case-study of mineworkers emphasize the role of poor living and working conditions, suggesting an alternative policy agenda that focuses on improving these conditions. However, as noted above, this has been resisted by mining companies (when they have engaged with this issue). More generally, this line of investigation directs attention to policy that engages with improving the material experiences of mobile populations. A second important issue that could be addressed by policy relates to reducing increasing income and wealth inequalities. This continues to be a challenging issue in the sub-Saharan context, and points to the need for comprehensive social policies directed towards reducing such disparities. Finally, policy related to HIV and migration cannot be separated from the need to engage with, and address, gender inequalities (Deane *et al.* 2018). Whilst a full review of competing perspectives on how to reduce income and gendered inequalities in the context of HIV is beyond the scope of this chapter, highlighting this problematic illustrates how political economy approaches promote an understanding of the 'causes of the causes'. However, it must also be noted that political economy approaches do not always lead to the formulation of neat policy responses. For example, improvements in working conditions will be shaped by class struggle, whilst long-term women's empowerment may require broader social emancipatory movements that are beyond the scope of public health policymakers alone.

Conclusion

This chapter has discussed the limitations of social epidemiology that continue to draw on the standard risk-factor approach. These critical reflections have been illustrated with the case-study of migration, mobility and HIV in the sub-Saharan context, demonstrating the shortcomings of the quantification of a range of abstract mobility variables. Conversely, an alternative political economy approach has been briefly sketched: drawing attention to how the relationship between capital and labour, the influence of national and international capital and the historical evolution of capitalism have all shaped migratory flows and experiences, embedded gender inequalities and livelihood insecurities and created a socio-political context within which HIV thrives. Future work on political economy, as an important counterpoint to epidemiological and standard public health approaches, must continue to highlight such factors to demonstrate the ways in which capitalism produces and reproduces poor health (O'Laughlin 2013, 2015).

Notes

1 There are some exceptions, such as HIV prevalence in much of sub-Saharan Africa.
2 The term 'inequities' is used here in distinction from 'inequalities' to focus on the character of avoidable health inequalities.

References

Avery, C., Bossert, W., Clark, A., Ellison, G. and Ellison, S.F. 2020, 'An economist's guide to epidemiology models of infectious disease', *Journal of Economic Perspectives*, 344, pp. 79–104.
Bracken, M.B. 2003, 'The first epidemiologic text', *American Journal of Epidemiology*, 15(79), pp. 855–6.
Camargo Jr, K.R.d., Ortega, F. and Coeli, C.M. 2013, 'Modern epidemiology and its discontents', *Revista de Saúde Pública*, 47, pp. 984–91.
Campbell, C. 1997, 'Migrancy, masculine identities and AIDS: The psychosocial context of HIV transmission on the South African gold mines', *Social Science and Medicine,* 45(2), pp. 273–81.
Campbell, C. and Williams, B. 1999, 'Beyond the biomedical and behavioural: Towards an integrated approach to HIV prevention in the Southern African mining industry', *Social Science and Medicine*, 48(11), pp. 1625–39.
Carswell, J.W., Lloyd, G. and Howells, J. 1989, 'Prevalence of HIV-1 in East African lorry drivers', *AIDS*, 3(11), pp. 759–61.
Colander, D., Follmer, H., Hass, A., Goldberg, M., Juselius, K., Kirman, A., Lux, T. and Sloth, B. 2008, *The Financial Crisis and the Systemic Failure of Academic Economics*, Kiel Institute for the World Economy, Kiel.
Colebunders, R. and Kenyon, C. 2015, 'Behaviour, not mobility, is a risk factor for HIV', *The Lancet HIV,* 2(6), pp. e223–4.

Crush, J., Williams, B., Gouws, E. and Lurie, M. 2005, 'Migration and HIV/AIDS in South Africa', *Development Southern Africa*, 22(3), pp. 293–318.

CSDH. 2008, *Closing the Gap in a Generation: Health Equity Through Action on the Social Determinants of Health*, Final Report of the Commission on Social Determinants of Health, World Health Organization, Geneva.

Deane, K.D., Johnston, D. and Parkhurst, J.O. 2013, 'Migration as a tool in development policy: Caution ahead?' *The Journal of Development Studies*, 49(6), pp. 759–71.

Deane, K.D., Parkhurst, J.O. and Johnston, D. 2010, 'Linking migration, mobility and HIV', *Tropical Medicine and International Health*, 15(12), pp. 1458–63.

Deane, K.D., Samwell Ngalya, P., Boniface, L., Bulugu, G. and Urassa, M. 2018, 'Exploring the relationship between population mobility and HIV risk: Evidence from Tanzania', *Global Public Health*, 13(2), pp. 173–88.

Deane, K., Stevano, S. and Johnston, D. 2019, 'Employers' responses to the HIV epidemic in sub-Saharan Africa: Revisiting the evidence', *Development Policy Review*, 37(2), pp. 245–59.

Frérot, M., Lefebvre, A., Aho, S., Callier, P., Astruc, K. and Aho Glélé, L.S. 2018, 'What is epidemiology? Changing definitions of epidemiology 1978–2017', *PLOS ONE*, 13(12), p. e0208442.

Galea, S. and Link, B.G. 2013, 'Six paths for the future of social epidemiology', *American Journal of Epidemiology*, 178(6), pp. 843–9.

Hickel, J. 2012, 'Neoliberal plague: The political economy of HIV transmission in Swaziland', *Journal of Southern African Studies*, 38(3), pp. 513–29.

Kaplan, G.A. 2004, 'What's wrong with social epidemiology, and how can we make it better?' *Epidemiologic Reviews*, 26(1), pp. 124–35.

Khan, M.R., Patnaik, P., Brown, L., Nagot, N., Salouka, S. and Weir, S.S. 2008, 'Mobility and HIV-related sexual behavior in Burkina Faso', *AIDS Behaviour*, 12(2), pp. 202–12.

Kishamawe, C., Vissers, D.C., Urassa, M., Isingo, R., Mwaluko, G., Borsboom, G.J., Voeten, H.A., Zaba, B., Habbema, J.D., and de Vlas, S. J. 2006, 'Mobility and HIV in Tanzanian couples: Both mobile persons and their partners show increased risk', *AIDS*, 20(4), pp. 601–8.

Krieger, N. 1994, 'Epidemiology and the web of causation: Has anyone seen the spider?', *Social Science and Medicine*, 39(7), pp. 887–903.

Lagarde, E., Schim van der Loeff, M., Enel, C., Holmgren, B., Dray-Spira, R., Pison, G., Piau, J.P., Delaunay, V., M'Boup, S., Ndoye, I., Coeuret-Pellicer, M., Whittle, H. and Aaby, P. 2003, 'Mobility and the spread of human immunodeficiency virus into rural areas of West Africa', *International Journal of Epidemiology*, 32(5), pp. 744–52.

Last J.M. (ed) 2001, *Dictionary of Epidemiology*, Oxford University Press, New York.

Lawson, T. 2009, 'The current economic crisis: Its nature and the course of academic economics', *Cambridge Journal of Economics*, 33(4), pp. 759–77.

Lurie, M.N., Williams, B.G., Zuma, K., Mkaya-Mwamburi, D., Garnett, G., Sturm, A.W., Sweat, M.D., Gittelsohn, J. and Abdool Karim, S.S. 2003, 'The impact of migration on HIV-1 transmission in South Africa: A study of migrant and nonmigrant men and their partners', *Sexually Transmitted Diseases*, 30(2), pp. 149–56.

Lydie, N., Robinson, N.J., Ferry, B., Akam, E., De Loenzien, M. and Abega, S. 2004, 'Mobility, sexual behavior, and HIV infection in an urban population in Cameroon', *Journal of Acquired Immune Deficiency Syndrome*, 35(1), pp. 67–74.

Magadi, M. and Desta, M. 2011, 'A multilevel analysis of the determinants and cross-national variations of HIV seropositivity in sub-Saharan Africa: Evidence from the DHS', *Health and Place*, 17(5), pp. 1067–83.

Marmot, M. 2005, 'Social determinants of health inequalities', *The Lancet*, 365(9464), pp. 1099–104.

Marx, K. 1976 [1867], *Capital: Volume One*, Penguin Books, London.

McGrath, N., Eaton, J.W., Newell, M.-L. and Hosegood, V. 2015, 'Migration, sexual behaviour, and HIV risk: A general population cohort in rural South Africa', *The Lancet HIV*, 26, pp. e252–9.

McMichael, A.J. 1999, 'Prisoners of the proximate: Loosening the constraints on epidemiology in an age of change', *American Journal of Epidemiology*, 149(10), pp. 887–97.

Msimang, S. 2003, 'HIV/AIDS, globalisation and the international women's movement', *Gender and Development*, (11)1, pp. 109–13.

O'Laughlin, B. 2013, 'Land, labour and the production of affliction in rural Southern Africa', *Journal of Agrarian Change*, 13(1), pp. 175–96.

O'Laughlin, B. 2015, 'Trapped in the prison of the proximate: Structural HIV/AIDS prevention in Southern Africa', *Review of African Political Economy*, 42(145), pp. 342–61.

Olawore, O., Tobian, A.A., Kagaayi, J., Bazaale, J.M., Nantume, B., Kigozi, G., Nankinga, J., Nalugoda, F., Nakigozi, G., Kigozi, G. and Gray, R.H. 2018, 'Migration and risk of HIV acquisition in Rakai, Uganda: A population-based cohort study', *The Lancet HIV*, 5(4), pp. e181–9.

Palk, L. and Blower, S. 2015, 'Mobility and circular migration in Lesotho: Implications for transmission, treatment, and control of a severe HIV epidemic', *Journal of Acquired Immune Deficiency Syndrome*, 68(5), pp. 604–8.

Petros, G., Airhihenbuwa, C.O., Simbayi, L., Ramlagan, S. and Brown, B. 2006, 'HIV/AIDS and "othering" in South Africa: The blame goes on', *Culture, Health and Sexuality*, 8(1), pp. 67–77.

Ramjee, G. and Gouws, E. 2002, 'Prevalence of HIV among truck drivers visiting sex workers in KwaZulu-Natal, South Africa', *Sexually Transmitted Diseases*, 29(1), pp. 44–9.

Rosen, S. and Simon, J.L. 2003, 'Shifting the burden: The private sector's response to the AIDS epidemic in Africa', *The International Journal of Public Health*, 812, pp. 131–7.

Schooling, C.M. and Jones, H.E. 2018, 'Clarifying questions about 'risk factors': Predictors versus explanation', *Emerging Themes in Epidemiology*, 15(1), p. 10.

Skrabanek, P. 1994, 'The emptiness of the black box', *Epidemiology*, 5(5), pp. 553–5.

Sprague, L., Simon, S. and Sprague, C. 2011, 'Employment discrimination and HIV stigma: Survey results from civil society organisations and people living with HIV in Africa', *African Journal of AIDS Research*, 10(sup1), pp. 311–24.

Stampfer, M.J., Ridker, P.M. and Dzau, V.J. 2004, 'Risk factor criteria', *Circulation*, 109(25), pp. suppl IV 3–5.

Stillwaggon, E. 2002, 'HIV/AIDS in Africa: Fertile terrain', *Journal of Development Studies*, 38(6), p. 1.

Vissers, D.C., Voeten, H.A., Urassa, M., Isingo, R., Ndege, M., Kumogola, Y., Mwaluko, G., Zaba, B., de Vlas, S.J. and Habbema, J.D.F. 2008, 'Separation of spouses due to travel and living apart raises HIV risk in Tanzanian couples', *Sexually Transmitted Diseases*, 35(8), pp. 714–20.

Wemrell, M., Merlo, J., Mulinari, S. and Hornborg, A.-C. 2016, 'Contemporary epidemiology: A review of critical discussions within the discipline and a call for further dialogue with social theory', *Sociology Compass*, 10(2), pp. 153–71.

Zuma, K., Gouws, E., Williams, B. and Lurie, M. 2003, 'Risk factors for HIV infection among women in Carletonville, South Africa: Migration, demography and sexually transmitted diseases', *International Journal of STD and AIDS*, 14(12), pp. 814–7.

Zuma, K., Lurie, M.N., Williams, B.G., Mkaya-Mwamburi, D., Garnett, G.P. and Sturm, A.W. 2005, 'Risk factors of sexually transmitted infections among migrant and non-migrant sexual partnerships from rural South Africa', *Epidemiology and Infection*, 133(3), pp. 421–8.

16

DIGITAL HEALTH AND CAPITALISM

Olivia Banner

At one of many memorable early COVID-19 daily press briefings in the US, Dr. Deborah Birx – then leading the Trump administration's pandemic response – held up a poster board with the title 'Coronavirus Testing' and the subtitle 'New Options for Consumers', while explaining that Google would be triaging COVID tests. The dissonance of posing the solution to the novel coronavirus within a market framework ('consumer options'), especially at a moment when the questions the public had were about how the government would intervene to alleviate a major epidemiological and social crisis, was striking. A visit to the website, hastily set up by Google, revealed the hollowness of this promise: the tests were available for a select subset of high-risk people in a small Northern California region. Nonetheless, the emptiness of this system of signification – the poster board framing citizens as 'consumers', and the reference to 'Google' as some kind of salve in the face of a virus – amidst a public health crisis was illuminating. It clarified that the health of capitalism in the country would not only take preference over actual human health, but that it was the preferable societal route. Amidst a floundering governmental response to the pandemic, a flowchart backed by the semiotic power of the word 'Google' was considered sufficient to soothe the public. More likely, however, its actual intention was to soothe jittery financial markets.

The academic literature on health and capitalism has long understood the trajectories that led to this strange moment, and more recent considerations of the conjuncture between digital health and capitalism also made it somewhat predictable. This chapter summarizes the historical developments that continue to produce such events, centering on the entanglement of legislative, biomedical, biotechnological, informatic, and medical-professional historical shifts. It outlines how these shifts have contributed to the contemporary figuring of health through digital means, and it contextualizes these shifts as they arise out of neoliberalism. I define neoliberalism here as a pervasive ideology that frames all social domains and human relations under the reigning discourse of 'the market', and is characterized by a mode of governance that prioritizes privatization, austerity, marketization, securitization, and ultimately constructing human subjects as marketized and responsible for managing risk. Certainly, Birx's press briefing – with its rhetorical gestures toward volatile markets and a consumer empowered to manage disease risk – is emblematic of digital health's reliance on neoliberal ideology and its market logic. Moreover, her appearance on the lawn of the White House is emblematic of the US health system's saturation by such ideologies

DOI: 10.4324/9781003017110-18

and logics. After consideration of the historical political-economic trajectory leading to this contemporary moment in the US, the chapter ends by gesturing to the penetration of neoliberal models for digital health and capitalist accumulation globally.

Digital health: origins

Currently, digital health constitutes a massive site of capital investment. Encompassing technologies ranging from large (*e.g.* data mining for massive datasets; whole-hospital-system electronic health records) to small (*e.g.* consumer products such as Fitbits; implantable devices), the digital health industry consistently posts a yearly rise in venture capital investment. In 2021, global investment in digital health technologies increased 260 percent above 2016 levels (Haydon 2021), spurred partly by the pandemic's turn to digital platforms for care; the privatization of Britain's NHS, which turned London into a global hub for technological innovation in health; and legislation supporting high technology biomedical research. This confluence of events – a crisis in health/healthcare; state investment in capital accumulation through biomedicine and technology; and a neoliberal reorganization of public services – all plays a role in the multiple historical transformations that led to our current embrace of digital health.

The origins of digital health in the US lie in post-World War Two efforts to computerize the country's science and technology, a venture supported by researchers and corporations alike. For example, beginning in 1959, IBM organized a yearly Medical Symposium conference. Experts in life science and medical research spoke alongside public health administrators about the significance of informatic and computational technologies to their administrative and research practices, advancing IBM's goal that its computers would dominate the developing market. By the 1960s, there was a robust industry in medical technologies and computer systems to support them. Whether used in the examining room, the surgical theater, and hospital administration, or for patient scans and tests, medical technology had become integral to the practice of modern medicine. Yet, as scholars and activists noted early on, these technologies and their corporations thrived within the expansion of an 'American Health Empire' (Ehrenreich and Ehrenreich 1971) – namely, the shift of medical practice from the single-family physician to large institutions, including hospitals connected to medical schools and university research facilities. Because new, expensive technologies were necessary for the latest in medical diagnosis and care, physicians could only deliver adequate care when attached to facilities with access to such technologies.

At the same time, burgeoning computing companies – not just IBM, but also its competitors, Technicon and Control Data Corporation – were actively marketing their mainframe computers to medical and psychiatric institutions, claiming that computers could modernize older practices. Historians of computers in biomedicine note that between World War Two and the 1960s, policy turned to support computing-based research, as Congress made increasing appropriations for the National Institute of Health (NIH), which awarded federal grants within large medical institutions. Conferences held in the early-1960s trumpeted computers for advancing new medical discoveries, while academic and scholarly work became more prominent – supported by the NIH Advisory Committee on Computers in Research (Kaplan 1995; November 2011; see also: November 2012). Indeed, influential pieces published by two medical professionals on the NIH's committee reveal more than mere commentary on sectoral developments. One viewed computerization as imperative not because computers could improve diagnosis, but because their use would force all medical subfields to conform to standards and quantitative methods, ultimately leading to automated and optimized diagnoses. Further, both authors argued that computerization would offer the added benefit of addressing the federal government's rising healthcare costs.

It was the 1965 *Medicare Act*, and its almost immediate effect of granting millions of Americans new access to healthcare, that ultimately stimulated the language of healthcare emergency. The increase in the number of people seeking healthcare led the Department of Health, Welfare, and Administration to warn of the system's imminent collapse – a warning then voiced by President Richard Nixon at a presidential briefing in 1969. While the US federal government primarily framed this crisis as arising from increased costs, an additional crisis narrative circulated within the managerial sectors of the medical professions: hospitals experienced information overload, information that they were incapable of organizing, transmitting, or harnessing in any manner that made sense. As historians of medical informatics have shown (Plotnick 2010), medicine looked to other industries experiencing similar information overload – including aerospace, airlines, and Wall Street – for methods to address this supposed crisis. In tandem, these industries turned to a systems approach. A total information system would organize and make efficient a healthcare system that many claimed was breaking. As one proponent put it, 'The systems approach, if it is used wisely, is, at the least, a cure for chaos. Either we take the systems-approach route and perform well, or we accept absolute and utter confusion and chaos' (Ramo 1969; quoted in Plotnick 2010: 1282). The mid-century paradigm of rationalization and management here stretched from the business world to the healthcare world. Yet, early attempts to introduce computers in hospitals were not always greeted with applause by physicians and other healthcare professionals, including nurses. Medical computing professionals did not often take physician's values and work habits into account when they designed information systems. Those in medical computing framed this as a technology 'lag' and attributed it to physicians' obstinacy (Kaplan 1995).

Still, discourse that positioned healthcare as an issue of cost containment, stemming from a lack of managerial rationalization, permeated public policy health discourse. When Paul Ellwood (long an innovator in the area of health insurance cooperatives) consulted with the Nixon Administration on the *Health Maintenance Organization Act* (HMO) of 1973, he joined with Alain Enthoven (previously a US Secretary of Defense, and then a healthcare economist at Stanford). Enthoven viewed healthcare as desperately in need of managerial reform similar to what he had overseen at the Department of Defense. The resulting *HMO Act* was a legislative act that, over the next 20 years, would 'rationally' align health insurance and care with market imperatives. Following the logic of this *Act*, if insurance companies could introduce efficiency metrics into all levels of care, out-of-control spending could be reined in. Not surprisingly, it was Ellwood and Enthoven who would direct the 'managed-care' discourse into healthcare reform efforts that would last into the Clinton administration. The market rationale that dominated subsequent efforts to reform the administration of healthcare sometimes had backing from medical professionals (*e.g.* Schwartz 1970), but was often contested by those who viewed managed care and other insurance industry-friendly policies as an unwelcome intrusion into their professional authority (Tomes 2016).

Concomitant with these 'rationalization' measures, medical computing experts worked to design systems that would allow information to flow freely among institutional boundaries (Kaplan 1995). As early as 1964, in his innovation of the Patient-Oriented Medical Record (POMR), physician Lawrence Weed argued that standardizing how medical records were kept would make possible future biomedical breakthroughs (Weed 1969). More urgent for Weed, though, was that the POMR did exactly what its name indicated: it oriented the medical record around the patient, ensuring that record-keeping documented changes specific to that patient's condition and ongoing treatments. It was not until the late-1970s and 1980s – once computerization had become more generalized – that the field of 'medical informatics' emerged, laying the groundwork to realize

Weed's ultimate vision of data mining, as implied very clearly in his grander vision for the future of medicine (Kaplan 1995; see also Collen and Ball 2015).

Thus, by the 1980s, the dominant rhetoric surrounding computer technology in medical care no longer positioned it as a means to improve patient care (Kaplan 1995). Instead, this technology was envisioned as a method to rein in costs through management and administration. Throughout the decade, federal legislation provided the impetus for this shift in the role of computers from ameliorating patient care to ameliorating patient costs. For example, amendments to the *Social Security Act* in 1983 changed reimbursement to hospitals from a retrospective to a prospective method. Rather than reimbursing hospitals after medical procedures, the Center for Medicare and Medicaid began to distribute funds to hospitals based on diagnostic categories of patient groups, and structuring payments around predicted future costs. This kind of actuarial approach to resource management would, across the sector, be a boon to computer manufacturers, who could then market their technologies to a range of actors as predictive optimizers of treatment.

'Bioeconomies' and digital health development

It is, of course, no surprise that the years of accelerating calls for cost-cutting in healthcare coincided with the tenure of the Reagan administration, when neoliberalism – privatizing public goods and governing through austerity – emerged as a panacea in policy-making. Indeed, it was also during this decade that life itself – tissues, DNA, organs – became subject to commodification. Melinda Cooper (2008: 3) argues that the so-called neoliberal revolution of the 1980s tightly wove together 'state-funded research, the market in new technologies, and financial capital'. As healthcare became increasingly financialized, the possibilities for biodata – data about biological components of life – becoming marketized also emerged forcefully (see also: Waldby and Mitchell 2006; Vora 2015). A prominent example of this was the advent of the Human Genome Project (HGP). First discussed by leading research figures at conferences in 1986, the HGP received $13 million in government funding in the 1987 US budget (and an unprecedented $3 billion planned by the early-1990s). As Rodney Loeppky (2005) has argued, when no other actor could or would step forward, the US state supplied the research infrastructure to make possible nationally coordinated work on a 'map' of the complete human genome, thereby supplying the foundation for future industrial development.

With such an infrastructure in place and genome science as a potential site of capital accumulation established, the new 'bioeconomy' was borne. For instance, genome science forms the basis not only for contemporary for-profit genetic testing platforms, such as the direct-to-consumer DNA company 23andMe, but also for the more recent mRNA vaccines aimed at COVID-19. In this regard, the industrial form of medicine is constituted by the generation of data, catalyzing medical informatics as both a biological and a managerial roadmap.

No industrial development, however, emerges naturally from technological development. Rather, it requires concerted political action. During these decades, as medical informatics matured, patient records continued to frustrate biotech innovators, who viewed them as a treasure trove of information that could accelerate medical breakthroughs. Yet, as indicated in an influential Institute of Medicine 1991 special issue advocating for electronic health record systems, problems continued to plague their pervasive take-up (Dick and Steen 1991). In addition to physicians' reluctance to use them – they required more time on the part of physicians than paper record-keeping – both healthcare professionals and patient advocates raised concerns about privacy and the security of electronic health records. While the federal *Health Insurance Portability and Accountability Act*, passed in 1996, addressed concerns about privacy and security, integration of electronic record-keeping systems was still lacking.

By the 2000s, with continued public debate over the crisis in national healthcare, the US administration incentivized the use of electronic record-keeping systems. Introduced as part of the economic stimulus package of 2009, the *Health Information Technology for Economic and Clinical Health Act* tied technological development explicitly to 'economic health'. The law allowed incentive payments to be extended to healthcare professionals who could demonstrate 'meaningful use' of electronic record-keeping systems. One component of 'meaningful use' was that health information could be easily exchanged among healthcare entities. More recently, the *21st Century Cures Act*, passed in 2016, transformed the policy carrot into a stick, fining records vendors who 'blocked' the exchange of certain information in their programs.

Such interoperability and the massive datasets it could generate would be of use in other heavily funded research projects, all of them couched in stimulating new biomedical and technological investments and innovation. For example, in 2010, the National Institute of Mental Health (NIMH) announced a new funding stream, the Research Domain Criteria Project, which aims to harness genetic information for neuroscientific research while simultaneously using cell phones to gather data on affective states. The overall goal is to advance new forms of pharmaceutical innovation through the model of 'precision psychiatry'. In 2015, the NIH announced the Precision Medicine Initiative (PMI), overseen by the then Director of the NIH Francis Collins (Collins and Varmus 2015), which mobilized tropes of 'self-fashioning' and 'self-care' ('individualized medicine, tailored to you'). The initiative explicitly utilizes consumer-facing data gathering devices as a means to enable the next stage in individualized medical knowledge production. In 2018, the NIH opened enrollment in its All of Us study, in which one million people would share their electronic medical records and Fitbit data (if they had the device). The enrollment announcement indicated that its researchers would integrate data from other devices, once it could be made to match the study's protocols. Apple quickly announced a new platform for digital health development, CareKit, and its next model of the Apple Watch included atrial detection systems, designed specifically to make it attractive to the NIH's research. Importantly, the *21st Century Cures Act* ensured greater flows of big datasets among biomedical researchers. As described by NIH officials, the *Act* allows for immediate data-sharing among researchers funded through the NIH, 'giving all scientists the opportunity to use these data as quickly as possible to advance biomedical research' (Hudson and Collins 2017: 112).

Each of these endeavors harnesses biomedical research and clinical healthcare to technology use and development, conceived within a framework of future profits for medical industries (Clarke *et al.* 2003). Increasingly, these projects tether research to mobile consumer devices, ensuring capital investment in technology corporations. The announcement of the PMI, which expressly gestured to the Fitbit (now owned by Google), prompted Apple and Google – which had been working for a decade to enter the profitable medical records arena – to announce new platforms for their operating systems. These, in turn, allowed programmers to develop health-related applications that could be synced to ongoing biomedical research. Engaging with the sector more fully, Google's health-related technology spinoff, Verily Life Sciences, announced in 2015 that it would conduct its own 10,000-person study – Project Baseline – using its new prototype wearable Study Watch to track individual and group biodata (Maxmen 2017). As with the HGP, the US state (particularly via the NIH) generated research infrastructure – in this case, mandating technical features for data-sharing – that sparked continued capital investment in biotechnologies and biomedical innovation.

The neoliberal subject of digital health

A broader analysis of the complex ecosystem of health, in which such projects are embedded, would rightfully interrogate how health is framed – that is, whether these studies pursue knowledge of health as a field of merely digitized biological data, or whether it is also understood as (at least in part) environmentally produced. For the All of Us project, while documents gesture toward the importance of environmental factors, even here the rhetorical and conceptual frames in which these are situated place the burden squarely on the individual to navigate with enhanced knowledge of their biological data. For instance,

> [p]articipants with asthma could wear sensors to detect environmental pollutants and use mHealth apps to record their ease of breathing, leading to both new knowledge and the potential to take action to modify their exposure. This information may promote healthier behavior, reduce unnecessary testing, and improve medication compliance.
>
> (Precision Medicine 2015: 23)

In this way, the utilization of digital health is tightly bound to neoliberal doctrine, whereby individuals operating within a market terrain are equipped with both technology and knowledge in order to maximize individual responsibility and rational action.

How health insurance companies view digital health tools further exemplifies the accelerating presence of neoliberal dogma surrounding austerity and individual responsibility. For example, some insurance companies now incentivize wearables within policies, in effect rewarding the insured if they submit to constant surveillance, while allowing those with expendable wealth to opt out (easily paying the premium instead). Here, digital technology is used to transform health from a complex array of life circumstances into a matter of personal choice and self-regulation. This reward-punishment system of health governance obscures the social and political-economic structures that have been demonstratively shown to impact health far more than individual 'choices' (Fotopoulou and O'Riordan 2017; Elman 2018; Gidaris 2019).

It is here, too, where digital health dovetails with neoliberal constructions of the self-responsible subject, and we see that the often-lauded rise of the e-Patient remains more complicated than its superficial portrait suggests (*e.g.* Miah and Rich 2008). While heralded as an active participant in efforts to involve patients in determining research and care, the e-Patient is simultaneously a subject within a system of austerity, which validates behavior that makes denial of care more widespread. The e-Patient, now actively responsible for educating themselves regarding health status, treatment, and possible avenues for care, was even promoted in a provision of the *21st Century Cures Act*, which mandated opening electronic health records to patients. This was with an eye to patients managing their own care, and it has been brought home in the recent case of extraordinary activism on the part of 'COVID Longhaulers', who defined their own condition and terminology through gathering and analyzing available data (Callard and Perego 2021).

Conclusion

The history narrated above – focused on legislative, professional, and biomedical shifts – proceeded, of course, within a broader socio-historical context. It is important to note that each moment of so-called crisis in healthcare costs occurred in tandem with an expansion of healthcare access to new populations. Moreover, the intersection of 'fiscal crisis' with the active restriction of healthcare access to marginalized groups remains not-so-coincidental. It might also be important to note that neoliberal policies formed a major part of the response to social unrest and radical challenges to the capitalist order. For example, the Reagan administration's racism, which redirected popular anger at extant political-economic conditions, also undergirded its moves to de-fund public health measures for communities of color via an austerity logic.

The latest darlings of digital health, artificial intelligence and machine learning, remain in lockstep with (but also somewhat oblivious to) such austere and problematic outcomes. The claim to increase efficiency and decrease costs parallels the denial of care for those who need it most (Benjamin 2019). Disability activists have argued that the use of algorithmic logic, for instance in triaging scarce resources during public health crises, was designed to assess disabled life as that least-worth saving (*e.g.* DREDF 2020). One provision in the *21st Century Cares Act* mandates that Medicaid-receiving states use Electronic Visit Verification Systems for home-based personal assistance and care services, in order to root out fraud. Such measures amount to surveillance of the lives of poor, racialized, and disabled people, as well as the primarily poor female workers of color who provide such services (Gallopyn and Iezzoni 2020). In these and other instances, digital health under capitalism portends only restriction of services and a punitary health regime for those with the least political voice.

This chapter has focused on the US case, but digital health development now spans the globe. In the West, disaster capitalism (Klein 2007) provided the means for US corporations Google and Palantir to push into Britain's NHS (Powles and Hodson, 2017; Cox 2020; Kitchin 2020). Simultaneously, development discourse around healthcare access in the Global South both promotes and problematizes digital tools as a means to achieve universal healthcare (*e.g.* Kickbusch *et al.* 2021). Western, primarily American, corporations seek entry into these new global health markets, including through extraction of value via 'data colonialism' (Couldry and Meijas 2019). Across multiple jurisdictions and cultures, these corporations have seized on the prevailing notion of healthcare 'crisis' to harness political momentum toward privatization: identifying ways in which data can be used as an avenue of accumulation, regardless of the actual health outcomes. Regrettably, this illustrates, once again, that digital health is a primary site for capital investment across neoliberal systems of governance.

References

Benjamin, R. 2019, 'Assessing risk, automating racism', *Science*, 366(6464), pp. 421–2.

Callard, F. and Perego, E. 2021, 'How and why patients made long COVID', *Social Science and Medicine*, 268, p. 113426.

Clarke, A.E., Shim, J.K., Mamo, L., Fosket, J.R. and Fishman, J.R. 2003, 'Biomedicalization: Technoscientific transformations of health, illness, and US biomedicine', *American Sociological Review*, 68(2), pp. 161–94.

Collen, M, and Ball, M. 2015, *The History of Medical Informatics in the United States*, Springer, New York.

Collins, F. and Varmus, H. 2015, 'A new initiative on precision medicine', *New England Journal of Medicine*, 372(9), pp. 793–5.

Cooper, M. 2008, *Life as Surplus: Biotechnology and Capitalism in the Neoliberal Era*, University of Washington Press, Seattle.

Couldry, N. and Mejias, U. 2019 'Data colonialism: Rethinking big data's relation to the contemporary subject', *Television and New Media*, 20(4), pp. 336–49.

Cox, D. 2020, 'Alarm bells ring for patient data and privacy in the COVID-19 goldrush', *British Medical Journal*, 369, m1925.

Dick, R. and Steen, E. (eds) 1991, *The Computer-Based Patient Record*, Institute of Medicine, National Academy Press, Washington, DC.

Disability Rights Education and Defense Fund (DREDF). 2020, 'Preventing discrimination in the treatment of COVID-19 patients: The illegality of medical rationing on the basis of disability', accessed 25 March 2022, <https://dredf.org/the-illegality-of-medical-rationing-on-the-basis-of-disability/>.

Ehrenreich, B. and Ehrenreich, J. 1971, *The American Health Empire: Power, Profits, and Politics,* Knopf Doubleday, New York.
Elman, J. 2018, '"Find Your Fit": Wearable technology and the cultural politics of disability', *New Media and Society*, 20(10), pp. 3760–77.
Fotopoulou, A. and O'Riordan, K. 2017, 'Training to self-care: Fitness tracking, biopedagogy and the healthy consumer', *Health Sociology Review*, 26(1), pp. 54–68.
Gallopyn, N. and Iezzoni, L. 2020, 'Views of electronic visit verification (EVV) among home-based personal assistance services consumers and workers', *Disability and Health Journal,* 13(4), p. 100938.
Gidaris, C. 2019, 'Surveillance capitalism, datafication, and unwaged labour: The rise of wearable fitness devices and interactive life insurance', *Surveillance and Society*, 17(1–2), pp. 132–8.
Haydon, P. 2021, 'Record investment in global healthtech sees 280% increase on 2016 levels', mobihealthnews, 23 November, www.mobihealthnews.com/news/emea/record-investment-global-healthtech-sees-280-increase-2016-levels.
Hudson, K.L. and Collins, F.S. 2017, 'The 21st century cures act: A view from the NIH', *New England Journal of Medicine*, 376(2), pp. 111–3.
Kaplan, B. 1995, 'The computer prescription: Medical computing, public policy, and views of history', *Science, Technology, and Human Values*, 20(1), pp. 5–38,
Kickbusch, I., Piselli, D., Agrawal, A., Balicer, R., Banner, O., Adelhardt, M., Capobianco, E., Fabian, C., Gill, A., Lupton, D. and Medhora, R. 2021, 'The Lancet and financial times commission on governing health futures 2030: Growing up in a digital world', *The Lancet*, 398(10312), pp. 1727–76.
Kitchin, R. 2020, 'Civil liberties or public health, or civil liberties and public health? Using surveillance technologies to tackle the spread of COVID-19', *Space and Polity*, 24(3), pp. 362–81.
Klein, N. 2007, *The Shock Doctrine: The Rise of Disaster Capitalism*, Macmillan, New York.
Loeppky, R. 2005, *Encoding Capital: The Political Economy of the Human Genome Project*, Routledge, New York.
Maxmen, A. 2017, 'Google spin-off deploys wearable electronics for huge health study', *Nature*, 547(7661), pp. 13–4.
Miah, A. and Rich, E. 2008, *The Medicalization of Cyberspace*, Routledge, New York.
November, J. 2011, 'Early biomedical computing and the roots of evidence-based medicine', *IEEE Annals of the History of Computing*, 33(2), pp. 9–23.
November, J. 2012, *Biomedical Computing: Digitizing life in the United States*, Johns Hopkins University Press, Baltimore.
Plotnick, R. 2010, 'Computers, systems theory, and the making of a wired hospital: A history of technicon medical information system, 1964–1987', *Journal of the American Society for Information Science and Technology*, 61(6), pp. 1281–94.
Powles, J. and Hodson, H. 2017, 'Google deepmind and healthcare in an age of algorithms', *Health and Technology*, 7(4), pp. 351–67.
Precision Medicine Initiative (PMI) Working Group Report to the Advisory Committee to the Director, NIH. 2015, 'The precision medicine initiative cohort program – Building a research foundation for 21st century medicine', accessed 25 March 2022, <https://www.nih.gov/sites/default/files/research-training/initiatives/pmi/pmi-working-group-report-20150917-2.pdf>.
Ramo, S. 1969, *Cure for Chaos: Fresh Solutions to Social Problems Through the Systems Approach*, David McKay, New York.
Schwartz, W. 1970, 'Medicine and the computer: The promise and problems of change', *New England Journal of Medicine*, 283(23), pp. 1257–64.
Tomes, N. 2016, *Remaking the American Patient: How Madison Avenue and Modern Medicine Turned Patients into Consumers*, University of North Carolina Press, Chapel Hill.
Vora, K. 2015, *Life Support: Biocapital and the New History of Outsourced Labor*, University of Minnesota Press, Minneapolis.
Waldby, C. and Mitchell, R. 2006, *Tissue Economies: Blood, Organs, and Cell Lines in Late Capitalism*, Duke University Press, Durham.
Weed, L. 1969, *Medical Records, Medical Education, and Patient Care: The Problem-Oriented Record As a Basic Tool*, Case Western Reserve University Press, Cleveland.

17

THE POLITICAL ECONOMY OF HEALTH AND PLACE

From the Great Compression to COVID-19

Clare Bambra[1]

'Health inequality' refers to the systematic differences in health that exist according to socio-economic status (SES) (usually measured in terms of income, education, occupation, or area-level deprivation), region, or country. Inequalities in health are 'systematic differences in health between different socio-economic groups within a society. As they are socially produced, they are potentially avoidable and widely considered unacceptable in a civilized society' (Whitehead 2007: 473). Inequalities in health by SES are not restricted to differences between the most privileged groups and the most disadvantaged, but exist across the entire social gradient (Marmot 2005). The social gradient in health runs from the top to the bottom of society, and 'even comfortably off people somewhere in the middle tend to have poorer health than those above them' (Marmot 2005: 2). Across Europe, people with higher occupational status (*e.g.* professionals such as teachers or lawyers) have better health outcomes than those with lower occupational status (*e.g.* manual workers) (Eikemo *et al.* 2017). Similarly, people with a higher income or tertiary-level education have better health outcomes than those with a low income or no educational qualifications (Bambra 2016). Such inequalities are also evident between regions and between countries. For example, Americans live three years less than their counterparts in France or Sweden. People in the northern regions of England live two years less than people in the rest of England, and there is a 25-year gap in life expectancy across the suburbs of New Orleans (Bambra 2016).

Health inequalities have been increasing over the last 40 years. For example, while average life expectancy at birth in the European Union (EU) increased from 79.4 years in 2008 to 81.0 years in 2016, these increases were smaller among men and women with a lower level of education (Forster *et al.* 2018). To illustrate, in Denmark, the difference in life expectancy at age 30 between men with a low education and men with a tertiary education rose from 4.8 years to 6.4 years during this period. The respective gap for women increased from 3.7 years to 4.7 years (Forster *et al.* 2018). Similarly, in England, the gap in life expectancy for women between the most and least deprived areas increased from 6.8 years in 2010 to 7.1 years by 2015 (Department of Health and Social Care 2017). In Scotland, analysis of data up to 2017 found that deaths under 65 years had actually increased in recent years, reflecting worsening mortality rates among the most socio-economically disadvantaged populations (Walsh *et al.* 2020). In the US, there was a marked increase in the all-cause mortality of middle-aged white non-Hispanic men and women – particularly those in lower-income groups – between 1999 and 2013 (Case and Deaton 2020).

DOI: 10.4324/9781003017110-19

Box 17.1 Place

Place can be comprehended in simple geometric terms as 'a portion of space in which people dwell together' (*e.g.* latitude, longitude, elevation). Alternatively, it may be grasped in a more experiential sense as 'a milieu that exercises a mediating role on physical, social and economic processes and which effects how such process operate' – or, put more concisely, 'a distinctive coming together in space' (Agnew 2011: 318). Places are not, though, bounded and static, so much as fluid and relational – nodes within social, economic, and political networks (Cummins *et al.* 2007). Place does, though, require membership of communities, cities, or states. Rather, place both creates and contains social, economic, and political relations, as well as physical resources (Bambra 2016).

In sum, more privileged groups have benefited the most from any improvements in health over the last few decades, leading to increased health inequalities in some countries (Mackenbach *et al.* 2016). Further, the COVID-19 pandemic has also been experienced unequally, with death rates twice as high among the most socially excluded social groups (Bambra *et al.* 2020). There is also emerging evidence that COVID-19 is reducing life expectancy gains – with, for example, life expectancy falls of around one year on average in England and Wales between 2019 and 2020 as a result of the pandemic (Aburto *et al.* 2021). These immediate COVID-19–related decreases in life expectancy are likely to be higher in the most deprived areas and groups – once again, potentially increasing health inequalities into the future (Bambra *et al.* 2021).

This chapter examines the causes of these substantial inequalities in health at different geographical scales – between individuals, neighborhoods, cities, regions, and countries. It outlines how the discipline of health geography has traditionally explained these health divides – in terms of the effects of *compositional* and *contextual* factors, and the *relational* interaction of people with the wider environment (Bambra 2016). It outlines the analytical limits of these traditional approaches in terms of advancing our understanding of the relationship between health and place (see: Box 17.1) through outlining an alternative *political economy approach* – which scales up our conceptualization of context to also include the influence of national and international political and economic factors (Bambra *et al.* 2019). It then applies the political economy approach to explain international trends in health inequalities over the last 70 years – from the *Great Compression* to *COVID-19.*

Traditional explanations

This section outlines how the discipline of health geography has traditionally explained these health divides – in terms of the effects of compositional and contextual factors and the relational interaction of people with the wider environment (Bambra 2016).

Compositional approach

The compositional view argues that the health of a given place (be it a neighborhood, region, or country) is determined largely by the characteristics of the individuals who live within it. In turn, the health of individuals is shaped by their health behaviors (smoking, alcohol, physical activity, diet, drugs) and their socio-economic status (income, education, occupation). In this view, smoking, alcohol, physical activity, diet, and drugs are considered as individual lifestyle factors or risky health behaviors. These significantly influence the health of people and, therefore, places (Jarvis and Wardle 2006). Therefore, on average, areas (countries, regions, cities, neighborhoods) with higher rates of these unhealthy behaviors among their populations will experience poorer health than others, all things being equal.

The socio-economic status of people living in an area is also of substantial importance to health. Socio-economic status is a term that refers to occupational class, income, or educational level (Bambra 2011). As noted above, people with higher occupational status (*e.g.* professionals such as teachers or lawyers) have better health outcomes than non-professional workers (*e.g.* manual laborers). Having a higher income, or being educated to a degree level, can also have a protective health effect, whereas having a lower income or no educational qualifications can have a negative health impact. SES influences health through a variety of mechanisms. These include the following: cultural-behavioral (the link between SES and health is a result of differences according to SES in health-related behavior), materialist (inequalities in income and what it enables – such as access to health-promoting or health-damaging goods and services, and exposure to physical and psycho-social risk factors – shape health inequalities), and psycho-social (concerned with how social inequality makes people feel and the biological consequences of these feelings on health) (Bartley 2017).

Contextual approach

The contextual approach explains geographical inequalities in health by building on the compositional approach. However, it highlights that the nature of a *place* itself also matters for the health of that place – that is, not only individual factors matter, but also their collective, *placed* experience (Bambra 2016). In this view, health differs geographically according to place because the economic, social, and physical environment in which we live also determines our health. The contextual approach argues that *place* mediates the way in which individuals experience the social, economic, and physical determinants of health: places can be salutogenic (health-promoting) or pathogenic (health-damaging) environments. These place-based effects can, therefore, be seen as the collective effects of the social determinants of health.

There are three contextual aspects to place that have traditionally been considered as important to health: economic, social, and physical. Area-economic factors that influence health are often summarized as economic deprivation. They include area poverty rates, unemployment rates, wages, and types of work and employment in the area. Area-level economic factors, such as poverty, are a key predictor of health outcomes – including cardiovascular disease, all-cause mortality, limiting long-term illness, and health-related behaviors (Macintyre 2007).

Places also have social aspects that influence health. Opportunity structures are the socially constructed and patterned features of the area that may promote health through the possibilities they provide (Macintyre *et al.* 2002). These include the services provided, publicly or privately, to support people in their daily lives, such as childcare, transport, food availability, or access to a family physician or hospital, as well as the availability of health-promoting environments at home (*e.g.* good housing quality, access, and affordability), work (good-quality employment), and education (such as high-quality schools). Another social aspect of place is collective social functioning. Collective social functioning beneficial to health might, for instance, include high levels of social cohesion and social capital within the community. Some studies have found that areas with higher levels of social capital have better health, such as lower mortality rates, more positive self-rated health mental health outcomes, and beneficial health behaviors (Hawe and Shiell 2000). More negative collective effects can also arise from the reputation or history of an area (Halliday *et al.* 2021).

For its part, the physical environment of a place is also widely recognized as an important determinant of health and health inequalities (World Health Organization 2008). There is a sizable literature on the positive health effects of access to green space, as well as the negative health effects of waste facilities, brownfield or contaminated land, and air pollution (Bambra *et al.* 2014). Awareness of how such facets of the physical environment differ geographically has led to the development of the concept of 'environmental deprivation': mortality is lowest in areas with the least environmental deprivation, and highest in areas experiencing the greatest environmental deprivation (Pearce *et al.* 2010).

Relational approach

The contextual and compositional approaches are not mutually exclusive, and it has been acknowledged that their separation amounts to an oversimplification, ignoring the interactions between these two dimensions (Macintyre *et al.* 2002). Composition and context should not, therefore, be seen as separate or competing explanations – rather, they are entwined. Both contribute to the complex relationship between health and place that, in turn, lead to geographical inequalities in health. Place should be considered as an ecosystem comprising people, systems, and structures, such that 'there is a mutually reinforcing and reciprocal relationship between people and place' (Cummins *et al.* 2007: 1826). As such, Cummins *et al.* subsequently developed the *relational approach*, which suggests that compositional and contextual factors interact to produce geographical inequalities in health.

The relational approach helps us to understand how the health behaviors and SES characteristics of individuals are influenced by the various features of the area. By way of example, the occupational class can be determined by local school quality and the availability of jobs in the local labor market. In the same vein, children might not play outside for various reasons: the lack of a private garden (a compositional resource); a dearth of public parks or transport to reach them (a contextual resource); or a prevailing sense of inappropriateness for them to do so (contextual social functioning) (Macintyre *et al.* 2002). Finally, areas with more successful economies (*e.g.* more high-paid jobs) will, logically, have smaller proportions of low socio-economic status residents (Bambra 2016). Ultimately, these interrelational dimensions of compositional and contextual attributes substantially influence health outcomes. In fact, a study conducted in England on mental wellbeing noted how compositional factors (*e.g.* health behaviors and SES such as employment) relationally interacted with more contextual factors in the physical and social environment to produce inequalities (Bhandari *et al.* 2017; Akhter *et al.* 2018).

The political economy approach

From a political economy viewpoint, the traditional compositional, contextual, and relational approaches to understanding health inequalities are analytically limited, mostly because they only focus on individual characteristics or localized neighborhood effects. In this way, much geographical research misses the bigger picture: namely, that these compositional and contextual determinants of health are themselves shaped by wider political and economic factors (Bambra 2016). The relationship between health and place – and the health inequalities that, thereby, exist between places – is largely politically and economically determined (Bambra *et al.* 2005). That is, place matters for health, but political economy matters for place (Bambra 2016). This insight has led to the development of the political economy of health approach within health geography (Bambra *et al.* 2019). It argues that, to properly understand how place relates to health, we need to 'scale up' our analytical approach by applying insights from the wider political economy of health literature to consider the more fundamental causes of geographical inequalities in health.

The political economy approach to health has a long pedigree – arguably dating back to the Nineteenth Century (*e.g.* Virchow), with further influential work conducted in the late-1970s (*e.g.* Doyal and Pennell 1979). More recently, it has made a resurgence in social epidemiology and medical sociology, particularly in relation to the examination of cross-national differences in health (Schrecker and Bambra 2015), and within analyses of health inequalities between socio-economic groups (*e.g.* Krieger 2003; Bambra *et al.* 2005). Most notably, there is a substantial body of work that examines the impact of different welfare state arrangements on the patterning of population health and health inequalities (see: Beckfield 2018), which highlights how individual and local influences on health and wellbeing relate to broader social, economic, and political conditions operating at national and international scales (Bambra 2016).

In 2014, the Lancet-University of Oslo Commission on Global Governance for Health put forward the concept of the 'political determinants of health', insisting that 'construing socially and politically created health inequities as problems of technocratic or medical management depoliticizes social and political ills' (Ottersen *et al.* 2014: 636). The political economy approach argues that the contextual-level social determinants of health are, themselves, shaped by macro-level structural determinants: politics, the economy, the (welfare) state, the organization of work, and the structure of the labor market (Bambra 2011). Relatedly, population health is shaped by the social, political, and economic structures and relations that are often outside the control of the individuals, and the places, they affect (Krieger 2003). Individual and collective socio-economic factors, such as housing, income, and employment – indeed, many of the issues that dominate political life – are key determinants of health and wellbeing (Bambra *et al.* 2005). Accordingly, health inequalities between people and places are deemed politically determined, with patterns of disease

> [p]roduced, literally and metaphorically, by the structures, values and priorities of political and economic systems [...] Health inequities are thus posited to arise from whatever is each society's form of social inequality, defined in relation to power, property and privilege.
> (Krieger 2013: 245)

Thus, the consistent privileging of some places and people, and perennial marginalization of others, is a political choice: it is related to where power lies and in whose interests that power is exercised (Bambra *et al.* 2019). Political choices can, thereby, be seen as the *causes of the causes of the causes* of geographical inequalities in health (Bambra 2016).

By way of example, consider stroke or heart disease (Bambra 2016). The immediate clinical cause of such conditions could be hypertension (high blood pressure). The proximal cause of the hypertension itself could be compositional lifestyle factors such as poor diet, of which the contextual cause might be living in a low-income neighborhood. The causes of the latter are arguably political in nature – low-income neighborhoods exist because the political and economic system allows them to exist (Bambra 2016). Wages could be regulated so that they are higher (*e.g.* the living wage), or food prices could be controlled/subsidized (*e.g.* in the US, it is meat and corn oil that receive government subsidies, not fruit and vegetables; likewise in the EU, farmers are encouraged to produce dairy). Moreover, neighborhood food provision does not have to be left to the vagaries of the market, which leads to clustering of poor food availability in impoverished neighborhoods (Schrecker and Bambra 2015).

In this sense, geographical patterns of health and disease are produced by the structures, values, and priorities of political and economic systems (Krieger 2003). Area-level health is determined, at least partly, by the wider political, social, and economic system. It is also configured by actions by the state (government)- and international-level actors – including supra-national government bodies, such as the European Union; interstate trade agreements, such as the Transatlantic Trade and Investment Partnership [TTIP]; or large corporations. Quite literally, politics can make us sick or healthy (Schrecker and Bambra 2015). Politics and the balance of power between key political groups – notably labor and capital – determine the role of the state and other agencies in relation to health, whether there are collective interventions to reduce health inequalities across populations and place, and resolving whether those interventions are individually, environmentally, or structurally focused. In this way, politics is the fundamental determinant of the relationship between health and place, because it shapes the wider social, economic, and physical environment and, thus, the social and spatial distribution of salutogenic and pathogenic factors on both a collective and an individual level (Bambra 2016).

The political economy of health inequalities: from the Great Compression to COVID-19

This section applies the political economy approach to help understand trends in health inequalities over the last 70 years: from the Great Compression of the 1950s to 1970s, via the neoliberal turn of the 1980s and 1990s, through austerity after the Global Financial Crisis (GFC) of 2008 to the COVID-19 pandemic.

Health inequalities in the Great Compression: 1950s to 1970s

After the Second World War, welfare states were established in many high-income countries, including those in Western Europe, North America, and Australasia. These led to significant improvements to public housing, healthcare, and other major social determinants of health, including the highest ever share of national income distributed to workers (Eikemo and Bambra 2008). This period is known as the Great Compression (Scheidel 2017). The post-war welfare states represented a new form of political economy, and health inequalities – between socio-economic classes and by place – decreased substantially in this period (Bambra 2022).

In the 1960s, US President Lyndon B. Johnson announced his administration's 'Great Society' program, which would led to a series of substantial programs to address inequalities in medical care, civil rights, education, and poverty (Andrew 1998). For instance, the Medicare (universal health insurance for all those aged over 65 years) and Medicaid (limited healthcare costs coverage for welfare recipients) programs were introduced under this initiative. These substantially increased access to healthcare for the poor and elderly. Similarly, the 'War on Poverty' included various initiatives to address urban and rural poverty; increased educational opportunities (including significant increases in Federal funding for the education system); expanded the Federal food stamp program; increased the value of the state pension; and expanded the scope of the main Federal welfare program – Aid for Dependent Children – to cover black mothers (Karger and Stoesz 1990). The *1964 Civil Rights Act* formally outlawed racial discrimination (abolishing the racially discriminatory 'Jim Crow' legal system in 21 southern states and the District of Columbia), in requiring the desegregation of schools and public accommodation (including hospitals), as well as equalized voting rights (Beardsley 1986). An analysis by Krieger and colleagues (2008) examined the impact of these anti-poverty and civil rights reforms on health inequalities. They found that the influence of racial and income inequalities in premature mortality (deaths under age 75) and infant mortality rates (deaths before age 1) declined between 1966 and 1980.

Neoliberalism, enduring austerity, and health inequalities

The Great Compression and 'golden age' of the welfare state effectively ended with the stagflationary economic crisis of the 1970s and subsequent emergence of neoliberal economics. Initially, this development occurred predominantly in Anglo-American countries, but spread rapidly across continental Europe in the 1980s and 1990s (Bambra *et al.* 2010). Neoliberalism led to the erosion of the post-war welfare model of political economy, and resulted in an increase in poverty and health inequalities (Schrecker and Bambra 2015).

For example, health inequalities in the US increased between 1980 and 2002, during which time consecutive administrations cut public welfare services (including healthcare insurance coverage) and funding of social assistance, froze the minimum wage, and shifted the tax base from the rich to the poor, leading to increased income polarization (Krieger *et al.* 2008). These findings are mirrored in studies of welfare state reductions in New Zealand, where inequalities in all-cause mortality increased during the 1980s and the 1990s, as the country underwent major neoliberal structural reforms. The latter included the following: a less redistributive tax system; targeted social benefits; introduction of a regressive tax on consumption; privatization of major utilities and public housing; user charges for welfare services; and a more deregulated labor market (Shaw *et al.* 2005). In the UK, Thatcherism (1979–90) deregulated the labor and financial markets, privatized utilities and state enterprises, restricted social housing, curtailed trade union rights, marketized the public sector, significantly cut the social wage via welfare state retrenchment, accepted mass unemployment, and implemented large tax cuts for the business sector and most affluent (Scott-Samuel *et al.* 2014). During this period, while life expectancy increased and mortality rates decreased for all social groups, the climb was greater and more rapid among the most affluent social groups and places, thereby exacerbating existing inequalities.

More recent research into the fiscal austerity policies pursued in some European countries (including the UK, Greece, Spain, Italy, and Portugal) after the GFC has demonstrated their pernicious impact in augmenting health inequalities (Niedzwiedz *et al.* 2016). Across Europe, reductions in public spending adversely affected the mental health of disadvantaged social groups (Niedzwiedz *et al.* 2016). To illustrate, in the UK, it was estimated that austerity policies exerted pressure on key social and healthcare services, which resulted in up to 10,000 additional deaths in 2018 compared to previous years. Moreover, as child poverty rates increased between 2010 and 2020 (the decade of austerity), inequalities in infant mortality rates also increased (Robinson *et al.* 2019; Taylor-Robinson *et al.* 2019). The gap in mental health and wellbeing between deprived and affluent areas increased, as the former bore the brunt of rising rates of mental ill-health (Barr *et al.* 2015). In general, socio-economically and spatially concentrated increases in unemployment since 2007/08 have engendered increases in inequalities in both morbidity and mortality (Moeller *et al.* 2013). More particularly, austerity has disproportionately affected the health of vulnerable groups, especially individuals and families receiving low incomes or in receipt of welfare benefits (MacLeavy 2011). For instance, under the auspices of austerity, mortality rates among low-income women increased in the most deprived areas of the UK (ONS 2015).

In the wake of such deleterious health effects arising from the implementation of austerity, considerable evidence has accumulated in relation to substantial inequalities arising from the impact of COVID-19. During the early years of the pandemic, deaths were at least twice as high in the most deprived neighborhoods than in the most affluent; among people with low incomes; and disparities exist between urban and rural areas (Bambra *et al.* 2021). Inequalities also followed ethnicity and race, with the death rates of minority ethnic communities in England, Canada, and the US being more than double that of majority white communities. In addition to inequalities in the disease itself, the economic crisis resulting from government responses to the pandemic (such as lockdowns and social distancing) had unequal impacts – most adversely affecting those on low incomes or living in disadvantaged places (Bambra *et al.* 2020). While many governments implemented additional social protections to support people unable to work during the pandemic, these varied in generosity – being more extensive in the Nordic and continental European countries, and less so in the UK and US. It is too early to reflect on the long-term impacts of the pandemic on trends in health inequalities. However, it seems likely that such inequalities will only increase without increased governmental social protection. Indeed, there are signs in the UK that inequalities in life expectancy between the most and least deprived neighborhoods have increased since the pandemic (ONS 2022).

This overview of changes in political economy and trends in health inequalities suggests that expansion of social welfare and reduction of poverty levels engender reductions in health inequalities. Conversely, reduction of welfare provision begets increased poverty and health inequalities (Simpson *et al.* 2021; Bambra 2022). This has clear implications for the politics and policies needed for a more equitable and socially just recovery after the COVID-19 pandemic. Ultimately, the turn from the Great Compression to neoliberal and austerity politics has affected people and places in detrimental and unequal ways: widening spatial disparities and undermining previous gains in equality. Health inequalities were bound to follow suit, and the post-pandemic period will tell us much about whether governments have learned any lessons from this.

Conclusion

To date, health geography has conventionally presented three interlinked explanations for why there are such stark place-based inequalities in health: compositional, contextual, and relational. However, because of the analytical limitations inherent in these approaches, a political economy alternative has been developed and adopted within the discipline. As this chapter has shown, this latter approach offers a more structural, scaled-up understanding of geographical inequalities in health and how they change over time in relation to the political and economic context. As the world recovers from the COVID-19 crisis, there is a need for further political-economic analysis of the impacts of the pandemic on geographical inequalities in health and how they can be reduced in the future.

Note

1 This research was funded by the Wellcome Trust (reference: 221266/Z/20/Z) and the Norwegian Research Council (reference: 288638).

References

Aburto, J.M., Kashyap, R., Schöley, J., Angus, C., Ermisch, J., Mills, M.C. and Dowd, J.B. 2021, 'Estimating the burden of the COVID-19 pandemic on mortality, life expectancy and lifespan inequality in England and Wales: A population-level analysis', *Journal of Epidemiology and Community Health*, 75(8), pp. 735–40.

Agnew, J. 2011, 'Space and place', in Agnew, J. and Livingston, D. (eds), *The SAGE Handbook of Geographical Knowledge*, Sage, London, pp. 316–30.

Akhter, N., Bambra, C. and Mattheys, K. 2018, 'Inequalities in mental health and well-being in a time of austerity: Longitudinal findings from the Stockton-on-Tees cohort study', *SSM Population Health*, 6(6), pp. 75–84.

Andrew, J. 1998, *Lyndon Johnson and the Great Society*, Ivan R Dee, Chicago.

Bambra, C. 2011, *Work, Worklessness, and the Political Economy of Health,* Oxford University Press, Oxford.

Bambra, C. 2016, *Health Divides: Where You Live Can Kill You*, Policy Press, Bristol.

Bambra, C. 2022, 'Levelling up – Global case studies in reducing health inequalities', *Scandinavian Journal of Public Health*, 50(7), pp. 908–13.

Bambra, C., Fox, D. and Scott-Samuel, A. 2005, 'Towards a politics of health', *Health Promotion International*, 20(2), pp. 187–93.

Bambra, C., Lynch, J. and Smith, K.E. 2021, *The Unequal Pandemic: COVID-19 and Health Inequalities*, Policy Press, Bristol.

Bambra, C., Netuveli, G. and Eikemo, T. 2010, 'Welfare state regime life courses: The development of Western European welfare state regimes and age related patterns of educational inequalities in self-reported health', *International Journal of Health Services*, 40(3), pp. 399–420.

Bambra, C., Riordan, R., Ford, J. and Matthews, F. 2020, 'The COVID-19 pandemic and health inequalities', *Journal of Epidemiology and Community Health*, 74(6), pp. 964–68.

Bambra, C., Robertson, S., Kasim, A., Smith, J., Cairns-Nagi, J., Copeland, A., Finlay, N. and Johnson, K. 2014, 'Healthy land? An examination of the area-level association between brownfield land and morbidity and mortality in England', *Environment and Planning A*, 46(2), pp. 433–54.

Bambra, C., Smith, K. and Pearce, J. 2019, 'Scaling up: The politics of health and place', *Social Science and Medicine*, 232(1), pp. 36–42.

Barr, B., Kinderman, P. and Whitehead, M. 2015, 'Trends in mental health inequalities in England during a period of recession, austerity and welfare reform 2004–2013', *Social Science and Medicine*, 147(2), pp. 324–31.

Bartley, M. 2017, *Health Inequality: An Introduction to Concepts, Theories and Methods*, 2nd edn, Polity, London.

Beardsley, E.H. 1986, 'Good-bye to Jim Crow: The desegregation of Southern hospitals, 1945–70', *Bulletin of the History of Medicine*, 60(3), pp. 367–86.

Beckfield, J. 2018, *Political Sociology and the People's Health*, Oxford University Press, New York.

Bhandari, R., Akhter, N., Warren, J., Kasim, A. and Bambra, C. 2017, 'Geographical inequalities in general and physical health in a time of austerity: Baseline findings from the Stockton-on-Tees cohort study', *Health and Place*, 48(1), pp. 111–22.

Case, A. and Deaton, A. 2020, *Deaths of Despair and the Future of Capitalism*, Princeton University Press, Princeton.

Cummins, S., Curtis, S., Diez-Roux, A. and Macintyre, S. 2007, 'Understanding and representing "place" in health research: A relational approach', *Social Science and Medicine*, 65(9), pp. 1825–38.

Department of Health and Social Care. 2017, *Annual Report and Accounts 2016–17*, Department of Health and Social Care, London

Doyal, L. and Pennell, I. 1979, *The Political Economy of Health*, Pluto Press, London.

Eikemo, T. and Bambra, C. 2008, 'The welfare state: A glossary for public health', *Journal of Epidemiology and Community Health*, 62(1), pp. 3–6.

Eikemo, T.A., Bambra, C., Huijts, T. and Fitzgerald, R. 2017, 'The European Social Survey (ESS) rotating module on the social determinants of health: The first pan-European sociological health inequalities survey', *European Sociological Review*, 33(1), pp. 137–53.

Forster, T., Kentikelenis, A. and Bambra, C. 2018, *Health Inequalities in Europe: Setting the Stage for Progressive Policy Action*, Foundation for European Progressive Studies and Action on Social Change, Dublin.

Halliday, E., Brennan, L., Bambra, C. and Popay, J. 2021, '"It is surprising how much nonsense you hear": How residents experience and react to living in a stigmatised place – A narrative synthesis of the qualitative evidence', *Health and Place*, 68(3), p. 102525.

Hawe, P. and Shiell, A. 2000, 'Social capital and health promotion: A review', *Social Science and Medicine*, 51(6), pp. 871–8.

Jarvis, M. and Wardle, J. 2006, 'Social patterning of individual health behaviors: The case of cigarette smoking', in Marmot, M. and Wilkinson, R. (eds), *The Social Determinants of Health*, Oxford University Press, Oxford, pp. 224–37.

Karger, H. and Stoesz, D. 1990, *American Social Welfare Policy*, Longman, New York.

Krieger, N. 2003, 'Theories for social epidemiology in the 21st century: An ecosocial perspective', International Journal of Epidemiology, 30(4), pp. 668–77.
Krieger, N. 2013, *Epidemiology and the People's Health: Theory and Context*, Oxford University Press, Oxford.
Krieger, N., Rehkopf, D., Chen, J., Waterman, P., Marcelli, E. and Kennedy, M. 2008, 'The fall and rise of US inequities in premature mortality: 1960–2002', *PLoS Medicine*, 5(2), pp. 227–41.
Macintyre, S. 2007, 'Deprivation amplification revisited; Or, is it always true that poorer places have poorer access to resources for healthy diets and physical activity?' *International Journal of Behavioral Nutrition and Physical Activity*, 4(32), pp. 1–7.
Macintyre, S., Ellaway, A. and Cummins, S. 2002, 'Place effects on health: How can we conceptualise, operationalise and measure them?' *Social Science and Medicine*, 55(1), pp. 125–39.
Mackenbach, J.P., Kulhánová, I., Artnik, B., Bopp, M., Borrell, C., Clemens, T., Costa, G., Dibben, C., Kalediene, R., Lundberg, O. and Martikainen, P. 2016, 'Changes in mortality inequalities over two decades: Register based study of European countries', *British Medical Journal*, 11(353), pp. 1732–3.
MacLeavy, J. 2011, 'A "new politics" of austerity, workfare and gender? The UK coalition government's welfare reform proposals', *Cambridge Journal of Regions Economy and Society*, 4(3), pp. 355–67.
Marmot, M. 2005, 'Introduction', in Marmot, M. and Wilkinson, R. (eds), *Social Determinants of Health*, Oxford University Press, Oxford, pp. 1–5.
Moeller, H. 2013, 'Rising unemployment and increasing spatial health inequalities in England: Further extension of the North South divide', *Journal of Public Health*, 35(2), pp. 313–21.
Niedzwiedz, C.L., Mitchell, R.J., Shortt, N.K. and Pearce, J. 2016, 'Social protection spending and inequalities in depressive symptoms across Europe', *Social Psychiatry and Psychiatric Epidemiology*, 39(1), pp. 1–10.
ONS (Office for National Statistics). 2015, *Inequality in Healthy Life Expectancy at Birth by National Deciles of Area Deprivation: England, 2011 to 2013*, Office for National Statistics, London.
ONS (Office for National Statistics). 2022, *Inequality in Healthy Life Expectancy at Birth by National Deciles of Area Deprivation: England, 2015 to 2020*, Office for National Statistics, London.
Ottersen, P., Dasgupta, J. and Blouin, C. 2014, 'The Lancet-University of Oslo commission on global governance for health', *The Lancet*, 383(9917), pp. 630–67.
Pearce, J., Richardson, E., Mitchell, R. and Shortt, N. 2010, 'Environmental justice and health: The implications of the socio-spatial distribution of multiple environmental deprivation for health inequalities in the United Kingdom', *Transactions of the Institute of British Geographers*, 35(4), pp. 522–39.
Robinson, T., Brown, H., Norman, P., Barr, B., Fraser, L. and Bambra, C. 2019, 'Investigating the impact of New Labor's English health inequalities strategy on geographical inequalities in infant mortality: A time trend analysis', *Journal of Epidemiology and Community Health*, 73(3), pp. 564–8.
Scheidel, W. 2017, *The Great Leveler: Violence and the History of Inequality from the Stone Age to the Twenty-First Century*, Princeton University Press, Princeton.
Schrecker, T. and Bambra, C. 2015, *How Politics Makes Us Sick: Neoliberal Epidemics*, Palgrave Macmillan, London.
Scott-Samuel, A., Bambra, C., Collins, C., Hunter, D., McCartney, G. and Smith, K. 2014, 'The impact of Thatcherism on health and well-being in Britain', *International Journal of Health Services*, 44(1), pp. 53–71.
Shaw, C., Blakely, T. and Atkinson, J. 2005, 'Do social and economic reforms change socioeconomic inequalities in child mortality? A case study: New Zealand 1981–1999', *Journal of Epidemiology and Community Health*, 59(8), pp. 638–44.
Simpson, J., Bambra, C., Bell, Z., Albani, V. and Brown, H. 2021, 'Effects of social security policy reforms on mental health and inequalities: A systematic review of observational studies in high-income countries', *Social Science and Medicine*, 272(6), p. 113717.
Taylor-Robinson, D., Lai, E., Wickham, S., Rose, T., Bambra, C., Whitehead, M. and Barr, B. 2019, 'Assessing the impact of rising child poverty on the unprecedented rise in infant mortality in England, 2000–2017: Time trend analysis', *BMJ Open*, 9(10), p. e029424.
Walsh, D., McCartney, G., Minton, J., Parkinson, J., Shipton, D. and Whyte, B. 2020, 'Changing mortality trends in countries and cities of the UK: A population-based trend analysis', *BMJ Open*, 10(11), p. e038135.
Whitehead, M. 2007, 'A typology of actions to tackle social inequalities in health', *Journal of Epidemiology and Community Health*, 61(3), pp. 473–8.
WHO. 2008, *Commission on the Social Determinants of Health: Closing the Gap in a Generation*, World Health Organization, Geneva.

PART III

Contemporary political-economic dimensions of healthcare

18

COMMODIFIED HEALTHCARE, PROFITS, PRIORITIES AND THE DISREGARD FOR LIFE UNDER CAPITALISM

Isaac Christiansen

One of the most critical discussions regarding the political economy of healthcare is whether it should be treated as a right or as a commodity. Those who argue that it should be treated as the latter insist that healthcare is a commodity like any other, and that supply and demand signals are all that are needed to allocate human and technological resources to sufficiently address healthcare. In this view, people are not 'entitled' to access healthcare, but their health and ability to access healthcare services are seen as a personal, individual-level responsibility (Beauchamp 2013). According to this logic, the population's access to healthcare services should be determined by the ability to pay for direct out-of-pocket expenses, insurance premiums, copays and deductibles.

Further, proponents of this view argue that healthcare should be delivered through the market: via privately owned firms, and financed through for-profit insurance. They support this position by claiming that markets are the most effective and efficient tools to organize all economic activity; that private ownership provides incentives for innovation and long-term cost reduction; and that, by its very nature, private enterprise and management are more efficient than state enterprise, since private, profit-oriented owners (and consumers) will be responsive to market signals. Finally, in their view, healthcare markets offer 'choice' to the 'consumer' (Shleifer 1998; Haislmaier 2008). These arguments form part of an overall set of neoliberal arguments against any form of government ownership, regulation or 'intervention' in the economy. They also depend on untenable assumptions of 'perfect markets', with complete consumer knowledge of products, and tend to systematically exclude variables such as class, and the disparity between absolute need and effective demand. These capture precisely the structural ways in which capitalism foments inequality and the dynamics of monopoly formation.

In contrast, this chapter argues that healthcare is fundamentally a human right that should not be treated as a commodity. It contends that claims regarding the innate superiority of private owners and management relative to state ownership and management are false, and it insists on the difference between the nature of healthcare and most other commodified goods. In this context, the chapter suggests that commodification of healthcare delivery promotes health inequalities – both in the broader context outside of the healthcare system and in terms of healthcare provision itself. The market-oriented view fails on the basic premises of human justice, compassion and ethics, as

 DOI: 10.4324/9781003017110-21

it invariably excludes access to preventative and curative care to large segments of humanity and, thus, furthers unnecessary human suffering. Ultimately, it is imperative to articulate healthcare as a human right that is a social and collective responsibility (state, community and individual), as has been declared in Article 25 of the *Universal Declaration of Human Rights* (United Nations 1948), and in the *Declaration of Alma Ata* (1978).

To understand this phenomenon in more depth, the chapter begins with a brief discussion that positions healthcare as a human right rather than a commodity. Following this, it explores the prevailing commodification of healthcare in practice. Here, the bulk of evidence necessarily emerges from the US, where the logic of capital as a political-economic and ideological system so thoroughly dominates society. Finally, the argument explores the manner in which commodification and capital accumulation lead to contradictions within healthcare systems, as well as on a global level. In this regard, healthcare has become the subject of overt inequality and injustice around the world, leading to the necessity to consider alternative, socialistic possibilities for the future.

Healthcare as a human right

Interestingly, even some mainstream economists accept that, on some level, it is necessary to distinguish healthcare from other 'services', although they may also argue that public provision is still inferior to markets or that healthcare is an 'exception' to the general rule of the superiority of economic organization along capitalist lines. In contrast, the Marxist analysis presented here places class dynamics as central to political-economic processes, and it explores how these inform ideologies around healthcare delivery. Further, a Marxist approach perceives the challenges in obtaining a meaningful transformation to public financing and provision in any society where a market logic currently prevails. As such, healthcare is seen as part of the social wage, and an essential component of the value of labor power, such that a healthy (but exploitable) workforce should be essential to the smooth functioning of capitalism. After all, healthcare is a fundamental element of societal reproduction.

Nevertheless, there is no doubt that workers' essential needs for healthcare remain the subject of contestation, in spite of its central role in producing the goods and services from which capital profits. Capitalism simultaneously seeks to expand into new sectors like healthcare, seeking profits and raising costs, while also not hesitating to push wages below their value. Across the board, then, barriers to healthcare for the working-class are equivalent to reducing the means of subsistence for workers and, ultimately, are an attack on social reproduction.

With this understanding of health as a matter of social reproduction in mind, Hans Ulrich Deppe (2009: 31) presents five qualities of healthcare that underscore how and why it must be fundamentally treated as a right and not as a commodity. First, 'health is an existential good'. Without access to healthcare, our quality of life is severely diminished through increased likelihood of untreated illness and premature death from preventable causes, leading to unnecessary suffering for ourselves and our loved ones. Second, 'one cannot choose to be sick, as one can choose to consume, or not consume a commodity in the market', but rather 'illness is a general life risk'. These first two aspects clearly characterize healthcare access – like access to adequate nutrition and shelter – as a basic, generalized, common need. An individual can potentially avoid or postpone acquisition of most other commodities if they lack the means to obtain them. In cases where required healthcare is postponed or avoided, the consequences can range from developing serious health complications to premature death and, in the case of infectious diseases, put the larger society at risk.

Third, Deppe (2009) shows that healthcare needs are 'non-specific'. This refers to patients' often-minimal information surrounding the cause of their malaise. One has little or no control over the necessary diagnostic tests and treatments, and such decisions can be affected by rising costs that threaten access to critical care or impose severe financial hardship. Fourth, patients are in a 'vulnerable' position characterized by 'dependency and need, often combined with fear and shame'. Finally, those with the greatest need for care typically 'come from the lower social classes', and 'have the least financial resources'. This final point dovetails with Tudor Hart's (1971) argument that an inverse care law effectively operates in commodified healthcare systems, allocating more healthcare resources to those less in need and too little care to those in greater need. Hart emphatically stressed that the inverse care law operates more fully in societies where healthcare is treated as a commodity, but that it applied even in the UK, due to the broader inequalities produced by capitalism that surrounded the National Healthcare Service (NHS) model.

The commodification of healthcare

The more commodified a healthcare system's financing, biomedical research and pharmaceutical production, and the further a system moves from a well-resourced, fully public, integrated national healthcare system with active community participation, the further it moves from a rights-based approach. The more profoundly commodification penetrates different segments of the system, the more equitable access is eroded; the more costly and inefficient care generally becomes; and the more unequal health outcomes are amplified (Navarro 1976; Christiansen 2017). Healthcare systems based on private insurance, regardless of their form (whether managed care organization, consumer-driven care or accountable care organizations), have an economic incentive to avoid covering sicker and poorer populations to minimize risk and, instead, search for ways to deny covering expensive procedures or medications (Gaffney *et al.* 2018). Accordingly, the distribution of care by effective demand (those who are insured, and can afford the copays, deductibles and other cost-sharing arrangements) does not correspond to populations' healthcare needs.

Out-of-pocket expenditure is a known disincentive to seek medical care. In addition to the costly nature of obtaining private insurance, high deductibles and copays (which continue to characterize US healthcare under the *Affordable Care Act*) are also shown to increase forgone care, especially when contrasted with single-payer and national healthcare models (Dickman *et al.* 2017; Gaffney *et al.* 2018; Waitzkin and Hellander 2018). Further, having insurance does not guarantee that a needed treatment or intervention will be covered. Insurance company profits are determined by the difference between the income from premiums and the costs of care, taxes and administration. To remain profitable in a context of rising healthcare costs, many insurance companies require ample cost sharing, a phenomenon that undermines the ability of private, profit-oriented insurance to make healthcare truly accessible.

Improved accessibility to care is associated with better health outcomes. Christiansen and Mazur (2018) found that measures of accessibility, such as the government's share of total health expenditure,[1] physician density, vaccination coverage, and access to improved water and sanitation, were inversely associated with infant mortality in cross-sectional multivariate regression models. Conversely, increases in costs to patients through direct out-of-pocket payments, deductibles and cost sharing decrease accessibility, increase forgone care and, thereby, likely make healthcare more expensive (through more costly subsequent treatments) and worsen health outcomes (Dickman *et al.* 2017). In this light, having already accrued medical debt, or reasonably expecting it in the future, can provide sufficient incentive for individuals to forgo needed healthcare.

In the US, healthcare financing has serious negative financial and health impacts. For example, Ramsey *et al.* (2016) showed that cancer treatment often results in bankruptcies and that the latter resulted in an increased likelihood of mortality from treatable cancers. In this regard, it behooves us to have some pictures of the level of health debt in the US. In a July 2020 survey of 1,186 people conducted by Debt.com, almost half of all respondents (45.87 percent) had medical debt. Of the survey's respondents, 31 percent had medical debt between $1,000 and $4,999; 14.9 percent, between $5000 and $9,999; 15.3 percent, between $10,000 and $49,999; 3.1 percent, between $50,000 and $99,999; 0.96 percent, between $100,000 and $149,999; and 1.5 percent, with over $150,000 (Debt.com 2020).

Regardless of this perilous situation, the formation of a powerful complex of interests of private insurers, providers, medical technology firms and pharmaceutical corporate interests ensures that private, for-profit entities maintain a lock-hold over the healthcare system. Their dominance of this market recalls the words of Baran and Sweezy (1966) in *Monopoly Capital*, who suggested that monopolies are price makers rather than price takers. Healthcare in the US is so expensive relative to European countries, in part, due to consolidation among hospitals and providers, where growing private monopolies demand higher prices from insurance payers. Add to this the high cost of administering billing and payments when compared to the simplicity (and low cost) of single-payer or national healthcare administration. Arguing the cost advantages of single-payer systems, Gaffney *et al.* (2018: 208) indicate that '[i]n particular, the global budgeting of hospitals would permit the essential elimination of hospital billing activities, which currently consume 25% of hospital expenditures, almost double that of single-payer nations'.

In response to this situation, insurance companies have sought their own monopoly position, as a means to force hospitals and other providers to reduce costs. In turn, hospitals have merged 'to gain better bargaining power and become "too big to fail". In the ultimate move, some hospitals have started to become insurance companies' (Burlage and Anderson 2018: 77). For their part, pharmaceutical companies seek monopoly power through intellectual property rights (IPRs) and niche-busting. Since the length of time devoted to patents is limited, pharmaceutical companies exert influence (through leverage obtained by user fees) on regulators to accelerate the approval process for new drugs, and lobby policymakers and governments to extend the time for patents without compulsory licensing.[2] In the absence of government monopsony power that exists in a single-payer system, or nationalization of the pharmaceutical industry, these political-economic dynamics inflate healthcare costs and reduce accessibility.

The power of large pharmaceutical corporations does not just affect the question of healthcare access within countries, but property rights agreements among countries tie the hands of sovereign government that wishes to extend access to critical pharmaceuticals to populations in need. The imposition of IPRs by corporations through multi- and bilateral trade agreements often results in a situation in which poorer countries with high disease burdens are unable to access needed medication (Lexchin 2018; Sell and Williams 2020). The World Trade Organization's *Agreement on Trade Related Intellectual Property Rights* (TRIPs) was a major victory for capital over public health. The pattern is quite pernicious when viewed from the perspective of healthcare as a human right. For example, under TRIPs, corporations have filed Investor-State Dispute Settlement lawsuits against countries for having granted compulsory licensing (so that a generic version of the drug can be produced).

In one pertinent case, countries in the Southern African Development Community during the 1990s HIV/AIDS crisis could not access antiretroviral medications (ARVs), due to patents that made brand-name medications prohibitively expensive and prevented the use of generic versions. When South Africa passed a law to allow for the import of generic ARVs, bypassing IPRs, powerful multinational pharmaceutical corporations and the US government sued South Africa for TRIPs violations. Grassroots and international resistance led to the defeat of the lawsuit and the passing of the Doha *Declaration on the TRIPs Agreement and Public Health*. This allowed for greater flexibility in TRIPs applications for least-developed country (LDC) member-states for *certain* 'essential medicines', and compulsory licensing given certain criteria until 2033 or until a country 'graduates' from LDC status (George 2011; Lexchin 2018; 't Hoen *et al.* 2018). The push for free trade agreements such as CAFTA (Central American Free Trade Agreement) seeks further to erode hard-fought minimal protections for generic medicines, and further strengthens investor rights in so-called TRIPs-plus measures at the expense of population health (Castro and Westerhaus 2007). The outlandish nature of such agreements, with their predictably deleterious health impacts on the world's most vulnerable populations, could not be clearer:

> Agreements with countries in Asia and Latin America have conditioned 'free' trade on the expansion of intellectual property rights for multinational pharmaceutical companies holding ARV patents, among other medicines. Specifically, these agreements extend patent rights beyond the 20-year period, freeze generic manufacturing of ARVs in the country, protect the manufacturers' drug testing data for five years – known as data exclusivity – and limit options for compulsory licensing. Additional measures include a reduction in the number of inventions, such as 'diagnostic therapeutic and surgical methods' that can be excluded from patent law, the allowance of known substances to be patented again for each new use, and provisions requiring national drug regulatory authorities to block registration of generic medications.
>
> (Castro and Westerhaus 2007: S90)

There is a visible, sharp antagonism between public health and pharmaceutical corporate interests. Corporations seek to maximize profits and extend IPRs to maintain a monopoly position. The justification offered by pharmaceutical corporations for IPRs is that they need to recoup research and development expenses, a claim that appears dubious. Public funding of drug research at universities, as well as exaggerated accounts of pharmaceutical corporations' R&D expenses through the inclusion of marketing costs under the R&D rubric, seriously calls into question the validity of these claims (Castro and Westerhaus 2007; Lexchin 2018). On an international level, contrary to the rosy predictions of free-market fundamentalists, the bulk of pharmaceutical research and investment tends to ignore infectious diseases that affect countries and populations of the Global South, leaving them with high disease burdens and high poverty levels. In these resource-poor settings, there simply does not exist effective demand adequate to guarantee profitable investments by capital (Trouiller *et al.* 2001).

Capitalism and the contradictions of inequality and health

The essence of fundamental cause theory is that those who occupy higher class positions can translate their advantaged position into higher social-economic status, and their greater resources and status will also mean better health. Greater income and wealth inequality means uneven resources available for individuals and groups to obtain better nutrition; avoid unhealthy work and living conditions; and access knowledge pertaining to health and obtain higher quality care – all scenarios that contribute to greater inequality in population health. Critically, US wages have largely stagnated since the early-1970s, associated with a decline in unionization levels, and a rise in income and wealth inequality. In this context, Wilson (2009) contrasts the US and Canada in terms of the relationship between income and health. She finds that the steep income gradient in the US significantly increases the likelihood of experiencing a preventable disease (cardiovascular disease) versus a non-preventable disease (cancer), whereas in Canada, universal healthcare has softened the impact of inequality on health. Similarly, Decker and Remler (2004) provide evidence for a steeper income gradient related to self-reported negative health in the US than in Canada. Like Wilson, they found that the harmful impact of inequality is buffered by Canada's single-payer healthcare system.

Inequalities in accessibility, healthcare provision and outcomes are clearly visible within the US and have been exacerbated by neoliberal processes (Dickman *et al.* 2017; Gaffney and Muntaner 2018). While disparities in physician distribution are not as severe in the US, 'market forces' tend to increase rural-urban disparities in the distribution of primary care physicians (Petterson *et al.* 2013) and specialists (Aboagye *et al.* 2014). Moreover, disparities in class- and race-related health outcomes abound in the US health system. Racialized capitalism in the US is characterized by severe spatial, income, and wealth inequalities that fuel racialized inequalities in health access, morbidity and mortality (Laster Pirtle 2020). While the overrepresentation of Black Americans among the working-class and working poor accounts for a portion of the racialized health gap, a significant quantity of the disparity cannot be explained by traditional predictors, reflecting the persistent significance of race itself (Williams and Collins 2013). All of this has been telescoped in the context of COVID-19, where economic and racial health disparities have exacerbated the impact of the pandemic on communities of color throughout the US. For example, African-Americans experienced a disproportionately higher incidence of diseases that interact with COVID-19, are overrepresented in occupations characterized by an inability to telecommute, and are being disproportionately subject to incarceration – all of which elevated the risk of contracting COVID-19 (Laster Pirtle 2020).

Perspectives that favor private ownership and management of health also tend to shy away from comparative studies that contradict their central claims. A study financed by the Commonwealth Fund compared how the more commodified US healthcare system performs in comparison with its European counterparts. It showed that the US far outspends countries such as Denmark, Sweden, Norway, France, New Zealand, Canada, Germany, Switzerland, Australia, the Netherlands and the UK, only to perform *worse than all of them* on accessibility, equity, efficiency and 'healthy lives' (Davis *et al.* 2014).[3] Subsequent studies reflect similar inefficiencies in the capitalist organization of care. In a follow-up study, Schneider *et al.* (2017) observed the same phenomenon when the US was again compared to developed European countries on a host of important indicators in terms of accessibility, quality of care, equity, administrative efficiency and health outcomes. Once more, the hyper-commodified US healthcare system performed poorly despite its high levels of health expenditure.

Even Cuba, a country that has endured an extremely aggressive US economic war dating back to the beginning of the 1960s, has outperformed the US –in terms of not only human resources for health density (measured by the number of physicians relative to the population), but also accessibility (in Cuba, there is universal provision of state-financed and publicly provided universal healthcare). According to World Bank (2020b) data, Cuba has achieved slightly lower infant mortality than the US (in 2019, the Cuba figure was 5.0[4] per 1000 live births, while the corresponding US figure was 5.6[5]), and Cuba and the US are virtually tied for life expectancy (Cuba sits at 78.7 years, and the US at 78.5 years). Critically, the island nation spends a tiny fraction of that expended by the US on health. According to the World Health Organization (WHO 2020), as a proportion of its GDP, the US (with a much larger GDP) far outspent Cuba on healthcare in 2017 (US, 17.06 percent versus Cuba, 11.71 percent), while also expending more than all other rich developed countries. Whether the US healthcare system is compared to Cuba or to West European countries, ample empirical evidence greatly undermines the claim that organizing healthcare along capitalist lines enhances efficiency or leads to better outcomes.

On a global level, as Hart (1971) long ago indicated, healthcare tends to be inversely distributed relative to need. There are several empirical indicators that reflect this set of global contradictions, from geographic variation in hospital bed density to physician density, both between and within countries. Regarding the latter, according to the WHO (2020), at least 45 percent of countries had less than one doctor for every thousand people, with many countries in sub-Saharan Africa reporting fewer than one doctor for every 10,000 of their population. While there are many determinants of physician density, including training, retention, emigration and immigration of professionals, and population growth, brain drain remains a disturbing trend. Doctors tend to move from the public to the private sector, from impoverished rural areas to wealthier urban ones, and from poorer to richer countries.

The severity of healthcare system shortages of overexploited countries in the periphery or underdeveloped countries (particularly in sub-Saharan Africa) cannot be overstated. WHO Global Observatory data regarding physician density shows that in 2016, Togo reported 78,125 people for every doctor, and Malawi reported one doctor for every 60,606 people (WHO 2020). By 2018, the situation had improved, where in Malawi, an additional 365 physicians improved the ratio to 1:27,942, while in Togo, the increase in physicians from 96 to 611 reduced the ratio to 1:12,920. Yet, such trends are not uniformly encouraging: both the DRC and Tanzania, for instance, registered recent declines in physician density. In 2009, the ratio was 1:10,706 in the DRC, but by 2017, it had fallen to 1:13,513 people, while Tanzania shifted from 1:42,918 in 2002 to 1:71,429 in 2016.

Economic imperialism and global capitalism produce enormous economic inequalities, often through global labor arbitrage and unfair trade. This occurs through direct investment and arms-length production (Smith 2016). To comprehend just how unequal our world has become, Oxfam (2019) reported that there were 3.4 billion people living on less than $5.50 per day, while the 26 wealthiest billionaires held as much wealth as the poorest 3.8 billion people combined. Concomitantly, the super-rich have accrued approximately US$7.6 trillion hidden in offshore tax havens. The impact of such astronomical inequalities on global population health is severe. Thus, if we acknowledge that inequality is harmful to societal health, we must determine the root causes of such high levels of inequality, both between and within countries. This line of questioning would need to move beyond the work of scholars such as Pickett and Wilkinson (*e.g.* 2010, 2015), instead shining a critical light on capitalism (and imperialism) as a system that exacerbates health inequality through the commodification of care, while validating heightened economic inequality more generally (Muntaner *et al.* 2014).

Due to the acute nature of inequalities between countries, exacerbated by fiscal evasion, trade imbalance based on dependency, mismanagement, capital flight, costly development projects and economic crises, many countries have felt obliged to turn to international financial institutions (such as the World Bank and the International Monetary Fund) for loans. These IFIs often impose conditions through 'structural adjustment' that include financial deregulation, currency devaluation to stimulate exports and control inflation, reduction or elimination of tariffs, and a reduction of government spending on health and education (Gershman and Irwin 2000; Schoepf *et al.* 2000). Thus, structural adjustment represents the imposition on loan recipient nations of a more neoliberal form of capitalism, under the ideological imperative that trade liberalization, deregulation and privatization all lead to economic growth and development.

The external imposition of austerity in healthcare has not been confined to countries of the Global South, but has notably been applied to Greece, Spain and England. Gaffney and Muntaner

(2018) argue that neoliberalism in health has four key axes: (1) health system austerity, (2) a retreat from universalism, (3) a rise in cost sharing, and (4) health system privatization. In general, IFI-imposed austerity measures essentially strip countries of the sovereignty to select their own political-economic development strategy, and thereby subordinate population health to the needs of capital accumulation and debt repayment.

The health impacts of austerity and structural adjustment are well documented. Handa and King (2003) demonstrate how sudden currency devaluation and the elimination of food subsidies reduced Jamaican purchasing power in the early-1990s, disproportionately impacting poor urban families due to the rising cost of imported food and general inflation. These phenomena, in turn, led to a decline in the weight of preschool children and an increase in malnutrition. Using regression analysis of a 34-year period of cross-national panel data for 139 developing countries, Forster and colleagues (2019) found that structural adjustment conditionalities reduced health system access (defined as a composite measure of DPT3 and measles vaccination levels, antenatal care coverage, hospital beds and skilled birth coverage) and increased neonatal mortality rates. Similarly, Pandolfeli *et al.* (2014) analyzed time series longitudinal data on 37 sub-Saharan African countries and found that states that had undergone structural adjustment had higher maternal mortality rates than those that did not.

More generally, considering the widely recognized harmful relationship between inequality and health – whether through psychosocial mechanisms as argued by Pickett and Wilkinson (2015), or through a fundamental cause relationship or some combination – we must recognize that capitalism is a source of enormous duress, in that it generates inequality through a wide variety of mechanisms. Primary among these are the fundamental class antagonism between sellers of labor power and capital, the domination of industrial capital by commercial and financial capital, fiscal evasion, tax cuts for the wealthy, and the immense power of IFIs to impose austerity on indebted countries.

Thus, moving beyond capitalism toward a more equitable political-economic and social system, where production, commerce and finance are not controlled by major shareholders and boards of directors, is a necessary condition to address the forms of social inequality that plague society and contribute significantly to negative health outcomes. When healthcare is subjected to the logic of capital, as a means to seek profitable outlets for investment, treatment of healthcare as an essential human right is violated. The distribution of health personnel and resources then follows principles of market demand and not societal need, where centralization of capital into monopoly formation follows, and a general neglect of preventative and public health measures tends to emerge. This process is accompanied by a host of other problems, including political capture by insurance and pharmaceutical industries, rising costs, and greater disparity between access to care and those with the greatest need for that care. This commodification of healthcare profits from people's vulnerabilities and their most essential human needs, often threatening either denial of critical care or imposed financial hardship or bankruptcy, itself a source of stress and greater health risk. Though we have never been further from doing so, it remains necessary to reassert the importance of the *Alma Ata Declaration*, insisting on 'health for all' as a fundamental human right. The only viable path to such a scenario will involve separating healthcare from processes of commodification and capital accumulation.

Conclusion

This chapter argued that contrary to the predictions of neoclassical economics, healthcare quality and access are not improved when ownership and management are in private hands and when the distributive mechanism is left to the market. To the contrary, I contended here that access to healthcare is a fundamental human right, and that the greater the influence of commodification in healthcare, the more we find health inequalities. Further, capitalism in general (outside of healthcare) tends to augment inequality to obscene levels. In the future, it behooves us to examine health under different political, social and economic arrangements – particularly socialist-oriented societies – with seriousness. Following Navarro (1993: 8), we should keep in mind that 'the socialist experience always invokes enormous hostility, economic blockade, and even military intervention'. Even under such strained conditions, socialist societies have generally done quite well when contrasted to marketized healthcare systems, certainly in terms of health outcomes. Further research, for example, should examine the different levels of success obtained by these different societies in confronting the COVID-19 pandemic, compared to the disastrous prevalence and mortality rates within the US. At all levels, however, researchers must continue to expose the contradictions inherent in processes of commodification and capital accumulation, which underwrite a political economy of healthcare rife with inequality and injustice.

Notes

1 If government share were 0, that would mean 100 percent of the burden of healthcare financing would fall on individuals, who would either obtain care through private insurance or pay for care directly out of pocket. Moving closer to 100 percent sees a declining percentage expended on both of these options. Nevertheless, it is important to see how this is distorted in the US, with major public subsidies going to private insurance corporations, in addition to Medicare and Medicaid (Himmelstein and Woolhandler 2016).
2 This extends the time in which the pharmaceutical company can extract monopoly powers over medication.
3 In the Commonwealth Fund studies, 'healthy lives' is a composite measure of life expectancy, infant mortality and 'mortality amenable to health care' (Davis *et al.* 2014).
4 This figure comes from Cuba's 2019 Statistical Yearbook, compiled by Cuba's Ministry of Health, with data ratified by the Pan-American Health Organization, World Health Organization, UNICEF and United Nations Population Fund. This figure is higher than the 3.9 figure reported by the World Bank for Cuba in the same year.
5 This figure comes from the World Bank (2020a).

References

Aboagye, J.K., Kaiser, H.E. and Hayanga, A.J. 2014, 'Rural-urban differences in access to specialist providers of colorectal cancer care in the United States: A physician workforce issue', *JAMA Surgery*, 149(6), pp. 537–43.

Baran, P. and Sweezy, P. 1966, *Monopoly Capital: An Essay on the American Economic and Social Order*, Monthly Review Press, New York.

Beauchamp, D.E. 2013, 'Public health as social justice', in Donohoe, M.T. (ed), *Public Health and Social Justice: A Jossey-Bass Reader*, Jossey-Bass, San Francisco, pp. 11–9.

Burlage, R. and Anderson, M. 2018, 'The transformation of the medical-industrial complex: Financialization, the corporate sector and monopoly capital', in Waitzkin, H. (ed), *Health Care Under the Knife: Moving Beyond Contemporary Capitalism*, Monthly Review Press, New York, pp. 69–82.

Castro, A. and Westerhaus, M. 2007, 'Access to generic antiretrovirals: Inequality, intellectual property law, and international trade agreements', *Cadernos de Saúde Pública*, 23, pp. S85–96.

Christiansen, I. 2017, 'The commodification of healthcare and its consequences', *World Review of Political Economy*, 8(1), pp. 82–103.

Christiansen, I. and Mazur, R. 2018, 'Accessibility and health: An international analysis of government expenditure, socioeconomic development and infant mortality', *Journal of Critical Thought and Praxis*, 18(2), pp. 16–34.

Davis, K., Stremikis, K., Squires, D. and Schoen, C. 2014, *Mirror, Mirror on the Wall: How the Performance of the U.S. Health Care System Compares Internationally*, Commonwealth Fund, New York.

Debt.com 2020, 'Many Americans can't afford to pay off less than $5,000 in medical debt', accessed 3 January 2021, <https://www.debt.com/research/medical-debt-survey/>.

Decker, S.L. and Remler, D.K. 2004, 'How much might universal health insurance reduce socioeconomic disparities in health? A comparison of the U.S. and Canada', *National Bureau of Economic Research*, Working Paper No. 10715.

Declaration of Alma Ata. 1978, 'Declaration of Alma Ata', International Conference on Primary Health Care, Alma Ata, Union of Soviet Socialist Republics.

Deppe, H. 2009, 'The nature of health care: Commodification versus solidarity', in Panitch, L. and Leys, C. (eds), *The Socialist Register 2010: Morbid Symptoms – Health Under Capitalism*, Monthly Review Press, New York, pp. 29–38.

Dickman, S., Himmelstein, D.U. and Woolhandler, S. 2017, 'Inequality and the health-care system in the USA', *The Lancet*, 389(10077), pp. 1431–41.

Forster, T., Kentikelenis, A.E., Stubbs, T.H. and, King, L. 2019, 'Globalization and health equity: The impact of structural adjustment programs on developing countries', *Social Science and Medicine*, 346, p. 112496.

Gaffney, A., Himmelstein, D. and Woolhandler, S. 2018, 'The failure of Obamacare and a revision of the single payer proposal after a quarter century of struggle', in Waitzkin, H. (ed), *Health Care Under the Knife: Moving Beyond Contemporary Capitalism*, Monthly Review Press, New York, pp. 192–210.

Gaffney, A. and Muntaner, C. 2018, 'Austerity and health care', in Waitzkin, H. (ed), *Health Care Under the Knife: Moving Beyond Contemporary Capitalism*, Monthly Review Press, New York, pp. 119–35.

George, E. 2011, 'The human right to health and HIV/AIDS: South Africa and South-South cooperation to reframe global intellectual property principles and promote access to essential medicines', *Indiana Journal of Global Legal Studies*, 18(1), pp. 167–97.

Gershman, J. and Irwin, A. 2000, 'Getting a grip on the global economy', in Kim, J.Y., Millen, J.V., Irwin, A. and Gershman, J. (eds), *Dying for Growth: Global Inequality and the Health of the Poor*, Common Courage Press, Maine, pp. 11–43.

Haislmaier, E.F. 2008, *Health Care Reform: Design Principles for a Patient-Centered, Consumer-Based Market*, The Heritage Foundation, Washington.

Handa, S. and King, D. 2003, 'Adjustment with a human face? Evidence from Jamaica', *World Development*, 31(7), pp. 1125–45.

Hart, T. 1971, 'The inverse care law', *The Lancet*, 297(7696), pp. 405–12.

Himmelstein, D. and Woolhandler, S. 2016, 'The current and projected taxpayer shares of US health costs', *American Journal of Public Health*, 106(3), pp. 449–52.

Laster Pirtle, W.N. 2020, 'Racial capitalism: A fundamental cause of novel coronavirus (COVID 19) pandemic inequities in the United States', *Health Education and Behavior*, 47(4), pp. 504–8.

Lexchin, J. 2018, 'The pharmaceutical industry in the context of contemporary capitalism', in Waitzkin, H. (ed), *Health Care Under the Knife: Moving Beyond Contemporary Capitalism*, Monthly Review Press, New York, pp. 83–98.

Muntaner, C., Rai, N., Ng, E. and Chung, H. 2014, 'Social class, politics, and the spirit level: Why income inequality remains unexplained and unsolved', in Navarro, V. and Muntaner, C. (eds), *The Financial and Economic Crises and Their Impact on Health and Social Well-Being*, Baywood Publishing Company, Amityville, pp. 475–87.

Navarro, V. 1976, *Medicine Under Capitalism*, Prodist, New York.

Navarro, V. 1993, 'Has socialism failed? An analysis of health indicators under capitalism and socialism', *Science and Society*, 57(1), pp. 6–30.

New York Times. 2020, 'Coronavirus map: Tracking the global outbreak', *The New York Times*, accessed 17 December 2020, <www.nytimes.com/interactive/2020/world/coronavirus-maps.html>.

Oxfam 2019, 'Public good or private wealth', *Oxfam Briefing Paper*, Oxford.

Pandolfeli, L.E., Shandra, J. and Tyagi, J. 2014, 'The international monetary fund, structural adjustment, and women's health: A cross national analysis of maternal mortality in Sub-Saharan Africa', *The Sociological Quarterly*, 55(1), pp. 119–42.

Petterson, S.M., Philips, R.L., Bazemore, A.W. and Koinis, G.T. 2013, 'Unequal distribution of the U.S. primary care workforce', *American Family Physician*, 87(11). https://www.aafp.org/pubs/afp/issues/2013/0601/od1.pdf.

Pickett, K.E. and Wilkinson, R. 2010, *The Spirit Level: Why Equality Is Better for Everyone*, Penguin, London.

Pickett, K.E. and Wilkinson, R. 2015, 'Income inequality and health: A causal review', *Social Science and Medicine*, 128, pp. 316–26.

Ramsey, S.D., Bansal, A., Fedorenko, C.R., Blough, D.K., Overstreet, K.A., Shankaran, V. and Newcomb, P. 2016, 'Financial insolvency as a risk factor for early mortality among patients with cancer', *Journal of Clinical Oncology*, 34(9), pp. 980–6.

Schneider, E.C., Sarnak, D.O., Squires, D., Shah, A. and Doty, M.M. 2017, *Mirror, Mirror 2017: International Comparison Reflects Flaws and Opportunities for Better U.S. Health Care*, The Commonwealth Fund, accessed 16 July 2020, <https://interactives.commonwealthfund.org/2017/july/mirror-mirror/assets/Schneider_mirror_mirror_2017.pdf>.

Schoeph, B.G., Schoepf, C. and Millen, J. 2000, 'Theoretical therapies, remote remedies, SAPs and the political ecology of poverty and health in Africa', in Kim, Y., Jim, J.V., Millen, A., Gershman, I. and Gershman, J. (eds), *Global Inequality and the Health of the Poor*, Common Press, Monroe, pp. 91–125.

Sell, S.K. and Williams, O.D. 2020, 'Health under capitalism: A global political economy of structural pathogenesis', *Review of International Political Economy*, 27(1), pp. 1–25.

Shleifer, A. 1998, 'State versus private ownership', *Working Paper No. 6665*, NBER, Cambridge.

Smith, J. 2016, *Imperialism in the Twenty-First Century: Globalization, Super Exploitation and Capitalism's Final Crisis*, Monthly Review Press, New York.

't Hoen, E.F.M., Kujinga, T. and Boulet, P. 2018, 'Patent challenges in the procurement and supply of generic new essential medicines and lessons from HIV in the southern African development community (SADC) region', *Journal of Pharmaceutical Policy and Practice,* 11(1), p. 31.

Trouiller, P., Torreele, E., Olliaro, P., White, N., Foster, S., Wirth, D. and Pécoul, B. 2001, 'Drugs for neglected diseases: A failure of the market and a public health failure?', *Tropical Medicine and International Health*, 6(11), pp. 945–51.

United Nations. 1948, *Universal Declaration of Human Rights*, accessed 21 December 2020, <https://www.un.org/en/universal-declaration-human-rights/>.

Waitzkin, H. and Hellander, I. 2018, 'Obamacare: The neoliberal model comes home to roost – If we let it', in Waitzkin, H. (ed), *Health Care Under the Knife: Moving Beyond Contemporary Capitalism*, Monthly Review Press, New York, pp. 99–118.

Williams, D.R. and Collins, C. 2013, 'U.S. socioeconomic differences in health: Patterns and Explanations', in LaVeist, T.A. and Isaac, L.A. (eds), *Race, Ethnicity and Health*, Jossey-Bass, San Francisco, pp. 375–418.

Wilson, A.E. 2009, 'Fundamental causes of health disparities: A comparative analysis of Canada and the United States', *International Sociology*, 24(1), pp. 93–113.

World Bank. 2020a, 'Mortality rate, infant (per 1,000 live births) – United States, Cuba', accessed 16 December 2020, <https://data.worldbank.org/indicator/SP.DYN.IMRT.IN?locations=US-CU>.

World Bank. 2020b, 'Life expectancy at birth, total (years) – United States, Cuba', Accessed 16 December 2020, <https://data.worldbank.org/indicator/SP.DYN.LE00.IN?locations=US-CU>.

World Health Organization. 2020, 'Current health expenditure (% of GDP)', *Global Health Expenditure Database*, accessed 16 July 2020, <https://apps.who.int/nha/database/Select/Indicators/en>.

19

THE FINANCIALIZATION OF LONG-TERM CARE IN CANADA

The case of Ontario

Jackie Brown

Within the study of political economy, financialization has emerged as a concept to describe the growing influence, mainly over the course of the last four decades, of the financial sector on other parts of the economy. Financialization has been described as 'a structural transformation of economies, firms (including financial institutions), states and households' (Aalbers 2016: 2), where there is an increasing 'tendency for profit making in the economy to occur [...] through financial channels rather than through productive activities' (Krippner 2011: 4). While there is a lively debate concerning the 'status' of financialization within the overall domain of political economy, this chapter is concerned with its effects on social policies – specifically, long-term care. It argues that financialization, with its profit imperatives, constitutes an important underlying cause of the increasingly austere circumstances within long-term care. Moreover, the chapter explores the gender-specific nature of this relationship, arguing that the ultimate outcome of finance-driven austerity is an unrecognized, unpaid, and unjust burden placed on women to fill the care-gap.

The chapter begins by briefly presenting the wider debates around financialization and feminist political economy pertinent to the delivery of long-term care. Following this, it takes up the specific case of Ontario, Canada, as an illustrative example of the financialized and gendered effects of neoliberalism on long-term care. I begin by highlighting the dual process of privatization and financialization in the province's long-term care system, emphasizing its growing and dominant role in care provision. With the imperatives of financialization as the backdrop, the final section points to the role of long-term care in social reproduction, and the detrimental and gendered effects engendered by financialization. Ultimately, the incentives embedded in financialization are shown to be uniquely at odds with the provision of quality care and decent work in Ontario's long-term care homes.

Financialization and feminist political economy

With respect to the provisioning of housing, Leilani Farha (2017: 3) argues that financialization constitutes a mechanism by which 'capital investment [...] disconnects housing from its social function of providing a place to live in security and dignity'. This damaging separation is caused by the treatment of housing as an asset class by publicly traded companies, private equity firms, pension funds, and other investment vehicles designed to maximize returns for investors. In order

DOI: 10.4324/9781003017110-22

to generate higher returns, the financial sector uses tactics that compromise housing affordability and security of tenure by purchasing distressed properties, evicting long-term tenants, and raising rents (August 2020; Leijten and de Bel 2020). Such strategies negatively impact access to housing in general and, without a doubt, raise concerns for the provision of long-term care.

Land is particularly vulnerable to financialization. David Harvey has long insisted on the geographical dimension of capital, theorizing that the built environment serves as a 'spatial fix' for overaccumulation (Harvey 2001; Christophers 2011). This is achieved, in part, by 'fixing investments spatially, embedding them in the land, to create an entirely new landscape [...] for capital accumulation' (Harvey 2001: 28). Real estate is attractive to investors because it serves as an income stream in the present, via the collection of rent and, in the future, as a well-established form of collateral (Fernandez and Aalbers 2016; Aalbers *et al.* 2020). Key to financialization is the transformation of property from fixed and immobile land into a liquid and tradable asset (Gotham 2009). This not only permits investors to buy and sell shares in land without engaging in the complexities of direct ownership, but it also allows comparisons to be made across different asset classes. Processes of financialization have been observed in many sectors in which real estate plays an underlying role, including rental housing (Fields and Uffer 2016; August and Walks 2018; August 2020), student housing (Revington and August 2020), farmland (Fairbairn 2020), daycares (Gallagher 2021), and long-term care (Horton 2019; August 2021).

As such, financialization of housing must be understood as part of the overall change in the organization of the economy under neoliberalism. Neoliberalism is the product of broad political-economic restructuring, arising following the collapse of Bretton Woods and stagflation during the 1970s. These circumstances occasioned a shift in public policy toward a politics in which market priorities were (and continue to be) heavily foregrounded (Bresser-Pereira 2010). Neoliberal doctrine is based on the assumption that deregulation, the privatization of public goods, and the advancement of market-based solutions, with limited state intervention, form the ideal scenario for economic growth and societal well-being (Davis and Walsh 2017). The deregulation of financial markets and subsequent financialization of economic activity was a critical pillar of this political strategy, and it has proceeded simultaneously with other regulatory policies in ways that have demonstrably tightened the conditions of housing. For instance, a common effect of neoliberal policies has been the significant decline in affordable housing. In the UK, housing policy was changed to offer tenants the 'right to buy' their units, effectively converting homes from public to private housing by exposing them to, rather than protecting them from, the free market (Hodkinson *et al.* 2013). In Canada, the government cut back on the construction of public housing: declining from 20,000 to 30,000 new social housing units per year in the early-1970s to less than 3,000 per year in the late-1990s (Walks and Clifford 2015). Specific to long-term care, federal transfers to the provinces for healthcare were reduced beginning in the 1990s, which grossly affected available funds for the provision of long-term care (Armstrong *et al.* 2019). Through such determined withdrawal of state services, wherein governments create a gap in provision, a burgeoning financial sector is enabled to invest in and commodify long-term care.

While financialization is essential to understanding the provisioning of housing under neoliberalism, feminist political economy further elucidates its impact on long-term care. Women continue to shoulder more responsibility for unpaid care work than do men. They are also overrepresented in paid care occupations – comprising, for instance, 75 percent of care workers in Canada as of 2016 (Khanam *et al.* 2022). Feminist political economy is concerned with the devaluation of labor traditionally performed by women, including care work and domestic work. In particular, it highlights distinctions and overlap between paid and unpaid labor, and 'productive' and 'reproductive' work. As Nancy Folbre (2014: 5) observes, 'caregivers are typically expected to provide love as well as labor; "caring for," while also "caring about"'. In this sense, if political economy is concerned especially with reproduction of labor, feminist political economy demands that we consider social reproduction as a foundational element of both labor and overall societal well-being and functionality. The assumption that either devalued care professions or unrecognized care will prop up neoliberal social reproduction extends, of course, beyond long-term care. However, long-term care is certainly a critical site of our increasingly privatized and gendered forms of social provision, with a largely unjust set of conditions for both providers and recipients of care.

Financialization of long-term care in Ontario

The provision of long-term care in Canada falls mainly to individual provinces and territories, with significant variation across the country with respect to regulation and management. While the federal government distributes funds through the Canada Health Transfer for 'extended healthcare services', including long-term care, provinces are authorized to spend the money according to their own priorities. In Ontario, the provincial government subsidizes day-to-day care and new home construction. Funding for day-to-day care is distributed in four 'envelopes': nursing and personal care; program and support services; raw food; and other accommodations, which is intended for housekeeping services, building maintenance, dietary services, laundry, and other expenses to maintain or improve the care environment (Ministry of Health and Long-Term Care 2017). Money left unspent from the first three envelopes must be returned to the government, but providers are permitted to retain any surplus funds from the other accommodations envelope.

Long-term care home ownership may be public, non-profit, or for-profit. In Ontario, 16 percent of homes are municipally owned, while 27 percent are owned by non-profit organizations (CIHI 2021a). Ontario has the highest proportion of for-profit homes in Canada, at 57 percent of the province's 627 homes, compared to 29 percent of homes in the country as a whole. Prior to the 1970s, most for-profit long-term care homes were independently owned, often by a single individual or family. Today, they are increasingly part of larger chains, many of which are financialized. While the sector as a whole has experienced chronic issues of inadequate care and poor labor conditions, there is evidence that for-profit homes consistently produce worse outcomes than public or non-profit homes. For-profit homes in Ontario are associated with lower staffing levels (Berta *et al.* 2005) and higher hospitalization and mortality rates (Tanuseputro *et al.* 2015). In addition, for-profit homes under chain ownership provide less direct and indirect care per resident per day than other ownership types (Hsu *et al.* 2016). Moreover, seniors themselves appear to exhibit a preference for homes not under for-profit ownership, with 68 percent of individuals on the Ontario long-term care wait list ranking a not-for-profit home as their top choice (AdvantAge Ontario n.d.).

The COVID-19 pandemic raised further concerns around for-profit ownership. In total, nearly one in three long-term care homes in Canada experienced an outbreak in the pandemic's first wave, and a reported 14,739 residents died of the virus between March 1, 2020, and February 15, 2021 (CIHI 2021b). The first wave caught many homes unprepared, and in the system and staffing breakdown that followed, some residents died not of COVID-19, but of dehydration and neglect (Marrocco *et al.* 2021). In Ontario, Stall *et al.* (2020) found a correlation between for-profit ownership and COVID-19 mortality, which the authors determined was largely a factor of chain ownership and outdated design standards. Among homes that experienced an outbreak with at least one death, the mortality rate from COVID-19 at for-profit homes was found to be more than triple that of municipal homes, and nearly double that of non-profit homes (Cochrane and Sanger 2022). On an international level, a systematic review of 32 studies across five countries concluded that while for-profit ownership was not consistently linked to higher risk of outbreak, there was evidence of higher rates of COVID-19 infections and deaths at for-profit homes (Bach-Mortensen *et al.* 2021).

There has also been significant qualitative work conducted on the impact of for-profit ownership in Ontario. In particular, research by Pat Armstrong and others describes the consequences of privatization on workers and residents, including poor labor conditions experienced by predominantly female frontline care workers (Armstrong *et al.* 2009, 2019; Armstrong *et al.* 2016). Some of this work touches on financialization, observing that many for-profit chains are owned by investors whose returns are subsidized by public funding, and that the underlying real estate may be a primary attraction (Armstrong *et al.* 2019, 2021). Furthermore, the process of bidding for new licenses and the complexity of the regulatory regime work to the benefit of financialized chains, which are 'increasingly global in reach' and 'prepared to quickly sell, move or close nursing homes in the interests of profit making' (Armstrong and Baines 2020: 99).

For-profit ownership in the province expanded in the 1990s through a competitive bidding process, initiated by Mike Harris' Progressive Conservative government, which allocated two-thirds of new long-term care beds to for-profit companies (Armstrong *et al.* 2019). Several providers who benefited most from this process, including Extendicare and Sienna Senior Living, later transitioned into publicly traded companies. Harris was the chair of Chartwell's Board of Directors until 2022, a position that reflects what some have described as a 'revolving door' between Ontario's Progressive Conservative Party and for-profit long-term care (Helguero 2020). Other aspects of long-term care in the province have also been privatized, via the contracting out of food, laundry, staffing services, and more. This history of privatization facilitated financialization in the sector within the context of neoliberalism. The shift occurred largely in the 1990s and 2000s via a process of consolidation, whereby existing chains and new companies went public (August 2021). They partnered with institutional investors to finance acquisitions and established expertise in development and construction to build new homes. Today, the management and boards of directors of publicly traded long-term care companies are heavily dominated by individuals with a background in real estate development and investment or financial services.

Six of the ten biggest owners of long-term care beds in Canada were financialized as of 2020 (August 2021). The top four spots were all held by financialized companies: Revera (pension fund), Extendicare (publicly traded), Sienna Senior Living (publicly traded), and Chartwell (publicly traded). In total, financialized companies owned approximately 22 percent of long-term care beds across Canada, and as many as 32 percent in Ontario (August 2021). The impact of financialization extends beyond ownership, however, with some companies also offering management and consulting services. This creates additional layers of financialization when other financialized companies retain these services. For example, management of homes owned by the private equity firm Southbridge is contracted out to Extendicare. Financialized business practices can also permeate non-financialized homes when private management services are utilized by non-profit providers.

Financialized companies are distinct, in that they are embedded in a particular web of stakeholders that drives profit maximization. All financialized companies are beholden to a set of shareholders, investors, or fund holders, on whose behalf they are expected to generate returns. Publicly traded companies are listed on the stock market and distribute regular dividends to shareholders, who expect stable yields, if not steady growth. Such companies are also required to make quarterly financial disclosures to securities regulators. Members of the public can purchase stock in publicly traded companies; in contrast, investment in private equity firms is limited to institutional and accredited investors, and often requires a substantial minimum investment (for example, the minimum investment for Yorkville Asset Management, which owns Southbridge, is $500,000) (Yorkville Asset Management n.d.). Moreover, private equity firms are not required to make the same disclosures as publicly traded companies, making it difficult to obtain information on their corporate structure and financial status.[1]

Publicly traded companies are monitored by analysts at major banks who, along with investors, attend quarterly conference calls and earnings presentations, in order to report on financial performance. This information is used to forecast future returns and make recommendations to clients, who may purchase or sell shares on this basis. In turn, such ratings may impact decision-making by management. Analysts often pose questions about improving profit margins and mitigating unexpected costs. In Chartwell's Q1 2013 call, one analyst inquired as to when the company expected to increase dividends: 'The one thing that I find missing in all of your presentations is any mention of an increase in the payout to unitholders. Every month, I look at the press release and I see the dreaded 0.045' (S&P Capital IQ 2013a). The following quarter, the same individual commented:

> I do hope that the Board of Directors is being guided by management, as much as any Board of Directors ever is guided by management towards the need for a good, strong, for want of a better word, share price.
>
> (S&P Capital IQ 2013b)

The concern for steady returns and consistent growth is ubiquitous on such calls.

All for-profit long-term care providers operate as businesses with a profit incentive, which has led to the diversion of public funds for private gain. Financialized long-term care companies in Ontario cannot drive profits by increasing prices, as resident accommodation rates are set by the province and standardized across homes of all ownership types. As a result, they employ other means to extract profits, primarily government subsidies, growth, and cost minimization. Over the last decade, the amount of long-term care funding in Ontario extracted as profit has been estimated at nearly C$4 billion (Cochrane and Sanger 2022). In the case of publicly traded companies, profits are distributed as dividends: between 2010 and 2021, Chartwell, Extendicare, and Sienna Senior Living paid out a combined C$2.3 billion to their shareholders (Cochrane and Sanger 2022). Dividend totals reached record highs in 2020 and 2021, the first two years of the pandemic, at C$235 million and C$242 million, respectively.

During the first three quarters of 2020, the three aforementioned companies paid out nearly C$171 million to shareholders, while simultaneously receiving C$138.5 in emergency pandemic funding (Wallace *et al.* 2020). In one of its quarterly conference calls, a Sienna Senior Living executive maintained that the dividends were paid out of accommodation fees and revenues from the retirement business, rather than government aid (Sienna Senior Living 2021b). Beyond the fact that government aid likely enabled all three companies to circumvent a drop in dividend payouts, the funneling of accommodation fees to shareholders highlights a fundamental distinction between financialized companies and other providers. In contrast, municipal and non-profit providers reinvest all profits in their homes. In fact, they often supplement provincial subsidies with other sources of funding to raise the standard of care. In 2015, for instance, Ontario municipalities jointly contributed approximately C$350 million in tax revenues to their long-term care homes, equivalent to an additional $21,600 per bed (Association of Municipalities of Ontario 2019).

As noted above, land matters in financialization, and long-term care companies are predicated on a strategy of rapid growth via construction of new homes, acquisition of existing homes, and diversification into related businesses. Ongoing expansion can help generate additional revenue to offset unexpected costs and impending interest payments, as well as increase returns. It also permits companies to position themselves as dominant providers in the sector, which may give them more sway in lobbying and securing new licenses. Sienna Senior Living grew from 26 long-term care homes at the time of its initial public offering (IPO) in 2010, to 43 homes in 2021 (Leisureworld Senior Care Corporation 2010; Sienna Senior Living 2021a). Chartwell, which owned a combined total of 44 long-term care homes and retirement residences when it completed its IPO in 2003, had 130 properties by 2021 (179 when partially owned properties are included) (Chartwell 2003, 2021). Chartwell recently entered into an agreement to sell off 16 of its long-term care homes in Ontario in a C$446.5 million deal, framing the transaction as a 'strategic decision' to focus on its retirement business (Chartwell 2022). Extendicare went the opposite way, selling 11 retirement residences to expand its long-term care and home care offerings (RENX Staff 2022). Sales and acquisitions of this nature are demonstrative of the extent to which care facilities are treated as assets, and their centrality to a financialized company has less to do with 'care' and more to do with their capacity to produce a service commodity that procures return on investment.

Financialized chains are also distinguished by their comparatively easier access to capital, which facilitates growth. In particular, as a number of companies in the senior housing sector went public in the late-1990s and early-2000s, access to capital markets enabled them to finance major acquisitions, purchasing homes and even entire chains owned by smaller companies (August 2021). As financialized companies expand, they become increasingly dominant in the sector, furthering their ability to obtain new licenses and lobby for policies to their benefit. For example, in a 2019 conference call, an Extendicare executive stated that while they had received government approval to build new homes in Ontario, they intended to wait 'until the economics are more favorable' (Extendicare 2019). He predicted that the province would soon move ahead with the desired subsidy increase, in part because the long-term care bed shortage was putting pressure on public hospitals. In the context of overburdened hospitals and long wait lists for long-term care, such delay tactics give companies leverage to negotiate for more funding. Indeed, once such arrangements are in place and have reached a critical mass within the system, it is difficult to conceive how governments can transition away from them.

Financialized long-term care and social reproduction

Long-term care homes are, of course, more than real estate or service assets – they are residential facilities that provide assistance with activities of daily living and access to 24-hour nursing and personal care. In Canada, approximately 168,205 individuals live in long-term care homes, in addition to 86,145 in mixed long-term care/retirement homes (Statistics Canada 2016). The Province of Ontario represents a significant portion of this total, with more than 78,000 long-term care residents (Financial Accountability Office of Ontario 2019). While long-term care residents are *primarily* seniors, they also include many individuals with disabilities who require extra assistance with day-to-day tasks. In providing housing and round-the-clock care for seniors, long-term care homes potentially alleviate the implicit caregiving responsibilities of adult children, spouses, and other family members. Long-term care is, thus, implicated in the market economy in two ways: by permitting close relatives of seniors to participate more fully in the workforce, and by providing paid work in elder care. Furthermore, paid work in elder care, particularly the frontline work of personal support workers (PSWs), tends to be precarious and poorly compensated.

PSWs, many of whom are racialized and immigrant women, assist residents with personal care such as bathing, dressing, and toileting. They comprise 58 percent of employees in Ontario's long-term care homes (Long-Term Care Staffing Study Advisory Group 2020). PSWs experience low wages and limited opportunities for advancement (Zagrodney and Saks 2017), and are often subjected to aggression and physical violence from residents (Banerjee *et al.* 2012). Approximately 50 percent of PSWs are retained in the healthcare sector for less than five years, with burnout due to short-staffing listed as a common reason for departure (Long-Term Care Staffing Study Advisory Group 2020). Often working short-staffed and pressed for time, PSWs report regularly feeling inadequate because they are unable to deliver the quality of care and attention they suggest residents deserve (Armstrong *et al.* 2009: 112). Their reactions shed light on another dimension of Folbre's point above: many PSWs do, in fact, care *about* residents, but structural conditions such as understaffing leave them frustrated and exhausted.

Insufficient government funding leads to systemic staffing issues in long-term care homes of all ownership types, but the problem is particularly acute in for-profit and financialized homes. While the value proposition of real estate is an important driver of financialization, maintaining lower wages and staffing levels is a profit extraction strategy in what is a highly labor-intensive sector. As Amy Horton (2019: 145) observes in the UK context, investors and neoliberal governments treat frontline care workers as 'disposable' and 'a cost to be minimized'. Nevertheless, the presumption that PSWs are easily replaceable has recently been called into question, with the Ontario Minister of Long-Term Care acknowledging that improving working conditions is necessary to reduce attrition (Ministry of Long-Term Care 2020).

Ultimately, however, in the realm of social reproduction, the assumptions that underpin neoliberal ideology do not hold true; namely, that competition and consumer choice will lead to optimized efficiency (Corlet Walker *et al.* 2022). Not only is the long-term care sector entirely reliant on government subsidies, but the notion that residents dissatisfied with their care can simply 'exit' and go elsewhere is illusory. In fact, bed shortages and the overwhelming difficulty of relocating an ailing senior to a new institution mean that most residents will remain in homes with substandard care. As the individuals closest to the site of care, PSWs witness first-hand the effects of budget cuts on residents' quality of life, and often feel compelled to make up for shortfalls by putting in extra hours and advocating for better supplies. The consequences of underfunding are, thus, borne primarily by precarious workers and vulnerable residents.

By resituating elder care as wage labor in institutions instead of unpaid labor in the home, long-term care homes theoretically shift responsibility away from family members. In reality, however, many family members continue to be involved in care even after a senior enters long-term care, in order to pick up the slack in under-resourced homes (Long-Term Care Staffing Study Advisory Group 2020). In addition, it is not uncommon for individuals and families to hire private companions to assist with feeding and other activities in the long-term care home, provided they can afford to do so (Daly *et al.* 2015). This phenomenon not only results in an uneven distribution of care, but also creates an even more precarious class of workers and potentially papers over the severity of understaffing. Family members may also perform caregiving duties for their loved one in long-term care. This role disproportionately falls to women, who find time for this labor around their own busy work schedules. Women are also primarily responsible for the administrative work involved in selecting a home and making move-in arrangements – indeed, as a Chartwell executive noted, it is the daughter of the prospective resident to whom the company's marketing is directed (S&P Capital IQ 2019). By relying on low-paid and unpaid female labor, financialized companies can, thus, increase profits by keeping labor costs down.

There is significant pressure on and within the provincial government to build more long-term care homes, given the aging population and already high demand. As of May 2021, more than 38,000 people were on the wait list for long-term care in Ontario, with a median wait time of 171 days (Government of Ontario 2021). However, there is also ongoing advocacy in favor of alternatives to long-term care. According to one survey, 78 percent of Canadians want to age at home, but only 26 percent expect they will be able to do so (March of Dimes 2021). For many seniors, the transition to long-term care represents a loss of independence that isolates them from their families, friends, and communities. While this chapter addresses the particular issue of financialization, it also acknowledges the substantive critical assessments of long-term care more broadly as a predominant institution of senior housing and care. Long-term care has constituted a significant portion of social reproduction conventionally provided from other sources, but its delivery has, in many instances, procured less-than-adequate standards of care, with not nearly the required attention to seniors' needs and anxieties. Moreover, the industry's viability is premised on the gendered and racialized assumptions that low-cost care from demoralized PSWs suffices, and that family can shore up the rest.

Conclusion

Long-term care exists at the nexus of healthcare and housing and, as such, must be analyzed in a manner that accounts for dynamics in both sectors. Financialization of rental housing negatively impacts access to housing by reducing affordability and increasing precarity. In long-term care, the stakes are possibly even higher, as financialization threatens quality of care for vulnerable residents, as well as working conditions for staff. One of the most significant manifestations of financialization occurs in the built environment, as the proposition of stable yields and strong collateral make property an attractive investment, particularly when financial markets allow it to be packaged and traded as a liquid asset. As long as it remains profitable, finance capital will seek out investment in real estate – whether it be housing, farmland, or long-term care homes. Furthermore, in their ongoing drive for higher returns, financialized companies will continue to grow, capturing an increasing proportion of the market.

While Ontario regulates long-term care, the government also actively permits its financialization. As this chapter has shown, this has profoundly negative effects on the provision of care within institutions, and it does not necessarily 'alleviate' or seriously address largely gendered care responsibilities passed on to relatives. In other words, market imperatives may economize care, but they substantively generate the worst possible outcomes, where care is diminished *and* gender exploitation is renewed. Yet, as with any service provision in which financialization is already entrenched, the scale of disruption necessary to bring this about is large. Even if the Ontario government (like other governments) were not somewhat enamored by the 'benefits' of the market and private investment, it seems unlikely to undertake such disruption in the foreseeable future. Reaching a state in which long-term care or other services are perceived as public goods would require substantial political will to enact legal and policy maneuvers to shield them from capital markets. It would also necessitate proposals to reduce the scope of privatization; decrease or halt licenses to for-profit providers; build capacity among public and non-profit providers; and, importantly, increase funding and support for community-based care.

Note

1 For their part, pension funds are expected to maintain high and consistent returns on behalf of contributors and beneficiaries. By way of example, Public Sector Pension Investment Board (PSPIB), a crown corporation operating as a private company, is one of the biggest pension funds in Canada, with C$204.5 billion in assets under management as of March 31, 2021 (PSP Investments 2021). It manages the pension plans of federal public servants, and members of the Canadian Armed Forces, Royal Canadian Mounted Police, and Reserve Force. PSPIB owns Revera, a long-term care chain it purchased in 2007 by acquiring 100 percent of the shares in the then-publicly traded Retirement Residences Real Estate Investment Trust (PSP Investments 2007). Critically, while PSPIB lacks the public transparency of a public company, it retains the imperative of high returns on its investments, linked to pension fund growth expectations.

References

Aalbers, M.B. 2016, *The Financialization of Housing: A Political Economy Approach*, Routledge, London.

Aalbers, M.B., Fernandez, R. and Wijburg, G. 2020, 'The financialization of real estate', in Mader, P., Mertens, D. and van der Zwan, N. (eds), *The Routledge International Handbook of Financialization*, Routledge, Abingdon, pp. 200–12.

AdvantAge Ontario, n.d, *Challenges and Solutions*, The Difference Matters, accessed 10 October 2022, <https://thedifferencematters.ca/challenges-and-solutions>.

Armstrong, P, Armstrong, H. and MacLeod, K.K. 2016, 'The threats of privatization to security in long-term residential care', *Ageing International*, 41(1), pp. 99–116.

Armstrong, P., Armstrong, H., MacDonald, M. and Doupe, M. 2019, 'Privatization of long-term residential care in Canada: The case of three provinces', in Armstrong, P. and Armstrong, H. (eds), *The Privatization of Care*, Routledge, London, pp. 87–101.

Armstrong, P., Armstrong, H., Buchanan, D., Dean, T., Donner, G., Donner, A., Sholzberg-Gray, S., Himelfarb, A. and Shrybman, S. 2021, *Investing In Care, Not Profit: Recommendations To Transform Long-Term Care In Ontario*, Canadian Centre for Policy Alternatives, Ottawa.

Armstrong, P. and Baines, D. 2020, 'Privatization, hybridization and resistance in contemporary care work', in Baines, D. and Cunningham, I. (eds), *Working in the Context of Austerity: Challenges and Struggles*, Bristol University Press, Bristol, pp. 97–108.

Armstrong, P., Banerjee, A., Szebehely, M., Armstrong, H., Daly, T. and Lafrance, S. 2009, *They Deserve Better: The long-Term Care Experience in Canada and Scandinavia*, Canadian Centre for Policy Alternatives, Ottawa.

Association of Municipalities of Ontario. 2019, *A Compendium of Municipal Health Activities and Recommendations*, Reports and submissions, Association of Municipalities, Ontario.

August, M. 2020, 'The financialization of Canadian multi-family rental housing: From trailer to tower', *Journal of Urban Affairs*, 42(7), pp. 1–23.

August, M. 2021, 'Securitising seniors housing: The financialisation of real estate and social reproduction in retirement and long-term care homes', *Antipode*, 54(3), pp. 653–80.

August, M. and Walks, A. 2018, 'Gentrification, suburban decline, and the financialization of multi-family rental housing: The case of Toronto', *Geoforum*, 89, pp. 124–36.

Bach-Mortensen, A.M., Verboom, B., Movsisyan, A. and Degli Esposti, M. 2021, 'A systematic review of the associations between care home ownership and COVID-19 outbreaks, infections and mortality', *Nature Aging*, 1(10), pp. 948–61.

Banerjee, A., Daly, T., Armstrong, P., Szebehely, M., Armstrong, H. and Lafrance, S. 2012, 'Structural violence in long-term, residential care for older people: Comparing Canada and Scandinavia', *Social Science and Medicine*, 74(3), pp. 390–8.

Berta, W., Laporte, A. and Valdmanis, V. 2005, 'Observations on institutional long-term care in Ontario: 1996–2002', *Canadian Journal on Aging*, 24(1), pp. 71–84.

Bresser-Pereira, L.C. 2010, 'The global financial crisis, neoclassical economics, and the neoliberal years of capitalism', *Revue de la Régulation*, 7. https://journals.openedition.org/regulation/7729.

Chartwell. 2003, 'Initial public offering prospectus', accessed 21 March 2022, <https://sedar.com/>.

Chartwell. 2021, *Annual Report 2021*, Chartwell, accessed 10 February 2023, <https://s23.q4cdn.com/371771841/files/doc_financials/2021/ar/CHARTWELL_ANNUAL_REPORT_2021-final-LR.pdf>.

Chartwell. 2022, 'Chartwell enters into agreements to transition its interests in Ontario long term care platform', accessed 10 February 2023, <https://investors.chartwell.com/English/press-market-information/press-releases/news-details/2022/Chartwell-Enters-into-Agreements-to-Transition-Its-Interests-in-Ontario-Long-Term-Care-Platform/default.aspx>.

Christophers, B. 2011, 'Revisiting the urbanization of capital', *Annals of the Association of American Geographers*, 101(6), pp. 1347–64.

CIHI. 2021a, *Long-term Care Homes in Canada: How Many and Who Owns Them?*, Canadian Institute for Health Information, accessed 19 January 2023, <https://www.cihi.ca/en/long-term-care-homes-in-canada-how-many-and-who-owns-them>.

CIHI. 2021b, *The Impact of COVID-19 on Long-Term Care in Canada: Focus on the First 6 Months*, Canadian Institute for Health Information, accessed 21 January 2023, <https://www.cihi.ca/sites/default/files/document/impact-covid-19-long-term-care-canada-first-6-months-report-en.pdf>.

Cochrane, D. and Sanger, T. 2022, 'Careless profits: Diverting public money from long-term care in Ontario', *Canadians for Tax Fairness*, accessed 10 February 2023, <https://www.taxfairness.ca/en/resources/reports/report-careless-profits>

Corlet Walker, C., Druckman, A. and Jackson, T. 2022, 'A critique of the marketisation of long-term residential and nursing home care', *The Lancet Healthy Longevity*, 3(4), pp. e298–e306.

Daly, T., Armstrong, P. and Lowndes, R. 2015, 'Liminality in Ontario's long-term care facilities: Private companions' care work in the space "betwixt and between"', *Competition and Change*, 19(3), pp. 246–63.

Davis, A. and Walsh, C. 2017, 'Distinguishing financialization from neoliberalism', *Theory, Culture and Society*, 34(5–6), pp. 27–51.

Extendicare. 2019, 'Third quarter 2019 results', 8 November, accessed 19 September 2022, <https://www.gowebcasting.com/events/extendicare-inc/2019/11/08/third-quarter-2019-results/play>.

Fairbairn, M. 2020, *Fields of Gold: Financing the Global Land Rush*, Cornell University Press, Ithaca.

Farha, L. 2017, *Report of the Special Rapporteur on Adequate Housing as a Component of the Right to an Adequate Standard of Living, and on the Right to Non-Discrimination in This Context*, Digital Library, United Nations, accessed 10 February 2023, <https://digitallibrary.un.org/record/861179?ln=en>.

Fernandez, R. and Aalbers, M.B. 2016, 'Financialization and housing: Between globalization and varieties of capitalism', *Competition and Change*, 20(2), pp. 71–88.

Fields, D. and Uffer, S. 2016, 'The financialisation of rental housing: A comparative analysis of New York City and Berlin', *Urban Studies*, 53(7), pp. 1486–502.

Financial Accountability Office of Ontario. 2019, *Long-Term Care Homes Program: A Review of the Plan to Create 15,000 New Long-Term Care Beds in Ontario*, accessed 19 December 2022, <https://www.fao-on.org/en/Blog/Publications/ontario-long-term-care-program>.

Folbre, N. 2014, 'Who cares? A feminist critique of the care economy', *Rosa Luxemburg Stiftung*, accessed 10 February 2023, <https://rosalux.nyc/a-feminist-critique-of-the-care-economy/>.

Gallagher, A. 2021, '"A 'golden child' for investors": The assetization of urban childcare property in NZ', *Urban Geography*, 42(10), pp. 1440–58.

Gotham, K.F. 2009, 'Creating liquidity out of spatial fixity: The secondary circuit of capital and the subprime mortgage crisis', *International Journal of Urban and Regional Research*, 33(2), pp. 355–71.

Government of Ontario. 2021, *Ontario Building New Long-Term Care Home in Vaughan*, Newsroom, accessed 19 January 2023, <https://news.ontario.ca/en/release/1000949/ontario-building-new-long-term-care-home-in-vaughan>.

Harvey, D. 2001, 'Globalization and the "spatial fix"', *Geographische Revue*, 2, pp. 23–30.

Helguero, S. 2020, 'The "revolving door" between Ontario's PCs and the for-profit seniors care industry worst hit by coronavirus', *The Post Millennial*, 3 June, accessed 21 December 2022, <https://thepostmillennial.com/the-revolving-door-between-ontario-pcs-and-companies-running-seniors-homes-hit-worst-by-covid-19>.

Hodkinson, S., Watt, P. and Mooney, G. 2013, 'Introduction: Neoliberal housing policy – Time for a critical re-appraisal', *Critical Social Policy*, 33(1), pp. 3–16.

Horton, A. 2019, 'Financialization and non-disposable women: Real estate, debt and labour in UK care homes', *Environment and Planning A: Economy and Space*, 54(1), pp. 144–59.

Hsu, A.T., Berta, W., Coyte, P.C. and Laporte, A. 2016, 'Staffing in Ontario's long-term care homes: Differences by profit status and chain ownership', *Canadian Journal on Aging*, 35(2), pp. 175–89.

Khanam, F., Langevin, M., Savage, K., and Uppal, S. 2022, *Women Working in Paid Care Occupations*, Statistics Canada, accessed 19 January 2023, <https://www150.statcan.gc.ca/n1/pub/75-006-x/2022001/article/00001-eng.htm>.

Krippner, G.R. 2011, *Capitalizing on Crisis: The Political Origins of the Rise of Finance*, Harvard University Press, Cambridge.

Leijten, I. and de Bel, K. 2020, 'Facing financialization in the housing sector: A human right to adequate housing for all', *Netherlands Quarterly of Human Rights*, 38(2), pp. 94–114.

Leisureworld Senior Care Corporation. 2010, 'Initial public offering prospectus', accessed 7 January 2023, <https://sedar.com/>.

Long-Term Care Staffing Study Advisory Group. 2020, *Long-Term Care Staffing Study*, Ministry of Long-Term Care, accessed 9 January 2023, <https://www.ontario.ca/page/long-term-care-staffing-study>.

March of Dimes. 2021, 'National survey shows Canadians overwhelmingly want to age at home; just one-quarter of seniors expect to do so', accessed 21 December 2022, <https://www.marchofdimes.ca/en-ca/aboutus/newsroom/pr/Pages/Aging-at-Home.aspx>.

Marrocco, F.N., Coke, A. and Kitts, J. 2021, *Ontario's Long-Term Care COVID-19 Commission*, final report and progress on interim recommendations, Government of Ontario, accessed 10 February 2023, <https://www.ontario.ca/page/long-term-care-covid-19-commission-progress-interim-recommendations>.

Ministry of Health and Long-Term Care. 2017, *Policy: LTCH Level-of-Care Per Diem Funding Policy*, Government of Ontario, accessed 21 February 2023, <https://www.health.gov.on.ca/en/public/programs/ltc/archived_ltch.aspx>.

Ministry of Long-Term Care. 2020, *A Better Place To Live, A Better Place To Work: Ontario's Long-Term Care Staffing Plan*, Government of Ontario, accessed 21 December 2022, <https://www.ontario.ca/page/better-place-live-better-place-work-ontarios-long-term-care-staffing-plan>.

PSP Investments. 2007, 'Public sector pension investment board succeeds in bid for retirement residences real estate investment trust', accessed 9 January 2023, <https://www.investpsp.com/en/news/public-sector-pension-investment-board-succeeds-in-bid-for-retirement-residences-real-estate-investment-trust/>.

PSP Investments. 2021, 'Our performance', accessed 7 January 2023, <https://www.investpsp.com/en/investment-performance/>.

RENX Staff. 2022, 'Sienna, Sabra JV to acquire 11 Extendicare seniors homes', *Real Estate News EXchange*, accessed 27 November 2022, <https://renx.ca/sienna-sabra-jv-to-acquire-11-extendicare-seniors-homes>.

Revington, N. and August, M. 2020, 'Making a market for itself: The emergent financialization of student housing in Canada', *Environment and Planning A: Economy and Space*, 52(5), pp. 856–77.

Sienna Senior Living. 2021a, *Q3 Report to Shareholders*, accessed 7 January 2023, <https://www.siennaliving.ca/getmedia/7f9d8903-bec4-4a95-a188-b4e5f8c1b130/Combined-Final-LS-MD-A-and-FS.pdf>.

Sienna Senior Living. 2021b, 'Q4 2020 financial results conference call and slides', 19 February, accessed 7 January 2023, <https://www.siennaliving.ca/investors/events-presentations>.

S&P Capital IQ. 2013a, 'Transcript: Chartwell retirement residences, Q1 2013 earnings call, May 03, 2013', *MarketScreener*, accessed 7 January 2023, <https://www.marketscreener.com/quote/stock/CHARTWELL-RETIREMENT-RESI-1409600/news/Transcript-Chartwell-Retirement-Residences-Q1-2013-Earnings-Call-May-03-2013-39075656/>.

S&P Capital IQ. 2013b, 'Transcript: chartwell retirement residences, Q2 2013 earnings call, Aug 14, 2013', *MarketScreener*, accessed 7 January 2023, <https://www.marketscreener.com/quote/stock/CHARTWELL-RETIREMENT-RESI-1409600/news/Transcript-Chartwell-Retirement-Residences-Q2-2013-Earnings-Call-Aug-14-2013-38972840/>.

S&P Capital IQ. 2019, 'Transcript: Chartwell retirement residences, Q2 2019 earnings call, Aug 09, 2019', *MarketScreener*, <https://www.marketscreener.com/quote/stock/CHARTWELL-RETIREMENT-RESI-1409600/news/Transcript-Chartwell-Retirement-Residences-Q2-2019-Earnings-Call-Aug-09-2019-37919568/>.

Stall, N.M., Jones, A., Brown, K.A., Rochon, P.A. and Costa, A.P. 2020, 'For-profit long-term care homes and the risk of COVID-19 outbreaks and resident deaths', *Canadian Medical Association Journal*, 192(33), pp. E946–55.

Statistics Canada. 2016, 'Type of collective dwelling (16), age (20) and sex (3) for the population in collective dwellings of Canada, provinces and territories', 2016 Census, Government of Canada, accessed 19 December 2022, <https://www12.statcan.gc.ca/datasets/Index-eng.cfm?Temporal=2016&Theme=116&VNAMEE=&GA=-1&S=0>.

Tanuseputro, P., Chalifoux, M., Bennett, C., Gruneir, A., Bronskill, S.E., Walker, P. and Manuel, D. 2015, 'Hospitalization and mortality rates in long-term care facilities: Does for-profit status matter?' *Journal of the American Medical Directors Association*, 16(10), pp. 874–83.

Walks, A. and Clifford, B. 2015, 'The political economy of mortgage securitization and the neoliberalization of housing policy in Canada', *Environment and Planning A: Economy and Space*, 47(8), pp. 1624–42.

Wallace, K., Tubb, E. and Chown Oved, M. 2020, 'Big for-profit long-term-care companies paid out more than $170 million to investors through Ontario's deadly first wave', *The Toronto Star*, 26 December, accessed 19 December 2022, <https://www.thestar.com/news/gta/2020/12/26/big-for-profit-long-term-care-companies-paid-out-more-than-170-million-to-investors-through-ontarios-deadly-first-wave.html>.

Yorkville Asset Management. n.d., 'Yorkville health care fund', accessed 7 January 2023, <https://www.yorkvilleasset.com/en/investments-and-funds/yorkville-health-care-fund>.

Zagrodney, K. and Saks, M. 2017, 'Personal support workers in Canada: The new precariat?' *Healthcare Policy*, 13(2), pp. 31–9.

20
THE ANATOMY OF BIG PHARMA

Marc-André Gagnon

The global pharmaceutical sector has many layers of complexity. It is one of the most regulated sectors in terms of consumer safety; is dominated by monopolies and intellectual property protection over specific and sometimes life-saving products; but is also consistently one of the most profitable sectors year after year. Supply in the pharmaceutical 'market' is controlled by large global pharmaceutical companies, while demand is largely directed by large public drug plans. Complex power dynamics result from the workings of this 'market', involving the production of knowledge and beliefs, massive marketing toward patients and physicians, and constant lobbying to allow new drugs to enter the market – even when their benefits are unclear, their risks are mostly unknown, and their pricing is opaque.

This chapter provides a critical introduction to the global political economy of the pharmaceutical sector. After identifying its main structures, the chapter focuses on dominant pharmaceutical companies, often referred to as 'Big Pharma'. It then analyzes the evolution of the pharmaceutical sector, and how dominant pharmaceutical companies consolidated their structural power through specific dominant business models (from 'blockbuster drugs' to 'nichebuster drugs'). Finally, the chapter investigates 'ghost-management' strategies deployed by Big Pharma to shape knowledge, regulation, and social structures.

Structure of the pharmaceutical market

In 2021, sales of medication globally amounted to more than US$1.4 trillion (IQVIA 2022: 39). The US represents 4.2 percent of global population, and more than 40 percent of global sales in pharmaceuticals. Lower-income countries represent more than half of the global population, but only 4.9 percent of global sales (see: Table 20.1).

New drugs arriving on the market are normally brand-name patented products, developed and manufactured by large drug companies capable of marketing their products around the globe while dealing with diverse national regulations. New patented drugs normally benefit from a 20-year patent that gives the drug company market exclusivity over the product. Once the patent expires, the original brand-name drug usually continues to be sold, but must face the competition of generic versions of the drug (branded or not) manufactured at lower prices by competitors. Large

DOI: 10.4324/9781003017110-23

Table 20.1 Global drug spending and growth in selected countries, 2021 (or nearest year)

	2021 spending US$ billion	*Percent of global sales*	*2017–21 CAGR*** *(percent)*
Global	1,423.5	100	5.1
US	580.4	40.8	4.9
China	169.4	11.9	6.1
Japan	85.4	6.0	–0.5
Germany	64.6	4.5	6.2
France	42.0	3.0	3
UK	36.6	2.6	5.9
Italy	36.5	2.6	3
Brazil	31.6	2.2	11.7
Spain	29.8	2.1	5.4
Canada	27.4	1.9	5.2
India*	25.2	1.8	11.1
Russia	18.8	1.3	11.4
Lower-income countries (excluding India)*	43.6	3.1	N.A.

Source: Calculations based on IQVIA (2022) and OECD (2022).

* Lower-income countries include both low-income countries and lower-middle-income countries. India is usually included among lower-income countries, but is listed separately in the table. The list of lower-income countries is determined by the World Bank and can be found on their website: <https://data.worldbank.org/?locations=XN-XM>.

** Compounded Annual Growth Rate.

Table 20.2 Global medicine spending by product type, 2021

	Global	*Ten largest developed markets**
Original brands	888.7	708.3
Non-original brands	246.1	88.5
Unbranded generics	153.8	96.6
Other (*e.g.* vitamins, minerals)	132.7	41.8
Total	1,421.3	935.2

Source: IQVIA (2022).

*The ten largest high-income countries with pharmaceutical spending greater than US$10 billion are Australia, Canada, France, Germany, Italy, Japan, South Korea, Spain, the UK, and the US.

pharmaceutical companies associated with 'Big Pharma' normally produce original brand-name drugs, which represent the bulk of global sales (see: Table 20.2).

Non-original brands and unbranded generics are normally sold at lower prices than original brands. Among OECD countries, the share of generics (branded or not) in the total pharmaceutical market was 53 percent in terms of volume, and 24 percent in terms of value (OECD 2021: 243). Most medications are purchased as prescription drugs, which require the authorization of a healthcare professional, such as a prescribing physician. In OECD countries, on average, prescription drugs normally represent 79 percent of sales in purchased drugs, while over-the-counter drugs (which do not require a prescription) represent 21 percent of the total market (OECD 2021: 236).

The market for patented original brand-name drugs is characterized by its wide pricing bracket (for the same products) and its opacity. On average, the official listed price of the same patented drug sold at US$39 in Turkey is US$70 in Australia, US$82 in the UK, US$93 in Japan, US$100 in Canada, and US$349 in the US (Patented Medicines Price Review Board 2021: 47). This does not mean that poorer countries pay less for their drugs – on the contrary, existing evidence shows that poorer countries often pay higher prices for the same drugs in absolute terms or as a percentage of average income (Morgan *et al.* 2020). However, the official listed price is not the real price of these drugs, since confidential rebates are now the norm among high-income countries and can vary considerably between countries or between therapeutic areas (Morgan *et al.* 2017). National public drug plans covering the whole population of a country normally have greater bargaining power to negotiate higher rebates. Such national public drug plans exist in most high-income countries, with the important exceptions of the US and Canada.

Conversely, most lower-income countries do not benefit from such national public comprehensive drug coverage that would ensure better access and increase bargaining capacity. Accordingly, access to a limited basket of essential medicines is often impossible for most of the population. Thus, even if ensuring 'access to safe, effective, quality and affordable essential medicines and vaccines for all' is a vital component of the Sustainable Development Goals (SDGs) (United Nations 2019), nearly two billion people globally have no access to essential medicines, which results in greater pain and suffering, prolonged illness, inappropriate use, needless disabilities, and preventable deaths (Ozawa *et al.* 2019; Wirtz *et al.* 2017).

New drugs are approved by national health authorities based on their effectiveness relative to a placebo, not in relation to existing drugs. In fact, most newly patented drugs arriving on the market do not represent a therapeutic advance as compared to drugs that already exist. According to medical journal *Prescrire* (2021), among the 109 new patented drugs that entered the French market in 2020, only nine represented a clear therapeutic advantage compared to existing drugs, while 83 did not represent a significant therapeutic advantage – including ten of which were considered more harmful than beneficial. In Canada, the Patented Medicines Price Review Board (Patented Medicines Price Review Board 2021: 13) concluded that, between 2010 and 2019, only 17 percent of new patented drugs introduced in the Canadian market represented a therapeutic advantage, while 83 percent did not represent any significant therapeutic advantage over already marketed drugs. It might be argued that new drugs that are similar to older ones ('me-too' drugs) allow for greater price competition and reduce costs. Yet, this argument is flawed if we consider that, in Canada, these patented 'me-too' drugs not only represented 83 percent of all new marketed drugs between 2010 and 2019, but also represented more than 70 percent of all revenues (Patented Medicines Price Review Board 2021: 13).

The purchase of medications is mostly performed by private and public drug insurance plans, but patients often still have to shoulder the burden with co-payments, deductibles or premiums. Many drug plans use health technology assessment to limit patient reimbursement to drugs that provide value for money. However, some drug plans will reimburse any drug at any price, which creates flawed financial incentives for drug companies to produce expensive drugs with no additional therapeutic value. For example, Medicare Part D in the US, by law, does not have the capacity to discriminate between drugs or negotiate rebates (Gagnon and Wolfe 2015). According to data provided by the Centers for Medicare and Medicaid Services (CMS),[1] Medicare Part D spent US$183 billion in 2019 on prescription drugs, which represents around 13 percent of global sales in medicines.

In many ways, the purchase of drugs can be compared to a dinner for three at a restaurant: one person orders the food (the prescribing physician), one person eats the food (the patient), and a third person pays for the food (the insurer). Extending the metaphor, it could be added that the waiter embodies the drug company pushing for their most expensive products to be prescribed by the physician. This state of affairs creates complex power dynamics: demand is driven mostly by physicians' prescriptions where they do not have to pay for the products. As such, pharmaceuticals are one of the rare markets where demand is not directly limited by a budget constraint. In particular, this situation creates important incentives for drug companies to massively promote their drugs toward prescribers. For example, in the US, it has been estimated that while drug companies spent US$4 billion in advertising their drugs to patients each year, they also spent an impressive US$42.8 billion annually to promote their products to prescribing physicians (Gagnon and Lexchin 2008).

It is important to note that the existing literature shows no correlation between patented drug prices and research and development costs. In the words of Hank McKinnell, ex-CEO of Pfizer: 'It's a fallacy to suggest that our industry, or any industry, prices a product to recapture the R&D budget' (McKinnell 2005: 46). Claims that the prices of drugs are related to their level of therapeutic benefit or their degree of innovation remain unsubstantiated. It seems that the only logic behind drug prices is that drug companies charge what the market will bear, based on purchasers' willingness-to-pay. For example, in the US between 2009 and 2013, first-in-class cancer drugs were priced, on average, at $116,100 per year, while next-in-class cancer drugs were priced at $119,765 per year (Mailankody and Prasad 2015). Between 2010 and 2015, only 35 percent of new cancer drugs represented any therapeutic advance on existing drugs, but no relation could be established between the price of drugs and benefits to society and patients (Vivot *et al.* 2017). After analyzing 65 anti-cancer drugs in different countries, no significant association was found between monthly treatment costs and clinical benefits in all assessed countries (Vokinger *et al.* 2020). In terms of political economy, this raises an important question: how can pharmaceutical companies access markets and push for the reimbursement of expensive drugs when these drugs do not always represent a therapeutic advance? It is to such issues that the chapter now turns.

Identifying Big Pharma

'Big Pharma' is a term that refers to firms that dominate the global pharmaceutical sector. While dominant firms or core companies shape and drive the evolution of their business sector, they generally do not embody the whole sector, as a business sector comprises core companies alongside a *supporting nexus* of concatenated and complementary (rather than competitive) enterprises. This supporting nexus consists of small, medium, or large firms (or public research labs) that cooperate with core companies, but rarely do core companies evolve out of this nexus.

The business historian, Alfred D. Chandler, offers an interesting toolbox to identify the core companies of a sector and differentiate them from their supporting nexus. Chandler's basic concept is that the competitive strength of industrial firms in market economies rests on *learned organizational capabilities* (Chandler 2005: 6). Those organizational capabilities can be classified in three ways: (1) technical knowledge required for research; (2) functional capabilities that are product-related (development, manufacturing, and marketing), and (3) managerial capabilities. Only firms 'efficient' enough (in business terms) in building their organizational capabilities can become core companies of a sector. The first enterprises to develop an integrated set of capabilities essential to commercializing their products in a new business sector can be considered the 'first movers' (Chandler 2005: 7). They benefit from their learned organizational capabilities, which become their 'learning bases' (Chandler 2005: 8) to develop their control of the networks of production and distribution, to improve existing products and processes, or to adapt to new conditions. First movers and late entrants to the industry who managed to catch up become 'core companies' (Chandler 2005: 8) – also called dominant firms – that set the direction in which the whole business sector evolves (Chandler 2005).

In the case of the pharmaceutical sector, most core companies embodying *Big Pharma* remain first movers that have existed since at least the 1920s (Gagnon 2009). It is important to note that all core companies in the pharmaceutical sector are vertically integrated companies, and possess three common organizational features: significant research and development, large manufacturing capacities, and considerable marketing and promotional capabilities. A pharmaceutical company that specializes only in one of these three aspects can be an important player of the supporting nexus, but all Big Pharma companies possess these three core capabilities.

There can be no definitive list of the entities usually referred to as 'Big Pharma'. As a rule of thumb, one can consider the drug companies comprising Big Pharma as those included among the global 200 largest corporations in terms of market value. While this means that slight variations may occur in terms of which firms are considered members of Big Pharma, this listing has remained largely consistent over time (Gagnon 2009). In February 2019, 19 drug companies with market capitalization between US$64 billion and US$366 billion were listed among the world's 200 largest corporations in terms of market value, 13 of which were listed among the 100 largest corporations (see: Table 20.3).

Table 20.3 Pharmaceutical companies included among the world's 200 largest corporations in terms of market value, February 2019

Pharmaceutical company	*Country*	*Global rank in market value*	*Market capitalization (US$ billion)*	*Net profit on net sales in 2018 (percent)*
Johnson and Johnson	US	9	366	18.8
Pfizer Inc	US	21	245	20.8
Roche Hldg-Genus	Switzerland	24	235	18.5
Novartis Ag-Reg	Switzerland	26	230	23.7
Merck and Co	US	36	208	14.7
Abbott Labs	US	62	132	7.7
Eli Lilly and Co	US	64	130	13.2
Novo Nordisk-B	Denmark	71	124	34.5
AbbVie Inc	US	75	122	17.4
Amgen Inc	US	77	117	35.3
Sanofi	France	87	107	12.1
AstraZeneca Plc	UK	94	102	9.8
GlaxoSmithKline	UK	95	102	11.8
Gilead Sciences	US	126	87	24.7
Bristol-Myer SQB	US	128	84	21.9
Bayer Ag-Reg	Germany	152	72	21
Biogen Inc	US	169	65	32.9
Takeda Pharma	Japan	175	64	10.6
Celgene Corp	US	177	64	26.5

Source: Bloomberg Database.

Considering that global sales of medication in 2018 totaled US$1,205 billion (IQVIA 2019: 49), and that the combined sales in medications produced by these companies for that year were US$467.8 billion, Big Pharma thus represents almost 40 percent of global sales in medicines, and almost two-thirds of global sales of original brand-name drugs.

What distinguishes Big Pharma companies from core companies in other business sectors is their high rate of net profitability, which averaged 21 percent in 2019. This high rate of profitability is not due to an exceptional year, as it has been steady over time (Gagnon 2009; Ledley *et al.* 2020). Some analysts have even emphasized that Big Pharma is not only beating the average rate of profit, but is also actually 'beating the Hell out of the average' (Nitzan and Bichler 2021). Accordingly, Big Pharma is systematically doing better compared to core companies in other business sectors (Gagnon 2009; Ledley *et al.* 2020).

Standard economic theory normally contends that higher profitability in a specific sector will engender more investment, which will increase productive capacity and supply, and bring back the rate of profit toward the average. However, the pharmaceutical sector shows that dominant drug companies are not competing with newcomers that, instead, normally remain confined to the supporting nexus. Most of the investment in that sector is concentrated on acquiring existing productive capacity and consolidating dominant positions through mergers and acquisitions, instead of creating new productive capacities through gross fixed capital formation (Gagnon 2009; Montalban and Sakinc 2013). To understand the reasons behind the sustained high profitability in pharmaceuticals, it is important to understand the basis of the business models at work in the sector.

From 'blockbusters' to 'nichebusters': evolution of business models

The pharmaceutical sector has evolved a lot over time. In general, analysts tend to agree that most breakthrough therapeutic innovations happened between the 1940s and 1960s. This period is considered the age of 'therapeutic revolution' (Temin 1980), characterized by a 'cascade of discoveries' (Redwood 1988). In the 1960s, an important scandal shook the sector when thousands of babies were born deformed because of thalidomide, a drug used to reduce nausea during pregnancy. Stricter safety regulations were put in place in the 1960s and 1970s, making randomized controlled trials a fundamental factor in the approval process of new drugs. Until the beginning of the 1980s, dominant firms in the pharmaceutical sector enjoyed a level of profit on par with dominant firms in other sectors (Gagnon 2009). While the neoliberal turn of the 1980s significantly relaxed antitrust regulations in a way that fostered substantial waves of mergers and acquisitions in pharmaceuticals, the 1980s were also characterized by a substantial increase in the level of intellectual property protection in high-income countries, especially for brand-name drugs (Drahos and Braithwaite 2002). While the neoliberal agenda emphasized free markets and competition, regulatory reforms in the pharmaceutical sector led to increasing monopolistic capacities, which allowed Big Pharma to substantially increase their profits as compared to dominant companies in other industrial sectors (Gagnon 2009).

Since the 1980s, the justification for the increase of intellectual property rights in the pharmaceutical sector has been its relationship to therapeutic innovation. This narrative of 'more intellectual property means more innovation' remains ever-present, for example in the negotiation of international trade agreements (Correa and Hilty 2022; Gleeson *et al.* 2019; Lexchin and Gagnon 2014; Schram *et al.* 2018); in the debate over a *Trade-Related Aspects of Intellectual Property Rights* waiver to better address the COVID-19 pandemic (Etten 2022; Patnaik 2022); and in the opposition against regulating excessive pricing of patented drug products (Crowe 2022). Nevertheless, many now contend that the current high level of intellectual property protection has become detrimental to real therapeutic innovation because of the creation of patent thickets, patent trolls, evergreening strategies, or constant threats of litigation (Baker 2021; Boldrin and Levine 2013; Drahos and Braithwaite 2002; Freilich and Meurer 2021; Gold 2021; Heller and Eisenberg 1998; Zaitchik 2022). Indicative of this, increases in intellectual property protection since the 1980s have failed to deliver significant innovation in subsequent decades, instead delivering mostly 'me-too' blockbuster drugs, with little therapeutic advance (Gagnon 2009).

A 'blockbuster' drug is a drug marked by over US$1 billion in global sales. A 'me-too' drug is a structurally similar variant to already existing drugs, but for which a patent can still be obtained because it remains a new molecule. These 'me-too' drugs often have no real additional therapeutic value, but are priced 20 to 40 percent higher than the original drug (Collier 2011). The commercial success of 'me-too' drugs relies less on the quality of research and development or the capacity to innovate in therapeutic terms, and more on the companies' capacity to conduct massive promotional campaigns aimed at convincing physicians to prescribe. Disproportionate spending on promotion and large sales forces are key elements in facilitating the elevation of a new product to blockbuster status, even if it was therapeutically equivalent to other products. Products associated with the dominant blockbuster model of the 1990s and 2000s were evident in different therapeutic areas, such as cholesterol reducers, anti-hypertensive drugs, antipsychotics, antidepressants, proton-pump inhibitors, and psychostimulants.

In the 2000s, blockbuster business models became victims of their own success, in that they saturated the 'me-too' market. While governments were deploying austerity measures and trying to constrain health expenditure, drug costs (a large proportion of which were 'me-too' drugs) were growing faster than the gross national product in most OECD countries. The model was becoming unsustainable (Gagnon 2015). Medical insurance systems became more selective about which new drugs they would reimburse and began demanding more value for their money. Most governments started relying on health technology assessment (HTA) and began proactively managing their formulary of reimbursed drugs. Clinical superiority over placebo was no longer sufficient, and pharmaceutical companies had to justify the pharmaco-economic value of new drugs based on a cost-benefit analysis to secure reimbursement. The increasingly systematic use of health technology assessments in various member-states of the OECD in the 2000s was a fundamental factor leading to the crisis that hit the blockbuster model (Benoît 2020).

Big Pharma adapted to this new state of affairs in various ways, including rationalization (staff cuts and closing of research and development departments) and a wave of merger and acquisition deals (Montalban and Sakinc 2013). Other firms sought to diversify by moving into the generics or vaccines sector. However, the most promising route to maintain high levels of profitability in spite of the systematic use of HTA was to focus on specialty drugs that could be sold at much higher prices. Accordingly, a new dominant business model has emerged since the early-2010s, focusing on specialty drugs and orphan drugs developed for rare diseases. This new model constitutes a new business model – the 'nichebuster model' – where very expensive drugs sold to targeted populations can still achieve sales of more than US$1 billion (Dolgin 2010; Gagnon 2015; Gibson and Lemmens 2014).

New specialty drugs, often produced through biotechnology, are mainly intended for the treatment of chronic, complex, or rare diseases and various forms of cancer. Many laws and programs in Europe and the US are also aimed at promoting the development of such niche treatments through subsidies, tax credits, or extended market exclusivity (Marselis and Hordijk 2020). Crucially, by targeting specialty markets with a lower number of patients where no established therapy exists, companies can demand higher prices than what would be possible in already saturated markets. Under these conditions, the bargaining power of drug plans becomes more limited for these products.

A central characteristic of specialty drugs is their very expensive prices, as societies are normally willing to pay higher prices to treat cancer or rare diseases (Gagnon 2015). Specialty drugs represented around 20 percent of global spending on medications in 2010 and now constitute around 40 percent; their total share of spending is expected to continue to grow in the coming years by 1 percent a year at the global level and 2 percent a year in the largest developed markets (IQVIA 2022: 48). The increasing cost for reimbursing these drugs is making many drug plans unsustainable and sometimes forcing the imposition of restrictions on reimbursement (Charbonneau and Gagnon 2018). For example, the rise in the costs of anti-cancer drugs has been exponential, even when new anti-cancer drugs bring little or no new therapeutic value (Vivot *et al.* 2017). Analysis using HTA shows that in 1995, patients and insurers were paying on average (in constant 2013 US$) $54,100 for each year of life gained. In 2005, they were paying $139,100 for each year of life gained and $207,000 in 2013 (Howard *et al.* 2015). Because of our high willingness to pay for these types of products, even when a drug still brings little or uncertain therapeutic value to the market, this new 'nichebuster' business model keeps incentivizing inefficient development of expensive drugs with little therapeutic value (Prasad *et al.* 2018).

While the bulk of profitable drugs in 2005 were still blockbuster, 'me-too' chemical drugs intended for large populations, the most profitable drugs in 2020 were nichebuster biological drugs, intended for a more limited population. These include anti-cancer drugs, antivirals, and drugs against autoimmune diseases or against multiple sclerosis (see: Table 20.4).

Table 20.4 Top 30 drugs by global sales, 2020

Drug brand name (generic name)	*Manufacturer(s)*	*2020 sales (US$, billion)*	*Indication(s)*
Humira (adalimumab)	AbbVie	19.8	Rheumatoid and psoriatic arthritis, ankylosing spondylitis, Crohn's disease, ulcerative colitis
Keytruda (pembrolizumab)	Merck	14.4	Various cancers
Eliquis (apixaban)	Bristol Myers Squibb and Pfizer	14.1	Blood clots
Revlimid (lenalidomide)	Bristol Myers Squibb	12.2	Myelodysplastic syndrome, multiple myeloma, and mantle cell lymphoma
Eylea (aflibercept)	Regeneron Pharmaceuticals, Bayer	10.7	Age-related macular degeneration, macular edema, and diabetic retinopathy
Imbruvica (ibrutinib)	Pharmacyclics (AbbVie) and Janssen (Johnson and Johnson)	9.4	Chronic lymphocytic leukemia/small lymphocytic lymphoma with 17p deletion, Waldenström's macroglobulinemia

(*Continued*)

Table 20.4 (Continued)

Drug brand name (generic name)	*Manufacturer(s)*	*2020 sales (US$, billion)*	*Indication(s)*
Dupixent (dupilumab)	Sanofi Genzyme, Regeneron Pharmaceuticals	8.1	Atopic dermatitis, asthma, chronic rhinosinusitis with nasal polyps.
Stelara (ustekinumab)	Janssen (Johnson and Johnson)	7.7	Plaque psoriasis and psoriatic arthritis
Biktarvy (bictegravir, emtricitabine, and tenofovir alafenamide)	Gilead sciences	7.3	HIV
Opdivo (nivolumab)	Bristol Myers Squibb	7.0	Various forms of cancer
Xarelto (rivaroxaban)	Janssen (Johnson and Johnson)/Bayer	6.5	Reducing risk of stroke, deep vein thrombosis, pulmonary embolism, DVT prophylaxis following knee or hip replacement surgery
Prevnar 13 (pneumococcal 13-valent conjugate vaccine)	Pfizer	5.9	Pneumococcal vaccine
Ibrance (palbociclib)	Pfizer	5.4	HR-positive and HER2-negative breast cancer
Avastin (bevacizumab)	Roche	5.3	Colorectal, lung, glioblastoma, kidney, cervical and ovarian cancer
Januvia/Janumet (sitagliptin)	Merck and Co.	5.3	Type 2 diabetes
Trulicity (dulaglutide)	Eli Lilly	5.1	Type 2 diabetes
Enbrel (etanercept)	Amgen	5.0	Plaque psoriasis, rheumatoid arthritis, psoriatic arthritis, juvenile idiopathic arthritis, and ankylosing spondylitis.
Ocrevus (ocrelizumab)	Roche	4.6	Relapsing or primary progressive multiple sclerosis
Rituxan (rituximab)	Roche, Pharmstandard	4.5	Various autoimmune diseases and cancers
Xtandi (enzalutamide)	Astellas Pharma and Pfizer	4.4	Prostate cancer
Tagrisso (osimertinib)	AstraZeneca	4.3	Non–small-cell lung carcinomas

(*Continued*)

Table 20.4 (Continued)

Drug brand name (generic name)	*Manufacturer(s)*	*2020 sales (US$, billion)*	*Indication(s)*
Darzalex (daratumumab)	(Janssen) Johnson and Johnson	4.2	Multiple myeloma
Perjeta (pertuzumab)	Roche	4.2	HER2-positive breast cancer
Cosentyx (secukinumab)	Novartis	4.0	Plaque psoriasis, psoriatic arthritis, ankylosing spondylitis
Jardiance	Boehringer Ingelheim and Lilly	4.0	Type 2 diabetes, cardiovascular disease
Herceptin (trastuzumab)	Genentech (Roche)	3.9	Breast, stomach, and esophageal cancer
Gardasil/Gardasil 9 (human papillomavirus 9-valent vaccine)	Merck	3.9	Various cancers caused by human papillomavirus
Avonex/Plegridy (interferon beta-1a/ peginterferon beta-1a)	Biogen	3.9	Multiple sclerosis
Tecfidera (dimethyl fumarate)	Mylan (now Viatris)	3.8	Relapsing multiple sclerosis
Remicade (infliximab)	Janssen (Johnson and Johnson)	3.7	Crohn's disease, ulcerative colitis, rheumatoid arthritis, ankylosing spondylitis, psoriatic arthritis, plaque psoriasis

Source: Buntz (2021).

Considering the importance of financialization within the pharmaceutical sector, and its focus on maximizing shareholder value, it follows that new drugs are managed as financial assets for the purpose of maximizing shareholder returns (Haslam 2013; Izhar Baranes 2017; Montalban and Sakinc 2013; Roy 2020). Under such circumstances, it is no surprise that high profitability does not translate into more research and development, but rather into higher returns for shareholders, often achieved through share buybacks and mergers and acquisitions (Haucap *et al.* 2019; Tulum and Lazonick 2018). While the dynamics of financialization affects most industrial sectors, the pharmaceutical sector is also characterized by specific corporate strategies that increase Big Pharma's earning capacities in ways that render negative outcomes for population health and well-being.

Is ghost-management the core activity of Big Pharma?

At the beginning of the Twentieth Century, Thorstein Veblen (1904, 1923) asserted that dominant firms in a business sector are those for which the bulk of their capitalization is based on goodwill or intangible assets, which he defined as monopolistic capacities, or the capacity to gain something for nothing (see also: Gagnon 2007). As such, it is incumbent on analysts to understand what constitutes the main intangible assets for Big Pharma in the Twenty-First Century. An important body of literature exists detailing the abuses of pharmaceutical companies that frequently sell risky and overpriced drugs (Abraham and Davis 2013; Angell 2004; Gøtzsche 2013; Jureidini 2020; Lexchin 2018; Light 2010; Rajan 2017). Some authors identify the operation of 'ghost-management' in these processes: the systematic, behind-the-scenes strategy to shape knowledge, ideas, and narratives about specific products to increase demand, and exertion of effort to produce not only knowledge, but also selective ignorance or uncertainty through the dissemination of false, misleading, or contradictory information (Gagnon 2021; Sismondo 2018). In particular, Big Pharma's influence over the scientific narrative about their products is a central component of what Veblen (1904, 1923) would call their 'intangible assets'. The ways in which drug companies build their influence over science through conflicts of interests, non-disclosure of adverse clinical results, and publication planning are described in detail by Sismondo (2018).

While it is impossible to measure the amounts of financial resources deployed by Big Pharma to influence science, it is possible to account for amounts spent on other ghost-management strategies in the US pharmaceutical sector and contrast it to the amounts spent on research and development. According to the OECD, drug companies spent US$64.6 billion on research and development in 2016.[2] In contrast, it was estimated that US$54 billion was spent on promotional expenditures directed toward healthcare professionals in 2004, including US$42.8 billion toward prescribing physicians. Considering that there were 700,000 active physicians at the time, promotional expenditures for pharmaceutical products represented around US$61,000 per physician (Gagnon and Lexchin 2008). It is very conservative to estimate that at least a similar amount was also spent in 2016. In addition to promotion, drug companies also foster conflicts of interests with practicing physicians by paying them directly for their services (for research, education, or marketing purposes). CMS Open Payment Data shows that in the US, drug manufacturers paid US$10.86 billion (directly or through an institutional affiliation) to 624,000 physicians in 2019, which represents an average of US$17,400 per physician.[3] Drug companies also spent heavily in direct-to-consumer advertising in US media (excluding social media), with expenditures totaling US$6.5 billion in 2018 (Snyder Bulik 2019).

Lobbying is also a significant activity for drug companies. According to the Center for Responsive Politics, based on data from the Senate Office of Public Records, the pharmaceutical sector was the top lobbying industry in the US in 2018, with declared spending of US$282 million (Gagnon 2021: 171). Finally, it is important to note that patient advocacy organizations can help exert pressure on governments to force the reimbursement of new drugs at high prices. These organizations have become a central part of the communication strategies used by Big Pharma (McCoy 2018). It is estimated that drug companies spent US$932 million in 2017 in grants to patient organizations in the US (Gagnon 2021: 173).

Conclusion

By adding up the numbers in terms of dollars spent on ghost-management activities that do not contribute anything to improving health outcomes, and then contrasting this to amounts spent on research and development, it can be concluded that the core activity of Big Pharma in the US is ghost-management, rather than developing new, therapeutically significant products to improve the health of patients. The main 'intangible assets' of dominant drug companies lie not in their capacity to innovate, but in their capacity to shape knowledge, habits of thought, and social structures to artificially increase demand and scarcity for their products – as exemplified most recently by the abhorrently high levels of profit accruing to Big Pharma during the COVID-19 pandemic (Anderson 2022).

While the dominant business model in the sector evolved from a focus on 'blockbusters' to a focus on expensive 'nichebusters', this new model continues to incentivize the inefficient development of drugs with little or uncertain therapeutic value. Consistent with these observations, Big Pharma has succeeded in regularly maintaining higher annual levels of profitability than dominant firms in other business sectors. Given this structural position, the weight of this sector's business activities is evidently focused around market position much more than the health and well-being of patients.

Notes

1 CMS data is available here: <https://www.cms.gov/Research-Statistics-Data-and-Systems/Statistics-Trends-and-Reports/Information-on-Prescription-Drugs/MedicarePartD>.
2 See: <https://data.oecd.org/healthres/pharmaceutical-spending.htm>.
3 See note 1.

References

Abraham, J. and Davis, C. 2013, *Unhealthy Pharmaceutical Regulation: Innovation, Politics and Promissory Science*, Palgrave Macmillan, New York.

Anderson, T. 2022, 'From operation warp speed to TRIPS: Vaccines as assets', in Di Muzio, T. and Dow, M. (eds), *COVID-19 and the Global Political Economy: Crises in the 21st Century*, Routledge, London, pp. 122–35.

Angell, M. 2004, *The Truth About the Drug Companies: How They Deceive Us and What To Do About It*, 1st ed., Random House, New York.

Baker, D. 2021, 'The future of the pharmaceutical industry: Beyond government-granted monopolies', *Journal of Law, Medicine and Ethics*, 49(1), pp. 25–9.

Benoît, C. 2020, *Réguler L'accès aux Médicaments*, Libres cours, Presses Universitaires de Grenoble, Fontaine.

Boldrin, M. and Levine, D.K. 2013, 'The case against patents', *Journal of Economic Perspectives*, 27(1), pp. 3–22.

Buntz, B. 2021, '50 of 2020s best-selling pharmaceuticals', *Drug Discovery and Development*, accessed 13 January 2022, <https://www.drugdiscoverytrends.com/50-of-2020s-best-selling-pharmaceuticals/>.

Chandler, A.D. 2005, *Shaping the Industrial Century the Remarkable Story of the Modern Chemical and Pharmaceutical Industries*, Harvard University Press, Cambridge.

Charbonneau, M. and Gagnon, M-A. 2018, 'Surviving niche busters: Main strategies employed by Canadian private insurers facing the arrival of high cost specialty drugs', *Health Policy*, 122(12), pp. 1295–301.

Collier, R. 2011, 'Bye, bye blockbusters, hello niche busters', *Canadian Medical Association Journal*, 183(11), pp. E697–8.

Correa, C.M. and Hilty, R.M. (eds) 2022, *Access to Medicines and Vaccines*, Springer, Cham.

Crowe, K. 2022, 'After a 5-year fight to lower drug prices, Ottawa's pledge quietly falls apart', *CBC News*, accessed 26 May 2022, <https://www.cbc.ca/news/health/drug-prices-canada-regulations-1.6449265>.

Dolgin, E. 2010, 'Big pharma moves from "blockbusters" to "niche busters"', *Nature Medicine*, 16(8), p. 837.

Drahos, P. and Braithwaite, J. 2002, *Information Feudalism: Who Owns the Knowledge Economy?*, Earthscan, London.

Etten, M.V. 2022, 'Intellectual property waiver on COVID-19 innovation is unnecessary and harmful', accessed 26 May 2022, <https://catalyst.phrma.org/intellectual-property-waiver-on-covid-19-innovation-is-unnecessary-and-harmful>.

Freilich, J. and Meurer, M.J. 2021, 'Patent system often stifles the innovation it was designed to encourage', *The Conversation*, accessed 27 May 2022, <http://theconversation.com/patent-system-often-stifles-the-innovation-it-was-designed-to-encourage-148075>.

Gagnon, M-A. 2007, 'Capital, power and knowledge according to Thorstein Veblen: Reinterpreting the knowledge-based economy', *Journal of Economic Issues*, 41(2), pp. 593–600.
Gagnon, M-A. 2009, 'The nature of capital in the knowledge-based economy: The case of the global pharmaceutical industry', PhD Thesis, York University.
Gagnon, M-A. 2015, 'New drug pricing: Does it make any sense?' *Prescrire International*, 24(162), pp. 192–5.
Gagnon, M-A. 2021, 'Ghost management as a central feature of accumulation in corporate capitalism: the case of the global pharmaceutical sector', in Benquet, M. and Bourgeron, T. (eds), *Accumulating Capital Today: Contemporary Strategies of Profit and Dispossessive Policies*, Routledge, London, pp. 163–177.
Gagnon, M-A. and Lexchin, J. 2008, 'The cost of pushing pills: A new estimate of pharmaceutical promotion expenditures in the United States', *PLoS Medicine*, 5(1), p. e1.
Gagnon, M-A. and Wolfe, S. 2015, 'Mirror, mirror on the wall: Medicare Part D pays needlessly high brand-name drug prices compared with other OECD countries and with U.S. government programs', accessed 12 January 2022, <https://ir.library.carleton.ca/pub/18756>.
Gibson, S.G. and Lemmens, T. 2014, 'Niche markets and evidence assessment in transition: A critical review of proposed drug reforms', *Medical Law Review*, 22(2), pp. 200–20.
Gleeson, D., Lexchin, J., Labonté, R., Townsend, B., Gagnon, M-A., Kohler, J., Forman, L. and Shadlen, K.C. 2019, 'Analyzing the impact of trade and investment agreements on pharmaceutical policy: Provisions, pathways and potential impacts', *Globalization and Health*, 15(Suppl 1), p. 78.
Gold, E.R. 2021, 'The fall of the innovation empire and its possible rise through open science', *Research Policy*, 50(5), p. 104226.
Gøtzsche, P.C. 2013, *Deadly Medicines and Organised Crime: How Big Pharma Has Corrupted Healthcare*, Radcliffe Pub, London.
Haslam, C. 2013, *Redefining Business Models: Strategies for a Financialized World*, Routledge, London.
Haucap, J., Rasch, A. and Stiebale, J. 2019, 'How mergers affect innovation: Theory and evidence', *International Journal of Industrial Organization*, 63, pp. 283–325.
Heller, M.A. and Eisenberg, R.S. 1998, 'Can patents deter innovation? The anticommons in biomedical research', *Science*, 280(5364), pp. 698–701.
Howard, D.H., Bach, P.B., Berndt, E.R. and Conti, R.M. 2015, 'Pricing in the market for anticancer drugs', *The Journal of Economic Perspectives*, 29(1), pp. 139–62.
IQVIA. 2019, 'The global use of medicine in 2019 and outlook to 2023', IQVIA Institute for Human Data Science, accessed 15 January 2022, <https://www.iqvia.com/insights/the-iqvia-institute/reports/the-global-use-of-medicine-in-2019-and-outlook-to-2023>.
IQVIA. 2022, 'The global use of medicines 2022', IQVIA Institute for Human Data Science, accessed 9 January 2022, <https://www.iqvia.com/insights/the-iqvia-institute/reports/the-global-use-of-medicines-2022>.
Izhar Baranes, A. 2017, 'Financialization in the American pharmaceutical industry: A Veblenian approach', *Journal of Economic Issues*, 51(2), pp. 351–8.
Jureidini, J. 2020, *The Illusion of Evidence-Based Medicine: Exposing the Crisis of Credibility in Clinical Research*, Wakefield Press, Mile End.
Ledley, F.D., McCoy, S.S., Vaughan, G. and Cleary, E.G. 2020, 'Profitability of large pharmaceutical companies compared with other large public companies', *JAMA*, 323(9), pp. 834–43.
Lexchin, J. 2018, *Private Profits Versus Public Policy: The Pharmaceutical Industry and the Canadian State*, University of Toronto Press, Toronto.
Lexchin, J. and Gagnon, M-A. 2014, 'CETA and pharmaceuticals: Impact of the trade agreement between Europe and Canada on the costs of prescription drugs', *Globalization and Health*, 10(1), pp. 1–6.
Light, D. 2010, *The Risks of Prescription Drugs*, Columbia University Press, New York.
Mailankody, S. and Prasad, V. 2015, 'Five years of cancer drug approvals: Innovation, Efficacy, and costs', *JAMA Oncology*, 1(4), pp. 539–40.
Marselis, D. and Hordijk, L. 2020, 'From blockbuster to "nichebuster": How a flawed legislation helped create a new profit model for the drug industry', *British Medical Journal*, 370, p. m2983.
McCoy, M.S. 2018, 'Industry support of patient advocacy organizations: The case for an extension of the Sunshine Act Provisions of the Affordable Care Act', *American Journal of Public Health*, 108(8), pp. 1026–30.
McKinnell, H.A. 2005, *A Call to Action: Taking Back Healthcare for Future Generations*, Mcgraw-Hill, New York.
Montalban, M. and Sakinc, M.E. 2013, 'Financialization and productive models in the pharmaceutical industry', *Industrial and Corporate Change*, 22(4), pp. 981–1030.

Morgan, S.G., Bathula, H.S. and Moon, S. 2020, 'Pricing of pharmaceuticals is becoming a major challenge for health systems', *British Medical Journal*, 368, pp. 1–4.

Morgan, S.G., Vogler, S. and Wagner, A.K. 2017, 'Payers' experiences with confidential pharmaceutical price discounts: A survey of public and statutory health systems in North America, Europe, and Australasia', *Health Policy*, 121(4), pp. 354–62.

Nitzan, J. and Bichler, S. 2021, 'Pharmaceuticals: Beating the hell out of the average', working paper, accessed 13 January 2022, <https://www.econstor.eu/handle/10419/234557>.

OECD. 2021, *Health at a Glance 2021: OECD Indicators*, OECD, Paris, accessed 12 January 2022, <https://www.oecd-ilibrary.org/social-issues-migration-health/health-at-a-glance-2021_ae3016b9-en>.

OECD. 2022, 'Health resources: Pharmaceutical spending - OECD data', OECD, accessed 10 January 2022, <http://data.oecd.org/healthres/pharmaceutical-spending.htm>.

Ozawa, S., Shankar, R., Leopold, C. and Orubu, S. 2019, 'Access to medicines through health systems in low- and middle-income countries', *Health Policy and Planning*, 34(Supp. 3), pp. iii1–3.

Patented Medicines Price Review Board. 2021, *Annual Report 2019*, accessed 15 October 2021, <https://www.canada.ca/en/patented-medicine-prices-review/services/annual-reports/annual-report-2019.html>.

Patnaik, P. 2022, *The TRIPS Waiver Negotiations at the World Trade Organization (October 2020- June 2022): A Reportage from Geneva Health Files*, Geneva Health Files, Geneva.

Prasad, V., McCabe, C. and Mailankody, S. 2018, 'Low-value approvals and high prices might incentivize ineffective drug development', *Nature Reviews: Clinical Oncology*, 15(7), pp. 399–400.

Prescrire. 2021, *L'année 2020 du Médicament: Progrès de L'année 2020 par Rapport aux Progrès des 9 Années Précédentes*, accessed 12 January 2022, <https://www.prescrire.org/fr/3/31/60649/0/NewsDetails.aspx>.

Redwood, H. 1988, *The Pharmaceutical Industry: Trends, Problems and Achievements*, Oldwicks Press, Felixstowe.

Roy, V. 2020, 'A crisis for cures? Tracing assetization and value in biomedical innovation', accessed 16 January 2022, <https://direct.mit.edu/books/book/4848/chapter/625227/A-Crisis-for-Cures-Tracing-Assetization-and-Value>.

Schram, A., Ruckert, A., VanDuzer, J.A., Friel, S., Gleeson, D., Thow, A-M., Stuckler, D. and Labonte, R. 2018, 'A conceptual framework for investigating the impacts of international trade and investment agreements on noncommunicable disease risk factors', *Health Policy and Planning*, 33(1), pp. 123–36.

Sismondo, S. 2018, *Ghost-Managed Medicine Big Pharma's Invisible Hands*, Mattering Press, Manchester.

Snyder Bulik, B. 2019, 'Big spending from AbbVie, Pfizer pushes pharma's 2018 ad spend to $6.5B', *FiercePharma*, accessed 16 January 2022, <https://www.fiercepharma.com/marketing/kantar-tallies-6-5-billion-for-pharma-ad-spending-2018-abbvie-humira-ranks-as-top>.

Sunder Rajan, K. 2017, *Pharmocracy: Value, Politics, and Knowledge in Global Biomedicine*, Duke University Press, Durham.

Temin, P. 1980, *Taking Your Medicine: Drug Regulation in the United States*, Harvard University Press, Cambridge.

Tulum, Ö. and Lazonick, W. 2018, 'Financialized corporations in a national innovation system: The U.S. pharmaceutical industry', *International Journal of Political Economy*, 47(3/4), pp. 281–316.

United Nations. 2019, 'Take action for the sustainable development goals', *United Nations Sustainable Development*, accessed 26 May 2022, <https://www.un.org/sustainabledevelopment/sustainable-development-goals/>.

Veblen, T. 1904, *The Theory of Business Enterprise*, Transaction Books, New Brunswick.

Veblen, T. 1923, *Absentee Ownership and Business Enterprise in Recent Times: The case of America*, Allen and Unwin, London.

Vivot, A., Jacot, J., Zeitoun, J-D., Ravaud, P., Crequit, P. and Porcher, R. 2017, 'Clinical benefit, price and approval characteristics of FDA-approved new drugs for treating advanced solid cancer, 2000–2015', *Annals of Oncology*, 28(5), pp. 1111–6.

Vokinger, K.N., Hwang, T.J., Grischott, T., Reichert, S., Tibau, A., Rosemann, T. and Kesselheim, A.S. 2020, 'Prices and clinical benefit of cancer drugs in the USA and Europe: A cost–benefit analysis', *The Lancet Oncology*, 21(5), pp. 664–70.

Wirtz, V.J., Hogerzeil, H.V., Gray, A.L., Bigdeli, M., de Joncheere, C.P., Ewen, M.A., Gyansa-Lutterodt, M., Jing, S., Luiza, V.L., Mbindyo, R.M. and Möller, H. 2017, 'Essential medicines for universal health coverage', *The Lancet*, 389(10067), pp. 403–76.

Zaitchik, A. 2022, *Owning the Sun*, Counterpoint, Berkeley, accessed 27 May 2022, <https://www.penguinrandomhouse.ca/books/691699/owning-the-sun-by-alexander-zaitchik/9781640095069>.

21
AUTOMATING THE WELFARE STATE
The case of disability benefits and services

Georgia van Toorn[1]

Social services and benefits for disabled people have long served as fertile grounds for various forms of neoliberal statecraft. Since the 1980s, disability services have been radically transformed by the introduction of market mechanisms. This has included outsourcing arrangements that give private providers and people with disability a greater role in the direct management of their support (Pedlar and Hutchison 2000; van Toorn 2021). Disability pension regimes have similarly been 'neoliberalized' through the introduction of various technologies of (re)classification and social sorting for eligibility determination (Soldatic 2019). These developments have increased the numbers of disabled people deemed medically fit to work and, therefore, ineligible for benefits.

More recently, the neoliberal restructuring of disability provisioning has manifested in a shift toward automated decision-making (ADM). ADM refers to the use of rules, formulas, or a prescribed set of steps – often encoded in computer algorithms – to either assist or replace the judgment of human decision-makers. While ADM is now commonplace in the public sector, it is also widely used by private companies to whom governments have delegated the responsibilities for providing and administering social services (Collington 2021). This form of 'technological outsourcing', where decision-making is outsourced to automated systems designed and operated by the private sector, has important social implications – in terms of both service quality and government accountability (Crawford and Schultz 2019; Boughey 2021; Dickinson and Yates 2023). In disability services, outsourced ADM is particularly fraught given stark asymmetries of power and information between providers, recipients, and funders of disability services; the value placed on human interaction and person-centered services; and the real and perceived vulnerabilities of people with disability.

Outsourced ADM raises important questions about the power of corporations in an age of automation. Legal scholar Frank Pasquale (2017), a prominent critic of algorithmic tools, argues that digital capitalism is shifting the boundaries of 'functional sovereignty', as commercial digital platforms exercise powers and functions previously reserved for the territorial state. A parallel shift is underway in the social welfare sector. The automation of government decision-making is redrawing boundaries between state and market, giving private companies a much larger stake in public administration. There is a growing body of research on how, with the help of technology, governments are divesting themselves of functions once thought to be the exclusive preserve of sovereign states (Margetts 1995; Dunleavy *et al.* 2006; Crawford and Schultz 2019; Dencik and

 DOI: 10.4324/9781003017110-24

Kaun 2020; Tilley 2020; Collington 2021; Dickinson and Yates 2023). The literature on public sector automation, for example, points to the myriad ways in which ADM reproduces and deepens social inequalities by preventing the poor from accessing public assistance and criminalizing their behaviors (Benjamin 2019; Eubanks 2019; Park and Humphry 2019; Henman 2020). Yet within this body of critical literature, there is very little sustained empirical research on the economic dimensions of automation, particularly the intersection of automation and outsourcing in social services. Outsourced ADM raises important questions about political accountability and the privatization of public administration. These issues have hitherto received little scrutiny from critical political economists, despite warnings that 'the private sector is taking a leading role in designing, constructing, and even operating significant parts of the digital welfare state' (Alston 2019: 1).

This chapter takes up the call to consider seriously the enhancement of corporate power arising from social service automation, and the social justice implications of outsourced ADM. I explore how automation is reconfiguring the political economy of disability provisioning in the UK and the US. These case-studies were chosen for two principal reasons. First, the two countries exemplify a 'liberal' social policy orientation (Esping-Andersen 1990) and, therefore, can be fruitfully compared to reveal common patterns and variations in their respective policy trajectories. Second, both are relatively advanced in their adoption of automated technologies, particularly in the health and disability domains. Thus, they offer insights into possible futures of ADM in other countries. Taken together, the two case-studies provide a starting point for critical discussion of the (neo)liberal welfare state's outsourcing of ADM and the ways in which the global IT industry profits from the algorithmic social sorting of disabled bodies. They lend empirical support to claims that, under digital capitalism, citizens are 'increasingly subject to corporate, rather than democratic, control' (Pasquale 2017: n.p.). More specifically, they reveal the political-economic conditions in which corporate and digital agents are displacing health professionals and public officials as arbiters of how public resources are allocated (or not allocated) among people with disability.

To lay the foundations for this argument, the chapter begins with a discussion of the historical origins of automation in disability benefits and services. The following sections explore the reconfiguration of state-corporate-citizen relations in recent decades as private companies have accrued *de facto* decision-making powers under outsourced ADM arrangements.

The road to the digital poorhouse

Automation is commonly associated with modern, computer-based technologies. Yet, early attempts by states to classify and sort people based on impairment predate the emergence of the modern, post-war welfare state. Roulstone and Prideaux (2012: 6) locate 'the rise of [a] calculative logic', used to classify disability within evolving state-capital-labor relations in British factory work from the Eighteenth Century. Industrial capitalism demanded the segregation of disabled people from others who were more easily able to be integrated into the rhythms and discipline of factory work (Humpage 2007). There emerged a need to distinguish those whose bodies were amendable to the production process from those who were of limited value to the capitalist system. The 'sick', the 'insane', and the 'aged and infirm' would receive poverty relief in asylums and poorhouses – public or charitable institutions that provided housing for the poor and homeless – where little or no work was required of inmates. Their labor power was 'effectively erased, excluded from paid work' (Russell and Malhotra 2019: 3). In poorhouses, these groups were afforded social protection from the vicissitudes of market capitalism, though typically in highly crowded, unsanitary, and degrading conditions (Katz 1984). Virginia Eubanks (2019) argues that poorhouses were the precursor to the modern-day 'digital poorhouse', a metaphor for the ensemble of automated systems – encompassing ADM, algorithms, big data, and predictive analytics – used by governments to administer public services. Both brick-and-mortar poorhouses and their digital descendants, she argues, serve the purpose of removing the 'defective' classes from society and deterring the undeserving poor from accessing public resources (Eubanks 2019).

By the Nineteenth Century, poorhouses had spread to the US and parts of Western Europe. Public and religious authorities developed more complex ways of classifying people based on type and severity of impairment, to determine where they would be housed. This system of classification relied on official certifications and diagnoses made by doctors (Barnes 1991). As Barnes (1991) notes, this gave the nascent medical profession immense power, foreshadowing the medicalization of disability, which frames disability as an individual problem requiring medical treatment. It gave doctors authority in determining eligibility for public resources in ways that were, according to Oliver and Barnes (2012: 86), 'compatible with capitalist interests as [they] depoliticize[d] and individualize[d] social problems'.

Modern eugenics provided an added impetus for the development of tools designed to categorize and segregate disabled people and control their behaviors (Humpage 2007). In the US, the scientific charity movement advocated more systematic and supposedly scientific methods of poverty management (Eubanks 2019). Large-scale data collection was central to this endeavor. Information on poor families and individuals was collected to determine whether they were 'fit' to breed, based on the eugenic belief that by studying families, certain traits could be established as genetic in origin, thereby justifying policies aimed at removing people with socially 'undesirable' traits (Rafter 1992). Social scientists administered 'lengthy questionnaires, took photographs, inked fingerprints, measured heads, counted children, plotted family trees, and filled logbooks with descriptions like "imbecile," "feeble-minded", "harlot," and "dependent"' (Eubanks 2019: 23). These eugenicist methods of data collection were foundational to the welfare state's approach to poverty management. They gave scientific legitimacy to the state's use of diagnostic categories in determining access to education, employment, and poverty relief (Roulstone and Prideaux 2012). In New York State, the eugenics movement defined the first group of people – 'fertile, feeble-minded, female paupers' – to be officially recognized as 'dysgenic' (Rafter 1992: 17). This would provide the rationale for social policies of segregation and institutionalization for over a century, a clear example of the long-standing link between classification and control.

The second half of the Twentieth Century saw a shift from institutional to community-based care in many liberal welfare states (Roulstone and Prideaux 2012). Doctors, however, retained a gatekeeping role regarding disability benefits and services intended to support people to live independently in the community. Doctors' medical assessments determined who was, and who was not, entitled to public assistance: evaluating an individual's need for personal care and support with the tasks of daily living, as well as their capacity to work to support themselves financially (Humpage 2007). As Soldatic (2019) thoroughly documents, disability assessments and work tests became central to the neoliberal restructuring of disability welfare provisioning from the 1970s onward. These technologies were the main social policy levers used to limit public spending on disability programs and to enforce waged work (Grover and Soldatic 2013). As technologies of governance, they represented a relatively crude form of algorithmic decision-making. Typically, these assessments utilized decision criteria[2] and scoring systems, combined with information about an individual's functional capabilities, to determine work capacity. Though relatively unsophisticated by today's standards, these rule-based systems provide an early example of the application of algorithmic models in the welfare state's targeting of public resources to the neediest disabled citizens.

What emerges from this history is a dynamic in which 'disability', as a bureaucratic category, performs important work in determining how social welfare resources are distributed. Deborah

Stone (1984) refers to this as 'boundary work'. In her book, *The Disabled State*, she proposes that all societies face a 'fundamental distributive dilemma', owing to the co-existence of work-based and needs-based distributive systems (1984: 17). In the interests of fiscal discipline and accumulation, capitalist welfare states create strong incentives encouraging citizens to work, rather than claim benefits. Yet, not all citizens are able to satisfy their material needs through work, and some are excluded from the labor market altogether, due to age, illness, disability, or the absence of sufficient numbers of jobs to meet labor supply. The dilemma lies in the fact that states must provide some level of needs-based social assistance for those unable to work, which can undercut the incentive to work for those who can.

To resolve this tension, 'society must develop a set of rules to determine the boundaries of the two systems, rules that specify who is subject to each distributive principle and what is to be distributed within each system' (Stone 1984: 17). In most liberal welfare states, where disability benefits are highly targeted, these rules consist of eligibility criteria, which determine whether a person is disabled 'enough' to qualify for public assistance. These criteria are not fixed. They are subject to constant challenge and political contestation. The disability category, therefore, serves an important regulatory function for welfare states in maintaining the dominance of the work-based distributive system, while limiting needs-based social provisioning. By tightening criteria, states can control the relative numbers of people in each system, with obvious consequences for fiscal demands placed on the state and tax-transfer system. The incentive to tighten eligibility, therefore, is driven by an austerity agenda of preventing as many people as possible from claiming unemployment benefits in general, and disability benefits in particular, as the latter are typically worth more and are paid for longer periods (Grover and Soldatic 2013). Disability criteria have been progressively tightened over recent decades as part of the neoliberal trend toward increased welfare conditionality.

To sum up, the emergence of a calculative logic in disability services and welfare provisioning has conditioned capitalist welfare states to quantify, categorize, and classify disability as a means of managing the political economy of welfare and the economy more generally. More recently, states have begun to outsource the boundary work involved in governing the disability category. While governments set the rules determining eligibility for disability benefits and services, the application of those rules is increasingly the job of private companies who are contracted by government to carry out its assessments. Thus, it is no longer people's own GPs or public administrators who are the principal gatekeepers of disability social provisioning, but a profit-driven industry of multinational healthcare and, increasingly, IT companies who perform the regulatory work of the state with no democratic oversight. These companies are involved in all aspects of public administration, from the collection and processing of data on existing or potential welfare claimants, to decisions about who is entitled to public assistance and how much (Dencik and Kaun 2020). They are, in Benjamin's (2019: 53) words, 'governing without a mandate', meaning that 'people whose lives are being shaped in ever more consequential ways by automated decisions have very little say in how they are governed'. These shifts in power, and their contribution to unjust outcomes for people with disability, are exemplified in two case-studies to which we now turn.

UK: automating judgment, misjudging need

The UK was an early adopter of outsourced ADM in social security for unemployed people with disability. While its technologies of algorithmic decision-making were similar to those used in other (neo)liberal welfare states in the 1990s and early-2000s – namely, questionnaires and decision criteria – the UK was unique in its heavy reliance on external consultants and IT companies to design and deliver government administrative systems (Dunleavy *et al.* 2006). Over the past two decades, a handful of private companies have come to dominate decision-making around eligibility for disability benefits. These companies are funded to conduct assessments on behalf of the Department for Work and Pensions, typically through very large contracts worth hundreds of millions of pounds. The assessments generate data that are used to inform the final decision determining eligibility for disability benefit. Theoretically, the decision ultimately rests with a departmental administrator. In practice, decision-making power has been corporatized as public administrators have increasingly come to rely on computer-generated recommendations provided by private sector operators.

This privatization-automation nexus emerged when medical assessments were first introduced as part of the shift from the Invalidity Benefit to the Incapacity Benefit in 1995. The two decades prior had seen large increases in the number of people claiming long-term sickness and disability benefits, due partly to demographic shifts and high unemployment rates (Sainsbury *et al.* 2003: 7). Seeking to contain rising social expenditure by limiting access to these benefits, the UK government established the 'all-work test' as part of a new points-based method of assessing work capacity. Prior to the test, eligibility for the disability benefit was largely determined by the claimant's GP, who would conduct the assessment by taking into consideration a range of physical and socioeconomic factors affecting their patient's capacity to work (Gulland 2019: 71). Under the new Incapacity Benefit system, the all-work test became the main method of quantifying work capacity (Gulland 2019). Decision-making power was transferred to government-contracted health professionals, who assessed applicants' capacity to work in *any* job, regardless of their skills, interests, or prior work history.

The new assessment process was, according to Gulland (2019: 72), 'highly regulated and formulaic'. Through a self-completed questionnaire, it examined a range of activities, including walking, standing, sitting, bending, and lifting, with points awarded against different 'descriptors' of work-related activity (Corden and Sainsbury 2001). Depending on the number of points accumulated, the claimant would then usually be referred for a medical assessment, while these data would inform the decision made by the Benefits Agency Medical Service (then part of the Department of Social Security). It was envisaged that the all-work test would be more 'objective' and grounded in occupational health. It would restrict disability benefits to those who 'genuinely needed it' (Parliamentary Office of Science and Technology 2012: 1). In this sense, the quantification of work capacity, enabled by the all-work test, was an essential component of the neoliberal (re)regulation of the disability category based on hierarchies of moral deservingness (Soldatic 2019). Initiated by John Major's Conservative government, the targeting of disability benefits was later extended under Tony Blair's New Labor government. In 1998, the Blair government outsourced the medical administration of the Incapacity Benefit to the Sema group – a for-profit consulting firm-cum-IT services company (Killoughery 1999). Under the new regime, Sema would employ its own doctors to conduct medical assessments on the government's behalf (Gulland 2019). Three years later, the company was taken over and renamed Schlumberger Sema, but retained its government contract to assess 1.3 million Incapacity Benefit claimants each year (Committee on Public Accounts 2002).

The decision to outsource the medical assessment of work capacity was justified as a means of improving quality and addressing the backlog of Incapacity Benefit cases (Committee on Public Accounts 2002). Yet, outsourcing created the usual set of problems related to the prioritization of profit over human health and wellbeing. A series of parliamentary inquiries found that Schlumberger Sema had a financial incentive to complete as many assessments as possible quickly and with minimal resources (Committee on Public Accounts 2002). It was concluded that the aim of striking 'the right balance between incentives to cut costs, speed delivery and improve quality [...] had not been achieved in this case' (Committee on Public Accounts 2002: Para. 4). One inquiry found that Schlumberger Sema had a strategy of overbooking appointments for medical examinations, which resulted in 3 percent of applicants (over 17,000 a year) being turned away unseen (Committee on Public Accounts 2002: Para 5, viii). Over 40 percent of appeals made against eligibility decisions were successful, indicating systemic failure in the information-gathering and decision-making process (Committee on Public Accounts 2002: Paras 4–5). The problem was partly attributed to an overreliance on outmoded clerical administration systems. This was the impetus for the Department's subsequent plan to automate aspects of the assessment process, in the hope that 'computerized processes' would improve information communication between doctors and government (Sainsbury *et al.* 2003).

Over the next decades, the assessment process became increasingly technology-driven, and less grounded in medical opinion. A new work test called the Personal Capability Assessment was introduced in 2000, followed by the Work Capability Assessment (WCA) in 2008, when the current Employment and Support Allowance benefit was introduced. The WCA was designed to raise the threshold at which people would qualify for the new disability benefit. Digital technologies were enlisted to augment the process of regulating access to the disability category. A new questionnaire was introduced with descriptors designed to increase the number of points needed to reach the designated eligibility threshold (Litchfield 2013: 35). The process was designed so that the private sector assessment providers could complete the process cheaply and consistently, with minimal interference from 'the original experts' – that is, GPs (Litchfield 2013: 35). This was a priority for providers, as disability assessments were a lucrative industry and contractors were paid by results.

In 2004, Schlumberger Sema was acquired by a French company, Atos, and eventually renamed Atos IT Services. Soon after, the company's contract was extended by seven years at a value of £500 million (Williams 2011). With algorithmic technologies becoming a central feature of public sector governance, Atos adopted a new software program, called the Logic Integrated Medical Assessment (LiMA). Developed by the Department of Work and Pensions (DWP), LiMA's main function was to record data gathered through each medical assessment and generate a standardized report for DWP decision-makers who had the final say in determining access to benefits (Harrington 2010). The reports themselves had a monetary value, as Atos was paid for the number of assessments completed, regardless of their quality (Work and Pensions Committee 2011a). The digitization of assessments saved time and, therefore, money. Under the WCA system, each assessor had a target to complete their assessments in an average of 46 to 49 minutes. This time-based target affirms Soldatic (2013) insightful conceptualization of temporal measurement as a key technology in the social regulation of disability.

In recent years, eligibility rules have tightened further, and new categories have been created, with more stringent work conditionalities applied to those found to have 'limited capability' for work (Gulland 2019: 73). These changes have succeeded in their aim of making benefits harder to claim (Harrington 2010: 30). The increased obstructions to claiming benefits have been correlated with a marked increase in suicide among UK disability benefit applicants (Barr *et al.* 2016).[3] Numerous public inquiries, reviews, and media reports provide evidence of the complicity of the global IT industry in this 'techno-rationalist system', the purpose of which is to 'deny as many people as possible income-replacement benefits on the grounds of disability' (Grover 2014: 1325). A review of the WCA, for example, found that Atos relied on the LiMA to such an extent that the process was perceived to be driven by technology, rather than human judgment (Litchfield 2013). The test was 'impersonal and mechanistic' (Harrington 2010: 9), with assessors 'just asking the questions that are on the computer' (Work and Pensions Committee 2011b: n.p.). That a very high level of trust and authority was invested in technology is demonstrated by the fact that, in 98 percent of cases, DWP decision-makers followed the advice of the automated reports (Harrington 2010). This demonstrates that Atos played a major role in decision-making, since 'the Atos assessment is rarely questioned by the Decision Maker' (Harrington 2010: 48). Little has changed in the years since Atos was superseded by another outsourcing giant, Maximus, whose contract was recently extended at a value of £236.4 million, despite its track record of harmful and inaccurate decision-making (Bloom 2019). Other multinationals – including IBM, Tata Consultancy, and CapGemini – are striking lucrative deals with the DWP to develop machine learning for use in the Universal Credit system (Booth 2019).

The situation in the UK highlights the increasing power wielded by private companies in determining access to disability benefits. The dominance of these companies indicates that what Navarro (1976) theorized as a 'medical-industrial complex' has since metamorphosed into a medical-*technical* industrial complex, wherein technology and the global IT industry shape the medical management of disability in and by capitalist welfare states. These companies do not merely support government decision-making. Rather, they *are* the (*de facto*) decision-makers. As such, they wield a modern form of biopower, exercised through the systematic extraction, digital transformation, and commodification of disability and health data for governance purposes. This datafication of disability denotes a political economy in which disability as a category not only does 'boundary work', but in which disabled bodies are also valued as a source of profitable data. While profiteering from disability is not new, the role of technology companies in enabling this process is a more recent phenomenon. Outsourced ADM confers powers previously associated with the state onto private tech firms. As Dencik and Kaun (2020: 5) suggest, this outsourcing creates an 'intricate ecosystem between public and private entities taking shape through technological infrastructures in the public sector'. Public services, they suggest, are increasingly 'organizing themselves around the disruptive activities of technology companies that over time come to dictate societal arrangements' (Dencik and Kaun 2020: 5). The following case-study explores what happens when this dynamic intensifies through shifts to more complex forms of algorithmic decision-making.

US: pretending objectivity, obscuring responsibility

US states have generally lagged behind the UK in outsourcing the governance of disability welfare programs by means of automation. However, algorithmic decision-making has proliferated rapidly in the last decade or so, with 41 states now operating an automated disability governance system of some kind, often with the involvement of the private sector (Center for Democracy and Technology 2020). Many states have a patchwork of algorithmic tools and processes in-place across multiple service areas, spanning home care, mental health, and specialist behavioral and intellectual disability support programs. Consequently, there are not the same nation-wide monopolies in the disability assessment industry, as witnessed in the UK. Instead, outsourcing has been more piecemeal and uneven, with some states developing their own in-house eligibility assessment technologies and others outsourcing.

The state of Arkansas provides an illuminating case within a case of outsourced ADM in disability services. Arkansas is one of several states in which public authorities turned to automation to mitigate budgetary pressures arising from the expansion of Medicaid coverage for low-income Americans. Automated assessment tools have been introduced over the past decade across a range of human services, in part to control access to publicly funded care and support for sick, elderly, and disabled people (Bierman 2012). One particular algorithm, or set of algorithms, called interRAI, became one of the most widely used across the US (Center for Democracy and Technology

2020). The algorithm adopted in Arkansas's home care program utilized a relatively simple scoring system. Assessors would administer a lengthy, computer-based questionnaire covering 'everything from mental health to how much help [people needed] in daily activities like eating or doing their personal finances' (McCormick 2021: n.p.). The algorithm scored people's answers and sorted them into categories, assigning a standard number of home care hours to each category. Prior to the automation of this process, assessors (usually nurses) judged the number of home care hours required on a case-by-case basis; social workers and case managers would then create a needs-based individualized care plan (Lecher 2018). Arkansas state officials claimed that the system produced biased and 'arbitrary decisions', resulting in the need for less human discretion (Lecher 2018: n.p.).

Yet, the interRAI algorithm had its own arbitrary calibrations. A difference of one or two points on a particular question, for example, would see a person's benefit cut by dozens of home care hours each month (Lecher 2018). The system was also plagued by coding errors. In one example, a version of the interRAI software did not account for symptoms associated with diabetes. Almost one in five beneficiaries had their hours reduced due to the error (Administrative Rules and Regulations Subcommittee [hereafter, ARRS] 2018). A separate coding error meant that, for nearly two years, people with cerebral palsy received much less than they were entitled to: on average, a difference of 25 hours per month. It took years for these issues to be remedied, because DWP officials lacked the expertise to understand what had gone wrong and how to fix the software error. Meanwhile, people were left without vital home care support. They, too, were confounded by the automated decisions and had no comprehension of the criteria by which they were assessed (ARRS 2018).

As harmful as these technological errors were, they were apparently genuine errors in the way certain items were coded. The fundamental injustice built into the algorithmic system itself was its austerity-driven approach to service rationing, which was ultimately a political matter rather than a technical one. After the interRAI algorithm was introduced, many home care recipients had their care hours cut, without explanation of why their entitlement had changed despite their circumstances remaining the same (Lecher 2018). It emerged through a series of court cases and public hearings that the algorithm had been the vehicle for a significant reduction in Arkansas's public resourcing of home care. Prior to its use, the maximum number of hours per day of care for those aged under 65 was capped at eight, which was barely sufficient for people with acute care needs (ARRS 2018). Automation saw the daily cap reduced to five-and-a-half hours. This level of resourcing was insufficient to meet the care needs of people living with severe impairment, as was highlighted in one Senate committee hearing, which heard evidence of Arkansawyers 'lying in their own waste, going without food, going without any sort of community contact' (ARRS 2018: 17). When it was found that an algorithm was behind the drastic cuts to home care services, questions were raised about the state's accountability for the outcomes of algorithmic care planning. It was emphasized that 'while the algorithm sets the proportions for care […] it's the state's decision to decide how many hours to insert into the equation' (Lecher 2018: n.p.). This case exemplifies the ways in which algorithms can provide a veneer of objectivity to political decisions taken about the distribution of rights and resources among some of society's most socially disadvantaged groups. Indeed, it actually conceals the political origins of the algorithmically generated decisions that shape disabled people's lives in profound ways.

In 2018, after years of litigation and public controversy, the interRAI algorithm was abandoned by the Department of Human Services. It was soon replaced by a new tool called the Arkansas Independent Assessment (ARIA), and the entire assessment and care-planning process was outsourced to a multinational healthcare company, Optum. ARIA had a clear cost-cutting motive underlying its use. Under a directive from Arkansas's Republican Governor, Asa Hutchinson, Optum set out to achieve $835 million in Medicaid savings through 'program efficiencies', targeted at 'individuals with chronic, high-cost behavioral health, developmental and long-term care needs' (Optum 2019: 1). The algorithm designed for this purpose had been developed in Minnesota and adopted in Arkansas, despite widely reported software problems 'disrupt[ing] the delivery of vital services to tens of thousands of Minnesotans with physical and developmental disabilities' (Serres and Howatt 2019: n.p.).

The logic of ARIA was relatively simple. People were categorized according to their answers to a computerized questionnaire. Each category was then assigned a standard number of care hours (McCormick 2021). Unlike the scoring system utilized by Atos, however, Optum's method of weighting the answers was unknown to both assessors and the assessed. In fact, Optum's assessors seemingly had very limited input into the process, with the algorithm recommending the appropriate level of care and public officials merely 'authorizing' the determination (Optum 2017). In 2019, the year it was first used to assess eligibility for assisted living services, Optum's algorithm delivered drastic cuts to the social safety-net. Twenty-three percent of applicants lost support to which they were previously entitled (Davis 2019). Thirty-one percent were denied home care. As is often the case, the cuts disproportionately impacted the poorest and most disadvantaged communities, exacerbating the very social inequalities that systems of public health and disability care are tasked with addressing.

The case of Arkansas in the US indicates that outsourced ADM not only significantly reduces accuracy and accountability in the determination of how social welfare is distributed, but also obscures the political nature of decision-making processes themselves. In its more complex forms, the funneling of values-based decisions into algorithmic calculations can serve to pull a veil of objectivity and non-responsibility over what are, in fact, intentional strategies aimed at minimizing government welfare spending.

Concluding remarks

Well before the birth of the modern welfare state, disabled bodies and lives were measured, categorized, classified, and datafied. Although they have not been recognized as such, work tests and other data-driven tools of disability assessment were harbingers of the modern algorithmic technologies now widely deployed across the public sector. It is now broadly acknowledged that ADM poses numerous problems in terms of appropriateness, cost-effectiveness and, more fundamentally, social justice (Park and Humphry 2019; Bennett and Keyes 2020; Dencik and Kaun 2020). This chapter has contributed to this critical literature by documenting the changes that have occurred in the governance of disability benefits and services via mechanisms of automation. It has demonstrated that, rather than enhancing efficiency and fairness in public administration, ADM has been a vehicle for significant reductions in social spending and attempts by states to redraw the boundaries of the disability category.

In the current age of ADM, automation almost always involves outsourcing. It makes *prima facie* sense to suggest that government functions are being outsourced to algorithms. It is a common shorthand way of describing the ceding of political control to automated systems and processes. Yet, this shorthand obscures the political agency behind the algorithms. When governments outsource to automated technologies, they are outsourcing to the private companies who engineer and operate those technologies on the government's behalf. Automation, therefore, is opening new avenues through which political powers of decision-making are accrued by companies and organizations linked to, but distinct from, the welfare state. In the case of disability provisioning, access to public resources is increasingly subject to corporate rather than democratic oversight. Whereas it was previously the state's role to govern the boundaries of the disability category, that function is increasingly falling to the private sector, including the global IT industry. To the extent that these entities are motivated by private interests and the maximization of shareholder value, their automated systems serve private rather than public ends and, in so doing, undermine democratic accountability.

The ways in which automation is transforming welfare state decision-making warrant close academic and public scrutiny. Future research in this area should seek not only to document these developments, but also to critically analyze the ways in which ADM structurally reconfigures welfare relations, such that powerful state and corporate interests are advanced over the rights and wellbeing of citizens. Aside from outsourced ADM, there are many other socio-technical arrangements shaping the political economy of health and welfare that warrant further attention. These include public-private data-sharing partnerships, the privatization of digital, e-government and e-health infrastructure and assets, and forms of marketization that give private and civil society organizations a greater role in delivering social services via digital apps and platforms. These developments speak to core concerns of political economy: namely, to asymmetries of power and the colonization of the public domain by commercial technologies, logics, and practices. They point to the need for a deeper, critical engagement with ADM and the political-economic forces underpinning its deployment in public services.

Notes

1 This research was funded by the Australian Research Council Centre of Excellence for Automated Decision-Making and Society (grant number CE200100005).
2 Decision criteria are rules, standards, or, in this case, numerical thresholds (*e.g.* the number of hours one is capable of working per week) used to determine eligibility for public assistance.
3 Research by Barr *et al.* (2016) suggests that for every 10,000 people assessed through the WCA between 2010 and 2013, there were six associated suicides.

References

Administrative Rules and Regulations Subcommittee. 2018, 'Administrative rules and regulations subcommittee of the arkansas legislative council', Arkansas State Legislature, accessed 13 September 2021, <https://www.arkleg.state.ar.us/Calendars/Attachment?committee=040&agenda=648&file=A+Summary+Agenda+9-18-18.pdf>.

Alston, P. 2019, *Report of the Special Rapporteur on Extreme Poverty and Human Rights*, United Nations, accessed 29 September 2021, <https://digitallibrary.un.org/record/1648309?ln=en>.

Barnes, C. 1991, *Disabled People in Britain and Discrimination: A Case for Anti-Discrimination Legislation*, C. Hurst and Co. Publishers, London.

Barr, B., Taylor-Robinson, D., Stuckler, D., Loopstra, R., Reeves, A. and Whitehead, M. 2016, '"First, do no harm": Are disability assessments associated with adverse trends in mental health? A longitudinal ecological study', *Journal of Epidemiology and Community Health*, 70, pp. 339–45.

Benjamin, R. 2019, *Race After Technology: Abolitionist Tools for the New Jim Code*, Polity Books, Cambridge.

Bennett, C.L. and Keyes, O. 2020, 'What is the point of fairness? Disability, AI and the complexity of justice', *ACM SIGACCESS Accessibility and Computing*, 125, pp. 1–11.

Bierman, S. 2012, *ArPath: Advancing Electronic LTSS Systems in Arkansas*, Department of Human Services, accessed 13 September 2021, <https://www.hilltopinstitute.org/wp-content/uploads/hilltop/Symposium12/BiermanSlides.pdf>.

Bloom, D. 2019, 'DWP quietly hands private firms £600m extra to test disabled people for benefits', *Mirror*, 6 June, accessed 13 September 2021, <https://www.mirror.co.uk/news/politics/dwp-quietly-hands-private-firms-16243454>.

Booth, R. 2019, 'Benefits system automation could plunge claimants deeper into poverty', *The Guardian*, 14 October, accessed 11 September 2021, <https://www.theguardian.com/technology/2019/oct/14/fears-rise-in-benefits-system-automation-could-plunge-claimants-deeper-into-poverty>.

Boughey, J. 2021, 'Outsourcing automation: Locking the "black box" inside a safe', in Boughey, J. and Miller, K. (eds), *The Automated State: Implications, Challenges and Opportunities for Public Law*, The Federation Press, Alexandria, pp. 136–53.

Center for Democracy and Technology. 2020, 'Appendix B: States' use of algorithm-driven decision-making tools for benefits determinations', Center for Democracy and Technology, accessed 13 September 2021, <https://cdt.org/wp-content/uploads/2020/10/Screen-Reader-Friendly-Version-States-Use-of-Algorithm-Assisted-Decision-making-Tools-for-Benefits-Determinations.docx>.

Collington, R. 2021, 'Disrupting the welfare state? Digitalisation and the retrenchment of public sector capacity', *New Political Economy*, 27(2), pp. 312–28.

Committee on Public Accounts. 2002, *The Medical Assessment of Incapacity and Disability Benefits*, UK Parliament, accessed 13 September 2021, <https://publications.parliament.uk/pa/cm200102/cmselect/cmpubacc/683/68303.htm>.

Corden, A. and Sainsbury, R. 2001, *Incapacity Benefits and Work Incentives,* Department of Social Security Research Report, No.141, Corporate Document Services, Leeds.

Crawford, K. and Schultz, J. 2019, 'AI systems as state actors', *Colombia Law Review*, 119(7), pp. 1941–72.

Davis, A. 2019, '2 state panels vote to review vendor's medicaid-care assessments contract', *Arkansas Democrat Gazette*, 10 July, accessed 13 September 2021, <https://www.arkansasonline.com/news/2019/jul/10/benefits-eligibility-denials-draw-look-/>.

Dencik, L. and Kaun, A. 2020, 'Datafication and the welfare state', *Global Perspectives*, 1(1), p. 12912.

Dickinson, H. and Yates, S. 2023, 'From external provision to technological outsourcing: Lessons for public sector automation from the outsourcing literature', *Public Management Review*, 25(2), pp. 243–61.

Dunleavy, P., Helen, M., Bastow, S. and Tinkler, J. 2006, *Digital Era Governance: IT Corporations, the State, and e-Government,* Oxford University Press, Oxford.

Esping-Anderson, G. 1990, *The Three Worlds of Welfare Capitalism,* Princeton University Press, Princeton, NJ.

Eubanks, V. 2019, *Automating Inequality: How High-Tech Tools Profile, Police, and Punish the Poor*, Picador St Martin's Press, New York.

Grover, C. 2014, 'Atos healthcare withdraws from the work capability assessment: A comment', *Disability and Society*, 29(8), pp. 1324–8.

Grover, C. and Soldatic, K. 2013, 'Neoliberal restructuring, disabled people and social (in)security in Australia and Britain', *Scandinavian Journal of Disability Research*, 15(3), pp. 216–32.

Gulland, J. 2019, *Gender, Work and Social Control: A Century of Disability Benefits*, Palgrave Macmillan, London.

Harrington, M. 2010, *An Independent Review of the Work Capability Assessment*, Department for Work and Pensions, accessed 13 September 2021, <https://assets.publishing.service.gov.uk/government/uploads/system/uploads/attachment_data/file/70071/wca-review-2010.pdf>.

Henman, P. 2020, 'Governing by algorithms and algorithmic governmentality: Towards machinic judgement', in Schuilenburg, M. and Peeters, R. (eds), *The Algorithmic Society: Technology, Power, and Knowledge*, Routledge, London, pp. 19–34.

Humpage, L. 2007, 'Models of disability, work and welfare in Australia', *Social Policy and Administration*, 41(3), pp. 215–31.

Katz, M.B. 1984, 'Poorhouses and the origins of the public old age home', *The Milbank Memorial Fund Quarterly, Health and Society*, 62(1), pp. 110–40.

Killoughery, M. 1999, 'Disability and incapacity benefits: The role that doctors play', *Psychiatric Bulletin*, 23, pp. 260–3.

Lecher, C. 2018, 'What happens when an algorithm cuts your health care', *The Verge*, 21 March, accessed 13 September 2021, <https://www.theverge.com/2018/3/21/17144260/healthcare-medicaid-algorithm-arkansas-cerebral-palsy>.

Litchfield, P. 2013, *An Independent Review of the Work Capability Assessment – Year Four*, Department for Work and Pensions, accessed 13 September 2021, <https://assets.publishing.service.gov.uk/government/uploads/system/uploads/attachment_data/file/265351/work-capability-assessment-year-4-paul-litchfield.pdf>.

Margetts, H. 1995, 'The automated state', *Public Policy and Administration*, 10(2), pp. 88–103.

McCormick, E. 2021, 'What happened when a "wildly irrational" algorithm made crucial healthcare decisions', *The Guardian*, 2 July, accessed 13 September 2021, <https://www.theguardian.com/us-news/2021/jul/02/algorithm-crucial-healthcare-decisions>.

Navarro, V. 1976, *Medicine Under Capitalism*, Croom Helm, London.

Oliver, M. and Barnes, C. 2012, *New Politics of Disablement*, Palgrave Macmillan, Hampshire.

Optum. 2017, 'Arkansas independent assessment', *Optum*, accessed 13 September 2021, <https://medicaid-saveslives.files.wordpress.com/2017/08/ar-ind-assessments-080917.pdf>.

Optum. 2019, 'Independent assessments', *Optum*, accessed 13 September 2021, <https://www.optum.com/content/dam/optum3/optum/en/resources/case-studies/gov-arkansas-ia-case-study.pdf>.

Park, S. and Humphry, J. 2019, 'Exclusion by design: Intersections of social, digital and data exclusion', *Information, Communication and Society*, 22(7), pp. 934–53.

Parliamentary Office of Science and Technology. 2012, *Assessing Capacity for Work*, UK Parliament, accessed 13 September 2021, <https://researchonline.lshtm.ac.uk/id/eprint/2017894/1/POST-PN-413%20(2).pdf>.

Pasquale, F. 2017, *From Territorial to Functional Sovereignty: The Case of Amazon*, The law and political economy project, accessed 13 September 2021, <https://lpeblog.org/2017/12/06/from-territorial-to-functional-sovereignty-the-case-of-amazon/>.

Pedlar, A. and Hutchison, P. 2000, 'Restructuring human services in Canada: Commodification of disability', *Disability and Society*, 15(4), pp. 637–51.

Rafter, N. 1992, 'Claims-making and socio-cultural context in the first U.S. Eugenics Campaign', *Social Problems*, 39(1), pp. 17–34.

Roulstone, A. and Prideaux, S. 2012, *Understanding Disability Policy*, Policy Press, Bristol.

Russell, M. and Malhotra, R. 2019, 'Introduction: Capitalism and the disability rights movement', in Rosenthal, K. (ed), *Capitalism and Disability*, Haymarket Books, Chicago, pp. 1–10.

Sainsbury, R., Corden, A. and Finch, N. 2003, *Medical Evidence and Incapacity Benefit: Evaluation of a Pilot Study*, research report, Department for Work and Pensions Research Report, 189, Corporate Document Services, Leeds.

Serres, C. and Howatt, G. 2019, 'Disparities dog system to distribute disability services', *Star Tribune*, 31 October, accessed 13 September 2021, <https://www.startribune.com/disparities-dog-system-to-distribute-disability-services/563636552/>.

Soldatic, K. 2013, 'Appointment time: Disability and neoliberal workfare temporalities', *Critical Sociology*, 39(3), pp. 405–19.

Soldatic, K. 2019, *Disability and Neoliberal State Formations*, Routledge, London.

Stone, D. 1984, *The Disabled State*, Temple University Press, Philadelphia.

Tilley, S. 2020, 'In the name of "digital inclusion": The true cost of the automation and privatisation of Australia's social security system', *Social Alternatives*, 39(1), pp. 28–38.

van Toorn, G. 2021, *The New Political Economy of Disability: Transnational Networks and Individualised Funding in the Age of Neoliberalism*, Routledge, London.

Williams, Z. 2011, 'Disability assessment may be a farce, but it's not French', *The Guardian*, 29 December, accessed 13 September 2021, <https://www.theguardian.com/commentisfree/2011/dec/28/disability-benefits-government-procurement>.

Work and Pensions Committee. 2011a, *The Role of Incapacity Benefit Reassessment in Helping Claimants into Employment*, Sixth Report of the Session 2010–12, Vol. 1, House of Commons, London.

Work and Pensions Committee. 2011b, *Examination of Witnesses (Question Numbers 79–200)*, UK Parliament, accessed 13 September 2021, <https://publications.parliament.uk/pa/cm201012/cmselect/cmworpen/1015/11051802.htm>.

22

UNDERSTANDING THE HEALTH-POLITICS NEXUS IN THE SHADOW OF POPULISM

Toward a political science of, and for, health

Volkan Yilmaz

'Populism' has become a catch-all phrase to describe a wide range of contemporary political actors that almost all scholars employing this concept find politically undesirable. Health matters did not fall under the remit of populism literature until recently, except for a few studies on healthcare reforms. With the outbreak of the COVID-19 pandemic, health matters have become more salient, which has led to the proliferation of studies employing the notion of populism in examining health politics and policy (*e.g.* Ringe and Rennó 2023).

On the one hand, this is a welcome development for political science as it disregarded health matters, with only a few exceptions (*e.g.* Alford 1974), and thus contributed to the misperception of health as being free from politics (Bambra *et al.* 2005). On the other hand, the way this emerging literature approaches the health-politics nexus is not entirely satisfactory for two reasons. First, most scholars using the populism framework continue to ignore the political nature of health itself and, instead, view health as a playground for 'more important' political goals. Yet, health can be at the center of politics, and examining the relation between health and populism necessitates an appreciation of the distinctive features of health politics (Carpenter 2012), as well as various complex aspects of health policy. Second, because of the first problem, populism scholars end up reducing complex health politics to a dichotomy between 'bad' populists and others.

This chapter presents a review of the literature examining health within the framework of populism. Using a specific definition of populism as an inclusion criterion would unjustifiably restrict the scope of this review. Therefore, a broad inclusion criterion that uses populism as a lens to examine health politics and policy is employed. To this end, the chapter is organized into four sections. The next section provides an overview of the definitional debates surrounding populism. Following this, the third and fourth sections offer a critical account of the literature on the populism-health nexus in general, and during the COVID-19 pandemic in particular, respectively. The final section sets out the conditions for a new political science of, and for, health – a call that has been increasingly made within the discipline of public health (De Leeuw *et al.* 2014; Bekker *et al.* 2018) and identifies potential avenues for further research.

DOI: 10.4324/9781003017110-25

Populism as a contested concept

The literature on populism is dominated by definitional discussions. Candidates for the foundational form of populism are abundant. It has, so far, been characterized as a political strategy (Weyland 2017, 2001, 1999), a thin-centered ideology (Mudde 2004), a logic of political articulation (Laclau 2005a, b), a political style (Moffitt and Tormey 2014), a standalone ideology (Freeden 2017), a moment symbolizing destabilization of the existing hegemony (Mouffe 2018), a discursive frame (Aslanidis 2016; Norris and Inglehart 2019), and a mode of political action (Bickerton and Accetti 2021). Although a broad inclusion criterion of populism as a lens to comprehend health is used at the review stage, adopting a particular definition is necessary to offer a robust analysis. Inspired by Weyland's approach (2017), this chapter treats populism primarily as a majority-building political strategy, used in contexts where elections matter, that risks undermining non-electoral checks-and-balances institutions while aiming at monopolizing executive decision-making. It is not an ideology or a political orientation as it lacks a programmatic center.

One of the defining characteristics of the populism definition used in this chapter is that it is only applicable to contexts where political legitimacy originates primarily from general elections, and where public authority officially lies in the hands of elected representatives. This makes populism also applicable to competitive authoritarian contexts that fail to meet the standards of liberal democracy (Levitsky and Way 2002), as long as electoral competition and the weight of popular legitimacy are still largely present. This understanding of populism is different from its alternative use to characterize an ideological frame along with socialism and liberalism (*e.g.* Freeden 2017), and its application to full-fledged authoritarian regimes as a discursive frame (*e.g.* Duckett and Langer 2013).

The relationship between populism and democracy is complex (Canovan 1999). On the one hand, the relationship seems symbiotic. In electoral democracies, reaching out to citizens with a clear message to convince them that the sender of the message is better placed than rivals to deliver desired goals (Greve 2021a) is at the heart of the legitimate acquisition of political power. On the other hand, the nature of the relationship seems to be antagonistic. The populist tendency to unify and realize 'national will' creates tension with democracy. Therefore, populism can lead to an erosion of the limits imposed by non-electoral checks-and-balances institutions on the executive branch, as well as to the potential transition to non-democratic regimes (Mudde 2004; Norris and Inglehart 2019).

Defining populism necessitates responding to the question of when a political strategy becomes antithetical to democratic sustainability. Any answer to this question should consider two factors: scholars' understanding of democracy, which is partly exogenous to the phenomenon at hand, and the context within which this question is asked. First, scholars hold diverse understandings of democracy that range from elitist and technocratic to liberal constitutional, participatory, and reconciliatory. Therefore, the criteria they use in identifying the de-democratizing potential (or impact) of populist strategies differ. A major exception to this – one that will likely elicit broad agreement from most scholars on its populist character – is a political strategy that leads to a broader transition toward a neopatrimonial political system (Charrad and Adams 2011), where bureaucracy loses ground completely. Second, scholars have differing views on the compatibility of various non-electoral checks-and-balances institutions with democracy. These institutions range from the independence of the constitutional courts to that of central banks; from collective bargaining autonomy to professional autonomy. There is no standard for their availability across contexts. In addition, these institutions constitute a heterogeneous group, and the impact of each on decision-making in different policy sectors might vary. Therefore, whether the erosion of specific checks-and-balances institutions should be considered as evidencing de-democratization requires a nuanced examination of the limitations that these institutions impose on decision-making in a particular policy sector in a specific context.

Populism is a majority-building political strategy that aims at seizing political power. While it can work with different political orientations, it is not always clear whether a populist strategy has any political content other than achieving political power. In other words, drawing on De Certeau's (1988) distinction between tactics and strategies, no agreement has been reached on whether populism's relationship with certain political demands is merely tactical, or can also be strategic. On the one hand, some scholars (*e.g.* Schrecker 2017; Koltai *et al.* 2020; Felder *et al.* 2021) imply that populist appeals are often rooted in people's grievances that precede the emergence of these appeals. Alternatively, others (*e.g.* Laclau 2005b; Moffitt and Tormey 2014) emphasize the performative element of populism that can create its own constituency, sometimes based on non-issues and pure manipulation. This was evidenced during the Brexit referendum in the Leave campaign's use of the argument that European Union membership restricts the financial resources available to the NHS in the UK. Evaluating both within populism seems to be the best possible solution.

Populism is chameleonic in its compatibility with different political orientations. Political ideas that are associated with populist strategies vary across time and contexts. For instance, in terms of economic policies, it has incorporated economic étatist, as well as neoliberal, characters (Roberts 1995; Beauchamp 1997; Weyland 1999). The chameleonic nature of populism has led many scholars to qualify it with adjectives that hint at its particular political content. For instance, Mudde and Kaltwasser (2013) underline that populism can rest on inclusionary or exclusionary elements. Inclusionary populism is often used to refer to left-wing populisms observed mostly in Latin America (Clark and Patterson 2021) and Southern Europe (Kaltwasser and Zanotti 2021), while exclusionary populisms are mostly associated with the radical right in Western Europe (Rinaldi and Bekker 2021).

Despite the sophistication of the literature seeking to define populism, the empirical uses of the notion suffer from 'sloppy conceptualisation and, as a result, invalid inferences' (Rooduijn 2019: 362). One observation is that populism is usually associated with specific political actors (Canovan 1999; Barr 2009). Once an actor is defined as a populist, scholars do not give much information about what using the concept of populism adds to the analysis. Alternatively, the term has been operationally defined as a discursive frame (Aslanidis 2016). This approach enables comparative research by identifying the discursive components of populism, but it also risks uprooting populism from the political-economic context within which it emerges and functions, thereby reducing it to a universally available option of political communication.

Populism and health

The most important limitation of the literature on populism and health is that political orientation is erroneously considered as evidence for the impact of populism. One example is the study by Pavolini *et al.* (2018), which identifies populism as a threat to universal health coverage worldwide. Similarly, Speed and Mannion (2020) conclude that populists grant healthcare access only to those they consider as part of 'the people'. Another exemplary study is the scoping review by Rinaldi and Bekker (2021), which reduces populism to European populist radical right (PRR) parties, and suggests that it leads to the undermining of equity in healthcare and worsening health outcomes.

Populism is often associated with exclusionary forms of nationalism, nativism, and chauvinism. Therefore, international cooperation is another area in which scholars expect to see the negative impact of populism. This line of literature also suffers from the problem of attributing a certain political orientation to populism. Some authors (Speed and Mannion 2017; Mason 2020) equate populism with national protectionism, while simultaneously presenting globalization as a beneficial process for health. Nevertheless, the evidence (Cornia *et al.* 2009) shows that globalization has failed to improve health outcomes, especially in post-Soviet and sub-Saharan African countries. While right-wing populists' scapegoating of the World Health Organization during the COVID-19 pandemic (Sengul 2021), efforts to defund it, and reluctance to follow its guidance (Wilson *et al.* 2020) might be seen as factors contributing to the erosion of an internationally coordinated response (McLachlan 2020), such phenomena are products of these actors' political orientations rather than the populist strategies they deploy. Some Latin American populist actors' positive attitudes toward international solidarity demonstrate that populism is not intrinsically antithetical to international cooperation (Birn and Muntaner 2019).

Leaving aside the confusion of populism with political orientation, there is disagreement in the literature about the impact of actors deemed populist on health policies. For example, De Cleen and Speed (2021) find Rinaldi and Bekker's conclusion of the negative influence of PRR parties on welfare generosity unconvincing, and note that these parties sometimes prevent other coalition partners from implementing a welfare retrenchment agenda. Blum and Kuhlmann (2021) also maintain that European PRR party perspectives on social policy are heterogeneous, even though they are often grouped under the generic title of exclusionary populism. In addition, scholars often disregard some left-wing actors that rely on populist strategies to promote inclusionary and equitable healthcare systems (De Cleen 2018). Rather than conflating populist strategies with particular political orientations, some authors (De Cleen 2018; De Cleen and Speed 2021) call for explicitly naming the specific political orientations of these actors.

It is not easy to establish a link between populism and healthcare policy, as populism is never sufficient to describe the political direction adopted by governments (De Cleen and Speed 2021). In other words, 'there is no such thing as populist policies' (Kaltwasser and Zanotti 2021: 43.). In addition, in the literature on broader social policy dynamics, Kaltwasser and Zanotti (2021) suggest that the impact of populism on European welfare states is still largely unknown and, to the extent that it is examined, Greve (2021a, b) argues that it seems uneven and possibly overestimated. Therefore, the policy-level impact of populism is difficult to grasp (Powell 2017), and any study on this impact should be nuanced and context-specific: tasked with identifying how the interplay between populist strategy and political content influences healthcare policy, rather than the latter alone.

The health policy impact of populism might be a function of its impact on policy-making in health. When health becomes a platform within which populist strategies are deployed, examining how those strategies influence and shape policy-making becomes a worthwhile exercise. To examine populist strategies in health, one distinction that could be made is between public health and healthcare, as their policy-making environments often differ considerably. Another gateway into populist strategies in health could be to examine how these strategies frame the role of physicians, medical experts, other medical professionals, and their professional organizations in policy-making. To identify a health policy-making strategy as populist, it is crucial to consider the policy-making structure preceding the populist strategy, to make our understanding of health democracy explicit, and to clarify what role we think medical professionals and their organizations should play. The distinction that De Cleen (2018: 269) makes between 'the use of expertise in policy design' and 'expert-led technocratic decision-making' can be useful for the latter task.

In contexts where professional autonomy is present and effective, populist strategies in health might result in the questioning of its legitimacy, especially if and when this autonomy poses a barrier to the populist project. The study by Pavolini *et al.* (2018), for instance, finds that strong professionalism and the presence of physicians in health policy-making would restrict the negative impact of populism on health policy, which is defined as undermining universal health coverage. However, the US case – which is not included in this study – presents a falsifying example for this claim, as it fails to provide universal health coverage, although it meets both conditions. Agartan and Kuhlmann (2019) do not exclude the possibility that populists might work with individual physicians, provided that these physicians contribute to their desired ends. However, they suggest that this would not necessarily discredit the reverse relationship between populism and professionalism.

Another key mechanism through which populism might influence health policy-making is through its alleged disregard for scientific evidence. Speed and Mannion (2017), for instance, underline the post-truth element in some contemporary populisms, and expect this element to result in exclusionary and inequitable health policies. Alternatively, De Cleen (2018) highlights politicians' picking and choosing of which expert knowledge and scientific evidence they incorporate in policy-making, and concludes that there is not necessarily a connection between populism and distrust of expert knowledge.

One promising area for further study on the populism-health nexus is the influence of successful populist projects on health, regardless of the place of health – or its lack thereof – in their platforms. Health impacts may materialize due to the influence of populism on democracy (including non-electoral checks-and-balances between institutions) and social cohesion. This makes a good hypothesis because both democracy (Besley and Kudamatsu 2006) and social cohesion are found to be good for health (Wilkinson and Pickett 2010).

It is often assumed in the populism literature that political actors deploy populist strategies in health to achieve non–health-related broader goals (*e.g.* Kaltwasser *et al.* 2017). Nevertheless, as Lasco and Curato (2019) suggest, political objectives directly related to health sometimes take the center stage in populist projects. To describe these cases, they coin the term 'medical populism', which is defined as 'a political style based on performances of public health crises that pit "the people" against "the establishment"' (Lasco and Curato 2019: 1). Medical populism, therefore, represents a distinct and autonomous strategy, the ultimate goal of which is confined to the domain of public health policy (Lasco 2020; Lasco and Larson 2020).

One promising avenue for research on the populism-health nexus has focused on the link between the political saliency of health and healthcare system types. In a study of five European countries, Pavolini *et al.* (2018) suggest that the form of the healthcare system within countries influences whether healthcare becomes part of the populist discourses. They observe that populist discourses in Denmark and Germany do not explicitly refer to health policy, unlike those in Italy, Turkey, and the UK. They argue that higher spending on health and inclusion of physicians in policy-making act as a barrier against populist attention to health. In a study on the influence of PRR parties on welfare policies in European countries, Rinaldi and Bekker (2021: 147) maintain that tax-funded, public sector-led, universalistic healthcare systems are 'more susceptible to welfare chauvinistic appeals'.

Questions around healthcare benefits packages, especially in publicly funded systems, may be susceptible to populist strategies, as their relevance to the public makes them an attractive instrument for majority building. The Polish case exemplifies how a government could deploy a populist strategy that secures itself a majority by using a controversial health issue, like abortion (Lendvai-Bainton and Stubbs 2021). Yet, the high political saliency of abortion in the US, with a marketized health system, shows us the limits of this argument. That is, the high popular saliency of health matters in some societies, not the health system type, may make health attractive to those using populist strategies.

Populism and the COVID-19 pandemic

With the COVID-19 pandemic, health matters have gained more popularity in political science. Many scholars contributing to this emerging literature have chosen populism as the appropriate lens with which to examine the politics of pandemic responses. One line of this literature addresses whether the pandemic has created an opportunity for populists to concentrate more power in their hands. This focus has even resulted in broad conclusions that identify an elective affinity between the pandemic and populism. For example, McKee *et al.* (2021: 514) expect 'populism fueling the spread of COVID-19 and, in turn, COVID-19 stoking the fires of populism'. Other studies offer more nuanced accounts. One example is the study by Guasti (2020), which shows that the ability of populist leaders to use the pandemic for consolidating executive power varies across contexts. Based on a study of four Central European countries, Guasti (2020) concludes that populist leaders in Hungary and Poland used the pandemic to further consolidate executive power and undermine civil rights protections, while a similar de-democratization tendency was effectively contained by other democratic actors and checks-and-balances institutions in Czechia and Slovakia.

Another strand of the literature uses the COVID-19 pandemic as a case to help examine what happens when populists do not proclaim a public health crisis for political purposes but, nonetheless, face one in reality. The performance of populists in their responses to the pandemic is a particularly interesting topic, as previous studies (*e.g.* Moffitt and Tormey 2014; Rooduijn 2014) observe that actors using populist strategies often proclaim a crisis, or even 'fabricate a sense of crisis' (Brubaker 2021), and present themselves as well placed to resolve it. Lasco and Curato (2019: 1) also maintain that medical populism is manifested in 'the performances of public health crises', implying that the crises themselves are populist products. The COVID-19 pandemic has created a distinctive environment for populism, as it is a public health crisis, the emergence of which preceded its incorporation into populist strategies. In this regard, whether populists govern well during crises has been one of the key questions pursued in the literature.

Some researchers suggest that populists failed to deliver during the COVID-19 pandemic. For instance, McKee *et al.* (2021) observe a negative correlation between a populist presence in governments and country performance during the pandemic. Similarly, Weiffen (2020) argues that populist leaders with different political orientations in three Latin American countries shared a disdain for medical expertise and an inability to implement preventive measures that limited the prevalence of COVID-19. In contrast to earlier accounts suggesting that populism thrives only by spectacularizing crises (Lasco and Curato 2019), Brubaker (2021: 7) succinctly argues that during the pandemic, some populists were 'performing non-crisis, performing normality in the face of an establishment in full crisis mode'. While Lasco (2020) attempts to describe the populist performance of non-crisis amidst the pandemic using the notion of medical populism, this phenomenon does not correspond to his previous definition of this concept (Lasco and Curato 2019). The catastrophic implications of the denialist attitudes of some populist leaders were evident in high levels of COVID-19–related mortality following a period of government inaction in some populist-run countries. Bayerlein *et al.* (2021) observe an 8 percent excess mortality rate in populist-governed countries. Pereira *et al.'s* (2020) study shows that, when faced with irrefutable human casualties, Brazilian President Bolsonaro's core constituency adopted an increasingly negative attitude toward the government. Once a government's position is falsified by the everyday experiences of laypeople, scholars observed two reactions from populist leaders. First, most seemed to come to terms with reality and aligned their policies with scientifically backed guidelines (Kavakli 2020).

Second, some leaders, such as Bolsonaro and Trump, attempted to cover their failure by projecting an 'exaggerated phantasized threat' (Zienert-Eilts 2020: 985), and actively promoting a distorted explanation for the pandemic (Agnew 2020).

Other researchers found no shared pattern between populism and pandemic response performance. For instance, Clark and Patterson (2021) report that some Latin American populists based their policy response on medical expertise and introduced stringent restrictions on human mobility. Having conducted a policy mapping exercise amidst the pandemic, Katsambekis and Stavrakakis (2020: 6) observe that 'populist responses to the pandemic have been as heterogeneous and as context-dependent as the ideological profile and programmatic orientation of populist actors themselves'. Ringe and Rennó (2023: 11) also conclude their edited volume, featuring 22 country case-studies, by noting that 'there is more variation in populist responses to the pandemic than is often observed or acknowledged'. Finally, Kavakli (2020) shows that preventive measures adopted by populist governments matched those of non-populists over time, despite an initial divergence between these two. In other words, while populist governments were typically late in adopting necessary public health measures, their policies converged with others over time.

Finally, the relationship between politics and science has, once again, been scrutinized from the perspective of populism during the COVID-19 pandemic. Katsambekis and Stavrakakis (2020) challenge the assumption that medical experts often speak with a single technocratic voice by referring to the different positions that key epidemiologists took, as well as the resulting dissimilar policy directions adopted in Sweden and Greece during the pandemic. Bickerton and Accetti (2021) propose that health policy responses to the pandemic in many countries have demonstrated that politics and science stand not as rivals, but rather as complements. Challenging the view that populism and technocracy are inherently contradictory, they articulate the concept of 'technopopulism' to underline that the interlinkages between these two political logics were often used in combination during COVID-19 responses (Bickerton and Accetti 2021).

Conclusion

The COVID-19 pandemic has created a rare opportunity for political researchers to take a closer look at the health-politics nexus, and to move health matters from the margins to the center of the discipline. Although growing numbers of scholars have seized this opportunity and provided valuable descriptive accounts of the politics of pandemic response in diverse contexts, analyses using the populism lens often suffer from conceptual and interpretive ambiguities. The most commonly observed manifestations of this ambiguity are the confusion of populism with political orientations, and the portrayal of health politics as a conflict between 'bad populists' and others. Not only are these conclusions oversimplified, but they also contradict the insights from the broader populism literature, suggesting that political orientation is not a constitutive element of populism. The historical failure of political science to recognize and address the political nature of health can explain why the emerging literature on populism and health remains conceptually weak. To compensate, a new political science of, and for, health can emerge on these three research agendas.

First, little is still known about the health-politics nexus. Developing a political compass for health is necessary to move the field forward. This health politics compass will identify diverse political ideas about health, present this diversity in a systematic framework, and reveal the relations between health-related political ideas and general political orientations. Exploring public attitudes toward health policy issues, examining the health-related political orientations of contemporary actors, and philosophical studies of values related to health policy matters can inform this process. The adaptation of such a health politics compass will, potentially, accommodate the heterogeneity of health policy issues that constitutes healthcare and public health issues, as well as its diverse subsectors (*e.g.* sexual and reproductive health).

Second, the relationship between populism and health is complex, and the influence of populism on health and healthcare rarely lends itself to straightforward interpretations. This is because health neither occupies a significant place on the political agenda in all contexts, nor attracts the attention of all political actors using populist strategies. Therefore, one avenue for further research is to explore if, and when, health matters become salient and are incorporated into populist strategies. Previous research on the link between health system types and the attractiveness of health to populists has already presented a good start in this direction.

Third, the health impact of populism can be examined through the mediation of its influence on democracy, checks-and-balances institutions, and social cohesion. Given that previous research indicates a positive relationship between living in democratic and cohesive societies and health outcomes, one hypothesis might be that successful populist strategies – regardless of whether health is explicitly mentioned in populist projects or not – may worsen health outcomes. Yet, such generalizations may be misleading and require careful consideration, as the health impact of populism will depend on which checks-and-balances institutions are influenced by populist processes, as well as the previous impacts of these institutions on health outcomes.

These three research agendas on different dimensions of the health-politics nexus may contribute to advancing health toward the center of political science: not only as a subject of inquiry, but also as a valuable political objective.

References

Agartan, T.I. and Kuhlmann, E. 2019, 'New public management, physicians and populism: Turkey's experience with health reforms', *Sociology of Health and Illness*, 41(7), pp. 1410–1425.

Agnew, J. 2020, 'American "populism" and the spatial contradictions of US government in the time of COVID-19', *Geopolitica(s)*, 11, pp. 15–23.

Alford, R.R. 1974, *Health Care Politics: Ideological and Interest Group Barriers to Reform*, University of Chicago Press, Chicago.

Aslanidis, P. 2016, 'Is populism an ideology? A refutation and a new perspective', *Political Studies*, 64(1), pp. 88–104.

Bambra, C., Fox, D. and Scott-Samuel, A. 2005, 'Towards a politics of health', *Health Promotion International*, 20(2), 187–93.

Barr, R.R. 2009, 'Populists, outsiders and anti-establishment politics', *Party Politics*, 15(1), pp. 29–48.

Bayerlein, M., Boese, V.A., Gates, S., Kamin, K. and Murshed, S.M. 2021, 'Populism and COVID-19: How populist governments (mis)handle the pandemic', *Journal of Political Institutions and Political Economy*, 2(3), pp. 389–428.

Beauchamp, D. 1997, 'Public health, privatization, and market populism: A time for reflection', *Quality Management in Health Care*, 5(2), pp. 73–9.

Bekker, M.P., Greer, S.L., Azzopardi-Muscat, N. and McKee, M. 2018, 'Public health and politics: How political science can help us move forward, *European Journal of Public Health*, 28(suppl. 3), pp. 1–2.

Besley, T. and Kudamatsu, M. 2006, 'Health and democracy', *American Economic Review*, 96(2), pp. 313–8.

Bickerton, C.J. and Accetti, C.I. 2021, *Technopopulism*, Oxford University Press, Oxford.

Birn, A.E. and Muntaner, C. 2019, 'Latin American social medicine across borders: South-South cooperation and the making of health solidarity', *Global Public Health*, 14(6–7), pp. 817–34.

Blum, S. and Kuhlmann, J. 2021, 'Understanding the "welfare state" in the context of austerity and populism', Greve, B. (ed), *Austerity, Retrenchment and the Welfare State*, Edward Elgar Publishing, Cheltenham, pp. 81–93.

Brubaker, R. 2021, 'Paradoxes of populism during the pandemic', *Thesis Eleven*, 164(1), pp. 73–87.

Canovan, M. 1999, 'Trust the people! Populism and the two faces of democracy', *Political Studies*, 47(1), pp. 2–16.

Carpenter, D.P. 2012, 'Is health politics different?' *Annual Review of Political Science*, 15(1), pp. 287–31.

Charrad, M.M. and Adams, J. 2011, 'Introduction: Patrimonialism, past and present', *The ANNALS of the American Academy of Political and Social Science*, 636(1), pp. 6–15.
Clark, M.A. and Patterson, A. 2021, 'Populism and health policy in Latin America', *International Journal of Health Policy and Management*, 10(9), pp. 585–7.
Cornia, G.A., Rosignoli, S. and Tiberti, L. 2009, 'Did globalisation affect health status? A simulation exercise', *Journal of International Development*, 21(8), pp. 1083–101.
De Certeau, M. 1988, *The Practice of Everyday Life*, University of California Press, Berkeley.
De Cleen, B. 2018, 'Populism, exclusion, post-truth: Some conceptual caveats', *International Journal of Health Policy and Management*, 7(3), pp. 268–71.
De Cleen, B. and Speed, E. 2021, 'Getting the problem definition right: The radical right, populism, nativism and public health', *International Journal of Health Policy and Management*, 10(8), pp. 523–7.
De Leeuw, E., Clavier, C. and Breton, E. 2014, 'Health policy – Why research it and how: Health political science', *Health Research Policy and Systems*, 12(1), p. 55.
Duckett, J. and Langer, A.I. 2013, 'Populism versus neoliberalism: Diversity and ideology in the Chinese media's narratives of health care reform', *Modern China*, 39(6), pp. 653–80.
Felder, M., Wallenburg, I., Kuijper, S., and Bal, R. 2021, 'Taking the relationship between populism and healthcare seriously: A call for empirical analysis rather than moral condemnation', *International Journal of Health Policy and Management*, 10(9), pp. 598–601.
Freeden, M. 2017, 'After the Brexit referendum: Revisiting populism as an ideology', *Journal of Political Ideologies*, 22(1), pp. 1–11.
Greve, B. 2021a 'Reflection upon the development of, and the future for, welfare states', in Greve, B. (ed), *Austerity, Retrenchment and the Welfare State*, Edward Elgar, Cheltenham, pp. 396–400.
Greve, B. 2021b, 'Austerity and the welfare state: An introduction', in Greve, B. (ed), *Austerity, Retrenchment and the Welfare State*, Edward Elgar, Cheltenham, pp. 2–9.
Guasti, P. 2020, 'The impact of the COVID-19 pandemic in Central and Eastern Europe: The rise of autocracy and democratic resilience', *Democratic Theory*, 7(2), pp. 47–60.
Kaltwasser, C.R., Taggart, P.A., Espejo, P.O. and Ostiguy, P. (eds) 2017, *The Oxford Handbook of Populism*, Oxford University Press, Oxford.
Kaltwasser, C.R. and Zanotti, L. 2021, 'Populism and the welfare state', in Greve, B. (ed), *Austerity, Retrenchment and the Welfare State*, Edward Elgar, Cheltenham, pp. 41–53.
Katsambekis, G. and Stavrakakis, Y. 2020, *Populism and the Pandemic: A Collaborative Report*, POPULISMUS Interventions No. 7, POPULISMUS, Thessaloniki, accessed 1 June 2021, <http://populismus.gr/wp-content/uploads/2020/06/interventions-7-populism-pandemic-UPLOAD.pdf>.
Kavakli, K. 2020, 'Did populist leaders respond to the COVID-19 pandemic more slowly? Evidence from a global sample', Bocconi University, Milan, accessed 2 June 2021, <https://www.covidcrisislab.unibocconi.eu/wps/wcm/connect/861fb424-a490-46a6-ba1e-f871867aa40d/Kerim+Can+Kavakli.pdf?MOD=AJPERES&CVID=naYayF6>.
Koltai, J., Varchetta, F.M., McKee, M. and Stuckler, D. 2020, 'Deaths of despair and Brexit votes: Cross-local authority statistical analysis in England and Wales', *American Journal of Public Health*, 110(3), pp. 401–6.
Laclau, E. 2005a, 'Populism: What's in a name?', in Panizza, F. (ed), *Populism and the Mirror of Democracy*, Verso, London, pp. 32–49.
Laclau, E. 2005b, *On Populist Reason*, Verso, London.
Lasco, G. 2020, 'Medical populism and the COVID-19 pandemic', *Global Public Health*, 15(10), pp. 1417–29.
Lasco, G. and Curato, N. 2019, 'Medical populism', *Social Science and Medicine*, 221, pp. 1–8.
Lasco, G. and Larson, H.J. 2020, 'Medical populism and immunisation programmes: Illustrative examples and consequences for public health', *Global Public Health*, 15(3), pp. 334–44.
Lendvai-Bainton, N. and Stubbs, P. 2021, 'Austerity, populism and welfare retrenchment in Central and South-Eastern Europe', in Greve, B. (ed), *Austerity, Retrenchment and the Welfare State*, Edward Elgar, Cheltenham, pp. 207–20.
Levitsky, S. and Way, L.A. 2002, 'Elections without democracy: The rise of competitive authoritarianism', *Journal of Democracy*, 13(2), pp. 51–65.
Mason, A. 2020, *Europe's Future: The Impact of COVID-19 on Populism*, International Development Research Network, Paris, accessed 30 August 2021, <https://idrn.eu/democracy-and-civil-society/europes-future-the-impact-of-covid-19-on-populism>.
McKee, M., Gugushvili, A., Koltai, J. and Stuckler, D. 2021, 'Are populist leaders creating the conditions for the spread of COVID-19?' *International Journal of Health Policy and Management*, 10(8), pp. 511–5.

McLachlan, C.A. 2020, 'Populism, the pandemic and prospects for international law', *KFG Working Paper Series, No. 45*, Potsdam Research Group 'The International Rule of Law – Rise or Decline?', Berlin.
Moffitt, B. and Tormey, S. 2014, 'Rethinking populism: Politics, mediatisation and political style', *Political Studies*, 62(2), pp. 381–97.
Mouffe, C. 2018, *For a Left Populism*, Verso, London.
Mudde, C. 2004, 'The populist zeitgeist', *Government and Opposition*, 39(4), pp. 541–63.
Mudde, C. and Kaltwasser, C.R. 2013, 'Exclusionary vs. inclusionary populism: Comparing contemporary Europe and Latin America', *Government and Opposition*, 48(2), pp. 147–74.
Norris, P. and Inglehart, R. 2019, *Cultural Backlash: Trump, Brexit, and Authoritarian Populism*, Cambridge University Press, Cambridge.
Pavolini, E., Kuhlmann, E., Agartan, T.I., Burau, V., Mannion, R. and Speed, E. 2018, 'Healthcare governance, professions and populism: Is there a relationship? An explorative comparison of five European countries', *Health Policy*, 122(10), pp. 1140–8.
Pereira, C., Medeiros, A. and Bertholini, F. 2020, 'Fear of death and polarization: Political consequences of the COVID-19 pandemic', *Revista de Administração Pública*, 54(4), pp. 952–68.
Powell, M. 2017, 'This is my (post) truth, tell me yours', *International Journal of Health Policy and Management*, 6(12), pp. 723–5.
Rinaldi, C. and Bekker, M.P. 2021, 'A scoping review of populist radical right parties' influence on welfare policy and its implications for population health in Europe', *International Journal of Health Policy and Management*, 10(3), pp. 141–51.
Ringe, N. and Rennó, L. 2023, *Populists and the Pandemic: How Populists Around the World Responded to COVID-19*, Routledge, London.
Roberts, K.M. 1995, 'Neoliberalism and the transformation of populism in Latin America: The Peruvian case', *World Politics*, 48(1), pp. 82–116.
Rooduijn, M. 2014, 'The nucleus of populism: In search of the lowest common denominator', *Government and Opposition*, 49(4), pp. 573–99.
Rooduijn, M. 2019, 'State of the field: How to study populism and adjacent topics? A plea for both more and less focus', *European Journal of Political Research*, 58(1), pp. 362–72.
Schrecker, T. 2017, '"Stop, you're killing us!" An alternative take on populism and public health', *International Journal of Health Policy and Management*, 6(11), pp. 673–5.
Sengul, K. 2021, 'Never let a good crisis go to waste: Pauline Hanson's exploitation of COVID-19 on Facebook', *Media International Australia*, 178(1), pp. 101–5.
Speed, E. and Mannion, R. 2017, 'The rise of post-truth populism in pluralist liberal democracies: Challenges for health policy', *International Journal of Health Policy and Management*, 6(5), pp. 249–51.
Speed, E. and Mannion, R. 2020, 'Populism and health policy: Three international case studies of right-wing populist policy frames', *Sociology of Health and Illness*, 42(8), pp. 1967–81.
Weiffen, B. 2020, 'Latin America and COVID-19: Political rights and presidential leadership to the test', *Democratic Theory*, 7(2), pp. 61–8.
Weyland, K. 1999, 'Neoliberal populism in Latin America and Eastern Europe', *Comparative Politics*, 31(4), pp. 379–401.
Weyland, K. 2001, 'Clarifying a contested concept: Populism in the study of Latin American politics', *Comparative Politics*, 34(1), pp. 1–22.
Weyland, K. 2017, 'Populism: A political-strategic approach', in Kaltwasser, C.R., Taggart, P., Ochoa Espejo, P. and Ostiguy, P. (eds), *The Oxford Handbook of Populism*, Oxford University Press, Oxford, pp. 48–72.
Wilkinson, R. and Pickett, K. 2010, *The Spirit Level: Why Equality Is Better For Everyone*, Bloomsbury Press, London.
Wilson, K., Halabi, S. and Gostin, L.O. 2020, 'The International Health Regulations (2005), the threat of populism and the COVID-19 pandemic', *Globalization and Health*, 16(1), pp. 1–4.
Zienert-Eilts, K.J. 2020, 'Destructive populism as "perverted containing": A psychoanalytical look at the attraction of Donald Trump', *The International Journal of Psychoanalysis*, 101(5), pp. 971–91.

23

TRADE AND INVESTMENT

The re-ordering of healthcare and public health policy?

Deborah Gleeson and Belinda Townsend

Trade and health, often perceived as separate policy fields, are intrinsically and increasingly intertwined. Trade agreements form part of the economic and political architecture that shapes the distribution of power, money and resources at global and national levels. Accordingly, they also configure many determinants of health.

The broad aim of trade and investment agreements (TIAs) is to reduce barriers to the flow of trade in goods, services and investment across borders, often described as 'trade liberalization'. They include a complex set of rules to govern the flow of goods, services and investment between countries. They can be bilateral (between two countries), plurilateral (involving more than two countries) or multilateral (including a large number of countries). The proliferation of trade agreements and increasing commitment to trade liberalization over recent decades have been informed by neoliberal economic theory and intensified processes of globalization. While a contested term, neoliberal theory – which gained prominence in the 1980s and 1990s, and became globalized through international monetary institutions – refers to 'political, economic and social arrangements within society that emphasize market relations [and] re-tasking the role of the state', thereby extending a discourse of 'competitive markets into all areas of life' (Springer *et al.* 2016: 2).

According to neoliberalism, trade liberalization is necessary for national and global economic growth and aggregate social welfare gains. However, empirical studies find that trade-related growth is marginal on average and inequitably distributed within and between countries, with poorer countries potentially losing out under some agreements (Sundaram and von Arnim 2009; Tausch 2016; Stiglitz 2017). Moreover, as we will show, trade agreements have evolved over recent decades beyond commitments on trading goods to encompass wide-ranging rules intended to restrict state regulation of markets – often with consequences for public health.

In this chapter, we describe key changes in the global trade and investment regime over the last two decades in terms of several shifts: multilateralism and the World Trade Organization; the proliferation of bilateral trade agreements; and the negotiation of several 'mega-regional' trade agreements. We explore the linkages between TIAs and healthcare and public health policy. We outline how trade agreements are negotiated and the power dynamics involved therein, and also describe the potential role of social movements and public health advocates in shifting these dynamics in ways that mitigate health risks.

DOI: 10.4324/9781003017110-26

The changing landscape of trade policy: from the WTO to bilateral and regional TIAs

The *General Agreement on Tariffs and Trade* (GATT), established after the Second World War, marked the beginning of a global multilateral trading system with codified rules on trade, with particular emphasis on reducing tariffs on goods. Underpinned by the growing prominence of neoliberalism in global economic institutions and high-income countries, this agreement was replaced in the mid-1990s by the World Trade Organization (WTO). The creation of the WTO, intended to provide an intergovernmental forum for settling trade disputes between trading partners, was guided by commitments to progressive trade liberalization and non-discrimination between trading partners. The birth of the WTO also led to an expansion of multilateral trade rules beyond tariffs to encompass regulatory measures and binding obligations on trade-related topics including agriculture, trade in services, intellectual property rights, sanitary and phytosanitary measures, and technical barriers to trade (Labonté 2002). For example, the establishment of the *Agreement on Trade-Related Aspects of Intellectual Property Rights* (TRIPS) – a foundational agreement established at the time of the formation of the WTO – established global rules on intellectual property (IP) protection and enforcement to which countries had to agree in order to join the WTO. The role of multinational pharmaceutical and IP-intensive corporations in shaping TRIPS through lobbying high-income country (HIC) governments has been well documented, and the agreement has been widely criticized for restricting access to medicines (Sell 2003).

These and other critical reflections on the WTO's neoliberal agenda throughout the 1990s and 2000s led to disagreements between low- and middle-income countries (LMICs) and HICs over the rules governing world trade and the stalling of WTO trade negotiations. The WTO's Doha Round, which commenced in 2001, was intended to respond to the development needs of LMICs. The negotiations have since stalled and effectively ceased, however, due to the lack of agreement between countries. Particularly controversial have been several HICs continuing to provide domestic agricultural subsidies and refusing to liberalize in areas that could face increased market competition from LMICs.

With this stalling of multilateral trade negotiations at the WTO, there has been an increase over the past two decades in bilateral and regional trade agreements, often driven by the United States or European Union (Baldwin 2011; Gleeson and Friel 2013). These agreements focus less on preferential market access (although this remains a key element), and more on the regulatory regimes that underpin increasingly complex supply chains and trade in services and investment (Baldwin 2011; Ravenhill 2014). Characterized by power asymmetries between economically powerful states such as the US, and LMICs, these agreements have created new rules beyond those contained within WTO agreements ('WTO-Plus' provisions) that have progressively constrained the policy space available to governments in many policy areas, including health. 'Policy space' has been usefully defined by Koivusalo *et al.* (2009: 105) as 'the freedom, scope and mechanisms that governments have to choose, design and implement public policies to fulfil their aims'.

For example, the mega-regional Trans-Pacific Partnership (TPP), negotiated originally between 12 Pacific Rim countries, included WTO-Plus provisions in areas such as IP and technical barriers to trade. It also featured novel chapters not included in previous trade agreements, addressing issues such as state-owned enterprises and regulatory coherence, and annexes applying to specific products and sectors, many of which had health implications (Labonté *et al.* 2016). Other plurilateral agreements negotiated in recent years have continued to layer WTO-plus provisions that constrain policy space, thereby engendering public health concerns, which we explore in the following section.

The impact of trade agreements on healthcare and public health policy

In this section, we briefly outline the implications of TIAs for healthcare and public health policy, focusing on health services, access to pharmaceuticals and harmful commodities. It is important to note that TIAs can affect many other determinants of health, such as wage inequality, employment and labor rights, and environmental degradation (*e.g.* Gleeson and Labonté 2020). They may also influence government finances, including public health budgets (Barlow 2020). However, these issues remain beyond the scope of this chapter.

Health services

Services and investment, including health services, are an increasing focus of TIAs. The WTO *General Agreement on Trade in Services* (GATS), which came into force in 1995, was the first multilateral agreement to liberalize services. GATS covers four types of health services delivery: the cross-border supply of health services (*e.g.* e-health activities and health insurance claim processing), consumption abroad ('health tourism'), commercial presence (establishment of a service in a host country) and movement of natural persons (temporary movement of health workers from one territory to another) (Sauve *et al.* 2015). However, most WTO members did not commit to opening their health sectors under GATS (Smith *et al.* 2009).

Health services have also been addressed increasingly by regional TIAs, which tend to involve much more extensive liberalization than GATS (Mashayekhi and Tuerk 2015). Recently, TIAs have moved away from a 'positive list' approach (naming those sectors and modes that will be opened to competition) toward a 'negative list' approach (where services rules cover all sectors, modes and services except those explicitly excluded at the time of the agreement). Negative list approaches reduce policy flexibility and increase the risk of inadvertently opening up sectors and services that should have been excluded from services commitments (Mashayekhi and Tuerk 2015).

Liberalization of the health sector can improve the range and quality of health services and technologies, improve access to services for remote populations and, in some cases, may reduce health system costs (Sauve *et al.* 2015). However, many opportunities provided by increased trade in high-technology healthcare can only be exploited by developed countries (Smith *et al.* 2009; Sauve *et al.* 2015). These prospects can also be realized without entering into binding, potentially irreversible commitments in international treaties that necessitate sacrificing some degree of policy flexibility. Risks associated with health services liberalization include diversion of resources from public to private systems, and from primary care to export-oriented high-technology diagnostic and treatment services, as well as potentially augmenting inequities in access to care and exacerbating the 'brain drain' of health professionals from resource-poor settings (Missoni 2013; Sauve *et al.* 2015).

Trade in services commitments do not generally cover public health services that do not engage in commercial activities (Sauve *et al.* 2015), and do not force countries to privatize their health services. Yet, when governments do privatize services, binding commitments in TIAs can make it difficult to 'unwind' privatization and reconfigure health systems according to population need and governmental priorities (Smith *et al.* 2009). Services privatized by one government may not be able to be returned to governmental control by the next.

Access to pharmaceuticals

The negotiation of the TRIPS Agreement was a key development that has shaped access to medicines since the end of the Twentieth Century. Prior to TRIPS, patent terms varied between countries, with some – such as India – not granting pharmaceutical product patents before entering the

WTO ('t Hoen 2009). TRIPS set a standard of 20-year patent terms and introduced a number of other intellectual property rights (IPRs), which favored the research-based global pharmaceutical industry (Sell 2007).

TRIPS included a degree of flexibility for countries in designing their domestic IP regimes according to domestic priorities, provided certain standards were met. An illustrative example is the right to use compulsory licenses to bypass patents in certain situations, including emergencies. WTO members' rights to use compulsory licensing and other TRIPS flexibilities were affirmed by the Doha *Declaration on the TRIPS Agreement and Public Health* (WTO 2001). However, TRIPS has been criticized heavily for entrenching and expanding pharmaceutical monopolies and placing life-saving medicines beyond the reach of millions of people in LMICs (Sell 2007; 't Hoen 2009). TRIPS flexibilities, including compulsory licenses, have been rarely utilized, partly due to subsequent bilateral and regional trade agreements that include more onerous provisions, along with other forms of pressure exerted by the US, EU and global pharmaceutical industry ('t Hoen 2009).

The COVID-19 pandemic has highlighted the limitations TRIPS places on access to new pharmaceutical products. Monopoly rights enshrined in TRIPS have allowed a small number of companies to control production of COVID-19 vaccines and limit global competition, restricting the global supply of these life-saving products. By November 2022 – almost three years into the pandemic, with almost 13 billion vaccine doses administered globally – only 23.1 percent of people in low-income countries had received a dose, in comparison with 68 percent of the global population (Global Change Data Lab 2022). In October 2020, India and South Africa made a proposal to the WTO for a temporary suspension of certain IP provisions within the TRIPS Agreement for COVID-19 medical products during the pandemic (WTO 2020). Known as the 'TRIPS waiver', this suspension would have bolstered the global supply of critical products, such as COVID-19 vaccines, by allowing them to be manufactured by Latin American, African and Asian firms (Moon *et al.* 2021). While the 'TRIPS waiver' proposal gained the support of over 100 WTO member-states, the EU and several other high-income countries initially opposed, and then progressively watered down, the proposal to the point where it became a 'narrowly defined, time-bound and highly circumscribed exception to the rules' (World Health Organization Council on the Economics of Health for All 2022: n.p.).

Many bilateral and regional trade agreements, particularly those negotiated by the US and EU, have expanded IPRs beyond those in TRIPS (Sell 2007; Lopert and Gleeson 2013). 'TRIPS-Plus' IPRs, which have become standard features of US trade agreements, include patents for new uses and methods of using existing drugs, patent term extensions, data exclusivity (preventing generic manufacturers from using clinical data submitted to regulatory agencies for a period of time) and patent linkage mechanisms (linking marketing approval to patent status). A growing empirical literature links these TRIPS-Plus IPRs to reduced access to generic drugs and increased costs for governments and consumers, particularly in LMICs (Islam *et al.* 2019; Tenni *et al.* 2022).

More recently, TIAs (particularly those to which the US is party) have also targeted other aspects of pharmaceutical policy and regulation. For example, provisions targeting pharmaceutical pricing and reimbursement, and the regulation of direct-to-consumer advertising, were proposed by the country in its agreements with Australia and South Korea, along with the TPP (Lopert and Gleeson 2013). The *Comprehensive and Progressive Agreement on Trans-Pacific Partnership* (CPTPP) – the amended TPP that arose following the US' withdrawal from negotiations – targets procedures for assessing drug safety and efficacy. Its components have, in turn, been included in subsequent agreements, including the *United States-Mexico-Canada Agreement* (USMCA) renegotiation of the *North American Free Trade Agreement* (NAFTA) (Gleeson *et al.* 2019; Labonté *et al.* 2019).

Public health policy: regulating tobacco, alcohol and food

Global trade and the TIAs that facilitate it are integrally linked with rising rates of non-communicable diseases (NCDs), particularly in LMICs (Labonté *et al.* 2011). These agreements have facilitated trade in harmful commodities, as well as placing increasing constraints on the policy space available to countries to address rising rates of NCDs (Thow 2009; Friel *et al.* 2015; Schram *et al.* 2015; Barlow *et al.* 2017).

Liberalization of trade in tobacco, for instance, has resulted in lower tariffs, increasing availability and lower prices, along with increased advertising and promotion (Friel *et al.* 2015). A study of 42 countries using data from 1970 to 1995 (Taylor *et al.* 2000) found that trade liberalization drove increases in cigarette consumption over this period, particularly in LMICs.

The tobacco industry has simultaneously used TIAs to challenge countries' efforts to regulate tobacco packaging in line with the recommendations of the WHO's *Framework Convention on Tobacco Control* (FCTC). Australia faced complaints brought by Ukraine, Honduras, Indonesia, Dominican Republic and Cuba at the WTO over its tobacco plain packaging legislation (Australian Government Attorney-General's Department n.d.). Uruguay and Australia have also both been forced to defend their tobacco control measures against investor-state disputes where market actors, in this case, tobacco companies, have directly initiated claims of compensation (Mitchell 2016). The investor-state dispute settlement (ISDS) case against each was ultimately unsuccessful. The case against Australia was dismissed on jurisdictional grounds. The tribunal ruled that the claim was an abuse of rights – Philip Morris Asia had acquired an Australian subsidiary after the announcement that plain packaging would be introduced, in order to utilize the ISDS mechanism in a bilateral investment treaty between Australia and Hong Kong (Australian Government Attorney-General's Department n.d.). Philip Morris' claim against Uruguay under a bilateral investment treaty between Switzerland and Uruguay was rejected on the grounds that Uruguay's tobacco control measures did not breach the agreement (McCabe Centre for Law and Cancer 2016). While both cases were ultimately rejected, Australia was left to cover approximately A$12 million in arbitration costs (Hepburn 2019), and both cases took several years to resolve.

Moreover, trade liberalization increases the availability and affordability of alcoholic beverages, as well as facilitating their promotion and advertising (Zeigler 2009; Labonté *et al.* 2011; Friel *et al.* 2015; Schram *et al.* 2019). The alcohol industry has actively lobbied for increased market access through trade negotiations, including the WTO and bilateral and regional trade agreements (Zeigler 2009). Along with reducing tariffs on alcoholic beverages and increasing penetration of transnational corporations, TIAs include a range of other rules that can present obstacles to regulating the production, sale, labeling, licensing and marketing of alcoholic beverages (Zeigler 2009; Miller *et al.* 2021). For example, the WTO *Agreement on Technical Barriers to Trade* (TBT) aims to ensure that technical regulations and standards do not create unnecessary obstacles to trade. These rules apply to labeling requirements such as health warnings on alcohol containers. Under the TBT Agreement, WTO members are obliged to ensure that imported products are treated no less favorably than 'like' domestic products, and that technical regulations are not more trade restrictive than necessary, while also being encouraged to base measures on international standards (WTO 1995).

Proposals for alcohol health warnings (along with other alcohol, tobacco and food regulations) have also frequently faced challenges at the WTO TBT Committee (Barlow and Stuckler 2021). Therein, the arguments of member-state representatives often reflect well-established industry arguments against public health policies (Barlow and Thow 2021; Barlow *et al.* 2022). New rules on labeling for wine and spirits, first included in the TPP/CPTPP and subsequently incorporated into at least five further trade agreements, oblige importing countries to permit alcohol suppliers to use supplementary labels to display required information (O'Brien *et al.* 2017; Gleeson and O'Brien 2021). While these rules do not expressly prevent governments from mandating evidence-based health warnings, they may create additional obstacles to the introduction of the best-practice health warning schemes.

Trade agreements have accelerated the nutrition transition in LMICs through several pathways, including trade in ultra-processed foods, foreign direct investment in supermarkets, and increased advertising by transnational food companies (Friel *et al.* 2013). Evidence supporting this relationship includes studies of NAFTA and trade liberalization in Central America. Hawkes and Thow (2009), for example, showed that two decades of trade liberalization in Central America resulted in increased availability and consumption of products associated with obesity and chronic diseases, including meat and processed foods. NAFTA similarly led to major changes in the importation of unhealthy food in Mexico, along with increased foreign direct investment by food and beverage companies (Clarke *et al.* 2012).

A further case study is provided by the Pacific Islands, where trade liberalization has increased importation of processed foods, contributing to high rates of obesity and NCDs (Snowdon and Thow 2013), although recent studies have suggested a complex picture with increases in availability of both healthy and unhealthy imported foods (Ravuvu *et al.* 2017; Ravuvu *et al.* 2021). Recent quantitative studies based on natural experiments have added to the evidence base by tracing the effects of trade liberalization in increasing in sugar-sweetened beverage consumption (Stuckler *et al.* 2012), sales (Schram *et al.* 2015) and production (Baker *et al.* 2016).

TIAs can also reduce the policy space available for governments to reduce diet-related disease. Examples include Thailand's move away from a traffic-light nutrition labeling scheme following claims by other countries that the proposal breached the WTO's TBT agreement (Friel *et al.* 2015) and Samoa's removal of its ban on turkey tail imports during its accession to the WTO (Thow *et al.* 2015). Recently negotiated regional TIAs, such as the CPTPP and USMCA, have raised concerns about how these agreements engender additional constraints on policy interventions to address diet-related disease (Labonté *et al.* 2019; Labonté *et al.* 2020).

Power, politics and inequalities

The conditions under which TIAs are negotiated and the power relationships that shape trade negotiations are important in determining their effects on health. Trade negotiations involve trade-offs between different sectors and priorities: countries will often sacrifice outcomes in one sector or industry to secure desired objectives in others. In this context, health ambitions such as access to affordable medicines can be traded for access to markets, with the hope of bringing economic gains that offset the negative impacts.

Bilateral and regional TIAs are generally negotiated out of the public eye, and there is little if any public access to negotiating documents. This contrasts with the level of access afforded to business interests during discussions, particularly transnational corporations and industry associations. This imbalance is particularly prominent in the US, where trade policy is shaped by trade advisory committees, populated by leaders of large corporations and business associations (Gleeson *et al.* 2017).

Industry interests also tend to have close ties with trade officials and interact with them frequently (Gleeson *et al.* 2017). Shared neoliberal ideas around market competition and a reduced role for the state between government trade officials and industry actors tend to reflect industry priorities in trade policy. Because trade officials often see the purpose of trade agreements as being 'for industry' (Townsend *et al.* 2020), corporate actors frequently report greater satisfaction than public health and NGO actors with the mechanisms available to advance their interests during trade dialogues (Battams and Townsend 2019). These include processes 'inside' the trade policy system, such as attending official consultations, or lobbying government on the sidelines of negotiating rounds; as well as processes 'outside' the trade domain, like participating in parliamentary inquiries, or shaping public opinion through the media (Friel *et al.* 2019).

Differences in power exist also between government portfolios and departments. For example, in Malaysia, health officials reported a general lack of consultation with trade officials and reliance on leaked text to identify potential health concerns. Similarly, in Australia, health officials have reported power imbalances with trade officials, making them reliant on trade officials to identify whether a TIA might affect public health measures (Battams and Townsend 2019).

Simultaneously, while the WTO is a *prima facie* democratic institution (each member has one vote), dynamics behind the scenes work to undermine this appearance. An example is the informal invitation-only 'green room' meetings favored by HICs, which involve non-transparent discussions among an elite group to reach a consensus on key issues (Jawara and Kwa 2004). LMICs are also at a disadvantage in the WTO due to the size of their negotiating teams, with some lacking even permanent missions in Geneva (Jawara and Kwa 2004). Essentially, WTO negotiations reflect existing patterns of power and inequality.

Power asymmetries are even more prominent in bilateral and regional TIAs, where LMICs often need to make more concessions than their trading partners (Ravenhill 2014). This is particularly the case when LMICs enter trade negotiations with large economies such as the US and EU, which largely set the agenda for trade negotiations (Ravenhill 2014). Trade negotiations are expensive and skills-intensive, requiring infrastructure that small and poorer countries often struggle to secure (Walls *et al.* 2015).

Resistance and de-legitimation: WikiLeaks, social movements and public health advocacy

The efforts of wealthy countries and transnational corporations to use TIAs to advance their interests have not gone uncontested. The *Doha Declaration*, as mentioned earlier, represents one (albeit limited) 'win' for LMICs against a powerful coalition of wealthy countries and the global pharmaceutical industry (Drahos 2007). Attempts by the US and EU to secure corporate-friendly rules, IPRs and investor-state dispute settlement processes, have been greeted with robust opposition from community groups and NGOs in many countries. A particularly pertinent example may be found in the resistance of Thai HIV/AIDS groups to US pressures for elevated levels of IP protection and pharmaceutical monopolies in the then-proposed Thai-US free trade agreement (which arguably contributed to its ultimate derailment).

The TPP also sparked strong community and NGO responses in countries such as the US, Australia and New Zealand, which arguably contributed to the US' withdrawal from the agreement. A key catalyst of these community responses was the release by several civil society organizations, including WikiLeaks, of successive drafts of US proposals and other negotiating documents, which exposed the often-egregious nature of the proposals and undermined the reassurances offered by trade ministers to stakeholders. Kampmark (2016) describes how these revelations by WikiLeaks and others triggered extensive public debate on what would otherwise have been arcane and secret.

The TPP negotiations were also met with a vigorous response from public health groups, including the Public Health Association of Australia (PHAA) and its counterpart in New Zealand. For example, a health impact assessment of the proposed TPP led by the PHAA, based on leaked negotiating documents (Hirono *et al.* 2015), received extensive media coverage and catalyzed statements from parliamentarians that arguably contributed to mitigating some of the more extreme pharmaceutical provisions (Hirono *et al.* 2016). Analysis of Australia's participation in the TPP has illustrated that both material and ideational conditions were important in explaining why some health issues, such as access to medicines, received greater attention than others (Townsend *et al.* 2020). These conditions include the strength of country exporter interests; political will of Trade and Health Ministers; framing of health issues; political party support; exogenous influencing events, such as ISDS cases; strength of evidence regarding the health issue; and the presence of existing domestic and international treaties (Townsend *et al.* 2020).

Social movements continue to play an important role in challenging the codification and expansion of corporate power in new-generation trade agreements. Movements have brought together farmers, indigenous peoples, public health advocates, Internet and access advocates, and trade unions around shared public interest concerns. Collectively, such broad coalitions have defeated corporate trade deals, such as the proposed EU-India free trade agreement, and the regional *Anti-Counterfeiting Trade Agreement* (James 2014). Civil society movements have also 'broken-open' previously closed regional trade agreement negotiations, such that they were more receptive to public health evidence and analysis, while also advancing greater public attention to health issues in those negotiations – particularly around access to medicines (Townsend 2021).

One of the key structural changes needed, in order to support greater consideration of public health objectives during trade negotiations, is reform of the trade treaty-making processes. Ultimately, public health movements and advocacy have experienced several barriers, including a lack of transparency around trade agreements; little involvement and no substantive consultation on what is being negotiated; minimal involvement of parliamentarians in trade processes; and no independent health impact assessments of trade treaties before, during or after they are signed. By relying on leaks, framing strategies and the formation of networks, social movements have had some influence, as described above. Yet, a re-orientation of the purpose of trade agreements is urgently required: connecting these to wider social and public interests, as well as to reforms that will enable public health and public interest engagement and assessment.

Conclusion

The proliferation of TIAs in recent decades, deeply rooted in globalization and neoliberalism, has had serious consequences for health. While agreements can facilitate greater access to health-promoting goods, other binding commitments can 'lock-in' liberalization of health services, constrain access to generic medicines, and impede efforts to regulate products associated with NCDs, thus re-shaping both healthcare and public health policy. The risk that TIAs will undermine health is exacerbated by the dynamics of trade negotiations, wherein industry interests and wealthy countries wield the greatest influence. Social movements and activism, however, have been important in successfully countering or mitigating many of the worst excesses of the neoliberal trade and investment regime.

References

Australian Government Attorney-General's Department. n.d., 'Tobacco plain packaging: Investor-state arbitration', Australian Government Attorney-General's Department, Canberra, accessed 4 December 2016, <https://www.ag.gov.au/tobaccoplainpackaging>.

Baker, P., Friel, S., Schram, A. and Labonté, R. 2016, 'Trade and investment liberalization, food systems change and highly processed food consumption: A natural experiment contrasting the soft-drink markets of Peru and Bolivia', *Globalization and Health*, 12, pp. 1–13.

Baldwin, R. 2011, *21st Century Regionalism: Filling the Gap Between 21st Century Trade and 20th Century Trade Rules*, Graduate Institute, Geneva.

Barlow, P. 2020, 'Global disparities in health-systems financing: A cross-national analysis of the impact of tariff reductions and state capacity on public health expenditure in 65 low- and middle-income countries, 1996–2015', *Health and Place*, 63, p. 102329.

Barlow, P., Gleeson, D., O'Brien, P. and Labonté, R. 2022, 'Industry influence over global alcohol policies via the World Trade Organization: A qualitative analysis of discussions on alcohol health warning labelling, 2010–19', *The Lancet Global Health,* 10(3), pp. e429–37.

Barlow, P., McKee, M., Basu, S. and Stuckler, D. 2017, 'The health impact of trade and investment agreements: A quantitative systematic review and network co-citation analysis', *Globalization and Health*, 13, pp. 1–9.

Barlow, P. and Stuckler, D. 2021, 'Globalization and health policy space: Introducing the WTO health dataset of trade challenges to national health regulations at world trade organization, 1995–2016', *Social Science and Medicine*, 275, p. 113807.

Barlow, P. and Thow, A.M. 2021, 'Neoliberal discourse, actor power, and the politics of nutrition policy: A qualitative analysis of informal challenges to nutrition labelling regulations at the World Trade Organization, 2007–2019', *Social Science and Medicine*, 273, p. 113761.

Battams, S. and Townsend, B. 2019, 'Power asymmetries, policy incoherence and noncommunicable disease control – A qualitative study of policy actor views', *Critical Public Health,* 29(5), pp. 596–609.

Clarke, S.E., Hawkes, C., Murphy, S.M., Hansen-Kuhn, K. and Wallinga, D. 2012, 'Exporting obesity: US farm and trade policy and the transformation of the Mexican consumer food environment', *International Journal of Occupational and Environmental Health*, 18(1), pp. 53–65.

Drahos, P. 2007, 'Four lessons for developing countries from the trade negotiations over access to medicines', *Liverpool Law Review*, 28, pp. 11–39.

Friel, S., Baker, P., Thow, A.-M., Gleeson, D., Townsend, B. and Schram, A. 2019, 'An exposé of the realpolitik of trade negotiations: Implications for population nutrition', *Public Health Nutrition*, 22(16), pp. 3083–91.

Friel, S., Gleeson, D., Thow, A.-M., Labonté, R., Stuckler, D., Kay, A. and Snowdon, W. 2013, 'A new generation of trade policy: Potential risks to diet-related health from the trans pacific partnership agreement. ', *Globalization and Health*, 9, pp. 1–7.

Friel, S., Hattersley, L. and Townsend, R. 2015, 'Trade policy and public health', *Annual Review of Public Health*, 36, pp. 325–44.

Gleeson, D. and Friel, S. 2013, 'Emerging threats to public health from regional trade agreements', *The Lancet*, 381(9876), pp. 1507–9.

Gleeson, D. and Labonté, R. 2020, *Trade Agreements and Public Health: A Primer for Health Policy Makers, Researchers and Advocates*, Palgrave MacMillan, Singapore.

Gleeson, D., Lexchin, J., Labonté, R., Townsend, B., Gagnon, M.-A., Kohler, J., Forman, L. and Shadlen, K.C. 2019, 'Analyzing the impact of trade and investment agreements on pharmaceutical policy: Provisions, pathways and potential impacts', *Globalization and Health*, 15, pp. 1–17.

Gleeson, D., Neuwelt, P., Monasterio, E. and Lopert, R. 2017, 'How the transnational pharmaceutical industry pursues its interests through international trade and investment agreements: A case study of the Trans Pacific partnership agreement', in de Jonge, A. and Tomasic, R. (eds), *Research Handbook on Transnational Corporations*, Edward Elgar, Cheltenham, pp. 223–54.

Gleeson, D. and O'Brien, P. 2021, 'Alcohol labelling rules in free trade agreements: Advancing the industry's interests at the expense of the public's health', *Drug and Alcohol Review*, 40(1), pp. 31–40.

Global Change Data Lab. 2022, 'Coronavirus (COVID-19) vaccinations', *Our World in Data*, accessed 18 February 2022, <https://ourworldindata.org/covid-vaccinations>.

Hepburn, J. 2019, 'Final costs details are released in Philip Morris v. Australia following request by IAReporter', *Investment Arbitration Reporter*, accessed 7 April 2022, <https://www.iareporter.com/articles/final-costs-details-are-released-in-philip-morris-v-australia-following-request-by-iareporter/>.

Hirono, K., Haigh, F., Gleeson, D., Harris, P. and Thow, A.-M. 2015, *Negotiating healthy trade in Australia: Health impact assessment of the proposed Trans-Pacific Partnership Agreement*, Centre for Health Equity Training Research and Evaluation, UNSW, Sydney.

Hirono, K., Haigh, F., Gleeson, D., Harris, P., Thow, A.-M. and Friel, S. 2016, 'Is health impact assessment useful in the context of trade negotiations? A case study of the Trans Pacific Partnership Agreement', *BMJ Open*, 6(4), p. e010339.

Islam, M.D., Kaplan, W.A., Trachtenberg, D., Thrasher, R., Gallagher, K.P. and Wirtz, V.J. 2019, 'Impacts of intellectual property provisions in trade treaties on access to medicine in low and middle income countries: A systematic review', *Globalization and Health*, 15, pp. 1–14

James, L. 2014, 'The anti-counterfeiting trade agreement and european civil society: A case study on networked advocacy', *Journal of Information Policy*, 4, pp. 205–27.

Jawara, F. and Kwa, A. 2004, *Behind the Scenes at the WTO: The Real World of International Trade Negotiations – Lessons of Cancun*, Zed Books, London.

Kampmark, B. 2016, 'Radical transparency in geopolitical economy: WikiLeaks, secret diplomacy and the Trans-Pacific partnership agreement', *Journal of Global Faultlines,* 3(1), pp. 1–15.

Koivusalo, M., Schrecker, T. and Labonté, R. 2009, 'Globalization and policy space for health and social determinants of health', in Labonté, R., Schrecker, T., Packer, C. and Runnels, V. (eds), *Globalization and Health: Pathways, Evidence and Policy*, Routledge, New York, pp. 105–30.

Labonté, R. 2002, 'International governance and World Trade Organization (WTO) reform', *Critical Public Health*, 12(1), pp. 65–86.

Labonté, R., Crosbie, E., Gleeson, D. and McNamara, C. 2019, 'USMCA (NAFTA 2.0): Tightening the constraints on the right to regulate for public health', *Globalization and Health*, 15, pp. 1–15.

Labonté, R., Gleeson, D. and McNamara, C.L. 2020, 'USMCA 2.0: A few improvements but far from a "healthy" trade treaty', *Globalization and Health*, 16, pp. 1–4.

Labonté, R., Mohindra, K.S. and Lencucha, R. 2011, 'Framing international trade and chronic disease', *Globalization and Health*, 7, pp. 1–15.

Labonté, R., Schram, A. and Ruckert, A. 2016, 'The Trans Pacific Partnership: Is it everything we feared for health?', *International Journal of Health Policy and Management*, 5(8), pp. 487–96.

Lopert, R. and Gleeson, D. 2013, 'The high price of "free" trade: US trade agreements and access to medicines', *Journal of Law, Medicine and Ethics*, 41(1), pp. 199–223.

Mashayekhi, M. and Tuerk, E. 2015, 'Regional trade agreements and health services', in Smith, R., Blouin, C., Mirza, Z., Beyer, P. and Drager, N. (eds), *Trade and Health: Towards Building a National Strategy*, World Health Organization, Geneva, pp. 56–75.

McCabe Centre for Law and Cancer. 2016, *The Award on the Merits in Philip Morris v Uruguay: Implications for WHO FCTC Implementation*, McCabe Centre for Law and Cancer, Melbourne.

Miller, M., Wilkinson, C., Room, R., O'Brien, P., Townsend, B., Schram, A. and Gleeson, D. 2021, 'Industry submissions on alcohol in the context of Australia's trade and investment agreements: A content and thematic analysis of publicly available documents', *Drug and Alcohol Review*, 40(1), pp. 22–30.

Missoni, E. 2013, 'Understanding the impact of global trade liberalization on health systems pursuing universal health coverage', *Value in Health*, 16, pp. S14–8.

Mitchell, A.D. 2016, 'Tobacco packaging measures affecting intellectual property protection under international investment law: The claims against Uruguay and Australia', in Alemanno, A. and Bonadio, E. (eds), *The New Intellectual Property of Health: Beyond Plain Packaging*, Edward Elgar, Cheltenham, pp. 213–32.

Moon, S., Alonso Ruiz, A. and Vieira, M. 2021, 'Averting future vaccine injustice', *New England Journal of Medicine*, 385(3), pp. 193–6.

O'Brien, P., Gleeson, D., Room, R. and Wilkinson, C. 2017, 'Marginalising health information: Implications of the Trans Pacific Partnership for alcohol labelling', *Melbourne University Law Review*, 41(1), pp. 341–91.

Ravenhill, J. 2014, 'Global value chains and development', *Review of Political Economy*, 21(1), pp. 264–74.

Ravuvu, A., Friel, S., Thow, A.-M., Snowdon, W. and Wate, J. 2017, 'Monitoring the impact of trade agreements on national food environments: Trade imports and population nutrition risks in Fiji', *Globalization and Health*, 13, pp. 1–17.

Ravuvu, A., Lui, J.P., Bani, A., Tavoa, A.W., Vuti, R. and Win Tin, S.T. 2021, 'Analysing the impact of trade agreements on national food environments: The case of Vanuatu', *Globalization and Health*, 17, pp. 1–15.

Sauve, P., Blouin, C., Bhushan, A. and Cattaneo, O. 2015, 'Trade in health services', in Smith, R., Blouin, C., Mirza, Z., Beyer, P. and Drager, N. (eds), *Trade and Health: Towards Building a National Strategy*, World Health Organization, Geneva, pp. 76–91.

Schram, A., Aisbett, E., Townsend, B., Labonté, R., Baum, F. and Friel, S. 2019, 'Toxic trade: The impact of preferential trade agreements on alcohol imports from Australia in partner countries', *Addiction*, 115(4), pp. 1277–84.

Schram, A., Labonté, R., Baker, P., Friel, S., Reeves, A. and Stuckler, D. 2015, 'The role of trade and investment liberalization in the sugar-sweetened carbonated beverages market: A natural experiment contrasting Vietnam and the Philippines', *Globalization and Health*, 11, pp. 1–13.

Sell, S.K. 2003, *Private Power, Public Law: The Globalization of Intellectual Property Rights*, Cambridge University Press, Cambridge.

Sell, S.K. 2007, 'TRIPS-Plus free trade agreements and access to medicines', *Liverpool Law Review*, 28, pp. 41–75.

Smith, R.D., Chanda, R. and Tangcharoensathien, V. 2009, 'Trade in health-related services', *Lancet*, 373(9663), pp. 593–601.

Snowdon, W. and Thow, A.-M. 2013, 'Trade policy and obesity prevention: Challenges and innovation in the Pacific Islands', *Obesity Reviews*, 14(S2), pp. 150–8.

Springer, S., Birch, K., and MacLeavy, J. 2016, *The Handbook of Neoliberalism*, Routledge, London.

Stiglitz, J.E. 2017, 'The overselling of globalization', *Business Economics*, 52(3), pp. 129–37.

Stuckler, D., McKee, M., Ebrahim, S. and Basu, S. 2012, 'Manufacturing epidemics: The role of global producers in increased consumption of unhealthy commodities including processed foods, alcohol and tobacco', *PLoS Medicine*, 9(6), p. e1001235.

Sundaram, J.K. and von Arnim, R. 2009, 'Trade liberalization and economic development', *Science*, 323(5911), pp. 211–2.

Tausch, A. 2016, 'Is globalization really good for public health?', *The International Journal of Health Planning and Management*, 31(4), pp. 511–36.

Taylor, A., Chaloupka, F.J., Guindon, E. and Corbett, M. 2000, 'The impact of trade liberalization on tobacco consumption', in Jha, P. and Chaloupka, F.J. (eds), *Tobacco Control in Developing Countries*, Oxford University Press, Oxford, pp. 343–64.

Tenni, B., Moir, H.V.J., Townsend, B., Kilic, B., Farrell, A.-M., Keegel, T. and Gleeson, D. 2022, 'What is the impact of intellectual property rules on access to medicines? A systematic review', *Globalization and Health*, 18, pp. 1–40.

't Hoen, E. 2009, *The Global Politics of Pharmaceutical Monopoly Power: Drug Patents, Access, Innovation and the Application of the WTO Doha Declaration on TRIPS and Public Health*, AMB Publishers, The Netherlands.

Thow, A.-M. 2009, 'Trade liberalisation and the nutrition transition: Mapping the pathways for public health nutritionists', *Public Health Nutrition*, 12(11), pp. 2150–8.

Thow, A.-M. and Hawkes, C. 2009, 'The implications of trade liberalization for diet and health: A case study from Central America', *Globalization and Health*, 5, pp. 1–15.

Thow, A.-M., Snowdon, W., Labonté, R., Gleeson, D., Stuckler, D., Hattersley, L., Schram, A., Kay, A. and Friel, S. 2015, 'Will the next generation of preferential trade and investment agreeements undermine the prevention of noncommunicable diseases? A prospective policy analysis of the Trans Pacific Partnership Agreement', *Health Policy*, 119(1), pp. 88–96.

Townsend, B. 2021, 'Defending access to medicines in regional trade agreements: Lessons from the Regional Comprehensive Economic Partnership – A qualitative study of policy actors' views', *Globalization and Health*, 17, pp. 1–14.

Townsend, B., Friel, S., Schram, A., Baum, F. and Labonté, R. 2020, 'What generates attention to health in trade policy-making? Lessons from success in tobacco control and access to medicines: a qualitative study of Australia and the (comprehensive and progressive) Trans-Pacific Partnership', *International Journal of Health Policy and Management*, 10(10), pp. 613–24.

Townsend, B., Schram, A., Baum, F., Labonté, R. and Friel, S. 2020, 'How does policy framing enable or constrain inclusion of social determinants of health and health equity on trade policy agendas?', *Critical Public Health*, 30(1), pp. 115–26.

Walls, H.L., Smith, R.D. and Drahos, P. 2015, 'Improving regulatory capacity to manage risks associated with trade agreements', *Globalization and Health*, 11, pp. 1–5.

World Health Organization Council on the Economics of Health for All. 2022, *The New WTO Decision on the TRIPS Agreement*, World Health Organization, Geneva.

World Trade Organization. 1995, *Agreement on Technical Barriers to Trade*, accessed 21 January 2023, <https://www.wto.org/english/docs_e/legal_e/17-tbt_e.htm>.

World Trade Organization. 2001, *Declaration on the TRIPS Agreement and Public Health*, accessed 21 January 2023, < https://www.wto.org/english/thewto_e/minist_e/min01_e/mindecl_trips_e.htm>.

World Trade Organization. 2020, *Waiver from Certain Provisions of the TRIPS Agreement for the Prevention, Containment and Treatment of COVID-19: Communication from India and South Africa. Council for Trade-Related Aspects of Intellectual Property Rights, IC/C/W/669*, accessed 21 January 2023, <https://docs.wto.org/dol2fe/Pages/SS/directdoc.aspx?filename=q:/IP/C/W669.pdfandOpen=True>.

Zeigler, D.W. 2009, 'The alcohol industry and trade agreements: A preliminary assessment', *Addiction*, 104(S1), pp. 13–26.

24

UNIVERSAL HEALTH COVERAGE

A case-study of the political economy of global health

David G. Legge

Universal health coverage (UHC) is the leading slogan in global health policy today. It is also a social movement – albeit, one primarily populated by economists, academics, policy think tanks, global philanthropists, and transnational corporations. The outcomes promised by the slogan – access to essential healthcare and protection from catastrophic healthcare costs – are admirable. However, an exploration of the implementation pathways prefigured in the policy narrative reveals unacknowledged contradictions and silences which, in turn, cast doubt on its promises. They point, instead, to an agenda fostering the irreversible installation of marketized, privatized, multitiered healthcare.

In making this case, the chapter commences with a brief review of the outcomes and metrics that define UHC, followed by a brief history of its evolution as a concept, including an introduction to some of the main participants in the UHC conversation. I then trace likely implementation scenarios implied by the current policy narrative, starting with the funding and delivery of 'beyond-the-package' services. This analysis suggests that the prevailing policy narrative is leading toward two-tiered healthcare, underpinned by a residual safety net (called 'UHC'), while making space for the marketization of healthcare more generally.

A political economy analysis throws further light on the gap between the promises and likely outcomes of the prevailing UHC narrative. The framework for this analysis centers on the *points of articulation* between global health and the political economy of global capitalism. My purpose is to identify the *dynamics of stability and change* in relation to global health, which arise at these points of articulation. The significance of low- and middle-income countries (L&MICs) as a market for transnational healthcare supply industries (pharmaceuticals, electronics, and finance) is one such dynamic. The UHC entrepreneurs have assembled a phalanx of pharmaceutical, electronic, and financial corporations behind them – corporations that are hankering for the market opportunities promised by the privatization of health systems in L&MICs. In the context of a global crisis of overproduction, the healthcare markets of L&MICs offer much-needed virgin territory for corporate expansion.

This analysis has important implications for governments and civil society organizations in the Global South. I conclude with some broad suggestions regarding activist engagement around UHC and for the pursuit of 'Health for All' more generally.

DOI: 10.4324/9781003017110-27

UHC: definitions and metrics

UHC is included as Goal 3.8 in the United Nations' *Sustainable Development Goals* (SDGs), specifically pursuing 'universal health coverage, including financial risk protection, access to quality essential healthcare services and access to safe, effective, quality and affordable essential medicines and vaccines for all' (UN DESA Statistical Division 2017).

Two broad indicators are used by the UN for monitoring Target 8 (UHC) of SDG Goal 3 (Good health and wellbeing). SDG indicator 3.8.1, the *UHC Service Coverage Index* (SCI), is a composite indicator based on tracer interventions, including reproductive, maternal, newborn, and child health, infectious diseases, and non-communicable diseases (WHO 2019). It is a very basic indicator. A community could score well on this index and still have a level of service coverage well below public expectations in high- and middle-income countries. The indicator is heavily biased toward interventions that are supported by large vertical disease–focused development assistance programs (in part, because these have established indicators). There is no attempt to measure quality or efficiency for most components of the index (WHO and World Bank 2017b). There are wide differences in service coverage by household income for many of the separate indicators included in the SCI, which are obscured by their integration into a single index. 'Improved sanitation', for instance, varies from 20 percent to 90 percent by wealth deciles. Similarly, antenatal care coverage ranges from 40 percent to 80 percent from the poorest to the wealthiest deciles (WHO 2019).

SDG indicator 3.8.2, 'Financial protection', is an estimate of the proportion of the population experiencing catastrophic household expenditures on health (more than 10 percent or 25 percent of total household expenditure or income) each year. A second indicator, 'Healthcare impoverishment', refers to the number of people being pushed into poverty each year through household healthcare expenditure. Most measures of financial protection (3.8.2) show deterioration between 2000 and 2015 (WHO 2019). A growing number of people and an expanding share of the population incurred catastrophic health spending across this period.

History of UHC

In May 2004, a new item entitled 'Social Health Insurance' appeared on the agenda of the World Health Organization's Executive Board (at the request of Kenya), supported by a brief report from the Secretariat (WHO 2004). The subsequent debate was fierce, including an apoplectic outburst from the United States' delegate, Dr Steiger, who 'was disappointed with the deep-seated bias shown in WHO, including the Executive Board, against private enterprise' (Executive Board 2005, p. 73). The Board subsequently adopted a fairly bland draft resolution ('Sustainable health financing, universal coverage and social health insurance'), which was adopted by the Assembly in May 2005 as *WHA58.33* (WHA 2005).

The *World Health Report 2010* (*WHR 2010*) was a transition point in terms of crystallizing the UHC concept. The *Report* introduced the UHC cube (the three dimensions being the proportions of the population covered, services covered, and costs covered), and explored how resources might be mobilized to ensure everybody can access essential services without incurring excessive out-of-pocket costs. The political momentum for UHC continued with *WHA Resolution 64.9* in May 2011 (WHA 2011), followed by the 2012 *UN General Assembly Resolution on Global Health and Foreign Policy* (UN General Assembly 2012), which implored all countries to shift their health systems toward UHC. Finally, in the 2015 *UN General Assembly Resolution 70/1* ('Transforming Our World: The 2030 Agenda for Sustainable Development'), UHC was included in the SDGs as Target 3.8 (UN General Assembly 2015). The adoption of Target 3.8 was complemented by the

2019 *High Level Political Declaration on UHC*, endorsed in *UN General Assembly Resolution 74/2* (UN General Assembly 2019). During this period, WHO also published a number of technical documents including on fiscal space (WHO 2014; Cashin *et al.* 2017), strategic purchasing (WHO-SEARO 2017), and health benefits packages (WHO 2021a).

The World Bank has taken a prominent role in the UHC conversation, notwithstanding its long record of promoting user fees, restricting public expenditure on health, supporting commercial health insurance markets, and promoting the private sector in healthcare (Nuruzzaman 2007; Lindner *et al.* 2013). In 2013, the Bank published a review of UHC schemes in developing countries (Giedion *et al.* 2013), and since 2015, the Bank has worked with WHO on the periodic UHC global monitoring reports (WHO and World Bank 2015, 2017b). In 2017, WHO and the World Bank, as part of *UHC2030* (see below), co-authored a UHC 'vision document' (WHO and World Bank 2017a).

In addition to WHO and the World Bank, there is a wider network of organizations and partnerships describing themselves as part of the 'UHC movement'. These are largely based in the US, and many are supported by the Rockefeller Foundation. The activities and materials produced through the 'movement' are largely directed at the governments of L&MICs, including both health and finance ministries.

The entrepreneurs behind this movement have also invested heavily in recruiting corporate 'sign-ons', in particular, from pharmaceutical and medical electronics corporations. Presumably, these corporate strategists anticipate UHC benefiting their bottom line (particularly in terms of market access), and hope that partnering with the UHC movement would help to prevent any whittling away of their intellectual property privileges.

The third constituency targeted by the movement comprises the putative funders: the bilateral and multilateral donors and the philanthropists who are invited to contribute directly to the costs of UHC in low-income countries. They are requested to pool their funds, loosen their conditions, collaborate in the formal terms and procedures, and offer medium- to long-term predictability – that is, to realize the aid effectiveness principles of Busan and Addis Ababa, which they have been hitherto loath to do (see: Ogbuoji and Yamey 2019).

At the core of the UHC 'movement' are *UHC2030*, the Joint Learning Network (JLN) for UHC; the US think tank, Results for Development (R4D); and the Rockefeller Foundation.

The mission of *UHC2030* (2022) is 'to create a movement for accelerating equitable and sustainable progress towards universal health coverage' and 'provide a platform where the private sector, civil society, international organizations, academia and governmental organizations can collaborate together to create a movement for accelerating equitable and sustainable progress towards universal health coverage'. Its strategic focus is on 'mobilizing collective action' for UHC. The private sector members of *UHC2030* include many global pharmaceutical (*e.g.* Pfizer) and medical equipment companies (*e.g.* GE and Philips), as well as the IFPMA (International Federation of Pharmaceutical Manufactures and Associations).

The Joint Learning Network for Universal Health Coverage (JLN4UHC 2022b) 'is an innovative, country-driven network of practitioners and policymakers from around the globe who co-develop global knowledge products that help bridge the gap between theory and practice to extend health coverage to more than 3 billion people'. It has members – largely L&MICs – whose officials participate in learning activities, which are resourced by 'facilitators'. The latter comprise experts, primarily drawn from the World Bank and JLN 'partners' – a category that includes private sector consultancies (*e.g.* R4D and Abt), technical agencies (*e.g.* IHI and NICE), and bilateral donors (*e.g.* USAID and JICA). The JLN is funded by the Gates Foundation, the World Bank, and GIZ (German Cooperation).

A key program, offered through the JLN between 2016 and 2021, was the Private Sector Engagement Collaborative, which worked 'to advance international guidance on engaging the private sector to achieve PHC-oriented UHC' (JLN4UHC 2022a). This work was largely directed to health officials from L&MICs, providing 'practitioners, development agencies, and research institutes with practical guidance for public-private engagement to deliver primary health services for UHC'. The Collaborative was led by Abt Associates, who were contracted to USAID under the SHOPS Plus project (Sustaining Health Outcomes through the Private Sector) (SHOPS Plus 2022). From 2015 to 2020, the SHOPS Plus project worked in 29 countries 'to increase access to priority health information, products, and services through the private sector'.

Results for Development (R4D 2021) is a not-for-profit consultancy based in Washington D.C., which provides much of the technical materials supporting the JLN and UHC2030. R4D was inaugurated in 2008 by former World Bank Vice President, David de Ferranti. Its staff include economists and policy analysts, several with close links with the World Bank. Much of R4D's work on UHC is supported by the Rockefeller Foundation.

One of R4D's first projects was the *Role of the Private Sector in Health Systems*. A key output of this project was a paper on *Provider Purchasing and Contracting Mechanisms* (England 2008), which set the Rockefeller agenda in relation to UHC. Its starting position, regarding the need for reform is: 'An entrenched public service that absorbs almost all of the money governments make available, mostly in the salaries and wages of public service workers, and that is largely inefficient, unresponsive, and unaccountable to consumers'. The program of reform envisages several possible configurations: first, government becomes the payer/purchaser and reduces its role in direct service provision; second, government transfers its purchaser function to an autonomous national funding body, but remains provider; and third, government ceases both provider and purchaser functions. The paper considers the perceived benefits and drawbacks of these different configurations and explores the technical requirements for effective purchasing.

A 2009 report, commissioned under Rockefeller's *Transforming Health Systems Initiative,* focused on the role of government in regulating private providers in mixed health systems (Lagomarsino, Nachuk, and Kundra 2009). This report summarized the findings of research commissioned by the Rockefeller Foundation examining the role of the private sector in health systems in developing countries.

Contradictions and silences in the prevailing UHC policy narrative

In this section, the implementation of the standard UHC policy narrative is explored, starting with the 'basic benefits package' and the financing of 'beyond-the-package' services. This analysis highlights contradictions and silences in the prevailing policy narrative. It suggests that, far from delivering access and financial protection, implementation of the policy narrative will lead to a two-tiered, marketized healthcare system with a residual safety net ('UHC') and significant barriers to expanding the basic benefits package.

Reducing user charges

WHO has campaigned around abolishing user charges, particularly since *WHR 2010*, on the grounds that they create barriers to accessing care and carry significant risk of medical impoverishment. The need to reduce (or eliminate) user charges has been WHO's principal argument for UHC. However, all versions of UHC currently under discussion emphasize that coverage will only include 'essential services' (commonly referred to as the 'defined benefits package').

Accordingly, there will also be a sector of service delivery of 'non-essential services' (that is, non-UHC services or 'beyond-the-package' services), the cost of which will be met through user charges, in some cases supported by supplementary private insurance. People without supplementary private health insurance, who need services beyond the package, will face user charges which, in turn, will drive some into medical impoverishment. Others will go without.

Supplementary private health insurance

With a limited benefits package under UHC, there will be political demand from the wealthy for beyond-the-package insurance coverage and commercial demand from the financial sector to access this opportunity. Where there are pre-existing health insurance plans, the more basic plans will be absorbed into the UHC arrangements, but there will be strong pressures for the more generous plans to continue separately, and to offer beyond-the-package services to their customers along with the UHC benefits package.

The availability of private insurance will jeopardize the political solidarity needed to sustain UHC and progressively expand the basic benefits package. Where supplementary health insurance operates beside the UHC safety net, the pressure exerted on governments will be to encourage the private sector to expand its offerings and its coverage rather than to expand the UHC benefits package.

Purchasing and purchaser-provider separation

The term 'purchasing' is commonly used in descriptions of UHC, while reference to 'purchaser-provider separation' is less frequent, though generally implied. For this to work, publicly administered health service agencies, where the government owns the assets and staff are directly employed, will need to be somehow set adrift (autonomized, corporatized, and privatized in the language of the World Bank [Preker and Harding 2003]). Insofar as they are providing services within the UHC benefits package, health service agencies will now be funded via direct payments through the UHC scheme. Accordingly, if they are to manage their own revenues and pay their staff, public health service agencies will need to be corporatized. In such circumstances, a single government-owned program of services will be transformed into a decentralized fleet of corporatized service agencies.

Once publicly administered agencies have been corporatized as separate providers for the basic benefits package, the agencies will press to be allowed to provide beyond-the-package services (on a user-pays basis). Once these agencies are established as independent service providers – billing both the UHC payer and the private health insurers – there will be increasing pressure to privatize them. Once privatized, their focus will turn to the more profitable districts and more profitable items of service.

While 'purchasing' could be interpreted as including government budget transfers to publicly owned service agencies, the term is generally used to refer to purchasing from a range of arm's length providers. In view of the frequent affirmation that UHC providers may be public, voluntary, or private, the clear implication is that publicly owned providers will be 'separated' or corporatized so that they are in the UHC market selling services to the UHC payer.

The UHC single payer

The World Bank has long supported competitive private health insurance markets (Brunner *et al.* 2012), but it appears to have accepted WHO's insistence on the need for single-payer financing in relation to UHC (WHO and World Bank 2017a). Kutzin (2014) points out that the single-payer function will require specialized data systems for managing and disbursing funds, as well as for monitoring service delivery, and that this will require a dedicated agency with significant autonomy, freed of many of the routine disciplines of the public service. There will be strong arguments for this agency to be corporatized in the process of emancipating it from routine public finance management controls. Once the corporatized agency has achieved stability and its systems are working smoothly, there will be pressure from the financial markets for further privatization.

In countries with multiple existing health insurance plans, the path to single-payer healthcare financing would involve the progressive amalgamation of different insurance plans, often with very different revenue flows and benefit packages, as well as different constituencies. This is always highly political and very difficult (for instance, as exemplified in the experience of the BRICS countries [Marten *et al.* 2014]). Such challenges can be avoided by treating UHC as a residual safety net (providing the minimum benefits package), while accommodating the more generous funds in a pluralist market for beyond-the-package services.

Capitation

Most of the expert documents regarding UHC tread cautiously around mode of payment, the unit which is to be purchased. However, budget funding has been precluded by the insistence on bringing the private sector into the UHC market, and the challenges of regulating fee-for-service payment are generally acknowledged. Output funding may be considered for in-patient care (although it involves complex and information-rich systems), but there are no such systems for ambulatory care. In this context, there will be strong arguments for capitation payment, particularly for primary care.

Capitation payment raises questions about the size and competence of the provider agency: whether it is derived from agencies previously in government service, or from voluntary or private agencies. Moreover, how solo practitioners and street vendors would fit into such a scheme has not been explained. Promoting quality and efficiency under capitation is a regulatory challenge, even in well-funded settings. Poorly regulated, privately operated managed care carries significant risks of underservicing.

Quality

The UHC marketplace considered by this analysis would comprise a corporatized single-payer disbursing funds to hospitals and to geographically based managed care organizations (MCOs) for services within the basic benefits package. Both hospitals and MCOs will also provide beyond-the-package services for which users will be charged, in some cases covered by supplementary private health insurance. Regulating for quality, efficiency, and equity in such markets would be particularly challenging.

WHR 2010 estimated that up to 40 percent of healthcare is ineffective or worse. Putting in place the systems and culture needed for effective clinical governance is critical for quality and safety at the agency and program level (Scally and Donaldson 1998; Halligan and Donaldson 2001). These systems are difficult to establish and manage in publicly administered health systems in wealthy countries, and more so in mixed healthcare delivery systems, but the challenges in the kind of healthcare markets being proposed for low-income countries under the rubric of UHC would be much greater.

The various technical papers about UHC do not address the challenge of inter-sectoral collaboration for better health, as highlighted in the *Alma-Ata Declaration* (1978) and the report of the *Commission on the Social Determinants of Health* (2008). *Alma-Ata* describes a model of comprehensive primary healthcare with local practitioners and agencies accountable to their communities for service delivery, and working with their communities to act upon the social and political determinants of health (Nandi and Schneider 2014). This is hard to achieve in publicly administered health systems. It has been virtually removed from the UHC agenda.

Efficiency

The meaning of technical efficiency in relation to healthcare is contested (Morgan 2016). Many health economists prefer to deal with the cost of interventions rather than the cost of outcomes, because measurement of the latter is fraught. However, conceptually, technical efficiency is fundamentally about the cost of outcomes. In publicly administered systems, the assessment of technical efficiency lies with agency and system managers who can deploy experience and judgment in integrating information about the cost *and* efficacy of interventions, even if they do not have comprehensive metrics for outcomes. However, the assessment of efficiency in the marketplace rests with regulators, who generally have more limited data and no personal engagement in the clinical world.

Allocative efficiency, understood as referring to investment choices between different programs (or levels of care, or options for improvement), calls for a capacity to compare the marginal benefits associated with different allocation choices and to direct resources accordingly. In publicly administered agencies and systems, these choices involve managerial judgment exercised in the context of budgeting. However, in the UHC model, the scope for such decisions is limited to adjusting the benefits package, with only crude indicators to estimate need, waste, and equity.

Equity

Equity is about fairness in the distribution of both resources and opportunities across geographic, gender, income, or ethnic differences (Morgan 2016). In publicly administered systems, distributional equity depends on budget decisions and political accountability. In market-based systems, healthcare providers are drawn to service the wealthy due to the higher likelihood of securing profitable outcomes.

In the current UHC model, services will be provided by private or voluntary providers and by erstwhile public sector agencies. As public sector agencies are progressively corporatized and privatized, they will also be drawn toward servicing urban areas and wealthier districts. There are, however, few levers in this model that encourage or require providers to locate in underserved districts.

The public sector alternative

Stratified competitive health insurance markets incorporate weak system-wide referral and support linkages, and provide for weak-to-no control of distributional equity, the efficient use of resources, or quality of care. Fee-for-service reimbursement encourages premium inflation and low-risk selection. Managed care schemes, based on capitation, carry substantial risks of underservicing. In contrast, publicly administered health systems provide policymakers with potent levers to promote efficiency, equity, and quality, and to realize primary healthcare principles (Kutzin 2001; García-Corchero and Jiménez-Rubio 2022). However, the public sector alternative has been effectively removed from the UHC agenda.

Questions arising

The analysis presented in this section, structured within a generic health systems framework, highlights a number of contradictions and silences in the prevailing UHC policy narrative. These are not explicable within this health systems framework and suggest the need for a wider frame of analysis – specifically, a political-economic analysis – through which we may clearly discern the political and ideological influences shaping the UHC narrative.

The political economy of global health and UHC

The framework for the analysis outlined in this section centers on critical points of articulation between global health and political economy, and explores the dynamics of stability and change at each point. Developing this framework has involved traversing insights arising from literature in both political economy (Robinson 2004; Stillwell 2012; Smith 2016; Patnaik and Patnaik 2021) and the history of global health over the last 200 years (Howard-Jones 1981; Rosen 1993 (1958); Stefanini 2008; Birn *et al.* 2009). The following discussion addresses only a selection of these points of articulation and their relevance for comprehending the structural significance of UHC in the context of contemporary capitalism.

Healthcare affordability and the price of medicines

Input prices clearly influence healthcare affordability for both the household and institutional payers, including government. However, pharmaceutical prices are a particular burden for low- and middle-income countries, since they generally reflect global market prices, whereas labor-intensive services reflect local wage and salary levels. The global average national pharmaceutical expenditure expressed as a proportion of total health expenditure is around 24 percent (Lu *et al.* 2011). Among high-income countries, a few spend more than this, including Qatar (32 percent), Greece (29 percent), and Czech Republic (27 percent). However, for many L&MICs, total pharmaceutical expenditure constitutes more than half of total health expenditure. Such countries include Papua New Guinea (50.3 percent), Kyrgyzstan (50.9 percent), Uganda (52.2 percent), India (56 percent), Ethiopia (56.6 percent), Pakistan (62.9 percent), and Tunisia (67 percent).

Monopoly pricing power under intellectual property protection is a major factor in sustaining high prices including for low-income countries. The *Agreement on Trade-Related Aspects of Intellectual Property Rights* (*TRIPS* 1994) includes provisions that, if codified through national legislation, can enable countries to issue compulsory licenses or to procure in foreign markets where prices are lower. However, many countries have been placed under heavy pressure (from the drug industry and from powerful countries) to adopt legislation, which precludes the use of TRIPS flexibilities.

The claim that high returns are needed to fund further research and development (R&D) is weak. Much of the R&D on which new drugs are based is publicly funded, and pharmaceutical R&D reflects profit expectations rather than public health needs. The global pharmaceutical industry generally spends more on marketing than on R&D. This is directed to increasing sales volumes (including overuse) and embedding brand consciousness in consumers and prescribers. Pharmaceutical profits are well above the norms in other industries, and fund high executive salaries, generous dividends, and share buybacks.

Generic pharmaceutical manufacturers should be able to enter the market once patents have expired, but it is common for generic manufacturers to be taken over by the large originator corporations. Industry consolidation (and increased monopoly) through mergers and acquisitions reflects the financialization of the modern capitalist economy.

The prices of imported healthcare supplies are also affected by barriers to local production. Trade liberalization and the emergence of huge transnational corporations managing far-reaching supply chains mean that the corporations can often market higher quality products more reliably than small local producers and have deep enough pockets to undercut local manufacturers.

Arrangements for large-scale joint procurement have the potential to negotiate lower prices through monopsonic purchasing power tied to scale. Joint country schemes require a common framework for regulatory approval, which can be complex to negotiate.

The issues of price transparency, *TRIPS* flexibilities, public sector production, and pooled procurement have been largely avoided by the policy entrepreneurs driving the UHC conversation. This undoubtedly reflects the political and financial support provided to the UHC 'movement' by powerful pharmaceutical corporations.

Health services as markets for transnational suppliers

The health sector globally, including the middle-classes of L&MICs, is a rich market for transnational suppliers, including pharmaceuticals, electronics, hospital chains, and health insurance. These industries are enthusiastic supporters of trade liberalization (including trade in services). The private sector constituencies of *UHC2030* and the JLN include big corporate names from pharmaceuticals, electronics, and finance. They are clearly aware of the market-forming potential of the UHC policy drive.

The increasing support for UHC among the G7 confederacy may reflect pressures from their healthcare supply industries for expansion of the healthcare market globally. In the context of a global crisis of overproduction and underconsumption in contemporary capitalism, healthcare is a market of great promise.

Macroeconomic crisis

The drive for UHC is shaped by wider macroeconomic dynamics. The global economic slowdown of the last several decades reflects a crisis of overproduction (and underconsumption). A growing mismatch has emerged between expanding productive capacity *vis-a-vis* slower growth in consumer demand, limited by the displacement of labor by technology, fossil fuels, and the spread of precarious employment.

Neoliberalism as a policy framework emerged in response to the evolving global economic crisis of stagnation that arose from the late-1970s. It constitutes a set of policies designed to protect the interests of the transnational capitalist class (Robinson 2004) from the effects of the macroeconomic crisis. Fiscal 'discipline' and policies of privatization and marketization, core elements of the neoliberal program, are of particular relevance to health service development and healthcare financing.

Global trade is increasingly conducted within global supply chains, which are commonly controlled by a small number of large transnational corporations and governed by trade rules designed to privilege the interests of the Global North. This is a regime of unequal exchange between North and South. Smith (2016) demonstrates how, when t-shirts made in Bangladesh or iPhones made in Shanghai are sold into Northern markets, the surplus value generated is captured by the TNCs, their Northern executives, and Northern governments in tax receipts. This regime greatly constrains fiscal capacity in L&MICs, including healthcare financing.

'Financialization' has been a core feature of this global crisis. As market demand has remained sluggish, the proportion of profit accruing to productive investment in people, infrastructure, and machinery has fallen. Concomitantly, profit has increasingly flowed into consumer lending to support debt-funded consumption; into the purchase of existing assets (housing, companies, stocks, and derivatives) for speculation on asset price inflation; into corporate mergers and acquisitions directed to concentrating control of global supply chains; and into expanding into new markets, including through the privatization of health services and health insurance. The explosive growth of the financial sector, while jobs and wages in other sectors have stagnated, has contributed to a significant widening of economic inequality.

The structural constraints on domestic resource mobilization

These macroeconomic dynamics impose sharp limitations on the capacity of L&MICs to mobilize domestic resources for healthcare, in particular because of the regime of unequal exchange arising from their location in the global value chains. Further constraints on fiscal capacity include the following: the burdens of debt servicing, tax competition, tax evasion, and the challenges of tax collection in the informal sector.

Constraints on domestic resources are complicated by widening inequality, which weakens community solidarity and contributes to increased resistance from the wealthier strata to the pooling of contributions for healthcare.

WHO (2021b) has sought to challenge doctrines of austerity in healthcare funding by pointing to the benefits to other sectors of the economy from local expenditure and employment in healthcare. However, in the absence of meaningful reform of neoliberal globalization, the scope for significant increases in domestic resources for healthcare in low-income countries appears limited.

Ecological crisis

Global warming and the loss of biodiversity constitute another face of the contemporary crisis of global capitalism, with myriad implications including: hunger from drought; deaths from heat stress; warming-induced storms, floods, and fires; and climate refugees facing displacement, migration, asylum-seeking, and war.

The threat of zoonotic illnesses and pandemics, arising from the continued human encroachment into natural environments, has implications for the contribution of UHC to 'global health security' (Wallace 2016). Rather than putting a brake on extractivism (minerals, forest products, agribusiness) and the heightened risk of pandemics, UHC promises a strengthening of disease surveillance and response capability. In particular, offering development assistance for UHC, while making this conditional on investing in health security, will help make the (rich) world safer for continued extractivism.

Global health governance

The wave of decolonization following the Second World War changed the make-up of the World Health Assembly, according developing countries a stronger voice in WHO decision-making. Issues where Assembly resolutions have caused corporate (and imperial) discomfort include: support for the 'New International Economic Order' in the *Alma-Ata Declaration*, the essential medicines list (Laing *et al.* 2003), the marketing of breast milk substitutes (Richter 2002), and the proposed medicines R&D treaty (Velásquez 2012).

However, while the rich countries are a minority in the Assembly, they can deploy the power of the purse. The freeze on mandatory contributions and tight earmarking of voluntary contributions have meant that today virtually all of WHO's operational expenditure is dependent on donor funding (Legge 2015). Accordingly, WHO's *de facto* budget is based on what the donors will fund rather than the priorities of the World Health Assembly.

Another major change has been the emergence of multiple global health initiatives (GHIs), where donor funding bypasses WHO and goes straight to the GHIs (such as Gavi, the Global Fund, and the Global Polio Eradication Initiative). Reframing global health governance in terms of multi-stakeholder partnerships rather than multilateralism is designed to ensure that the philanthropic foundations and the corporations have a formal voice in global health governance. The creation of the Access to COVID Tools Accelerator illustrates this multi-stakeholder model – including, in this case, the participation of the IFPMA in the design of the Accelerator and the COVAX facility (Legge 2020).

WHO has entered a Faustian pact with neoliberalism: WHO gets the credit for addressing healthcare access and financial protection in return for endorsing the neoliberal project of privatization and marketization of health services and healthcare financing.

The dance of legitimation

Perceived legitimacy plays a major role in maintaining political stability (Bexell 2014). The delegitimation/relegitimation cycle starts with policies that kill (structural adjustment, high prices for AIDS drugs, lack of access to vaccines) and the global opprobrium elicited by such policies. The perceived loss of legitimacy creates space for policy reform and contestation between ameliorative reform to restore legitimacy and more fundamental structural reform, thereby engendering the imperative for means to relegitimize the political-economic status quo.

The huge increase in development assistance for health following the launch of the *Millennium Development Goals* in 2000 was a massive investment in the relegitimation of the neoliberal regime, which had been tarnished by the use of TRIPS by large pharmaceutical corporations to defend impossibly high prices for antiretrovirals in South Africa (1997–2001). TRIPS was widely seen as bestowing privileges on the global pharmaceutical industry, which had the effect of denying large numbers of already-impoverished people the right to healthcare.

However, by the mid-2000s, the legitimacy of the MDGs and GHIs was already being questioned, as the adverse effects of narrow vertical programs were increasingly clear: internal brain drain, health system fragmentation, transaction cost burden, barriers to access, and medical impoverishment (WHO 2011). The rise of UHC and its inclusion in the SDGs was, to some extent, a response to the delegitimation of the MDGs and vertical disease management.

The COVID-19 pandemic has, since 2020, led to a new round in the dance of legitimation, due to the lack of solidarity manifest in the vaccine nationalism of the rich world and insistence of the G7 on protecting large pharmaceutical corporations from any accountability for price gouging and limits imposed on production volumes. At a time when vaccine coverage in Africa was less than 4 percent, Europe and parts of the US had achieved vaccination rates of around 80 percent and were introducing booster doses (de Bengy Puyvallée and Storeng 2022). The G7 and its corporate elites suffered a further loss of legitimacy in the eyes of the Global South as a consequence of their rejection of the South African and Indian proposal for a waiver of certain *TRIPS* provisions to enable expanded vaccine production in the Global South (TWN 2021). The promises of UHC contribute, to some degree, to shoring up the legitimacy of neoliberal globalization.

Conclusions: the promises of UHC

For poor people facing financial barriers to care and the risk of medical impoverishment, UHC promises access and financial protection, but the promise may be hollow. Widening inequality and multi-tiered health funding compromises solidarity and revenue raising and, therefore, the promise of progressively expanding the benefits package. The marketized health system that UHC will deliver will have very limited provisions for quality, efficiency, or equity. The problems that UHC purports to address – barriers to access and medical impoverishment in L&MICs – reflect the widening of economic inequality associated with the crisis of overproduction (including a regime of unequal exchange and financialization). As argued in the preceding discussion, however, the UHC narrative offers no prospect of reform to address such structural concerns.

For politicians, officials, and activists concerned about health development, UHC promises a pathway to health system strengthening, but skepticism is called for. UHC, as currently promoted, will lock in two-tiered health funding and two-tiered service delivery. Weak cost control in the private sector is likely to lead to premium inflation and political pressure to subsidize private insurance rather than expanding the basic package.

For the corporate strategists, UHC promises new markets for healthcare supply and finance. For the strategists of transnational capitalism, UHC will also contribute to the relegitimation of the global neoliberal regime, demonstrating that it is not so heartless after all.

Notwithstanding its money, institutions, and armies, the transnational capitalist class is vulnerable to delegitimation in the eyes of the Global South (and of some domestic constituencies in the Global North). The challenges for health equity activism include infusing health policy analysis with political economy; working on the specific and immediate health issues in ways that also address the larger structural causes; promoting an alternative vision of what a decent health system would look like; and working in ways that deepen solidarity across difference in building a better world.

References

Bexell, M. 2014, 'Global governance, legitimacy and (de)legitimation', *Globalizations*, 11(3), pp. 289–99.

Birn, A.-E., Pillay, Y. and Holtz, T.H. 2009, 'The historical origins of modern international health', in Birn, A.-E., Pillay, Y. and Holtz, T.H. (eds), *Textbook of International Health: Global Health in a Dynamic World*, Oxford University Press, New York, pp. 17–60.

Brunner, G., Gottret, P., Hansl, B., Kalavakonda, V., Nagpal, S. and Tapay, N. 2012, *Private Voluntary Health Insurance: Consumer Protection and Prudential Regulation*, World Bank, Washington, DC.

Cashin, C., Bloom, D., Sparkes, S., Barroy, H., Kutzin, J. and O'Dougherty, S. 2017, *Aligning Public Financial Management and Health Financing: Sustaining Progress Toward Universal Health Coverage*, World Health Organisation and Results for Development, Geneva.

Commission on Social Determinants of Health. 2008, *Closing the Gap in a Generation: Health Equity Through Action on the Social Determinants of Health*, WHO, Geneva.

de Bengy Puyvallée, A. and Storeng, K.T. 2022, 'COVAX, vaccine donations and the politics of global vaccine inequity', *Global Health*, 18(1), Article 26.

England, R. 2008, *Provider Purchasing and Contracting Mechanisms, Technical partner papers: The Rockefeller Foundation–Sponsored Initiative on the Role of the Private Sector in Health Systems in Developing Countries*, R4D, accessed 1 November 2022, <https://r4d.org/wp-content/uploads/Provider-Purchasing-and-Contracting-Mechanisms.pdf>.

Executive Board. 2005, *Executive Board, January 2005, Summary Records*, WHO, accessed 1 November 2022, <https://apps.who.int/gb/ebwha/pdf_files/EB115/B115_REC2-en.pdf#page=91>.

García-Corchero, J.D. and Jiménez-Rubio, D. 2022, 'How do policy levers shape the quality of a national health system?' *Journal of Policy Modeling*, 44(1), pp. 203–21.

Giedion, U., Alfonso, E.A. and Díaz, Y. 2013, *The Impact of Universal Coverage Schemes in the Developing World: A Review of the Existing Evidence*, World Bank, Washington DC.

Halligan, A. and Donaldson, L. 2001, 'Implementing clinical governance: Turning vision into reality', *BMJ*, 322(7299), pp. 1413–7.
Howard-Jones, N. 1981, 'The world health organization in historical perspective', *Perspectives in Biology and Medicine*, 24(3), pp. 467–82.
JLN4UHC. 2022a, 'Private sector engagement', accessed 14 November 2022, <https://www.jointlearningnetwork.org/what-we-do/private-sector-engagement/>
JLN4UHC. 2022b, 'What we do', <https://www.jointlearningnetwork.org/>.
Kutzin, J. 2001, 'A descriptive framework for country-level analysis of health care financing arrangements', *Health Policy*, 56(3), pp. 171–204.
Kutzin, J. 2014, 'Health financing for UHC: Why the path runs through the Finance Ministry and PFM rules', Fiscal space, public finance and health financing, Montreux, Switzerland.
Lagomarsino, G., Nachuk, S. and Kundra, S.S. 2009, *Public Stewardship of Private Providers in Mixed Health Systems*, Results for Development Institute, Washington, DC.
Laing, R., Waning, B., Gray, A., Ford, N. and 't Hoen, E. 2003, '25 years of the WHO essential medicines lists: Progress and challenges', *Lancet*, (361)9370, pp. 1723–9.
Legge, D.G. 2015, 'WHO shackled: Donor control of the world health organisation', *Third World Resurgence*, 298/299, accessed 16 June 2020, <http://www.twn.my/title2/resurgence/2015/298-299/cover01.htm>.
Legge, D.G. 2020, 'COVID-19 response exposes deep flaws in global health governance', *Global Social Policy*, 20(3), pp. 1–5.
Lindner, M.E., Preker, A.S. and Chernichovsky, D. 2013, *Scaling Up Affordable Health Insurance*, World Bank, Washington, DC.
Lu, Y., Hernandez, P., Abegunde, D. and Edejer, T. 2011, *The World Medicines Situation 2011: Medicine Expenditures*, WHO, Geneva.
Marten, R., McIntyre, D., Travassos, C., Shishkin, S., Longde, W., Reddy, S. and Vega, J. 2014, 'An assessment of progress towards universal health coverage in Brazil, Russia, India, China, and South Africa (BRICS)', *The Lancet*, 384(9960), pp. 2164–71.
Morgan, R, Ensor, T. and Waters, H. 2016, 'Performance of private sector health care: Implications for universal health coverage', *The Lancet*, 388(10044), pp. 606–12.
Nandi, S. and Schneider, H. 2014, 'Addressing the social determinants of health: A case study from the Mitanin (community health worker) programme in India', *Health Policy and Planning*, 29(suppl 2), pp. ii71–81.
Nuruzzaman, M. 2007, 'The world bank, health policy reforms and the poor', *Journal of Contemporary Asia*, 37(1), pp. 59–72.
Ogbuoji, O. and Yamey, G. 2019, 'Aid effectiveness in the sustainable development goals era', *International Journal of Health Policy and Management*, 8(3), pp. 184–6.
Patnaik, U. and Patnaik, P. 2021, *Capitalism and Imperialism: Theory, History and the Present*, Monthly Review Press, New York.
Preker, A.S. and Harding, A. 2003, *Innovations in Health Service Delivery: The Corporatisation of Public Hospitals*, The World Bank, Washington.
R4D. 2021, *Results for Development: Universal Health Coverage*, R4D, accessed 12 September 2021, <https://r4d.org/health/universal-health-coverage/>.
Richter, J. 2002, *Codes in Context: TNC Regulation in an Era of Dialogues and Partnerships*, The Corner House, Newton, Dorset, UK.
Robinson, W.I. 2004, *A Theory of Global Capitalism: Production, Class, and State in a Transnational World*, Johns Hopkins University Press, Baltimore, MD.
Rosen, G. 1993 [1958], *A History of Public Health (Expanded Edition)*, Johns Hopkins University Press, Baltimore, MD.
Scally, G. and Donaldson, L.J. 1998, 'Clinical governance and the drive for quality improvement in the new NHS in England', *BMJ*, 317, pp. 61–5.
SHOPS Plus. 2022, 'Accelerating private sector engagement', accessed 14 November 2022, <https://www.shopsplusproject.org/EOPseries>.
Smith, J. 2016, *Imperialism in the Twenty-First Century: Globalization, Super-Exploitation, and Capitalism's Final Crisis*, Monthly Review Press, New York.
Stefanini, A. 2008, 'From Alma-Ata to the global fund: The history of international health policy', *Social Medicine*, 3(1), pp. 36–48.
Stillwell, F. 2012, *Political Economy: The Contest of Economic Ideas*, 3rd edn., Oxford University Press, Melbourne.

TWN. 2021, 'Waiver from certain provisions of the TRIPS agreement for the prevention, containment and treatment of COVID-19', *Third World Network*, Penang, accessed 15 November 2022, <https://www.twn.my/title2/intellectual_property/trips_waiver_proposal.htm>.

UHC2030. 2022, *Taking Action for Universal Health Coverage*, accessed 14 November 2022, <https://www.uhc2030.org/>.

UN DESA Statistical Division. 2017, *SDG Indicators: Revised List of Global Sustainable Development Goal Indicators*, UN, accessed 1 November 2022, <https://unstats.un.org/sdgs/indicators/indicators-list/>.

UN General Assembly. 2012, *Global Health and Foreign Policy*, UN, New York.

UN General Assembly. 2015, *Transforming Our World: The 2030 Agenda for Sustainable Development*, United Nations, New York.

UN General Assembly. 2019, *Political Declaration of the High-Level Meeting on Universal Health Coverage, Resolution 74/2*, United Nations, New York.

Velásquez, G. 2012, 'Rethinking the r&d model for pharmaceutical products: A binding global convention', *Policy Briefs*, South Centre, Geneva, accessed 1 November 2022, <http://www.southcentre.int/policy-brief-8-april-2012/#more-1995>.

Wallace, R. 2016, *Big Farms Make Big Flu: Dispatches on Infectious Disease, Agribusiness, and the Nature of Science*, Monthly Review Press, New York.

WHA. 2005, *Sustainable Health Financing, Universal Coverage and Social Health Insurance*, WHO, Geneva.

WHA. 2011, *Sustainable Health Financing Structures and Universal Coverage*, WHO, Geneva.

WHO-SEARO. 2017, *Provider Payment Methods and Strategic Purchasing for UHC*, World Health Organization, Regional Office for South-East Asia, New Delhi.

WHO. 1978, *Declaration of Alma-Ata*, International Conference on Primary Health Care, Alma-Ata, USSR, 6–12 September, accessed 1 November 2022, <https://www.who.int/publications/almaata_declaration_en.pdf>.

WHO. 2004, *Social Health Insurance* WHO, Geneva.

WHO. 2010, *The World Health Report - Health Systems Financing: The Path to Universal Coverage*, WHO, Geneva.

WHO. 2011, *Health System Strengthening: Current Trends and Challenges*, WHO, Geneva.

WHO. 2014, *Fiscal Space, Public Finance and Health Financing*, WHO, Montreux, Switzerland.

WHO. 2019, *Primary Healthcare on the Road to Universal Health Coverage: 2019 Monitoring Report*, WHO, Geneva.

WHO. 2021a, *Principles of Health Benefit Packages*, World Health Organization, Geneva.

WHO. 2021b, *Working for Health: Five-Year Action Plan for Health Employment and Inclusive Economic Growth (2017–2021)*, WHO, Geneva.

WHO and World Bank. 2015, *Tracking Universal Health Coverage: First Global Monitoring Report*, WHO, Geneva.

WHO and World Bank. 2017a, *Healthy Systems for Universal Health Coverage - A Joint Vision for Healthy Lives, UHC2030 International Health Partnership*, WHO and World Bank, Geneva.

WHO and World Bank. 2017b, *Tracking Universal Health Coverage: 2017 Global Monitoring Report*, WHO and WB, Geneva.

WTO. 1994, *Agreement on Trade-Related Aspects of Intellectual Property Rights*, accessed 1 November 2022, <https://www.wto.org/english/docs_e/legal_e/27-trips_01_e.htm>.

PART IV

Geographical varieties of health and healthcare

25

CRITICAL POLITICAL ECONOMY OF LATIN AMERICA'S HEALTHCARE SYSTEMS

A century of struggles

Laura Nervi and Anne-Emanuelle Birn

Critically analyzing healthcare systems (HCS) in Latin America (LA) is both a fraught and illuminating undertaking. In general terms, most HCS within the region may be characterized as fragmented, segmented, inequitable, and extremely unequal. Their dynamics reflect, and are reflected in, broad – if uneven – political and social struggles at both national and international levels. At times, these movements have led to greater equity and inclusion; at others, they have been marked by profoundly reactionary, conservative, and/or neoliberal capitalist forces in the opposite direction, often-coopting discourses of universality and equity.

HCS in most Latin American countries are comprised of three subsystems: ministries of health providing a patchwork of services (of uneven quality and comprehensiveness) for people who are uninsured and impoverished; social security for the formal workforce; and the private (for-profit and non-profit) sector for the wealthy and those lacking access to the other subsystems. LA social security arrangements vary widely: for instance, Argentina has approximately 300 social security schemes that are largely governed by unions, El Salvador has a three-tier system, and Costa Rica has a single, unified social security system.

From a funding perspective, Latin American HCS mostly operate through multi-payer arrangements, with numerous channels (general tax revenues, employee/employer contributions, charities, international donors, private insurance, out-of-pocket payments) financing healthcare. These are generally segmented, with the population stratified into distinct schemes according to socio-economic categories, such as labor market insertion (formal, informal, self-employed, retired), industry, ability to pay, income level, and/or social class (Göttems and Mollo 2020). Provision is also mixed and fragmented, whereby uncoordinated delivery arrangements 'increase transaction costs and hinder the capacity to guarantee equitable access to and delivery of health services' (Pan American Health Organization 2005: 23).

Accordingly, fragmentation – both within the poorly regulated private sector and across overlapping municipal, provincial, and federal public programs – generates neither comprehensive nor coordinated outcomes, ultimately failing to provide continuity of care. Although mainstream literature portrays fragmentation and segmentation as technocratic matters, critical political economy approaches reveal the exclusion, or inequitable treatment, of different social groups, and consider

DOI: 10.4324/9781003017110-29

the associated inequities in access, quality, health outcomes, and costs as deeply political issues. This chapter presents a range of these century-long HCS struggles – entailing both advances and setbacks – and shows why the current depiction of HCS in LA as unidirectionally advancing toward universalism is wrongheaded.

Historical trajectories and political struggles

Although healthcare and social security systems in LA are often depicted as both derivative of European developments and uniformly incomplete, they arose from a remarkable mix of activism by a range of actors and struggles, pioneered by progressive and/or deal-making policymakers, and involving interchange and multidirectional learning within and beyond the region (Cueto and Palmer 2015).

Prime contextual impulses for early-Twentieth Century social security schemes were state-building efforts, which emerged from the ashes of Nineteenth Century instability, civil and regional wars, post-colonial reconfiguration of borders and creation of new nation-states, foreign (economic) infiltration and occupation, and conflict among land-owning oligarchies, industrialists, urban liberals, the Catholic Church, political actors, workers, Indigenous peoples, immigrants, and others. As in many settings circa 1900, workers – especially industrial laborers (and unions) in the region's burgeoning extraction, transport, and manufacturing industries – played a protagonistic role in mobilizing around health and social protections that began to take shape in the 1920s. Nascent social security schemes covered workers in particular unions or industrial sectors, while excluding most of the population – from agricultural workers to the informal sector, Indigenous populations, and dependents. Amidst this strife, shifting alliances of liberal elites and others sought to dislodge existing healthcare efforts, including: public, last resort institutions for the destitute; charity-based, usually Catholic, welfare (*beneficencia*) schemes and institutions, often with notable participation by women elites (Lavrin 1998); and incipient immigrant-driven mutual aid (friendly) societies (*mutualistas*), organized to protect against infirmity and unemployment, support strikes, and pay for healthcare and funerals.

Mesa-Lago (2005) famously categorizes Latin American social security systems into early, mid-century, and late phases. Each of these yielded different forms of social protection, and variously reflected German (Bismarck's 1880s carrot of worker protection against old age, sickness, and disability, against the stick of order) and more extensive British social security legislation (which unfolded gradually until Beveridge's post–World War Two workers' compact). Other influences were also important, including those of neighboring countries and the USSR, whose comprehensive health and social security model devised under Health Commissar, Nikolai Semashko, in the 1920s was studied by scores of Latin American visitors in subsequent decades (Birn 2020).

As amply studied, Chile is a *prima facie* case of a country's HCS mirroring both domestic and global political-economic vicissitudes. In 1924, a brief military takeover of a divided Parliament enabled passage of statutory social insurance for industrial workers, the *Caja del Seguro Obrero Obligatorio* (CSO), along with labor and sanitary codes and a newly created Ministry of Health. Social insurance, covering workers' compensation, pensions, and healthcare, and financed by a worker-employer-state triad (the approach advocated by the International Labour Organization), was initially opposed by unions, which – in a context of revolutionary agitation opposing any measures seen to be aiding capital – considered the CSO to be wage theft and, instead, favored investment in housing and education. Although CSO critics of all stripes abounded, it survived into the 1950s, covering some four-fifths of industrial workers (but not their families), albeit marred by fragmentation and the existence of dozens of sector-specific parallel social security schemes (Illanes 1993; Molina Bustos 2010; Singleton 2013).

After the Popular Front (a coalition of leftist parties) won national elections in 1938, Dr. Salvador Allende – a socialist and former medical student activist – became Health Minister. Allende sought to replace the CSO with a truly socialized unified healthcare system that would appropriately set priorities based on population needs and ensure universal access to healthcare. However, fears of added costs, physician opposition to perceived government interference in medical practice, and mounting anti-communism thwarted this effort (Pieper Mooney 2020). It was not until 1952, with Allende now a Senator, that a more circumscribed version of Chile's National Health Service (SNS) passed. Although the state was charged with responsibility for public health and eligibility expanded markedly to the poorest sectors, the SNS's envisioned universality was watered down by legislators: rural, self-employed, and white-collar workers were excluded, and private practice was not eliminated.

Chile's dozens of overlapping insurance arrangements and welfare institutions were rationalized, but the SNS was not merely a technocratic success. Decades of struggle by unions and social movements, allied with like-minded politicians and health professionals, had a major bearing on this effort, flaws notwithstanding, toward equity. In turn, it became an inspiration for the fight for universal health systems in Costa Rica, among other countries (Martínez Franzoni and Sánchez Ancochea 2016). Over the ensuing decades, the SNS evolved in fits and starts, with the formation of a publicly subsidized medical insurance system once again generating inequities. During Allende's campaign for President in 1970, his plan to create a unitary, publicly financed and operated HCS was so opposed by elites and physicians that it was left out of his overall platform of nationalization and redistribution. Upon election, his new administration soon met with a physician strike protesting the Popular Unity Party's 'popular power' approach to health. After Augusto Pinochet's CIA-backed military coup deposed Allende in 1973, the country's efforts toward health justice swung into reverse: the dictator turned Chile into a neoliberal experiment with its social protection systems at the vanguard of these reforms worldwide.

Health and social security systems underwent distinct, if parallel, trajectories in other settings. In Mexico, the 1917 *Constitution* established a national Department of Public Health and envisioned a social security system. However, the revolutionary years' instability impeded the latter until the 1940s, even as unionized workers in particular sectors (*e.g.* military, oil workers, rail workers) realized their own schemes earlier. Under Lázaro Cárdenas's 1930s leftist Presidency, goals of universal, equitable social rights were stymied by entrenched domestic elites and foreign investors. Scaled-back and targeted efforts, nonetheless, responded to popular mobilization: most prominently, rural health services partially staffed by medical and nursing trainees doing mandatory social service, and integrated medical and social services (funded by peasant contributions along a sliding scale) on traditional agricultural cooperatives (*ejidos*), whose revival was central to Cárdenas's land reform (Carrillo 2005). The passage of social security legislation exclusive to industrial workers further institutionalized segmentation, with informal and rural workers perennially left to the inadequate reach of the health ministry (Block 2018).

At the other end of LA, Argentina's first health minister, Ramón Carrillo, pushed by the region's most militant and powerful labor movement, led an extensive reorganization of the public subsystem in the late-1940s and early-1950s. For instance, he oversaw a massive public hospital expansion, more than doubling the number of beds in just eight years. He also led the implementation of large-scale disease campaigns and preventive (public health) measures that helped diminish or eliminate malaria and other endemic infectious diseases, and drastically reduced infant and tuberculosis mortality. Such measures were all undergirded by substantial improvements in living and working conditions during Juan Perón's government (Alzugaray 1998; Ramacciotti 2009).

Just a few countries managed to defy the triple constraints of exclusion, segmentation, and fragmentation to enable more propitious outcomes. Costa Rica, a Latin American leader in universal social protections and government services, marshaled the resources opened up by the abolition of the military after a divisive civil war in the 1940s to invest in education, nutrition, and healthcare. Its pioneering expansion of social insurance reversed the typical trickle-down approach by starting with the lowest-income blue-collar workers and expanding upward through the occupational ladder, with a unified system covering the entire population by the 1970s (Martínez Franzoni and Sánchez Ancochea 2013).

Nowhere has health reform (and political change) transpired as dramatically as in Cuba. Preceding the 1959 revolution, political parties had cleverly used public health to attract voters, and Cuba was early to establish a social security system marked by all of the aforementioned flaws. It is, thus, not surprising that healthcare was atop the revolutionary agenda, with investment enabled by nationalization of production and assets. Consulting Czechoslovakia – considered the Eastern Bloc country with the best health and healthcare organization – Cuba pursued centralized health planning and decentralized service delivery via a polyclinic model, prioritizing underserved and remote settings, as well as physician training given the mass exodus of doctors. By the 1970s, Cuba developed a solid primary health care (PHC)–based approach, reaching the entire population with free, high-quality healthcare services (Danielson 1979).

At bottom, the historical struggles for Latin American health justice reveal heterogeneous trajectories across the ups and downs of people's mobilizations, shifting political alliances, and powerful domestic and international forces, struggles still playing out today.

The rise of neoliberalism and its HCS effects

The hopeful period of LA's welfare state-building abruptly ended after 1980, when the global economy took a tempestuous turn sparked by soaring oil prices (starting in the 1970s) and spiraling interest rates. These shocks unleashed a debt crisis – first in LA and then across low- and middle-income countries (LMICs) that saw debt mount by 700 percent in just ten years (from US$70.2 billion in 1970 to US$579.6 billion in 1980). In LA, debt more than doubled in three years, and several countries defaulted, starting with Mexico in 1982 (Economic Commission for Latin America and the Caribbean 1996; Prashad 2012). The International Monetary Fund (IMF) and World Bank (WB) became engineers of LMIC state policies (in both economic and social domains) through strings-attached loans that constrained debtor countries in order to protect high-income country private banking sector creditors from bankruptcy. The strings, or conditionalities, on the loans took shape as structural adjustment programs, which obliged extensive economic reforms that shifted the economic development paradigm from state-led to market-led growth according to the so-called Washington Consensus. Measures included the following: elimination of public deficits; drastic reductions in public spending (particularly in social sectors); elimination of subsidies; regressive tax reforms; currency devaluation; massive privatization of public enterprises; elimination of both trade tariffs and barriers to foreign direct investment (FDI); and deregulation of environmental and public health protections. These instruments were all implemented alongside the enactment of new regulations favoring markets, FDI, and corporate capital (Birn *et al.* 2016).

The attack on the welfare state – one pillar of a neoliberal agenda favoring and globalizing (financial) capital – had initially unfolded in Margaret Thatcher's United Kingdom and Ronald Reagan's United States of America (with Chile as an experimental outpost). Yet, the debt crisis triggered a far deeper and faster transformation across the Third World, with LA serving as an incubator. By the mid-1980s, amidst large-scale capital flight, inflation rose to a staggering 1500 percent and poverty levels reached almost 50 percent, provoking worse infant mortality rates and school attendance, among other social indicator declines. The 1980s became branded as LA's 'Lost Decade', but since it took until 2004 for poverty rates to return to 1970s levels, a better characterization is the 'lost quarter century'. The international financial sector justified its interference in LA economies as a necessary response to the debt crisis, but terminating the region's post-War economic model of state-led development and import substitution policies –which were accompanied by the growing power of labor and other social groups (checked by authoritarian regimes at various points) – was the underlying driver (Birn *et al.* 2016).

Country by country, neoliberal structural transformation began with 'first-generation' reforms to minimize the size of the state, followed by 'second-generation' reforms that deepened the first phase and shifted the emphasis toward achieving efficient, 'modernized' states, including by overhauling social protection systems (Jacobs 1999). Reflecting these policies, health sector reforms also underwent two waves.

The prescriptions for the first wave of health reforms were issued in the WB's 1993 *World Development Report* (WDR), titled 'Investing in Health'. Defining health as a private good, the WDR: promoted privatization of public health/sanitation services; endorsed a limited package or 'basket' of interventions funded with public resources and delivered by private or public health services (US$12 per capita per year for the lowest-income, and US$21.50 for middle-income countries); and invited private investment, among other recommendations that became conditionalities to obtain health sector reform loans. Despite denunciations from activists, academics, and part of the World Health Organization's (WHO) staff, the WHO ultimately supported these neoliberal policies.

The first phase was implemented across LA during the 1990s, except in Cuba, Costa Rica, and Brazil. It started with drastic cutbacks in public expenditures on healthcare and a reduction of state responsibility for financing health services. In turn, health was redefined as an individual responsibility and a commodity to be bought in the marketplace (overturning the existing principle of health as a human right to be realized through the welfare state). The first phase also led to separation of the previously unified trio of health system functions: administration of funds/purchasing of services (public or private); provision/delivery of private or public services; and regulation. This separation of functions was key to imposing market competition between the private and public sectors; regulation was meant to control the excesses and abuses of the market, fraud, and non-compliance with contracts. This separation worked for (those who could afford) individual healthcare services, while debilitating the public health and preventive services that remained the responsibility of the state (Laurell 2016). During this phase, many countries also underwent decentralization processes that promised greater efficiency and accountability, but resulted in smaller budgets and more financial responsibility at local levels without concomitant power and policy-making latitude. With LA's still sizable middle-class, compared to other LMICs, neoliberalism thrived in another domain: infiltration of FDI into pension and insurance markets covering formal sector workers via social security systems. In the 1990s, US investment in health insurance and private pensions skyrocketed (Iriart et al. 2001).

The second phase of reforms was also launched in the 1990s and focused on 'structured pluralism', whose advocates later proclaimed that universal health coverage (UHC) could be achieved. It is important to clarify that the concept of UHC was coopted from a prior progressive 'health for all' agenda. UHC soon became a euphemism for neoliberal policies applied to the health sector, and stands in contrast to universal health systems (UHS) – that is, comprehensive, publicly funded, universal, and equitable HCS (in marked opposition to UHC's market-oriented, segmented approach) (Birn and Nervi 2019).

Advocates of structured pluralism view population health as an input to economic development (not the reverse). This approach establishes enrollment-based insurance schemes through the pooling of public and private funds, subsidizing demand among low-income populations to purchase insurance. Structured pluralism embraces market competition, both among and between public and private entities.

UHC (with the aforementioned flaws) became a policymaking battle cry of the Rockefeller Foundation, WHO, WB, and government officials in the early-2000s. To reiterate, UHC coopts progressive aspirations of public, universal healthcare systems into public subsidies for private health insurance covering a circumscribed set of needs. The worst consequences of neoliberal policies (no access to care and bankruptcy due to healthcare spending) are, thus, addressed, but the rationale of health as a profitable commodity remains intact. UHC, resoundingly adopted as a key target of the United Nations' 'Sustainable Development Goal 3' (Good Health and Well-Being), reduces the constellation of political, commercial, and other societal determinants of health to an insurance-centered effort to 'cover' as many people as possible. In turn, it fails to tackle the ingredients of good health or of well-functioning, comprehensive HCS, or even the assurance of healthcare provision. In sum, the UHC model, as envisioned by its champions, offers 'hypothetical' access – that is, 'nominal, not necessarily effective or realizable, access to healthcare' (Birn and Nervi 2019: 6).

Overall, the most important forms of commoditization have been: the contracting of private hospitals and providers using public funds, resulting in a massive transfer of resources from the public to the private sector; outsourcing of the most profitable aspects of service delivery (*e.g.* laboratories and pharmacies) and support services (such as cleaning, food services, and patient transportation); outsourcing of health services management, public sector human resources recruitment, and administration (including payroll); privatization of publicly funded health services, with incentives to private providers to purvey these services; introduction of user fees in public services to increase revenues and reduce utilization; insurance schemes reducing coverage to defined packages of services that exclude diagnostics and treatment of complex, chronic, and/or expensive services, thus leading to rising out-of-pocket expenses or lack of care; and promotion of individual private health insurance, and the introduction/increase of deductibles, co-payments, and co-insurance in public insurance plans (Ferreira and Mendes 2018; Birn and Nervi 2019).

Additionally, health policies in LA (as in most of the world) have largely overlooked the crucial role of the health workforce. Indeed, under neoliberal reforms, the health workforce has been a target for downsizing, deregulation, and labor precarization that – combined with repression and a reduced formal sector workforce – has led to the loss of union power. This has added to the longstanding critical issue of scarcity of nurses, physicians, and other health workers, particularly in rural and inner-city areas, and at the PHC level. With few exceptions, physicians' simultaneous employment in two or all three subsystems is a perennial problem for accountability and planning.

Although neoliberal governments have all implemented neoliberal health reforms, even progressive-leaning governments have had limited policy space to dismantle them.

Healthcare neoliberalism on the ground: from Chile to Brazil

Many Latin American countries, as illustrated here, swiftly adopted the WB's 1993 prescriptions and privatization processes. Chile was the earliest policy laboratory for disassembling the welfare state, anticipating – and informing – the Washington Consensus by nearly a decade. In the early-1980s, the pension system was privatized, followed by a legal and operational dismantling of the SNS a decade later. A two-tier system was designed to replace the SNS: relatively wealthy, young, and healthy people were incentivized to join ISAPREs (private insurance), while those of lower income, older age, and/or poorer health remained under the public FONASA scheme. FONASA was left chronically underfunded and overcrowded, and of poor quality. By 2000, ISAPREs' per capita spending was double FONASA's, despite demographic asymmetries: less than 25 percent of the population accounted for almost half of overall healthcare spending (Homedes and Ugalde 2005).

In Colombia, structured pluralism was adopted wholesale from the early-1990s. Healthcare financing and delivery underwent hyper-privatization, based on competition among public and mostly private (both non-profit and for-profit) Health Promoting Agencies (EPSs). Capitation-based health insurance, organized through a 2-tier structure of contributory and subsidized regimes, became compulsory and nominally universal, currently covering almost 98 percent of the population (though actual access to quality healthcare services is far lower). EPSs administer funds and offer a package of services via over 5,000 largely (over 70 percent) private Service Providing Institutions (IPSs). The government's 'subsidy' also shores up private EPSs facing bankruptcy. Although there has been progress in reducing the gap between the contributory and subsidized schemes, inequities persist. Colombia's HCS has experienced recurrent crises, most notably in 2007, when legal challenges forced a host of administrative adjustments that ultimately did not resolve access barriers and quality problems (South American Institute of Government in Health 2012; Uribe-Gómez 2017).

Neoliberal healthcare reform in Mexico represents a reversal of once-promising efforts toward equity. Building on the social security system for industrial workers (IMSS, founded in 1943) and another for civil servants (ISSSTE, launched in 1959), the 1980s saw the extension of social security–supported coverage to agricultural and informal workers through a succession of solidarity schemes. These established a large network of IMSS-administered and IMSS-subsidized rural health clinics and hospitals where no public facilities existed. However, neoliberal reforms – from decentralization to budget-cutting – then started tearing the system apart. The paradoxical culmination of the rhetoric of universality within institutionalized inequity was Mexico's 2004 Seguro Popular (SP) insurance. This scheme, targeted at the country's 50 million uninsured persons (almost half of its 2004 population of 105 million people), offered voluntary health insurance for a defined package of interventions. Rather than building on prior solidarity efforts, the SP program exacerbated Mexico's already fragmented and segmented system. Specifically, it created yet another separate system with premiums financed by the federal and state governments and participating families (with some exemptions, and a crudely administered sliding-scale arrangement for the poorest 20 percent), and public and private providers contracted to provide services. By 2012, the Health Secretariat and its allies asserted that UHC had been attained (Knaul *et al.* 2012) – a claim contradicted by national survey and census data (Laurell 2015). As envisioned by the WDR's 1993 prescriptions, the SP's package of services was far from equivalent to social security benefits: its defined set of covered interventions (rather than covered diseases) excluded such common causes of illness and premature death as complications related to diabetes (Mexico's leading cause of death), cerebrovascular diseases (strokes), many types of cancer, and trauma or burns. Moreover, because SP expansion was not accompanied by substantial infrastructure and human resources investments, barriers to both access and quality persisted, particularly in rural areas (Laurell 2016). Although out-of-pocket expenses declined by 10 percent in the last 20 years, according to the most recent data from 2019, out-of-pocket expenses still accounted for over 42 percent of total healthcare spending, and disproportionately affected low-income families (OECD 2017; WHO 2022).

Peru, whose HCS is less known, provides the most paradigmatic case of deregulated commoditization in LA. In 2009, over a decade after the passage of a new constitution, wholesale pension privatization, and a new health law, Peru issued its *Universal Health Insurance Framework Law*, which mandated the separation of functions and protected segmented insurance schemes based on labor market insertion and income level. Various public and private financing entities administer healthcare funds and purchase goods and services. The Comprehensive Health Insurance System (SIS) is responsible for approximately 60 percent of the population, and offers two types of coverage: a semi-contributory regime (less than 1 percent of affiliates), and a subsidized regime for impoverished persons. SIS contracts with the Ministry of Health, and regional governments for affiliates, to receive services in public facilities. Although SIS negotiates reimbursement rates, its debt is enormous and constantly growing. Due to the Ministry of Health and regional governments' limited capacity to meet demand, access to healthcare is inadequate and affiliates often resort to the unregulated informal, for-profit private sector, which now has triple the number of clinics, medical offices, and pharmacies as the public sector. Formal workers and their dependents – almost 30 percent of the population in 2019 – are covered by social security. The latter, in turn, was partially privatized in 1997 when for-profit insurance companies were established and funded through the transfer of 25 percent of total worker and state contributions to social security. Roughly 7.5 percent of the population, mostly economic elites, use voluntary private insurance companies, which are currently undergoing 'vertical integration' with networks of clinics, pharmacies, and laboratories (Brito 2020; WHO 2022).

As in Colombia, neoliberal healthcare reforms in Peru also spawned a range of public and private service delivery entities, resulting in myriad contract modalities between private and public sectors. As elsewhere, private entities have systematically failed to fulfill their contractual obligations and, due to minimal regulation, are rarely held accountable (Brito 2020). Although out-of-pocket expenses have been reduced, they still accounted for over 28 percent of national health expenditures in 2019 (WHO 2022).

Notwithstanding the overall aims of neoliberal healthcare reforms, they have not always been linear. In Chile, when post-Pinochet progressive administrations governed, important efforts were made to strengthen the public sector, even as conservative administrations sought to deepen privatization (Laurell 2016). Neoliberal reforms have also encountered resistance: Chile's recent uprisings, for example, incorporated equitable healthcare policies within larger movements for social justice, which contributed to the 2021 election of progressive candidate, Gabriel Boric, to the Presidency. Likewise, in Colombia, there has been widespread mobilization against 1990s healthcare reforms, resulting in the 2015 *Statutory Health Law* that recognizes health as a fundamental human right, explicitly including the right to healthcare access, and requiring EPSs and IPSs to provide the requisite services. In 2022, the historic win of Gustavo Petro and Francia Márquez's progressive coalition was accompanied by health justice advocates' ambitious call for a complete transformation of the healthcare system based on publicly funded and delivered, unified, decentralized, intercultural, intersectoral, and equitable principles. Whether these aspirations are realized remains to be seen.

In Mexico, the 2018 Presidential election victory of Pink Tide candidate, Andrés Manuel López Obrador, ushered in plans for an integrated national healthcare system funded by general taxes, featuring recentralized procurement, access to services at any institution regardless of insurance affiliation, and integration of financing and delivery functions. Reduction of the private sector's role was envisioned through an increase in public funding, jump-started by replacement of the SP with the Institute of Health for Wellbeing (INSABI) (Reich 2020). Although INSABI's initial plans to eliminate out-of-pocket expenses were well received, the overall reform was slowed down by the COVID-19 pandemic.

Similarly, in Peru, the 2021 election of Pedro Castillo's progressive government brought expectations of major change in the health sector, starting with a project to integrate public healthcare under a single umbrella, expand PHC, and assure the right to obtain healthcare without being enrolled in a plan. Given Castillo's removal from power in 2022, an anti-neoliberal healthcare reform is no longer on the table.

Neoliberal health reforms have an instructive counter-example that materialized at the height of 1980s/90s neoliberalism. Brazil was the only country in LA to introduce a public, universal, unified, equitable HCS approach in this period, amidst the government's adoption of market-oriented economic reforms. A health movement that brought together academics, administrators, activists, and a range of social movements during the larger anti-dictatorship struggle played a crucial role in driving the country's 1988 *Constitution* to recognize the right to health. The *Constitution* delineated the government's responsibility in guaranteeing this right, established the Unified Health System (SUS), and circumscribed the private sector's role as complementary (Machado and Azevedo e Silva 2019). SUS has been an inexhaustible source of inspiration for progressive policymakers, social movements, and academics within and beyond LA. In particular, it has been hailed for its integrated multi-professional, prevention-oriented, PHC-based model, as well as its decentralized approach that democratically redistributes decision-making power and resources to states and municipalities through a framework delineating the role of both the federal and local governments in health system governance, management, planning, financing, and delivery of services (Castro *et al.* 2019). Unlike the decentralization model advocated by the WB, in Brazil there has been bona fide sharing of power and resources, yielding improved responsiveness, quality, access, and equity.

SUS has dramatically increased access to healthcare at all levels (achieving nearly universal access to highly effective PHC), with notable morbidity and mortality improvements in conditions amenable to healthcare. SUS has reduced healthcare inequities and stimulated local decision-making capacity and participation in health planning, among many other achievements. Yet, it has also faced serious challenges: chronic underfunding (greatly exacerbated by a 2016 Constitutional amendment that freezes federal spending in health and education for 20 years); persistence of geographical inequities; increasing influence of the private sector in tertiary care provision and through outsourcing of services in public facilities; and the effects of a powerful insurance industry that benefits from huge government subsidies. In 2019, private health insurance premiums and out-of-pocket expenses accounted for, respectively, some 30 percent and 25 percent of national health expenditures, thereby putting the reach of SUS's model in jeopardy. Additionally, development of an integrated network of services that includes all levels of care and prevention remains a pending monumental task (Castro *et al.* 2019; WHO 2022).

In recent years, the most dangerous threat to SUS came from the radical right-wing Bolsonaro government, which imposed draconian austerity policies, along with renewed fragmentation. The regime also narrowed the scope of PHC (Azevedo e Silva *et al.* 2020) – eliminating the Mais Medicos partnership that brought thousands of Cuban physicians to underserved areas. Luiz Inácio Lula da Silva's return to the Presidency in 2023 is enabling a series of policies to strengthen the SUS.

Neoliberalism's intransigence and the Pink Tide

By the early-2000s, the neoliberal model started to unravel, with broad, ongoing people's resistance to its nefarious consequences across the world. In LA, demand for change materialized in elected progressive governments, from Argentina to Bolivia, Brazil, Chile, Ecuador, El Salvador, Uruguay, and Venezuela. The new administrations arising from this 'Pink Tide' of social democratic movements, alliances, and political parties soon channeled earnings from soaring commodity prices (based on a neo-extractivist model linked to significant environmental degradation) to an array of social policies targeting living and working conditions. This, in turn, served to improve health, especially for low-income urban workers. Measures included higher wages, cash transfer programs, renewed enforcement of labor and environmental laws, and expanded access (and, in some places, articulated rights) to healthcare – sometimes, as in the case of conditional cash transfers, heeding neoliberal logics of consumer (usually mothers') responsibility, without bona fide improvements in social services. Still, in Uruguay, an augmented anti-poverty program, progressive tax reforms, and a unified public health insurance financing pool led to a marked decline in the Gini (inequality) coefficient. Similar results were seen in Brazil, which introduced integrated nutrition and (non-conditional) cash transfer programs, and expanded PHC. Meanwhile, in Venezuela, South-South cooperation with Cuba (involving an oil-for-doctors exchange) enabled the establishment of neighborhood-based primary-care clinics; and in Bolivia, an inclusive intercultural HCS was introduced. To be sure, creation of Brazil's SUS predated the Pink Tide but, during most of the Workers' Party period in power, the federal government increased HCS funding.

Remarkable as many of these efforts were in bettering health and social conditions, and in generating unprecedented reductions in income inequality and extreme poverty, Pink Tide governments did not fundamentally change longstanding inequitable and deeply unjust societal structures, most egregiously affecting the lives, livelihoods, health, and ecology of Indigenous peoples whose territories faced heightened exploitation. This is because most of the social spending came not from income/wealth redistribution or tax code reforms addressing the extreme concentration of capital in corporations and wealthy individuals, but from commodity earnings.

Further, the failure to institutionalize redistributive reforms or redress longstanding power asymmetries engendered an appallingly swift reversal of Pink Tide investments once the commodity boom ended, with enormous negative consequences for HCS. After 2015, neoliberalism resurged in some countries in the context of new governments with right-wing and even authoritarian tendencies (Argentina, Bolivia, Brazil, Chile, Ecuador, El Salvador, Uruguay). Recent years have also witnessed some progressive administrations' return to power (Argentina, Chile, Bolivia, and Brazil), while others elected anti-neoliberal governments for the first time since the 1980s (Mexico, Peru, and Colombia). Still, other countries have stayed (unchanged) along a neoliberal path.

That said, a modicum of hope arises from a few settings. Costa Rica's HCS, despite certain reforms, has survived neoliberalism: fending off commodification, and continuing to pursue its aim of universal social security without barriers such as co-payment, and even reducing out-of-pocket expenses to about 22 percent of national health expenditures. Meanwhile, countries like Colombia, which have been extreme adherents to neoliberal health reforms, have had a sustained increase in public spending since the 2000s. Out-of-pocket expenses have remained low and stable, accounting for less than 15 percent of national health expenditures in 2019 (WHO 2022).

Other countries, such as El Salvador – which, after its bloody 1980s civil war, experienced two decades of neoliberal regimes – saw some notable advances under ten years of progressive FMLN governments. Although now threatened by a right-wing administration, FMLN reforms in short order spanned an increase in healthcare access, progress toward comprehensive PHC, intersectoral efforts, and an impressive reduction in out-of-pocket expenses. However, the planned building of a unified HCS, like Brazil's, was not viable, and its prospects have now dimmed. In El Salvador, as in many countries, the reform possibilities of even progressive governments were confined to the public subsystem, impeding truly redistributive and equitable policies that might have addressed the huge gap in per capita health spending between public and social security systems, not to mention the private sector.

Accompanying political struggles for health justice are resource issues: on average, LA per capita health spending is about one-quarter of the OECD average, and its public sector spending as a percentage of GDP is far lower than in OECD countries. Moreover, on average, private insurance and out-of-pocket expenses comprise 45 percent of total health spending in the region, while public spending accounts for less than 55 percent, far below the 74 percent average of OECD countries (OECD 2020).

Notwithstanding advances in some countries toward unified, publicly funded, universal, comprehensive, equitable, effective, and integrated HCS underpinned by the right to health – plus rising public investment in HCS – immense challenges remain throughout the region. This is due to an overall context of unfavorable international economic and trade conditions, combined with historical structural inequities under capitalism and the consequences of four decades of its neoliberal phase. Prior to the COVID-19 pandemic, HCS expansion – as part of larger, if temporary and uneven anti-poverty policies – translated into significant health gains. Yet, these improvements have remained highly inequitable within countries and markedly unequal across LA.

Conclusion: looking forward, not backward

HCS should be evaluated not only for what they address, but also for what they exclude or overlook. Both globally and in LA, such critical shortfalls span mental health, climate change, chronic diseases, long-term care, women's health, violence (gang and cartel killings; femicide), consideration of knowledge systems other than the biomedical, and the underlying structural determinants of health. One crucial issue stands out shamefully as an HCS failing in LA: very limited access to abortion.[1]

Moreover, the trends highlighted here need to be contextualized by the devastating impact of COVID-19 across the region. Not only have Argentina, Brazil, Peru, Uruguay, and other countries experienced among the world's highest total or per capita cases and deaths – either cumulatively or during different phases of the pandemic – but COVID-19 has also unleashed an unprecedented economic and social crisis. ECLAC (2020) projects that the crisis will lead to a 9 percent decline in GDP, together with sharp rises in unemployment and a poverty rate exceeding 37 percent (affecting over 230 million people), with some 96 million living in extreme poverty. Particularly affected are women, who account for most of the informal employment, Indigenous groups (10 percent of LA's population), Afro-descendant peoples (21 percent), and migrants. The collateral damage of COVID-19 (due to reduced or no access to healthcare services for acute or chronic conditions), and the impact of excess deaths, has once again revealed the longstanding structural problems of the region's HCS.

If historical experience is any guide, healthcare justice will require tax-based, solidly publicly financed HCS. However, in LA tax systems are regressive and raise insufficient funds, with hugely inequitable contributions by social class/tax bracket, and massive tax evasion by powerful elites and both domestic and transnational corporations. Without progressive tax reforms, universal HCS have no prospect of being sustainable. Yet, nostalgia for the days of 'solid' welfare states predating neoliberal claw-backs is misguided. Virtually all HCS in LA have long been plagued by inequities according to class, gender, race/ethnicity, location (urban vs rural), labor market insertion, and other factors. Ultimately, transformative anti-capitalist societies and deeply redistributive policies will require more: HCS based on principles of universal health justice, which are comprehensive, inclusive, participatory, single-tier (unitary/unified), publicly financed and delivered, and free from all forms of oppression.

Note

1 Criminalization has resulted in the exponential growth of illegal, unsafe abortions, accounting for a large proportion (over 30 percent in some countries) of pregnancy-related deaths, aggravated by suicide and intimate partner homicide (Fernández Anderson 2013; Berro Pizzarossa 2018). Currently, 4 of the 24 countries with an outright ban (including rape, and to save the life of the mother) are in LA: Dominican Republic, El Salvador, Honduras, and Nicaragua (Chile was among this group until 2018, when it partially decriminalized abortion). Despite vibrant feminist struggles for reproductive rights, the powerful influence of the Catholic Church, the US evangelical movement, and conservative political parties have impeded decriminalization and access to abortion services. Yet, change is afoot: abortion has been available on request in Cuba since 1965, and in recent years, it has been decriminalized in Argentina, Mexico, and Uruguay.

References

Alzugaray, R. 1998, *Ramón Carrillo, el Fundador del Sanitarismo Nacional*, Centro Editor de América Latina, Buenos Aires.

Azevedo e Silva, G., Giovanella, L. and Rochel de Camargo Jr., K. 2020, 'Brazil's national health care system at risk of losing its universal character', *American Journal of Public Health*, 110, pp. 811–2.

Berro Pizzarossa, L. 2018, 'Legal barriers to access abortion services through a human rights lens: The Uruguayan experience', *Reproductive Health Matters*, 26(52), pp. 151–8.

Birn, A.E. 2020, 'Alternative destinies and solidarities for health and medicine in Latin America before and during the cold war', in Birn, A.E. and Necochea, R. (eds), *Peripheral Nerve: Health and Medicine in Cold War Latin America*, Duke University Press, Durham, pp. 1–28.

Birn, A.E., Nervi, L. and Siqueira, E. 2016, 'Neoliberalism redux: The global health policy agenda and the politics of cooptation in Latin America and beyond', *Development and Change*, 47(4), pp. 734–59.

Birn, A.E. and Nervi, L. 2019, 'What matters in health (care) universes: Delusions, dilutions, and ways towards universal health justice', *Global Health*, 15(1), pp. 1–12.

Block, M.A. 2018, *El Seguro Social: Evolución Histórica, Crisis y Perspectivas de Reforma*, Universidad Anáhuac México Norte, Huixquilucan del Degollado.

Brito, P. 2020, *Los Mercados de la Salud y la Salud de los Mercados. Treinta Años de Mercantilización del Sistema Sanitario Peruano*, Unidad de Investigación de Políticas y Sistemas de Salud, Peruvian University Cayetano Heredia, Lima.

Carrillo, A.M. 2005, 'Salud pública y poder en México durante el Cardenismo, 1934–1940,' *Dynamis*, 25, pp. 145–78.

Castro, M.C., Massuda, A., Almeida, G., Menezes-Filho, N.A., Andrade, M.V., de Souza Noronha, K.V.M., Rocha, R., Macinko, J., Hone, T., Tasca, R. and Giovanella, L. 2019, 'Brazil's unified health system: The first 30 years and prospects for the future', *The Lancet*, 394(10195), pp. 345–56.

Cueto, M. and Palmer, S. 2015, *Medicine and Public Health in Latin America: A History*, Cambridge University Press, Cambridge.

Danielson, R. 1979, *Cuban Medicine*, Transaction, New Brunswick.

Economic Commission for Latin America and the Caribbean (ECLAC). 1996, *The Economic Experience of the Last Fifteen Years: Latin America and the Caribbean, 1980–1995*, United Nations, ECLAC, Santiago.

Economic Commission for Latin American and the Caribbean. 2020, *Health and the Economy: A Convergence Needed to Address COVID-19 and Retake the Path of Sustainable Development in Latin America and the Caribbean*, ECLAC, PAHO, Washington, DC.

Fernandez Anderson, C. 2013, 'The politics of abortion in Latin America', *Rewire News Group*, 17 July 2013, accessed 10 October 2021, <https://rewirenewsgroup.com/article/2013/07/17/the-politics-of-abortion-in-latin-america/>.

Ferreira, M.R.J. and Mendes, A.N. 2018, 'Commodification in the reforms of the German, French and British health systems', *Ciencia e Saude Coletiva*, 23(7), pp. 2159–70.

Göttems, L.B.D. and Mollo, M.L.R. 2020, 'Neoliberalismo na América Latina: Efeitos nas reformas dos sistemas de saúde', *Revista de Saúde Pública*, 54(74), <https://rsp.fsp.usp.br/artigo/neoliberalism-in-latin-america-effects-on-health-system-reforms/?lang=en>.

Homedes, N. and Ugalde, A. 2005, 'Las reformas de salud neoliberales en América Latina: Una visión crítica a través de dos estudios de caso', *Revista Panamericana de Salud Pública*, 17(3), pp. 210–20.

Illanes, M.A. 1993, *En el Nombre del Pueblo, del Estado y de la Ciencia. Historia Social de la Salud Pública. Chile, 1880–1973. Hacia una Historia Social del Siglo XX*, Fundación Interamericana (IAF) y ONG Colectivo Atención Primaria, Santiago.

Iriart, C., Merhy, E.E. and Waitzkin, H. 2001, 'Managed care in Latin America: The new common sense in health policy reform', *Social Science and Medicine*, 52, pp. 1243–53.

Jacobs, S.H. 1999, 'The second generation of regulatory reforms', paper prepared for delivery at the *IMF Conference on Second Generation Reforms*, 8–9 November 1999, OECD, accessed 28 September 2021, <https://www.imf.org/external/pubs/ft/seminar/1999/reforms/jacobs.htm>.

Knaul, F.M., González-Pier, E., Gómez-Dantés, O., García-Junco, D., Arreola-Ornelas, H., Barraza-Lloréns, M., Sandoval, R., Caballero, F., Hernández-Avila, M., Juan, M. and Kershenobich, D. 2012, 'The quest for universal health coverage: Achieving social protection for all in Mexico', *The Lancet*, 380(9849), pp. 1259–79.

Laurell, A.C. 2015, 'The Mexican popular health insurance: Myths and realities', *International Journal of Health Services*, 45(1), pp. 105–25.

Laurell, A.C. 2016, 'Las reformas de salud en América Latina: Procesos y resultados', *Cuadernos de Relaciones Laborales*, 34(2), pp. 293–314.

Lavrin, A.C. 1998, *Women, Feminism, and Social Change in Argentina, Chile, and Uruguay, 1890–1940,* University of Nebraska Press, Lincoln.

Machado, C.V. and Azevedo e Silva, G. 2019, 'Political struggles for a universal health system in Brazil: Successes and limits in the reduction of inequalities', *Global Health*, 15(1), pp. 1–12.

Martínez Franzoni, J. and Sánchez-Ancochea, D. 2013, *Good Jobs and Social Services: How Costa Rica Achieved the Elusive Double Incorporation*, Palgrave Macmillan, New York.

Martínez Franzoni, J. and Sánchez-Ancochea, D. 2016, *The Quest for Universal Social Policy in the South: Actors, Ideas and Architectures*, Cambridge University Press, Cambridge.

Mesa-Lago, C. 2005, *Las Reformas de Salud en América Latina y el Caribe: Su Impacto en los Principios de la Seguridad Social*, CEPAL, Santiago.

Molina Bustos, C.A. 2010, *Institucionalidad Sanitaria Chilena 1889–1989*, LOM Ediciones, Santiago.

Organization for Economic Co-operation and Development (OECD). 2017, 'Health at a Glance 2017: OECD Indicators', *OECD*, accessed 19 September 2021, <https://www.oecd.org/mexico/Health-at-a-Glance-2017-Key-Findings-MEXICO-in-Spanish.pdf >.

Organization for Economic Co-operation and Development. 2020, *Health at a Glance in Latin America and the Caribbean*, accessed 19 September 2021, <https://www.oecd.org/health/health-at-a-glance-latin-america-and-the-caribbean-2020-6089164f-en.htm>.

Pan-American Health Organization (PAHO). 2005, *Renewing Primary Health Care in the Americas*, Position Paper, PAHO, Washington, DC.

Pieper Mooney, J. 2020, 'From cold war pressures to state policy to people's health: Social medicine and socialized medical care in Chile', in Birn, A.E. and Necochea, R. (eds.) *Peripheral Nerve: Health and Medicine in Cold War Latin America*, Duke University Press, Durham, pp. 187–210.

Prashad, V. 2012, *The Poorer Nations: A Possible History of the Global South*, Verso, London.

Ramacciotti, K.I. 2009, *La Política Sanitaria del Peronismo*, Biblos, Buenos Aires.

Reich, M.R. 2020, 'Restructuring health reform, Mexican style', *Health Systems and Reform*, 6(1), p. e1763114.

Singleton, L. 2013, 'The ILO and social security in Latin America, 1930–1950', in Herrera León, F. and Herrera González, P. (eds), *América Latina y la Organización Internacional del Trabajo: Redes, Cooperación Técnica e Institucionalidad Social (1919–1950)*, Instituto de Investigaciones Históricas, Universidad Michoacana de San Nicolás de Hidalgo, Morelia, México, pp. 215–43.

South American Institute of Government in Health (ISAGS). 2012, *Health Systems in South America: Challenges for Universality, Comprehensiveness and Equity*, ISAGS, Río de Janeiro, Brazil.

Uribe-Gómez, M. 2017, 'Nuevos cambios, viejos esquemas: Las políticas de salud en México y Colombia en los años 2000', *Cadernos de Saúde Pública*, 33(suppl. 2).

World Health Organization (WHO). 2022, 'Health expenditure database', accessed 27 October 2022, <https://apps.who.int/nha/database/country_profile/Index/en >.

26

THE POLITICAL ECONOMY OF HEALTHCARE POLICY IN AFRICA IN THE AGE OF COVID-19

Jean-Germain Gros

Across much of Africa, healthcare policy produces systems that are ineffective, exclusive, and expensive (Peiffer and Rose 2016).[1] This was not supposed to be the case. Nearly every African country committed to making healthcare a social good at independence. Furthermore, except for the 1980s – when African countries were subject to the 'shock therapy' of structural adjustment programs – this commitment has been repeatedly reaffirmed at critical junctures: such as the *Alma Mata Declaration* of 1978, the Millennium Development Goals of 2000, the *Abuja Declaration* of 2001, and the Sustainable Development Goals of 2015 (Gros 2016). Hence, the problem is not policy adoption. What, then, ails healthcare policy in Africa? The main argument of this chapter is that politics and the economy in Africa, as they are currently embedded in the post-colonial state and primary commodity production, greatly hinder the implementation of the kind of effective, inclusive, and cost-efficient healthcare policy that Africa needs to face the health challenges of the Twenty-First Century. These challenges include rising morbidity from so-called 'rich man's diseases' (such as cancer and heart disease), pandemics (such as Ebola and COVID-19), and the endemic 'poor man's' diseases that continue to plague Africa (such as malaria, childhood diarrhea, cholera, and yellow fever).

The chapter theorizes healthcare policy in Africa from a political economy standpoint, in recognition of the fact that the larger social contexts in which policy is adopted and implemented matter. Social contexts, in turn, are influenced by history. Where Africa is concerned, that history is replete with external domination, starting with the transatlantic and Arab slave trades, which deprived much of the continent of its most able-bodied and healthiest members. The transatlantic slave trade alone is estimated to have extracted from Africa some 12 million people out of a population of 102 million in 1800 – just seven years before the abolition of the infamous trade (Cameron and Neal 2016). The colonial experience, though lasting less than 100 years (roughly 1885–1957), inflicted further damage by integrating Africa into the capitalist world economy as a primary commodity producer, with all of the vicissitudes this type of economy implies (discussed later in the chapter). Moreover, donor-imposed structural adjustment programs (SAPs) in the 1980s (in other words, neoliberalism) forced African governments to retrench, eroding the limited social gains made in the first decade or so of independence; in fact, neoliberalism may well have increased poverty across the continent (Schatz 1994).

DOI: 10.4324/9781003017110-30

Following the end of the Cold War, African countries did liberalize their political systems, by allowing opposition parties to contest elections and the press to operate more freely. *Ceteris paribus*, electoral democracy should produce inclusive social policy, including healthcare policy, as politicians and their parties compete for the votes of the demos, and as journalists are less constrained in reporting glaring social pathologies, which may shame elected officials into action. However, the sustainability of policy depends not only on the commitment of elected officials and vigilance of the fourth estate but, equally importantly, on the financial and human resources necessary to implement policy. In this sense, the future of healthcare policy in Africa is not dissociable from that of African economic and political institutions, although the agency of African leaders can palliate some of the worse side-effects of these institutions as they are presently configured.

The intersectionality of health, the economy, and politics

There is a great symbiosis between health and the economy, health and politics and, of course, the economy and politics. One consistent finding in comparative health policy studies is that as countries become prosperous, they spend more on the healthcare sector, which generally translates into improved health outcomes. Among OECD countries, only Britain spends less than 10 percent of its GDP on healthcare (9.6 percent) (Office for National Statistics 2019). In a now-famous study, Joseph P. Newhouse (1977) attributes well over 90 percent of the variations in healthcare spending among countries to variations in per capita GDP. Not surprisingly, health indices – from infant and maternal mortality rates to adult life expectancy and nearly everything in between – tend to be most impressive among wealthy countries, although there are exceptions (*e.g.* Cuba). While healthcare spending may not guarantee entry to the promised land of bountiful health, at the very least, it leads to the right path.

The relationship between health and the economy transcends macroeconomic conditions and fiscal spending. From a microeconomic perspective, a healthy population minimizes the number of working hours and days lost to sickness. In addition, it can more readily absorb new knowledge. Working time uninterrupted by illness and better technology translate into higher productivity, a key factor in economic development. Assuming productivity gains are shared with workers in the form of higher wages, rather than accruing primarily to the owners of capital – a phenomenon directly attributable to the ability of labor to organize – workers should experience the kind of living standard conducive to good health in an expanding economy. Specifically, they should be able to eat more nutritious food, live in decent houses, save (which decreases the mental stress wrought by uncertainty), and increase their purchase of medical care. In the latter connection, it is not just the governments of wealthy countries that spend more on healthcare; wealthy individuals also spend more on their health. An economy in which workers cannot make the most 'widgets' at the lowest cost per unit, due to ill-health, inevitably makes for a destitute population subsisting on low wages, which can only purchase the goods necessary for daily survival. In sum, a healthy workforce and a wealthy economy are mutually reinforcing.

What explains wealthy economies? Since the dawn of the industrial age, the strongest national economies have been those that have managed to add value to whatever endowments were bequeathed by nature. Primary commodity production without the value-added transformation wrought by industrialization has not been a source of the wealth of nations. Simply extracting resources from the ground or seabed and selling them overseas may earn countries foreign exchange – admittedly, lots of it in the exceptional case of fossil fuels in the age of the combustion engine – but does not necessarily make them developed. Volatility in the prices of most primary commodities does not make possible sustainable economic development which, as Thomas Piketty (2014) points out, requires moderate annual growth rates in the order of 3 to 4 percent over a generation (20 years). Economic performance in primary commodity-dependent countries tends to seesaw between brief periods of impressive growth rates, followed by longer periods of stagnation. Macroeconomic instability strains national budgets, undermining government commitments – not least in healthcare, which requires long-term planning, a non sequitur under conditions of uncertainty.

Yet, even when economies experience relatively lengthy periods of primary commodity-driven booms, these are unlikely to result in sustainable development and inclusive social policy for at least two reasons. A positive balance of trade may lead to a spending binge on private luxury goods, as elite arrivistes may be more concerned about displaying their newfound wealth than sharing it. In addition, an economy centered on commodity production (*matières premières*) tends to reinforce primary group identity, especially if foreign exchange earnings are associated with extraction from specific geographic areas, as illustrated by oil production in the Niger Delta region of Nigeria. Inclusive social policy here may be seen as a zero-sum proposition, a surreptitious way of robbing Peter to pay Paul. In the extreme, it may even lead to murmurs of secession, as disgruntled groups call for greater local control over 'their' resources.

In theory, it may be possible for an extractive political economy to generate inclusive social policy, if extractive activities are widely distributed across space and social classes. Alas, natural resource endowments are seldom so bestowed. Instead, they tend to be randomly concentrated. In the case of fossil fuels, the dinosaurs could not have chosen their final resting place so humans would not fight over their carbonized bodies, nor could they have anticipated the centrality of the combustion engine in modern transportation. An extractive economy generally dissipates large-scale social organization and does not foster the environment that produces inclusive social policy – which includes urbanization, labor unionization, competent public administration, strong political parties and, ultimately, democracy (Acemoglu and Robinson 2012). The history of healthcare policy unmistakably suggests that inclusive healthcare policy came about when Left parties were in power (*e.g.* Labor under Clement Richard Attlee in the UK after World War Two), or when Right parties and/or conservative leaders (*e.g.* Germany under Otto von Bismarck) co-opted inclusive policy to prevent Left parties from coming to power (Marmor *et al.* 2009). In both instances, the pressure for change was preceded by industrialization, the emergence of a more 'articulate' and concentrated workforce, the political empowerment of the masses through either enfranchisement or war, and an expanding economy.

If the economy and health exist in symbiosis, so too are politics and health strongly connected. Politics entails at least two things: conflict management and the allocation of things that are valued. Politics as conflict management is at its nadir when there is either no state to enforce the social contract, or the state itself becomes predatory by stripping people of their assets. Thus, life ceases to be 'nasty, brutish, and short', to reprise Hobbes' well-worn phrase, through politics – that is, when the people surrender a portion of their wealth to an overarching authority (the state) in return for effective protection (broadly understood to include social protection). Accordingly, it is no accident that the countries in which health indices are the poorest also happen to have weak, if not failed, states, which are often wracked by conflicts (Gros 1996). The absence of politics has deleterious consequences for health and, ultimately, life itself.

Yet, too much of the wrong kind of politics can be equally detrimental to health. The problem here is not the lack of resources or their predaceous appropriation by a malevolent Leviathan, but rather the legitimate use of legally sanctioned methods (lobbying, campaign contributions, media advertising) by private actors for ends that undermine the public good. The contradictions of politics as the production of valuable things are, perhaps, at their sharpest relief in regard to healthcare in the US, which spends a higher percentage of its GDP on healthcare than any other industrialized country (16.8 percent in 2019) (OECD 2021), but has the highest number of uninsured citizens among OECD countries (over 37 million Americans entirely lack health insurance and 41 million more have inadequate access to care) (Galvani *et al.* 2020). Healthcare spending in the US does not purchase inclusiveness or access but, rather, other things that are valued by special interest groups and the politicians who feed incessantly at the trough of campaign contributions. In sum, if the economy strongly influences how much countries are able to spend on healthcare, politics determines what they purchase: such as expensive medical equipment and procedures of questionable utility or low-cost prescription drugs.

What ails healthcare policy in contemporary Africa?

Healthcare policy in post-colonial Africa is hemmed in by the structure of African economies, which bode ill for the sustainability of inclusive healthcare systems in whatever variations they adopt – be it socialized medicine reminiscent of the UK, or social health insurance schemes in the mold of Germany, Canada, and Ghana. Dependence on primary commodity production for foreign exchange is antithetical to inclusive social policy in Africa, because of the twin menace of price fluctuation and demand volatility, as well as the uneven concentration of natural resources, which tend to stoke ethnic resentment in contexts of incomplete nationhood and lack of government transparency. The training of doctors requires at least seven years, while that of nurses takes three years. Therapeutic drugs and vaccines consume between three and five years from research and development to mass production. A mid-sized hospital in the West takes between 18 and 24 months to build, though longer in Africa where nearly everything, from electrical wires to bathroom fixtures, has to be imported (Gros 2016). In sum, returns-on-investment in healthcare have a long-term horizon, such that they require sustained commitment, which the vicissitudes of commodity production invalidate. Furthermore, prolonged periods of favorable terms of trade are no guarantee of fiscal solidarity, when countries have to play catch-up to previous years of stagnation and elites are eager to show off their new 'toys'.

International bonds are generally not an attractive source of financing healthcare capital projects in Africa (*e.g.* hospitals), because their yields (i.e. interest that African countries must pay to bondholders) are tied to risks, which are not abated by the volatility of commodity prices. Domestic bonds are unattractive to local investors for different reasons. Private health insurance schemes are an important source of hospital revenue in many countries, but they are limited in Africa, because of market distortions. Private healthcare financing in Africa follows the logic of actuarial fairness, rather than the principle of solidarity. This is because wealth is strongly influenced by age in Africa (Smith 2019). State power follows a similar pattern, hence the ubiquity of gerontocracy. The wealthy tend to be unhealthy because they are older and, therefore, susceptible to chronic illnesses requiring frequent medical care. The non-wealthy (the poor) tend to be healthier, because they are younger. The former can afford to pay for medical care out-of-pocket, which becomes a key line of social demarcation between 'big men' and 'small boys'. The latter cannot pay for healthcare out-of-pocket, nor do they have an urgent need to buy health insurance, which they do not expect to use (the optimism of youth). In sum, neither cohort has an incentive to pool resources and insure against medical risk. As is the case elsewhere, the poor and uninsured in Africa often use the hospital emergency room as the provider of first and last resort. This means that most hospitals in Africa likely operate at a loss, except those that cater to the über-rich, who tend to seek advanced, more expensive, care outside of Africa anyway. Local investors would be loath to hold hospital bonds in their investment portfolios under these conditions, in the absence of guarantees by the state.

The key thesis of the chapter can be substantiated in a straightforward fashion through examination of international trade – which earns countries foreign exchange – and government spending in general, with particular emphasis on healthcare. International trade and government spending should align in Africa, because taxes on cross-border exchange are relatively easy to collect, even by governments with limited extraction capacity. Thus, as foreign exchange earnings increase, so, too, should government spending in Africa generally point upward. Yet, what does the empirical evidence actually show? The focus here will be on merchandise trade since, with the exception of tourism, Africa does not derive significant revenue from trading in services (such as banking, insurance, and accounting).

Collectively, African countries account for a very low share of global merchandise trade: 2.4 percent in 2015. This is because Africa adds limited value to its exports: it simply extracts its abundant raw materials and sells them overseas. Measured as a proportion of global exports, the global trade powerhouses in 2015 were China (14 percent), the US (9 percent), and Germany (8 percent) – all of which are, of course, highly industrialized countries (Verter 2017).[2] Longitudinal merchandise trade data from the middle of the Twentieth Century to the present show that the nominal value of African exports rose from US$3.4 billion in 1948 to US$92 billion in 1993, surging to US$601 billion in 2013, before dropping precipitously to US$396 billion in 2015. Hence, if there was a *belle époque* in African merchandise trade since World War Two, it is situated between 1993 and 2013, when African exports increased by nearly 650 percent (Verter 2017). One might be tempted to conclude here that African trade performance is not hampered by its production profile – in other words, that it is possible for primary commodity producers to do well on the world market. There are strong reasons to suspect that the two decades in question were exceptional. More typical was Africa's experience in the decades before 1993 and the years after 2013.

African merchandise trade expanded at a much slower pace during the period between 1948 and 1993, which was also affected by steep inflation in 1973–74 and 1979, which reduced the real value of African exports. Between 2013 and 2015, African merchandise exports dropped by 33 percent, from US$601 billion in 2013 to US$552 billion in 2014 to US$396 billion in 2015 (Verter 2017). A simple, back-of-the-envelope calculation suffices to make the point. If 2013 is taken as the golden year of African merchandise exports, 54 African countries would each have earned, on average, US$11 billion from exports (601bn/54) – perhaps enough to make a difference in the fiscal outlook of the smaller African countries, but not the bigger ones. Yet, the more populous African countries (Nigeria, Egypt, South Africa, Angola, Democratic Republic of the Congo) received the lion's share of merchandise exports, since they also happened to be Africa's biggest producers of raw materials, especially minerals (Afreximbank 2019). Some of these same countries are legendary for their corruption. The export windfall, in turn, was unlikely to result in an increase in government spending to address social needs (as explored below). Even more concerning is what happened to Africa's top ten exporters from 2014 to 2018, as depicted in Table 26.1.

Table 26.1 supports the main contention of the chapter that primary commodity production is an unreliable source of revenue for governments in Africa. Between 2014 and 2018, three of the largest merchandise exporters in Africa experienced huge declines in their foreign exchange earnings: Nigeria (–46.7 percent), Algeria (–28.4 percent), and Angola (–31.1%). All three countries are, of course, oil producers, but the damage is not limited to them. In two other cases, the decreases were less dramatic, but still notable: Tunisia (–4.6 percent) and Ivory Coast (–8.9 percent). South Africa, Africa's largest exporter, saw a modest expansion (+2 percent) in its foreign trade earnings during this period. The statistic on Libya is surprising: income from trade increased 47 percent during the period. However, Libya's trade performance must be taken with a grain of salt (or two). Oil production collapsed almost completely after the death of Muammar Gaddafi in 2011.

Table 26.1 Top ten African exporters, 2018

Rank	*Country*	*2018 Exports (US$bn)*	*Percent of total*	*Percent change 2014–18*
1	South Africa	94.43	19.0	+2.0
2	Nigeria	52.92	10.6	–46.7
3	Angola	42.03	8.5	–28.4
4	Algeria	41.62	8.4	–31.1
5	Libya	30.68	6.2	+46.9
6	Egypt	29.33	5.9	+9.6
7	Morocco	29.33	5.9	+23.2
8	Ghana	17.00	3.4	No 2014 Data
9	Tunisia	16.00	3.2	–4.6
10	Ivory Coast	11.83	2.4	–8.9

Source: CIA (2020).

In turn, Libya started from a very low baseline in 2014. In addition, Libya is a collapsed state in the throes of a civil war. Renewed oil production is probably underwritten by a desire on the part of local warlords to capture the proceeds to pay for weapons and, increasingly, foreign mercenaries, rather than addressing the social needs of ordinary Libyans.

Concomitantly, the impact of political balkanization on the continent's international trade cannot be ignored in this chapter. On matters involving international trade, Africa does not speak with one voice. The African Continental Free Trade Area is the largest trade agreement to come into effect since the creation of the World Trade Organization itself, but it is not clear that it will accord African countries a unified voice in world trade negotiations. Whatever Africa earns from exporting to the rest of the world is divvied up among a relatively large number of countries that compete on world markets, thereby potentially driving commodity prices down and stymying government budgets. Policy coordination efforts by Ivory Coast and Ghana, the world's biggest producers of cocoa beans, point to the pernicious legacy effects of colonialism and inability of primary commodity producers in general to influence world prices. African merchandise exports reached an all-time high of $US998 billion in 2018. However, this figure accounts for only 2.7 percent of global merchandise trade – up from 2.4 percent in 2015, but well below the 7.4 percent share in 1948 (Verter 2017; Afreximbank 2019). Simply put, Africa is a lesser player in global merchandise trade than it was nearly 75 years ago. While parts of the world that used to be primary commodity producers industrialized their exports (such as Southeast Asia), Africa generally did not.

To be sure, African economies have changed internally, as have African societies, which are becoming more urbanized and 'wired'. The Gibeonite image of Africans as hewers of wood and drawers of water (Joshua 9:21)[3] must be challenged in all iterations, not least its underlying racism. Ethiopia is careening toward becoming a light manufacturing hub (EIU 2019). Rwanda has opted to become Africa's Silicon Valley (Forbes Africa 2023). Some African cities are already nascent high-tech enclaves (*e.g.* Lagos, Nairobi, and Johannesburg) (Siba and Sow 2017). Services now account for around 44 percent of GDP in Africa's largest economy, Nigeria (Statista 2022). Yet, these changes have yet to lead to a shift in Africa's position in the international division of labor. Oil and gas accounted for 95 percent of Nigeria's foreign exchange earnings in 2019 (Ziady 2021). South Africa, Algeria, Angola, and consorts are similarly reliant on their natural resource endowments for income. Africa's foreign exchange earnings remain stubbornly tethered to the extractive proclivities of dependent capitalism: that is, colonialism and neocolonialism. Meanwhile, other sectors (*e.g.* financial services) have become more significant in global trade than merchandise trade, at the volatile end of which Africa specializes (i.e. primary commodity production). Until Africa makes a decisive turn toward diverse economies roaring on all cylinders – including agriculture, industry, and services powered by innovative technologies – sustainable development will remain elusive, gravely problematizing the implementation of inclusive social policy.

We can now shift to African government spending which, again, might be expected to correlate strongly to international trade, a most important revenue source for governments on the continent. The *début de siècle* commodity boom was the longest in post-colonial African history (2000–13). It should have occasioned a rise in African government spending, even after accounting for the possibility that a portion of the trade windfall may have been allocated to debt servicing and repayment.[4] Concomitantly, the period should have seen a rise in African government spending on healthcare, since it coincided with the UN's Millennium Development Goals, which all African countries committed to implement. In Abuja in December 2001, they specifically pledged to spend at least 15 percent of government revenue on healthcare (see: WHO 2010). I dare go further: healthcare spending from all sources should have increased in Africa, based on historical trends elsewhere. As countries become wealthier, private sector spending on healthcare generally increases, not just government spending. The evidence is far from conclusive on each of these issues; if anything, it points the other way on some of the same issues (WHO 2010; Olalere and Gatome-Munyua 2020).

A caveat and some explanations are necessary here. Data on African government spending are relatively sparse; furthermore, they are published in national currencies, whose exchange rate convertibility is not easy to decipher, since currency values fluctuate daily. In some years, government spending data are not available, and for Ghana and Libya, data are not available at all. In Table 26.2, I examine government spending in 2000, 2006, 2012, 2013, and 2014 in the countries listed as the top 10 foreign trade earners in Table 26.1. The data reflect central government spending, as data concerning subnational governments are notoriously parsimonious and unreliable in Africa. In addition, of the top 10 African exporting countries, only Nigeria is an oil-rich federal republic – the others are unitary states. Accordingly, while spending on healthcare by state governments in Nigeria might be significant, this would not be reflected in the data. That is, total government spending on healthcare across Nigeria may be higher than 5 percent of GDP, or the state in Nigeria is exceedingly stingy! Conversely, central government expenditure in the remaining nine countries more than likely represents the lion's share of public sector spending on healthcare.

Table 26.2 reveals a mixed picture. During the first six years of the commodity boom of the early-Twenty-First Century, government spending as a percentage of Gross National Income in Africa seemed not to have appreciably changed (2000–06). This would seem to confirm the chapter's thesis. However, government spending increased markedly in the second half of the boom in South Africa, Angola, Algeria, Morocco, and Tunisia – that is, in half of the top 10 African exporters. This should have translated into increased healthcare spending by government during this period, which coincides with the UN's Millennium Development Goals. In reality, this did not happen.

Healthcare spending as a percentage of the national economy should have risen in Africa from 2000 to 2013, reflecting the improved fiscal outlook of the state and increased income for individuals and families. The figures below, again, show a mixed picture. Healthcare spending as a percentage of GDP in Africa was virtually identical at the beginning of the boom (2000) as its end (2013) – even declining slightly over the period (Figure 26.1). Meanwhile, it peaked in 2003 and 2004 at roughly 5.9 percent of GDP, after reaching a low of 4.9 percent in 2002. From

Table 26.2 Central government spending as a percentage of GNI in the top 10 African exporters, 2000–13

Rank	*Country*	*2000*	*2006*	*2012*	*2013*
1	South Africa	27.1	28.9	33.8	34.7
2	Nigeria	No data	7.9	5.1	5.0
3	Angola	21.8	23.8	26.3	30.8
4	Algeria	20.7	19.1	No data	29.5
5	Libya	No data	No data	No data	No data
6	Egypt	27.2	32.7	28.6	32.2
7	Morocco	24.1	26.5	No data	32.4
8	Ghana	No data	No Data	No data	No data
9	Tunisia	25.0	25.8	35.4	35.4
10	Ivory Coast	12.4	13.8	15.2	13.5

Source: Our World in Data (2020).

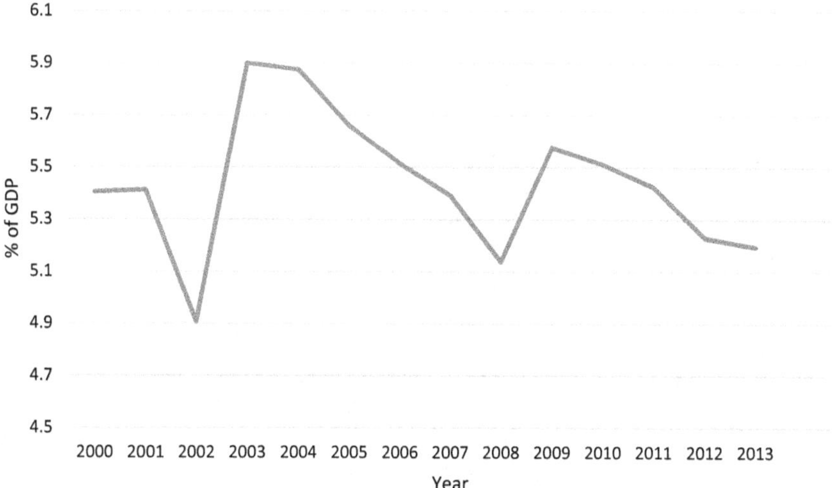

Figure 26.1 Healthcare spending as a percentage of GDP in Africa, 2000–13.

Source: Adapted from Macrotrends (2022), compiled from data in World Bank (n.d.).

a comparative perspective, Africa is well below average spending on healthcare across OECD countries, which stood at 9.7 percent of GDP in 2020, up from 8.8 percent in 2019 (OECD 2022). Per capita spending on healthcare in Africa more than doubled during the period, from around $US35 in 2000 to over $US97 in 2013 (Figure 26.2). This is well above the $US44 per annum threshold recommended by the World Health Organization, but still far below what is necessary to secure decent healthcare on the continent, especially in regard to chronic illnesses and advanced medicine (Gros 2016).

To summarize the data presented so far, expenditures on healthcare consume a comparatively modest portion of national economies in Africa. In countries outside the continent with inclusive healthcare policy – such as social healthcare insurance schemes and socialized medicine –

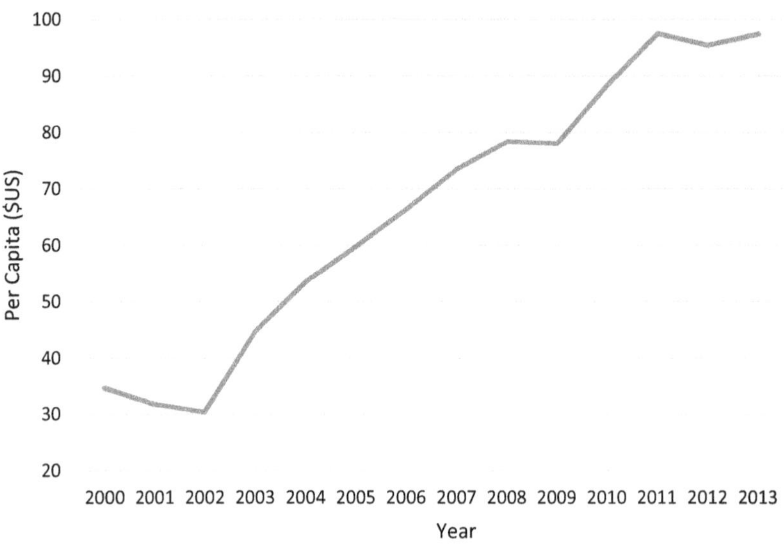

Figure 26.2 Healthcare spending per capita in Africa, 2000–13.

Source: Adapted from Macrotrends (2022), compiled from data in World Bank (n.d.).

expenditures on healthcare tend to consume closer to 10 percent of GDP. Generally, these are industrialized countries with much larger nominal GDPs than African countries. They have the technological capacity to make many of the inputs that go into healthcare and, thus, do not have to rely on foreign trade. African countries spend, on average, slightly more than 5 percent of GDP on healthcare. In 2013, average government spending in eight of the top ten export-earning countries in Africa was 26.6 percent of GDP (calculated from Table 26.2). The state in Africa does not tax enough and, therefore, cannot spend adequately on social goods. One reason for the paucity of revenue is the unreliability of one of its tax bases: foreign trade, which is exceedingly dependent on primary commodity production, the earnings from which fluctuate from year to year (as depicted in Table 26.1). In turn, annual GDP growth rates in Africa tend to be erratic, undermining the ability of government to honor commitments with a long-term horizon (such as healthcare).

The state, democracy, and healthcare policy in Africa: beyond ventral politics

In addition to the structure of African economies, healthcare policy is handicapped by the politics of the African state. Corruption is often identified as the bane of good government in Africa (Bayart 1993). This theme has given rise to a flowery (and often simplistic) literature in African studies (for instance, see: Szeftel 1998). There is more to the travails of politics in Africa than corruption, which every day is revealing itself to be common currency in countries that fashion themselves as role models for Africa. Not only does the state in post-colonial Africa not tax enough, but its control of territory is also often too tenuous to enable the implementation of the kind of social policy that is effective, efficient, and inclusive. The two conditions are, of course, interrelated. A state with an unreliable revenue base, as well as limited domination of space, will naturally have difficulties performing the tasks of modern statehood, which include the provision of social goods such as healthcare. All states, ultimately, are discriminating monopolists, because they are constrained by resource scarcity, law, customs, and other factors. The optimal allocation of their assets throughout the realm must be a sempiternal concern, as it directly impinges on their authority and legitimacy. This necessarily means that the state will broadcast power strategically – that is, unevenly – according to the circumstances. The African state is especially vulnerable in this regard. In its current configuration, it faces multiple, longstanding, more or less immovable, barriers, which are extremely difficult to overcome in the absence of African super-agency: such as regional, even continental, integration.

Almost 30 percent of African states are landlocked, yet 80 percent of global merchandise trade use maritime transportation. Adverse geography increases the costs of intercontinental trading for many African countries, decreasing potential revenue from trade for the state which, consequently, cannot spend as much on social services as might be necessary. To illustrate, Chad must pay Cameroon a transit fee of $US1.32 per barrel (as of 2018) to move crude oil from the Doba Basin Fields to the Atlantic port of Kribi. In 2019, Chad produced 130,000 barrels of oil per day, or 47,450,000 barrels annually.[5] Assuming, generously, that Chad kept half of its annual output for domestic consumption and shipped the rest to overseas market through the Chad-Cameroon pipeline, Chad would likely have paid a transit fee of $US31,317,000 to Cameroon in 2019. Annual per capita spending on healthcare in Chad is about $US30, at the time of writing. The conclusion should be readily apparent: absent the transit fee on oil, Chad could be spending more per capita on healthcare. Of course, it is not just Chad's main export earning that is impacted by bad geography. Chad imports nearly every consumer good imaginable, including staple food (flour, sugar, and rice), from which its Atlantic neighbors collect custom duties in various forms. Social spending in Chad is being squeezed not only by government corruption and military spending to attenuate conflict in the greater Lake Chad Basin, but also by various transaction costs wrought by physical isolation and Africa's political balkanization.

The inability of the African state to perform one of the crucial tasks of modern statehood (social services delivery) delegitimizes it in the eyes of citizens. This, in turn, opens it to challenge by religiously irredentist, anti-state forces, such as Boko Haram, Al-Qaeda in the Islamic Maghreb (AQIM), Islamic State. It is important to recall the history of this problem, as it is often mischaracterized as the terrorism of 'radical' Islam. The African state underwent privatization – in some instances, even criminalization – under the structural adjustment programs (SAPs) of the 1980s and early-1990s, as advocated by the World Bank and International Monetary Fund. Reduced to its simplest expression, as a result of SAPs, the state lost the contest for popular legitimacy to various groups which, through their networks of social services, were in some ways more penetrative and transformative of society. Some of these groups, with greater capacity to collect rent from extractive activities – such as illegal mining and logging – began to see themselves at the end of the Twentieth Century as alternatives to the state. More importantly, some ordinary Africans accepted their authority (Okolie and Nnamani 2019). In this respect, neoliberalism had deleterious effects on the ability of the African state to make inclusive social policy, shattering the narrative of an all-powerful, beneficent, Leviathan. The World Bank and International Monetary Fund could have played a more constructive role in social policymaking in Africa. This would have required strengthening the African state, which was anathema to the free-market dogmas of the Washington Consensus institutions.

Africa's democratic transition after 1990 could have been a defining moment for healthcare policy, as democracy should yield policy that is attuned to public needs. Yet, in practice, this only occurs under certain social conditions, which are not present in Africa at the moment.[6] In Africa, liberal democracy has yet to facilitate the formation of the kind of well-organized and 'articulate' pressure groups to which elected officials normally respond. Indeed, inasmuch as inclusive healthcare policy entails the creation and (or expansion) of public programs, this poses a problem in Africa where such programs are often stigmatized as inferior care and shunned by relatively well-to-do Africans (Gros 2016). Investigative journalism is still in its infancy in much of Africa. Even where it is not muzzled, the press is hardly equipped to speak truth to power and the larger public, especially in light of the complexity of healthcare. Most young people (*i.e.* under 40) in urban Africa likely get their news from social media – hardly a trusted source of in-depth, accurate information about important matters. Finally, liberal democracy in Africa has almost no footprint on social policy, as the rewards of democracy are distributed primarily in the form of private goods or patronage.

The African response to COVID-19

The preponderance of activities outdoors, instead of indoors – a practice aided by the (sub)tropical climate in much of Africa – a youthful population, the African approach to family,[7] and aggressive government-mandated mitigation measures in the cities spared Africa the worst of the COVID-19 pandemic during the early stages. Yet, this situation had changed by mid-2022, at which time over two-thirds of Africans were estimated to have been infected by the SARS-CoV-2 virus – due to the migration of more contagious variants of the virus to the rural areas, as well as the virus finding refuge in poor, overcrowded, urban neighborhoods (WHO 2022). African states found themselves ill-equipped to craft and implement sustainable policy throughout all corners of their territories in response to the pandemic. The internal resources were lacking to successfully instigate large-scale vaccination programs and provide comprehensive in-patient hospital treatment for the illnesses spawned by the virus, while developed countries failed to share sufficient and affordable quantities of vaccines with Africa to attenuate infection rates across the continent (see: Paquin and Plouffe-Malette 2023).

One of the few bright spots of healthcare policy during the colonial period was the emphasis on public health that, by definition, centered on preventive and promotive care (Gros 2016). After independence, African healthcare policy showed a marked preference for hospital-based curative care, resulting in the concentration of healthcare facilities in urban areas and expensive methods of treatment (*i.e.* biomedicine) that required significant importation of inputs. A sustainable healthcare system necessitates a strong public health component, inasmuch as such an approach tends to improve the health of the population at relatively low costs (hence the aphorism: an ounce of prevention is worth a pound of cure). Moving forward, the fight against COVID-19 is likely to have crowding-out effects on established public health initiatives, such as mass vaccinations against childhood diseases, unless African countries ramp up investment in all aspects of public health, including the manufacturing of mRNA and other vaccines.

Conclusion

Healthcare policy is inseparable from the broader social environment. Poor countries tend to have the worse healthcare systems and health outcomes (such as lower adult life expectancy, higher child mortality, and higher rates of infectious diseases), because of the structure of their economy and the politics of productive activities. At a micro-level, poor people tend to have worse healthcare treatments and health outcomes, as the COVID-19 pandemic has made abundantly clear in the US. There is a strong, not perfect, correlation, between wealth and power and health. This is why the political economy approach, along with the recognition that history matters, is an excellent tool in the study of healthcare policy. This epistemology is potentially vulnerable to the charge of structural determinism. To the extent that this criticism is valid, the lacuna can be addressed through incorporation of agency in ways that do not gainsay the political economy method. Policy, after all, implies an ability to choose under conditions of structural constraints, which can themselves be jettisoned by agency. It is not inevitable that poor countries have healthcare systems that are wanting across the entire spectrum of health needs, just as being poor and powerless in the international state system is not a matter of fate. Healthcare outcomes are not entirely dependent on wealth and power. Cuba proves the validity of this point. Some aspects of healthcare are more (or less) sensitive to resource scarcity than others. It is possible to achieve impressive healthcare results in some areas, even with modest investment. This is where smart policy comes in, which is to say: smart politics.

An intelligent healthcare policy can decide where scarce resources should be deployed to achieve the highest utility for the largest number of people. To illustrate, HIV/AIDS infection rates were lowered in the early-2000s, when governments across Africa – some with politically influential and deeply religious groups (such as the Tijaniyyah, Muridiyyah, Qadiriyyah, and Layene in Senegal) – promoted healthcare that stressed safe sex along with abstinence. Investment in billboards, radio spots, and the distribution of condoms was well worth the number of lives possibly saved. Even the weakest states have residual coercive and administrative capacity, which can be strategically deployed (such as in cities) at least some of the time. According to the International Center for Non-Profit Law (2020), during the early stages of the pandemic 146 measures were taken by African governments in response to COVID-19 – ranging from declarations of public health emergencies (the softest policy decision) to states of national disasters (the strongest). Sierra Leone imposed a year-long state of public health emergency before it recorded a single case of COVID-19, in an apparent lesson learned from the Ebola pandemic of 2014. State failure is seldom absolute and permanent; instead, it ebbs and flows. African leaders were not bashful in protecting their citizens against the spread of COVID-19, in spite of the fact that (a) Africa was not initially affected by the pandemic as much as other continents, and (b) African countries were the least likely to recover from the closure of their economy and that of the world, because of the susceptibility of African production to the chicaneries of international commodity trade.

In sum, although conditions subsequently changed as the virus disseminated across the continent, African leaders showed themselves capable of making tough choices without supplication for increased foreign aid, while many of their Western counterparts – with resilient economies and strong states – cowered in denial. In the interstice of the Afro-pessimism of the 1980s and the ‘Africa rising’ narrative of the 2000s, there is some hope that African leaders can, at last and against enduring structural odds, craft policy that produces healthcare systems that are effective, inclusive, and affordable.

Notes

1 Sub-Saharan Africa has 0.2 doctors per 1,000 people. The world average is 1.6 per 1,000 people. Inasmuch as contemporary healthcare is doctor-centric, this means most Africans do not have easy access to the most important providers of healthcare. In their pioneering study, Caryn Peiffer and Richard Rose (2016) have found that the poor in Africa tend to pay for government services that are, technically speaking, free. This, in turn, makes healthcare expensive for many Africans and, for those who cannot pay, inaccessible. The efficacy of Africa’s healthcare systems can be inferred from health outcomes, such as adult life expectancy (which is lower in Africa than other continents) and infant, child, and maternal mortality rates (which are higher in Africa than other continents).

2 This ranking remained unchanged by 2019.

3 See: <https://biblehub.com/joshua/9-21.htm>.

4 It is worth noting, however, that this possibility is unlikely, since some of Africa’s poorest countries had their debt cancelled under the International Monetary Fund’s Heavily Indebted Poor Countries Initiative.

5 The annual figure here is an estimate, not an official statistic. There are days of idleness in petroleum mining, just as there are also days when average daily production is exceeded. See: <https://www.petroleum-economist.com/articles/politics-economics/africa/2019/oil-price-recovery-eases-chads-gloom>.
6 Electoral accountability, of course, is not the only type of accountability. An authoritarian government that is afraid of being overthrown may try to blunt this outcome by implementing inclusive social policy.
7 In more than 30 years of visiting at least 15 African countries, some repeatedly (*e.g.* Ghana and Cameroon) for extended periods of time, I do not recall ever seeing a retirement home which, unfortunately, became human Petri dishes (so-called super-spreaders) during the early period of the COVID-19 pandemic. I am not suggesting that retirement homes do not exist in Africa, but they are extremely rare. Africans do not 'unload' the elderly on non-familial institutions. As Africa becomes more urbanized and prosperous, leading to more nuclear families, this could well change. Tradition, economic circumstances, and luck may have spared Africa the worst of COVID-19.

References

Acemoglu, D. and Robinson, J. 2012, *Why Nations Fail*, Crown Business, New York.

Afreximbank. 2019, *African Trade Report 2019*, Afreximbank, Cairo.

Bayart, J.-F. 1993, *The State in Africa*, Longman, London and New York.

Cameron, R. and Neal, L. 2016, *A Concise Economic History of the World*, Oxford University Press, London and New York.

CIA. 2020, 'Field listing: Exports', *World Factbook*, accessed 6 October 2020, <https://www.cia.gov/the-world-factbook/field/exports/country-comparison>.

EIU. 2019, 'Ethiopia: Africa's new manufacturing centre', *Economist Intelligence Unit*, 25 November, accessed 19 November 2021, <https://www.eiu.com/n/ethiopia-manufacturing/>.

Forbes Africa. 2023, 'Rwanda: Africa's Silicon Valley', 20 February, accessed 7 April 2023, <https://www.forbesafrica.com/contrarian/2023/02/20/rwanda-africas-silicon-valley/>.

Galvani, A.P., Parpia, A.S., Foster, E.M., Singer, B.H. and Fitzpatrick, M.C. 2020, 'Improving the prognosis of health care in the USA', *Lancet*, 395(10223), pp. 524–33.

Gros, J.-G. 1996, 'Towards a taxonomy of failed states in the new world order: Decaying Somalia, Liberia, Rwanda and Haiti', *Third World Quarterly*, 17(3), pp. 455–71.

Gros, J.-G. 2016, *Healthcare Policy in Africa: Institutions and Politics from Colonialism to the Present*, Rowman and Littlefield, Lanham.

ICNL. 2020, 'African government responses to Covid-19', accessed 18 April 2021, <https://www.icnl.org/.post/analysis/african-government-response-to-covid-19>.

Macrotrends. (2022), 'Sub-Saharan Africa healthcare spending, 2000–2020', *Macrotrends*, accessed 22 November 2022, <https://www.macrotrends.net/countries/SSF/sub-saharan-africa-/healthcare-spending>.

Marmor, T., Freeman, R. and Kieke, O. 2009, *Comparative Studies and the Politics of Modern Medical Care*, Yale University Press, New Haven.

Newhouse, J. 1977, 'Medical-care expenditure: A cross-national survey', *Journal of Human Resources*, 12(1), pp. 115–25.

OECD. 2021, 'Health spending', OECD Data Online, accessed 11 June 2021, <https://data.oecd.org/healthres/health-spending.htm>.

OECD. 2022, 'Health expenditure', accessed 21 November 2022, <https://www.oecd.org/els/health-systems/health-expenditure.htm>.

Office for National Statistics (UK). 2019, 'Healthcare expenditure, UK health accounts: 2017', 25 April, accessed 19 September 2020, <https://www.ons.gov.uk/peoplepopulationandcommunity/healthandsocialcare/healthcaresystem/bulletins/ukhealthaccounts/2017>.

Okolie, A.-M. and Nnamani, K.E. 2019, 'Neoliberal economic reforms and challenges of insecurity in Africa', *South East Journal of Political Science*, 3(1), pp. 300–32.

Olalere, N. and Gatome-Munyua, A. 2020, 'Public financing for health in Africa: 15% of an elephant is not 15% of a chicken', *Africa Renewal*, 13 October, accessed 11 October 2022, <https://www.un.org/africarenewal/magazine/october-2020/public-financing-health-africa-when-15-elephant-not-15-chicken>.

Our World in Data. n.d., 'Government spending', accessed 20 October 2020, <https://ourworldindata.org/government-spending>.

Paquin, S. and Plouffe-Malette, K. 2023, 'The WTO and the Covid-19 "vaccine apartheid": Big pharma and the minefield of patents', *Politics and Governance*, 11(1), pp. 261–71.

Peiffer, C. and Rose, R. 2016, 'Why are the poor more vulnerable to bribery in Africa? The institutional effects of services', *Journal of Development Studies*, 54(1), pp. 18–29.

Piketty, T. 2014, *Capital in the 21st Century*, Harvard University Press, Cambridge.

Schatz, S. 1994, 'Structural adjustment in Africa: A failing grade so far', *Journal of Modern African Studies*, 32(4), pp. 679–92.

Siba, E. and Sow, M. 2017, 'Smart city initiatives in Africa', *Brookings Institution*, 1 November, accessed 14 July 2021, <https://www.brookings.edu/blog/africa-in-focus/2017/11/01/smart-city-initiatives-in-africa/>.

Smith, S. 2019, *The Scramble for Europe*, Polity Press, Medford.

Statista. 2022, 'Nigeria: Distribution of gross domestic product (GDP) across economic sectors from 2011 to 2021', *Statista*, December, accessed 5 January 2023, <https://www.statista.com/statistics/382311/nigeria-gdp-distribution-across-economic-sectors/>.

Szeftel, M. 1998, 'Misunderstanding African politics: Corruption and the governance agenda', *Review of African Political Economy*, 25(76), pp. 221–40.

Verter, N. 2017, 'International trade: The position of Africa in global merchandise trade', in Ibrahim, M.J. (ed), *Emerging Issues in Economics and Development*, InTech, Croatia, pp. 64–89.

World Bank. n.d., 'World development indicators', *World Bank*, accessed 12 November 2022, <https://datatopics.worldbank.org/world-development-indicators/>.

World Health Organization. 2010, 'The Abuja Declaration: Ten years on', *WHO*, accessed 15 September 2021, <https://apps.who.int/iris/bitstream/handle/10665/341162/WHO-HSS-HSF-2010.01-eng.pdf?sequence=1>.

World Health Organization. 2022, 'Over two-thirds of Africans exposed to virus which causes COVID-19: WHO study', *WHO Africa*, 7 April, accessed 5 January 2023, <https://www.afro.who.int/news/over-two-thirds-africans-exposed-virus-which-causes-covid-19-who-study>.

Ziady, H. 2021, 'Nigeria is oil rich and energy poor – It can't wait around for cheaper batteries', *CNN Business*, 3 November, accessed 8 April 2022, <https://edition.cnn.com/2021/11/03/business/nigeria-clean-energy-transition/index.html>.

27

TRANSFORMATION OF HEALTHCARE IN CHINA

The pre- and post-Maoist eras

Rama V. Baru and Madhurima Nundy

The trajectories for growth and development among socialist countries are as varied as the capitalist world. The two major socialist powers, the Soviet Union and China, had different approaches to building socialism and economic development during the Twentieth Century. Thus, the differences in socialist praxis influenced socio-economic and welfare policies in both these countries. While the Soviet Union adopted the path of heavy industrialization, China focused much more on addressing rural inequalities. Prior to the socialist revolution in 1949, China was known as the 'Sick Man of Asia' since it was a country ravaged by poverty, disease, and socio-economic inequalities. Mao's concern was to address these basic needs through a system of guarantees colloquially referred to as the 'iron rice bowl'. This system guaranteed lifetime employment, food security, housing, and clothing, which had positive outcomes on health and well-being for a large section of the peasantry. The collectivization of agriculture provided its financial and institutional undergirding, and its ultimate dismantling began with the decollectivization process that would give rise to socio-economic and health inequalities.

Indeed, the rise of market socialism has had far-reaching consequences for the health sector. Global ideas of health sector reform and commercialization of health services restructured Chinese public hospitals. Through several waves of commercialization, beginning with public hospital reform and the rise of the private sector in provisioning, financing, medical devices, and pharmaceuticals, one can discern the rise of a medical-industrial complex in China.[1] The rise of this complex remains consistent with China's entry into global partnerships in the development of the 'for-profit' tertiary health sector for provisioning and medium- and high-end medical technology (Langwick 2010; Lin *et al.* 2016; Torsekar 2018; Baru and Nundy 2020; Daly *et al.* 2020).

In highlighting this political-economic trajectory of health in China, this chapter proceeds by first outlining the previous era of collectivization and health services under one-party rule. Following this, it turns to the introduction of decollectivization and market socialism. In terms of health, we highlight here the initiation of four distinct phases, the first of which (1978–2002) deals with transition. The next section tracks the second (2002–08) and third (2009–12) phases of reform, which realize both commercialization of health insurance and a growing tertiary and industrial sector, as well as the concomitant increase in unequal access and depreciated primary care. Finally, the chapter concludes by considering the current era (fourth phase), with its attendant incremental reforms that have failed to address commercial dominance and an over-reliance on curative care.

DOI: 10.4324/9781003017110-31

The Mao years: collectivization and health services (1949–80)

The relationship between improvements in socio-economic development and health status is well documented in several European countries (McKeown *et al.* 1972; PAHO 1988; Szreter 2002). These studies highlight the improvement in wages, food security, social welfare measures, and working conditions of the working classes. This resulted in a decline in mortality, due to the reduction in communicable diseases and improvement in life expectancy during the Nineteenth and early-Twentieth Centuries. Rapid industrialization in Western European countries was possible due to the extraction of surpluses from their colonies in Asia, Africa, and Latin America. As a result, colonial policies were exploitative –in terms of both expropriation of natural resources and unfair terms of trade that led to impoverishment of the peasantry and working classes in their respective colonies. As several post-colonial societies embarked on development, they faced resource and infrastructural constraints.

Approaching these challenges, varied forms of governmental organization prevailed, including different forms of democracy, military dictatorship, and one-party rule. The socialist revolution in China resulted in a government led by a single party: the Communist Party. It signified an approach to development that tried to address the extreme inequality and poverty in Chinese society, which was a shared challenge across post-colonial societies. Radical land reforms and guaranteed livelihoods with welfare support became the hallmark of the Chinese revolution, which led to improvements in the health and well-being of its population. The government's approach to public health was premised on the idea of the 'iron rice bowl', which provided guarantees to lifelong work, decent wages, food security, housing, and clothing. These guarantees ensured improvements in life expectancy, reductions in infant, child, and maternal mortality, and dramatic declines in deaths due to a host of communicable diseases (Acharya *et al.* 2001).

The public health approach after the revolution focused on preventive campaigns to eradicate pests via political mobilization by the Party cadre at the community level. In the first National Health Conference in 1950, guidelines were adopted for health service development that reflected socialist ideology. The most important among them was that health work was to combine with mass movements; promotion and preventive medicine were to take precedence over therapeutic medicine. The conference identified four guiding principles for healthcare: serve workers, farmers, and soldiers; prioritize preventive medicine over curative medicine; foster unity between traditional Chinese medicine (TCM) and allopathic medicine; and combine health efforts with mass mobilization (Wong and Chiu 1997: 77). As Hipgrave (2011: 225) notes:

> Early efforts in public health included work on vaccination, environmental sanitation and hygiene (including the early introduction of composting of night-soil to reduce the concentration of intestinal parasites) and the development of organized CDC programs. Incredibly, between 1950 and 1952, over 512 million of China's ~600 million people were vaccinated against smallpox, massively reducing case numbers; the last outbreak of smallpox in China occurred in 1960, 20 years before global eradication.

The early investments in health service infrastructure, especially in rural areas, were at the primary level of care in the form of Maternal and Child Health (MCH) centers and epidemiological prevention stations. The former focused on reducing new-born and puerperal infections by training traditional birth attendants and establishing 2,380 MCH centers by 1952 (Hipgrave 2011). The Epidemiological Prevention Stations were influenced by the Soviet model for disease control, and were mainly concerned with surveillance: monitoring the major communicable diseases that were responsible for morbidity and mortality.

It is well known in public health that preventive care is important, but there is also a role of curative services in preventing diseases. In the Chinese case, rural areas were given attention for prevention through Peoples' Campaigns and epidemiological prevention stations, but hospitals were almost non-existent. Thus, the rural population relied on practitioners of traditional Chinese medicine and other traditional healers through to the 1960s (Acharya *et al.* 2001; Hipgrave 2011). The training of doctors and expansion of hospitals, mostly in urban areas, only began in the mid-1960s. As such, health service provisioning differed in its structure, financing, and institutional arrangement between rural and urban areas. Simultaneously, the Great Leap Years (1958–62) constituted a setback to rural health improvement, due to famines that claimed many lives – a function of faulty policies to extract excessive surpluses from the peasantry. The effort to introduce course correction in the early-1960s could not easily undo the damage done to millions of lives who perished in the famines (Feng *et al.* 2017; Alvarez-Klee 2019).

In rural areas, the welfare system was an integral part of the collectivization process and institutional structure. In urban areas, arrangements were predicated on work settings in terms of financing and provisioning of welfare services. There were three major healthcare components, comprised of 'public medicine' for government employees, 'collective medicine' for workers in state-owned enterprises, and 'cooperative medicine' for rural residents (Burns and Huang 2017: 33). The relationship between the primary, secondary, and tertiary levels of provisioning was also established during this period of the Cultural Revolution (1966 onward).

Cooperative medicine was given top priority by Mao, especially during the Cultural Revolution. The main cadre of health workers in rural areas were the barefoot doctors, officially known as the 'informal rural medical worker'. They had basic training and knowledge in medicine, and their work would be established as national policy in 1968 (Alvarez-Klee 2019; Wang *et al.* 2019: 5). A three-tier rural health service delivery system under the cooperative medical scheme was developed in this period (as depicted in Figure 27.1). It included health institutions at three levels – village clinic, township health center, and county-level hospitals. These institutions provided preventive to rehabilitative services, along with training and research. From this foundation, the basic

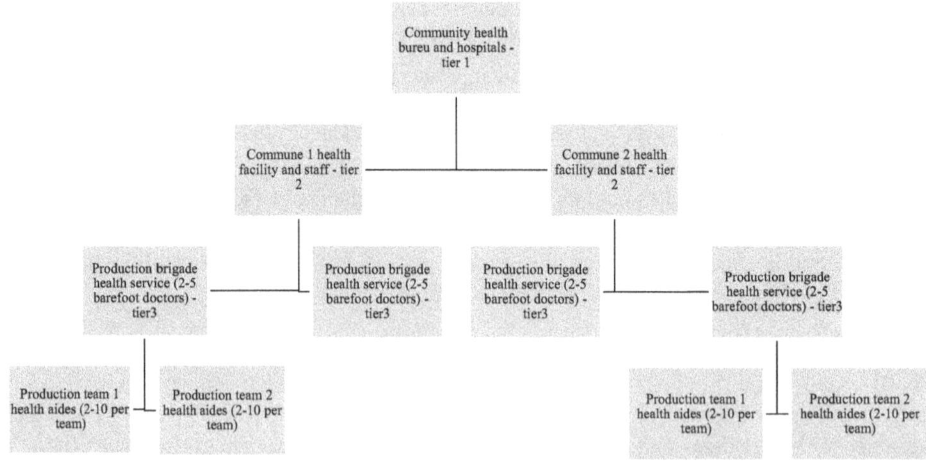

Figure 27.1 Rural government and health system in 1960s–70s China, depicting the three-tier network.
Source: Adapted from Hipgrave (2011: 227).

framework of Chinese health services emerged (Meng *et al.* 2015), with health financing occurring through risk-pooling and premiums, low reimbursements (especially for rural areas), and an emphasis on free preventive health services.

While the health status of the population improved by the late-1970s – largely due to equal wages, welfare services, food security, and preventive health – there were several anomalies that existed within health services. Specifically, there were insufficient numbers of health professionals, weak drug production, and inequity in the distribution of resources and services across rural and urban area (as well as across provinces). In fact, the inequities of this period form the basis for the contradictions and challenges of the post-reform period (Alvarez-Klee 2019).

Decollectivization and collapse of the cooperative medical scheme in rural areas

The shift from planned economy to socialist market economy brought in several changes in the 1980s. The political, economic, administrative and fiscal reforms all had far-reaching consequences for the health and health service systems (Meng *et al.* 2015). When China embarked on the opening of its economy in 1979, under Deng Xiaoping, it emphasized four modernizations – agriculture, industry, science and technology, and national defense. This was enshrined in the Constitution in 1977 by Zhou Enlai and Deng Xiaoping. Heavy investments were required to modernize agriculture and industries. Modernization of institutions was restricted mostly to urban areas.

With the shift to market socialism and dismantling of collectives, there was a breakdown in welfare services, including health. The decollectivization of agriculture, occurring in phases across provinces, led to the collapse of the institutional and financial frame for ensuring the four guarantees discussed above. This, in turn, led to the end of the guarantees retained under the 'iron rice bowl'. Health services were not the priority and were summarily neglected. By default, health institutions had to become self-reliant, as government subsidies were reduced considerably.

Economic reforms during this period resulted in massive layoffs (over 34 million) in state-owned enterprises (SOEs), leaving millions unemployed in urban areas. Health coverage in the past was linked to employment – whether as peasants in rural areas or workers in urban industries. As SOE reforms led to privatization, health insurance coverage was no longer available for workers in urban areas and, hence, no longer extended to dependents of the workers (Cao *et al.* 2012). Additionally, fiscal reforms in 1994 put pressure on local governments to increase expenditure despite reductions in revenue from the central government. Finally, administrative reforms focused on decentralization and more autonomy to local institutions, leaving them increasingly responsible for healthcare delivery in their region.

These reforms had negative consequences for the health sector, paving the way for commercialization of health services in rural and urban areas. The ultimate result was enhanced inequality in access to health – both on an inter-provincial and on a rural-urban basis. The separation of financing and provision of health services resulted in the breakdown of the institutional structures that had supported barefoot doctors and primary (and mobile) delivery of care. This opened the door for the large-scale privatization of health services in rural areas, as many barefoot doctors began to practice privately or gave up their role entirely. The integrated care linkages between primary and secondary or tertiary services were weakened, and thus, the three-tier healthcare system was no longer universal or comprehensive.[2] As central government revenue reduced, provinces had to generate their own revenue for financing health institutions, resulting in increased out-of-pocket expenditures. Income inequalities and inter-provincial inequalities in accessibility and affordability were already surfacing by the late-1970s, and only deepened over time. Public health also suffered, as epidemic stations – which were responsible for monitoring, surveillance, and management of communicable diseases – were no longer supplied the requisite funds to function effectively. At the county level, only 22 percent of these stations' budgets originated from government funds – the rest came from fee-for-service charges (Wang *et al.* 2019). Underlying all of this, of course, apart from the financial squeeze on health services, decollectivization resulted in growing socio-economic inequalities and increasing poverty across provinces, in both rural and urban areas. This increase in poverty intensified poor population health and, predictably, also led to a resurgence of communicable diseases (Acharya *et al.* 2001).

Public hospitals also underwent major reforms in phases that included institutional, financial, and administrative reforms. Baru and Nundy (2020) identify four distinct phases in the public hospital reforms, mainly focused on the secondary- and tertiary-level hospitals, while the primary-level infrastructure was weakened. The ideology and content of health reforms in China were influenced by global discourse being advanced through multilateral organizations like the Bretton Woods Institutions and World Health Organization. This involved the restructuring of public services and introduction of market principles within public institutions, where the tools of New Public Management were employed to commercialize health services. Among these, autonomization of public hospitals was utilized, whereby financing and administrative functions became the responsibility of each institution. In the first phase (1978–2002), financial autonomy was given to all hospitals when government funding declined. As a result, hospitals had to generate revenue by charging for medicines, diagnostic services and, in some cases, even consultation. This compulsion for revenue generation led providers to adopt problematic practices, such as over-prescription of medicines and unnecessary diagnostic testing, largely funded by out-of-pocket payments. By the late-1990s and early-2000s, out-of-pocket expenditure had climbed to 60 percent of total health spending in China, while government spending, on an average, was a mere 16 percent (NSBC 2018; Baru and Nundy 2020).

A major challenge to the reform process was the outbreak of the SARS (Severe Acute Respiratory Syndrome) epidemic in the early-2000s. The outbreak pointed to the fragmented, underfunded nature of health services, and made obvious that the primary level of services had been neglected. The epidemic stations that were responsible for monitoring communicable diseases were non-functional, due to long years of financial neglect. As a result, the burden of care fell on secondary and tertiary hospitals that had become inaccessible to many, especially rural residents.

Advancing commercialization and rising inequality

Generally, in the second phase of reform (2002–08), there was an ongoing push for commercialization in Chinese health services, with only mild efforts at course correction. At best, the Chinese government employed changes in financing strategies to contain rising costs. It also encouraged the growth of private hospitals and, subsequently, public-private partnerships in the health sector. These 'course corrections' largely addressed inequalities in access and strengthened primary-level care, in order to contain the rising costs of hospitalization and prevent the spread of infectious diseases. After the SARS debacle, China rebuilt its public health emergency response system and revived the primary health structure. However, disease prevention and control and curative services remained largely disconnected. The former was government-funded, while the latter was partly government-funded but mostly commercialized.

To improve access to healthcare, three different schemes of health insurance were introduced from 1998 to 2007. It commenced with insurance for urban employees in 1998 (the Urban Employee Basic Insurance Medical Scheme); followed by insurance for the rural population (the

National Rural Cooperative Medical Scheme), and then for urban residents who were not employed (the Urban Resident Basic Medical Insurance Scheme). Given the vast population of China, the insurance schemes resulted in improving coverage in terms of the breadth of the population, but the range of services available to beneficiaries and costs covered remained shallow. This nominal extension of coverage only managed to reduce out-of-pocket health expenditure from 60 percent in 2001 to 40 percent in 2008. This was mainly due to the success of the urban employee insurance scheme, while many rural residents and urban migrants and unemployed were still left out of the system, and had limited access to health insurance benefits (Cao *et al.* 2012; Baru and Nundy 2020). The administration of insurance schemes was complex, as different ministries were involved in each scheme – the Ministry of Health, Ministry of Social Security, and Ministry of Civil Affairs. These multiple actors further fragmented risk-pooling, and the urban employee scheme ultimately became the privileged scheme.

Apart from these financial reforms, public hospital reforms continued, as provinces and local governments experimented with various forms of autonomization. This followed the World Bank's approach, where ownership remained within the public sector, but agencies were transformed into independent entities, responsible for budgeting, services, and daily operations.

In the lead-up to the third phase of reform (2009–12), there was realization that the change in financing and provisioning had not addressed the challenges of equity and access. The Seventeenth Party Congress of 2007 emphasized the need for deepening reforms, stating that that public health and basic healthcare were public goods that should be accessible and affordable to all (Wang *et al.* 2019: 8). Around the same time, proposals were solicited from a diverse set of actors to address the issues of affordability and accessibility. These actors included a government think tank, two leading Chinese universities (Peking and Fudan), and external agencies – the World Bank, the WHO, and McKinsey and Co. (Yip and Hsiao 2015; Baru and Nundy 2020).

The proposals reflected the diverse ideological differences within and outside the government regarding the role of the state and market. The pro-government voices saw the National Health Service of the United Kingdom as the model, given its public finance and provision, while the pro-market voices preferred the insurance model for financing, accompanied by a competitive market of providers. After much deliberation – and mediation by Harvard University experts – a compromise was reached between deepening commercialization and a more paternalist model of health services (Yip and Hsiao 2015; Baru and Nundy 2020).

As such, the third phase of reform focused on four areas: wider coverage through insurance schemes; essential supply of drugs; strengthening of primary-level care; and public hospital reforms. Of particular note during these reforms is the last item, where government attempted to retain the social function of hospitals while curtailing irrational services. Essential lists of medicines were created across provinces, and the depth of insurance coverage was increased. In public hospitals, newer administrative and management reforms were introduced, leading to greater autonomization of public hospitals. These reforms included newer management models, separating governance and management from administration and supervisory functions within the hospital. The daily operations of hospitals, in other words, were kept separate from a management that was left to focus on the commercial development of the hospital. As Baru and Nundy (2020: 29) observe:

> There was a distinct transition in this phase from public hospitals as budgetary units in the past, when the hospital was run like a government organization and management personnel were essentially administrators, to autonomized organizations, where day-to-day management decisions were appropriated by managers and not bureaucrats. The separation of

government functions from those internal to the hospitals was done in order to reduce governmental control and surveillance. These separations presented two different patterns when implemented. In the first scenario, the management agency was under the jurisdiction of the health bureau. In a sense the goals of reforms were in line with those of the government. In the second one, the management institute was an independent agency and therefore independent of the health bureau.

Several provinces were selected for piloting these reforms, mainly in first- and second-tier cities, but there was no uniform model across the provinces. The separation in managerial functions further fragmented authority, and the net result was competition between public hospitals for public and private funds while attempting to retain the 'social function' of the hospital. This built-in contradiction of corporate aspirations for public institutions was emblematic of tensions evident across healthcare reform.

Finally, with a change in leadership in 2012, a fourth phase (2012 onward) of public reforms has witnessed a perceptible shift toward developing pro-market forces. The political report of the Nineteenth Party Congress in 2017 clearly sees the private sector as a major player. The policies during this period have facilitated the role of markets in public hospitals, and there has been an infusion of private capital into these institutions, based on their emerging business models (Navarro and Zhang 2014).

Indeed, much of the scholarly engagement with health reform in China has focused on public hospitals, but the rise of the 'for-profit' sector has also constituted a critical shift. Baru and Nundy's (2020) study on commercialization of medical care in China examines this movement of private capital – domestic and foreign – into financing, provisioning, pharmaceuticals, and health technologies since the 1980s. Here, the shift to market socialism opened up avenues for private capital in the economy and health sector, including a large domestic market in the pharmaceutical sector for Chinese medicines and the use of private practitioners at the primary, secondary, and tertiary levels. This history of foreign capital entry into health was primarily in the area of medical technology, driven in the 1980s by American entrepreneur Roberta Lipson. Setting up a company called Chindex, Lipson eventually partnered with Fosun, which was the largest Chinese pharmaceutical company, to establish the first chain of private hospitals called United Family Hospital Group (Baru and Nundy 2020). As such, the 1990s and early-2000s saw a growth of hospitals managed by domestic entrepreneurs in mostly urban areas in richer provinces, including '[the] high growth cities from the prosperous regions include Beijing, Shanghai, Guangzhou and Nantong', while this 'gradual expansion is now covering Tier II cities as well' (Baru and Nundy 2020: 53).

By 2011, then, private healthcare facilities accounted for 48 per cent of all health facilities in the country (Meng *et al.* 2015). During this period, the government has been actively promoting the development of the private health sector by encouraging more social investment in building healthcare facilities so that more players can be introduced into the health market. The market share of private hospitals increased from a mere 17 percent to nearly 56.4 percent between 2005 and 2016. In terms of actual beds in private hospitals, the increase has been more gradual from – 6 percent to 21.6 percent over the same period (Deng *et al.* 2018). Moreover, there is variation across provinces in the growth of private hospitals, with the eastern and southern regions having a higher number compared to the northern and western regions. In terms of utilization, about 86 percent of outpatient load is still in the public sector, exhibiting a drop from 2012, when over 90 percent was in the public sector. Similarly, for inpatient services, the load currently is about 82 percent, which has also seen a drop from 2012 (NBSC 2018).

The continuum of commercialization gained momentum from 2011 onward with deepening public hospital reform and encouraging the growth of private sector. In fact, the Twelfth Five-Year Plan sought to encourage 'the participation of private capital both in the form of greenfield investments and by reorganizing and restructuring public hospitals' (Baru and Nundy 2020: 62). With this reorientation of private capital in the health sector, there was an increase in public-private partnerships and the establishment of medical-industrial parks as a part of the larger strategy of Free Trade Zones (FTZs), which receive public subsidies and tax exemptions. This facilitated the emergence of a medical-industrial complex that involved 'partnerships between multiple sets of actors', including 'foreign and domestic investing firms, medical technology, pharmaceutical and insurance companies, real estate firms and hospital chains' (Baru and Nundy 2020: 63). Situated between pro-market and pro-government stances, this continuum was seen as a compromise: encouraging partnerships across provisioning and financing. This included joint ventures between tertiary public hospitals and private investor companies (pharmaceutical, medical device, private equity, and so on); multi-site practice by doctors, where a doctor from a public hospital could provide consultation for a private hospital; and reimbursement of health insurance in private hospitals, which further integrates private hospitals with the public healthcare system. Ultimately, the entry of foreign and domestic capital into medical care has rendered a complex system of healthcare, intermingling private capital with public provisioning; a burgeoning medical-industrial complex; and a hospital-dominated care system that blurs the boundaries between the public and private sectors (Baru and Nundy 2020).

Consequences of commercialization for provisioning and access

The continuum of commercialization in the Chinese health sector has brought in all the challenges and contradictions that exist between the role of market and state in health sectors across the world. Here, the core values of universality, equity, and comprehensiveness that typically inform public health systems have undergone a fundamental shift. The neoliberal proclivity for a split between public and private goods is deeply entrenched, and the power of markets to influence public policy is discernible across countries. Despite the gains made in China during the pre-reform era, in terms of both health outcomes and access to health services, the last five decades have witnessed a shift to a commercialized model of medical care. These trends are now here to stay, and opportunities to partner with foreign capital to bridge the financial gap in funding are actively sought. Several scholars have pointed to the fact that the Chinese health system is likely to face a crisis similar to that manifest in the United States. One already sees these tendencies, especially in the context of rising income inequalities, while the appetite among the rich and aspirational Chinese middle-class for private medical care only feeds a demand for growth in private insurance and hospitals. The utilization of health insurance more broadly has not proven especially effective in either financing or improving access to health services, leading to a general rise in medical costs. Despite the nominal efforts of the government to correct inequalities in access and rein-in out-of-pocket expenditures through the popular extension of health insurance, this strategy may not be sustainable in the long-run. China struggles to reorient the system based on primary care in a gatekeeper role, but secondary care and tertiary care remain overburdened. Resources are skewed toward curative (rather than primary and preventative) services, and the behavior of public hospitals at the secondary and tertiary levels reflects commercial imperatives that undermine a primary healthcare orientation.

As a consequence of this commercial dominance, major challenges facing the health system relating to inequalities in health insurance coverage, rising catastrophic expenditures (see: Figure 27.2), and unequal access to services across regions and rural-urban divides (Meng *et al.* 2015) are all-too-likely to be aggravated.

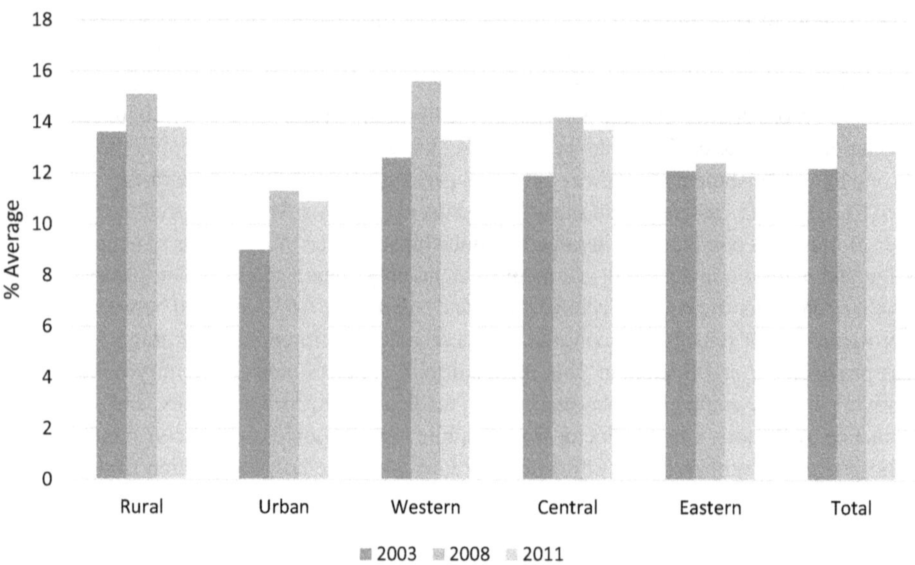

Figure 27.2 Average proportion of Chinese households with catastrophic health expenditure (percent).
Source: Adapted from Meng *et al.* (2015: 191).

In this context, China will face further challenges in the face of epidemiological and demographic transitions that continue to put demands on health provision. An aging population and high prevalence of chronic diseases call for effective health delivery that supplies not only curative approaches, but also preventive, promotive, rehabilitative, and palliative dimensions. A fragmented and commercialized health service system will deliver uneven outcomes in this regard, and this will almost certainly prove an impediment in addressing equity in access and rising costs.

Unfortunately, the diffused logic of market forces in the economy and health services now seems irreversible. While some adjustments have been made through financing and provisioning, the government's fine-tuning of policies is, at best, incremental. To deal with the many challenges of inequality and lack of broadly conceived, effective primary care, there is a need for coordination among key elements of the healthcare system. These include insurance schemes, provisioning of health services, essential medicines, creating referral structures, and enhancing human resources. Going beyond the public sector, there is a need to delineate and regulate the interests of private hospitals, along with the pharmaceutical and medical technology industries that are deeply entrenched in the Chinese system.

Notes

1 The notion of a medical-industrial complex was put forth by Relman (1980) with reference to the corporatization of health services in the United States.

2 'Comprehensive' primary health was defined by the *Alma Ata Declaration on Primary Health Care* in 1978. This was a holistic approach to health and well-being that encompassed all services through a range of services and programs that were accessible, equitable, safe, effective, and efficient (WHO 1978).

References

Acharya, A., Baru, R.V. and Nambissan, G.B. 2001, 'The state and human development: Health and education', in Deshpande, G.P. and Acharya, A. (eds), *Fifty Years of India-China: Crossing a Bridge of Dreams*, Tulika, New Delhi, pp. 203–67.

Alvarez-Klee, R. 2019, 'China: The development of the health system during the Maoist period (1949–76)', *Business History*, 61(3), pp. 518–37.

Baru, R.V. and Nundy, M. 2020, *Commercialisation of Medical Care in China: Changing Landscapes*, Routledge, London and New York.

Burns, L.R. and Huang, Y. 2017, 'History of China's healthcare system', in Burns, L.R. and Liu, G.G. (eds), *China's Healthcare System and Reform*, Cambridge University Press, Cambridge, pp. 31–74.

Cao, Q., Shi, L., Wang, H. and Dong, K. 2012, 'Report from China: Health insurance in China – Evolution, current status, and challenges', *International Journal of Health Services*, 42(2), pp. 177–95.

Daly, G., Kaufman, J., Lin, S., Gao, L., Reyes, M., Matemu, S. and El-Sadr, W. 2020, 'Challenges and opportunities in China's health aid to Africa: Findings from qualitative interviews in Tanzania and Malawi', *Globalization and Health*, 16(71).

Deng, C., Li, X. and Pan, J. 2018, 'Private hospital expansion in China: A global perspective', *Global Health Journal*, 2(2), pp. 33–46.

Feng, X.L., Martinez-Alvarez, M., Zhong, J., Xu, J., Yuan, B., Meng, Q. and Balabanova, D. 2017, 'Extending access to essential services against constraints: The three-tier health service delivery system in rural China (1949–1980)', *International Journal for Equity in Health*, 16(49).

Hipgrave, D. 2011, 'Communicable disease control in China: From Mao to now', *Journal of Global Health*, 1(2), pp. 224–38.

Langwick, S. 2010, 'From non-aligned medicines to market-based herbals: China's relationship to the shifting politics of traditional medicine in Tanzania', *Medical Anthropology: Cross-Cultural Studies in Health and Illness*, 29(1), pp. 15–43.

Lin, S., Gao, L., Reyes, M., Cheng, F., Kaufman, J. and El-Sadr, W.M. 2016, 'China's health assistance to Africa: Opportunism or altruism? *Globalization and Health*, 12(83).

Li Wang, Z.W., Ma, Q., Fang, G. and Yang, J. 2019, 'The development and reform of public health in China from 1949 to 2019', *Globalization and Health*, 15(45).

McKeown, T., Brown, R.G. and Record, R.G. 1972, 'An interpretation of the modern rise of population in Europe', *Population Studies: A Journal of Demography*, 26(3), pp. 345–82.

Meng, Q., Yang, H., Chen, W., Sun, Q. and Liu, X. 2015, *People's Republic of China Health Systems Review*, Health Systems in Transition, 5(7), Asia Pacific Observatory on Health Systems and Policies, WHO, Geneva.

National Bureau of Statistics of China (NBSC). 2018, *China Statistical Yearbook*, China Statistics Press, Beijing.

Navarro, V. and Wei, Z. 2014, 'Why hasn't China's high-profile health reform (2003–2012) delivered? An analysis of its neoliberal roots,' *Critical Social Policy*, 34(2), pp. 175–98.

PAHO (Pan American Health Organization). 1988, *The Challenge of Epidemiology: Issues and Selected Readings*, Scientific Publication no.505, PAHO, World Health Organization, Washington, DC.

Relman, A.S 1980, 'The new medical-industrial complex', *The New England Journal of Medicine*, 303(17), pp. 963–70.

Szreter, S. 2002, 'Rethinking McKeown: The relationship between public health and social change', *American Journal of Public Health*, 92(5), pp. 722–5.

Torsekar, Mihir. 2018 'China climbs the global value chain for medical devices', *Journal of International Commerce and Economics*, February, accessed 21 February 2021, <https://www.usitc.gov/publications/332/journals/final_china_and_medtech_gvc_jice_508_compliant.pdf>.

Wong, V.C.W. and Chiu, S.W.S. 1997, 'Health-care reforms in the people's republic of China: Strategies and social implications', *International Journal of Public Sector Management*, 10(1–2), pp. 76–92.

World Health Organization. 1978, *Declaration of Alma-Ata: International Conference on Primary Health Care*, WHO, Alma-Ata, accessed 7 December 2021, <https://www.who.int/publications/almaata_declaration_en.pdf>.

Yip, W. and Hsiao, W.C. 2015, 'What drove the cycles of Chinese health system reforms?, *Health Systems and Reform*, 1(1), pp. 52–61.

28

THE POLITICAL ECONOMY OF HEALTH AND HEALTHCARE IN INDIA

Shailender Kumar Hooda

The term 'political economy' has been variously defined and rediscovered over time and across disciplines since the Seventeenth Century. The roots of the political economy of 'health' can be traced back to Friedrich Engels' seminal work, *The Condition of the Working Class in England in 1844* (2009 [1845]; see also: Navarro 1985). Engels elaborated how social and working conditions produced by new industrial forms of capitalism resulted in widespread suffering and premature death among workers, while yielding untold wealth for the capitalist class who owned factories (Harvey 2021). He argued that high mortality and morbidity patterns in the working-class ultimately resulted from the organization of the productive relations of capitalism and its accompanying social environment, including poor housing, overcrowding, insufficient ventilation, chronic food shortage, excessive drinking, and the misdistribution of medical practitioners (Baer 1982). This doctrine highlights the social production of illness and disease in both advanced industrial and Third World countries, which finds its roots in the deterioration of social and natural processes, and is generally captured under the political economy of health/illness. The political economy of healthcare, however, is concerned with the impact that the capitalist mode of production has on the production, distribution, and consumption of health services, as well as how these processes reflect class relations within medical institutions and the larger societies in which they are embedded (Baer 1982). Thus, the political economy of health considers why and under what circumstances people become unhealthy, while healthcare addresses the activities associated with restoring this health and/or ameliorating discomfort and pain.

This chapter aims to understand these political-economic processes in the Indian context, with an eye to developing a historical perspective. It first describes the tensions and contradictions that have arisen with regard to health and the performance of the healthcare sector in terms of delivery, access, quality, and equality. It then explains how global neoliberalism has affected the role of the state in healthcare provisioning, and to what extent this has led to a divergence away from historically and culturally entrenched institutions in favor of a more neoliberal orientation. Ultimately, its aim is to discuss the key political-economic processes – both domestic and global – that have shaped healthcare in India in recent decades, as well as the central ideas, interests, and institutions that have informed this trajectory.

DOI: 10.4324/9781003017110-32

The political economy of work and well-being

Health is a desirable state in which the individual and/or population live well, work well, and enjoy their (physical, mental, and social) lives in the absence of disease or injury (WHO 1980). It is influenced both by internal and by external factors of the society in which people live. As noted above, in discussing the condition of the English working-class during the Industrial Revolution, Engels (2009 [1845]) described how hazardous work, working conditions, and environmental surroundings manifested themselves in injuries to the human body and, in extreme cases, severe disability or death. The condition of the Indian working-class, almost a century after the Engels work, had not especially changed. The Royal Commission of 1931 reported that working and living conditions among Indian labor were 'horrible' (Royal Commission on Labour in India 1931). The hazardous tasks and occupational and environmental conditions confronting workers resulted in severe disability and death in the 1960s (GOI 1969), and occupational health risks were identified as the tenth leading cause of morbidity (symptoms that included back pain, hearing loss, chronic obstructive lung disease, asthma, injuries, cancer, and leukemia) and mortality in the country (WHO 1998, 2002).

These risks have not yet abated. A recent estimate by the International Labor Organization (ILO 2019) reveals that, every year, occupational accidents and work-related diseases result in the deaths of 2.78 million workers globally. The construction industry faces disproportionately high rates of accidents. A recent Health and Safety Risk Index (HSRI) measured the levels of risk to occupational health and safety in 176 countries, and reported that among the BRIC nations (Brazil, Russia, India, and China) and nine other nations (including India), India was ranked in the 'extreme/high' risk category (GRP 2020). Bangladesh, Brazil, Colombia, Egypt, Honduras, India, Kazakhstan, the Philippines, Turkey, and Zimbabwe were reported to be the ten worst countries for workers in the world in 2020 (ITUC 2020). The risk of occupational injury in China and India is reported to be about two-and-a-half times higher than that found in Europe and North America (EMCONET 2007). Occupational health has largely been ignored for too long in India. Even after the Bhopal Gas Tragedy of 1984 – which resulted in the deaths of between 3,800 and 16,000 people, along with around 600,000 injuries – measures undertaken to meet minimal work standards have been inadequate (Mandal 2009). Such standards remained unresolved even in the newly introduced labor reform *Code-2019* (GOI 2019; Sood 2020).

Along with such severe working conditions, over 90 percent of the working-class in India are employed in the informal sector where work is insecure with low pay (GOI 2015). India is a country where informal labor is even rising in the formal sector through the utilization of temporary and contractual workers. The *Industrial Relations Code 2020* allows companies to directly hire workers on short-term contracts, rather than providing more stable employment (Sood 2020).[1] This helps to explain the increase in variable and insecure work, and how more and more workers are pushed into taking up hazardous and precarious work conditions while being left with low pay. The share of wages in gross value added has declined drastically in the formal sector over time (from 19.1 percent in 1990–91 to 9.9 percent in 2011–12), whereas the profit share increased substantially from 21.4 percent to 49.6 percent during the same period (Roy 2016).[2]

Thus, the driving force behind Indian corporate and industrial growth has been the desire for profit maximization, and Indian 'socialism' has merely supplemented and mystified this thrust. The search for higher profits has not only led to the neglect of workers' welfare, but has also created an increase in hazardous work and, unfortunately, high mortality. The availability of informal employment has not only failed to bring about a successful escape from poverty, but has contributed to existing vulnerabilities (GOI 2011; DGFAS n.d.). Additionally, class/caste is infused into the precarious conditions confronting labor. The *Labor Investigation Committee Report of India* (GOI 2002) highlighted the caste composition and social hierarchy prevalent in both industrial and agricultural sectors. It made clear that low-caste families and tribes, including Harijans, are predominantly engaged in low-level occupations – working as coolies, earth movers, rickshaw pullers, and so on – and that most are migrant laborers, arriving from low-income states (Mandal 2009).

Finally, industrialization and globalization are changing occupational morbidity drastically. Traditional labor-oriented markets have shifted toward greater automation and mechanization. New pathologies, such as cancer, stress, and heart diseases, are on rise. The health, safety, and well-being of employees across affected sectors are important for the country's development; however, only a fraction of workers are covered by health and safety legislation or social security measures (Hooda 2020a). As such, taking the formal industrialized and informal sectors together, working conditions provide ample health concerns. If we add to this occupational picture poor housing conditions, unhygienic sanitation and water conditions, and the disconcerting state of malnutrition in India, we are left with a situation that poses serious health risks and severe challenges to the healthcare system. Insecure workers and other people at risk necessarily look for health services that must be freely available in a public system, and it is to the realities of this challenge that the chapter now turns.

The political economy of healthcare: producing the providers

Since the time of independence, if one considers the production, distribution, and consumption of healthcare, it is notable that the quality of services rendered in India has been much higher for privileged classes than for the general population and poor. At the beginning of 1950s, social health insurance schemes – the Central Government Health Scheme (1954) for government employees, and Employees State Insurance Scheme (1952) for formal sector workers – were extended, with highly subsidized premiums to civil servants and formal sector workers (2–3 percent of the working population) (GOI 2011). Yet, the majority of the population and informal sector workers (90 percent of the total workforce) have been left with no such protection. The government, as a means of development, provides subsidized healthcare in the public system as an instrument to redistribute income and ensure the poor receive at least a minimum level of health services. In reality, however, whatever level of free (low-cost) public facilities are provided, the wealthiest people accessed them more than the poorest (Mahal 2001; GOI 2019a). In a way, wealthy households benefit more from the publicly provided services, because the rich consume and take advantage of public subsidy more than the poor, despite the latter having higher needs.

The structural distribution of the country's healthcare delivery system is such that it provides more and better healthcare facilities in cities, where more privileged social classes live, than in rural areas, which are predominantly inhabited by poor, landless laborers, and peasants. The evidence suggests that two-thirds of corporate, and over half of large, insurance-empaneled hospitals are located in cities of over five million people, state headquarters, or other select urban centers (Hooda 2020b). Because of the high concentration of privileged classes (civil servants/workers), three-quarters of total insurance claims are paid out within metro regions (Hooda 2020c). Moreover, rural areas have deficient or fragile health facilities, leading to inequitable access to healthcare. Across rural areas, there is great diversity in the distribution of health centers, which generally provide reproductive (maternal and child) healthcare, across and within states of India.

Human resources for health are critical for healthcare delivery, and the production and distribution of human resource development in India remains classed. The Bhore Committee in 1946 recommended that medical training institutions be spread across remote regions – at least one institute per 500,000 people. The state, however, has failed to create an adequate number of medical training institutions to meet growing health needs, opening considerable space for private players in the medical education field (Choudhury 2016). In most cases, those with political or corporate influence have access to medical colleges in the private sector, where doctors are trained only with the payment of additional capitation fees. There are instances where illegal payment of capitation fees paid by the students even exceeds Rs. 10–20 million (Pathak 2014; D'Silva 2015). The opportunities for medical training are largely availed by children of influential, wealthy, and privileged urban families. In other words, the medical education in private institutions is largely becoming the preserve of those who have the requisite economic and political resources, and where merit can also become a casualty (Jayaram 1995). Despite opposition by different stakeholders, and several judgments of the Supreme Court declaring that charging capitation fees is unfair and unjust, such practices continue unabated in India (Choudhury 2016).

Accordingly, the prevalence of capitation fees, high medical tuition, and other associated costs has resulted in medical education becoming inaccessible to low-income households. The medical education among these groups has reached abysmally low levels. In 2017–18, the number of people receiving medical education (graduate and above) was over 8 and 158 times higher among the general caste and the wealthy classes, when compared to the scheduled tribe (the lowest caste) and the poor, respectively (see: Figure 28.1). The richest rural and urban groups enjoyed acceptance rates around 203 and 38 times higher than their poorest rural and urban counterparts. A causal non-agricultural laborer is 795 times less likely to receive medical education than the regular wage/salary earner in a non-agricultural sector (Figure 28.1). Infused into these class realities, it is a widely recognized fact in India that elite higher education institutions engage in caste discrimination, as well (Thirumal 2021).

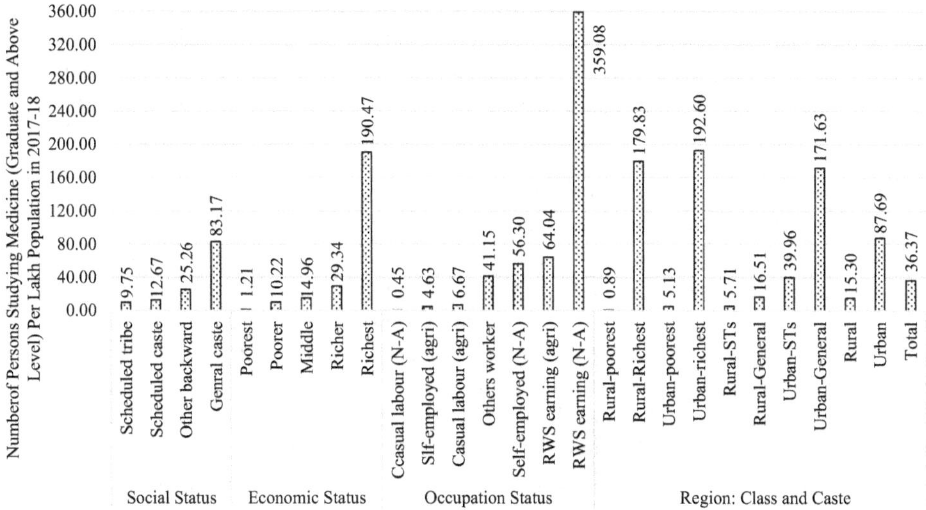

Figure 28.1 Medical education received according to status across class and caste.

Source: Author's estimates based on GOI (2019a).

Note: RWS = regular wage/salary in agriculture (agri.) and non-agriculture (N-A), while the 'agriculture' category represents only rural populations.

Importantly, the entry of the private sector into medical education has changed its orientation and content, leading to greater emphasis on the pursuit of specialization and super-specialization in clinical disciplines, as well as hospital-based dispensing of medicines. These changes influence the career choices and ethical values of medical graduates (Bajpayee and Saraya 2018), such that elite urban trainees exhibit almost no willingness to serve among rural poor population. They (physicians) generally regard medical skills as a valuable commodity and seek to market it largely in urban areas. This imbalance complicates the political economy of care, specifically how the state determines the distribution of resources and for whom, in the face of contradictions in delivery, access, quality, and equality.

The political economy of healthcare: arranging the system

Healthcare in India is provided by myriad organizations and institutions, and through arrangements in both public and private settings. The public system is vertically fragmented around primary, secondary, and tertiary care, while the private sector is fragmented across solo practitioners, independent medical clinics, and corporate-run hospitals, which provide a highly mixed and heterogeneous range of healthcare services (Hooda 2017). The public system was built on the premise that no citizen should be left behind due to her/his inability to pay, and the state will take primary responsibility to provide free or low-cost care. The public system continues to be relevant in citizens' lives, but has been confronted with several challenges relating to inefficiency in resource utilization and under-utilization of services, largely due to persistent gaps in health personnel and infrastructure. These gaps include deteriorating or absent infrastructure, inappropriate staffing, weak diagnostic and therapeutic services, non-availability of drugs, and poor referral services across a range of government, voluntary, and private hospitals. Alongside this, the system exhibits low coordination between public and private sectors, sub-optimal inter-sectoral coordination, emerging public health challenges of communicable and non-communicable diseases, escalating costs of healthcare, and ever-widening gaps of accessibility (Hooda 2021). Such inefficiencies result in a *de facto* denial of care for patients who would have otherwise sought treatment in a well-resourced system (Cylus *et al.* 2016). Even for those who do seek care, the fragmented, disorganized, and disaggregated healthcare ecosystem results in gaps in access, quality, and affordability, where patients are left to fend for themselves and seek treatments from multiple service providers, without any continuity in service provision (Baeza *et. al* 2019).

There exist massive inequities in access to healthcare and mortality outcomes across the rural-urban and poor-rich spectrums (Zodpey and Negandhi 2018). The absolute gap in life expectancy at birth between the richest and bottom poorest quintile groups remains 7.6 years (Selvaraj *et al.* 2021). Moreover, there is a marked difference in skilled birth attendance, where the richest experience 84.9 percent such attendance and the poorest quintile only 23.6 percent. There is a high concentration of untreated morbidity among vulnerable (the poor and elderly) populations, including poor, illiterate, and rural women who are less likely to receive antenatal care. Across income quintiles, there are disparities in health outcomes, access, and utilization of services, where the poor have the least access and endure the poorest outcomes (Selvaraj *et al.* 2021). Importantly, while high-income individuals avail themselves of the most modern and expensive health services, the poor – especially in rural areas – struggle to gain access to even rudimentary care. As per recent estimates, hospitalization rates among the well-off were three to six times higher than hospitalization rates for the poor (GOI 2019a).

In addition, while access to safe, effective, and quality medicines and vaccines has been made one of the targets of the Sustainable Development Goals, around two-thirds of the Indian population lack access to essential drugs and medicines (JSA 2006). The paradoxical situation is that the Indian pharmaceutical industry exports medicines across the globe and is known as the pharmacy to the world, while millions of Indian people are pushed into poverty due to the high cost of medicine (Selvaraj *et al.* 2014).

To address the quality, efficiency, and gaps in mortality and morbidity, several commitments have been made to raise public spending on health to 2–3 percent of GDP. The current spending level (1.18 percent of GDP) amounts to less than half of this spending target (Hooda 2021). The lack of access, availability, affordability, and quality of care has resulted in sub-optimal health outcomes, even comparing unfavorably in relation to many of India's peer countries. This inadequacy in the public system has even compelled the poor to utilize costly care from private providers. The poorest spend one-eighth of their total income on healthcare, while the government spends less and less. This has resulted in one of the most privatized healthcare systems in the world, where individuals frequently pay 62 percent of total health expenditure from their own pocket. Due to this situation of high out-of-pocket payments, the poor are financially squeezed and easily fall below the poverty line, while borrowing unmanageable amounts to meet healthcare expenditures (Hooda 2017). Even worse, the proportion of people unable to access any form of treatment, due to inability to pay, is large and growing (JSA 2006) – a situation only exacerbated by the COVID-19 pandemic.

Processes reshaping healthcare: modernization and neoliberalism

Every medical system has its own pattern of consumption, which is often based on the prevailing cultural understanding of disease and its causes (Hsiao 2003). Modern practice sometimes demands a sophisticated intervention, while proponents of traditional methods believe in mitigating and preventing disease by understanding its causes and advocate for improving the social environment. Allopathic advocates argue that Western medicine treats all types of disease better and faster than traditional healers. The first World Health Assembly of WHO in 1978 at Alma Ata, however, recognized the importance of preventive and traditional measures for improving the health in developing countries. In a debate about how a country's health system should be designed, it was argued that medical practices in Western industrial states and societies emphasize the curative elements of healthcare services in hospitals, medical practice, and pharmacies, centered on medical technology. Preventive care (prevention of diseases) and social medicine, it was argued, gained relatively little traction in these societies, and they did not take seriously the traditional views of developing countries regarding experiences of diseases, health, and spiritual healing (WHO 1978). It emerged from the Alma Ata that health services in the so-called developing countries should not be interpreted through the lens of Western medical practice. This is because the medical apparatus from industrial states was largely unaffordable and ill-suited to developing countries in terms of both price and utility, and because patterns of disease prevalence in these countries were different from developed countries. Even beyond costs and differential disease patterns, a lack of specialists (health personnel) in high-tech medicine would mean that such systems could not be easily replicated.

Instead, the central concept that emerged at Alma Ata – the Primary Healthcare (PHC) approach – was heavily concerned with people, and oriented around principles of social justice, accessibility, appropriateness, and social acceptance of medical services, with an eye to the needs of communities and their participation in health services. The PHC approach emerged as a central concept for attaining the goal of 'health for all' (HFA) by 2000. It strongly affirms health as a state of complete physical, mental, and social well-being, and not merely the absence of

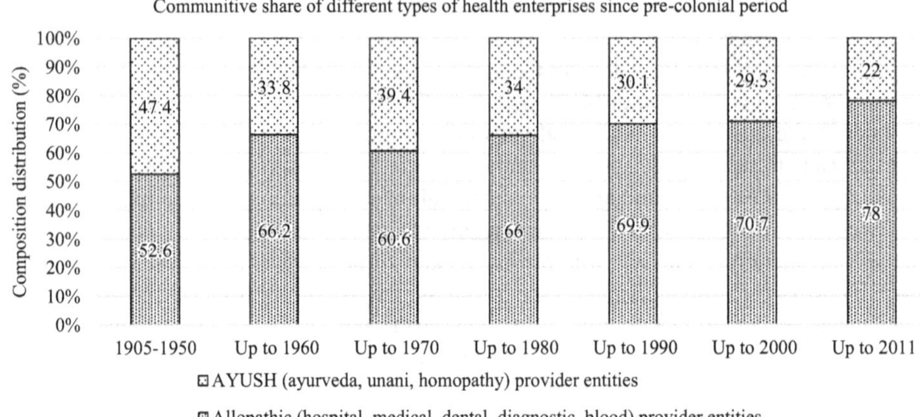

Figure 28.2 Toward modernization of health and medical care.

Source: Author's estimates, based on NSS Service Sector Enterprises (2010–11).

disease or infirmity. HFA involved a holistic framework of comprehensive healthcare provision to achieve *health for all* through state intervention. For better health system design, it called for more integrated and comprehensive health provision. Most of the participant countries, including India, signed and supported the HFA vision. India encompassed most of the HFA tenets (equity, universalism, comprehensiveness, government responsibility, community participation) in its *First National Health Policy* announced in 1983 (Hooda 2021). This policy, and several since, has called for greater public investment to promote primary healthcare alongside the development of the AYUSH (Ayurveda, Yoga, Unani, Siddha, and Homeopathy) system in the country.

From the precolonial to the post-Independence period, especially until early-1980s, the state was the main provider of healthcare, with increases in public health investment at both the national and the state level. This trend in rising public investment, however, was ended prior to the liberalization of the Indian economy during the 1990s (Hooda 2021). While a significant number of non-state players had established large charitable hospitals since the colonial period, medical education in post-graduation, specialization, and super-specialization led to dramatic changes in medical practice by the 1980s. Specialists began setting up private nursing homes, and the corporate sector began showing an interest in entering the hospital sector. Development in medical technology also hastened the process of commercialization and made for-profit hospitals a lucrative proposition (Duggal 2005). By the latter part of 1980s, the state's investments in the hospital sector started decelerating (Hooda 2021). It was during this liberalization phase that India underwent macro-economic policy restructuring, guided by Structural Adjustment Programmes (SAP) enforced by international agencies. The fiscal stringency induced by these measures affected central and state finances, squeezing social sector spending, especially on healthcare (Hooda 2015). For the private sector, this was a clarion call to increase its presence in the sector, and this agenda was reinforced by international agencies. Since this time, the Indian healthcare system, which had been largely dominated by AYUSH during the pre-colonial period, gradually moved toward the establishment of modern hospital-based allopathic medicine. Allopathic providers now dominate, with a 78 percent share of the healthcare market (see: Figure 28.2).

Over time, not only did for-profit hospitals become dominant, but privatization also emerged via user-charges and state utilization of contracts and outsourcing. In this regard, it is important to highlight the role of international agencies, like the World Bank, in pushing the agenda of privatization and limiting the role of the public sector in health. The Bank centered its 1993 *World Development Report* on 'Investing in Health', which highlighted the global improvement of life expectancy in the past 40 years (rising from 40 years in 1950 to 63 years in 1990). Child mortality was reduced significantly, and smallpox, which killed more than five million annually in the early-1950s, had been eradicated entirely. Moreover, vaccines had drastically reduced the occurrence of measles and polio (World Bank 1993). The Report acknowledged the role of the state, but simultaneously argued that public healthcare systems in developing nations were confronted with several challenges of efficiency and equity. As such, it insisted on limiting government involvement, rejecting the idea of healthcare as a public good and, instead, viewing it as a matter of free choice for individuals and families, who exhibited strikingly varied health needs.

Viewing healthcare as a private good, the Report consistently proposed a strategy for promoting both private insurance and delivery. It argued that when a country develops, a section of its population becomes able and willing to spend its own money on healthcare. At such a point, the state should not retain sole responsibility for health, and it should be shared with the private sector (World Bank 1993). Thus, between the late-1990s and early-2000s, India initiated several reforms imposing user fees in government hospitals (Ghosh 2010). Though these reforms were piecemeal in nature, they predictably led to extensive changes in organizational structure, financing, and delivery of healthcare services. The SAP and bank-proposed reforms became a guiding instrument in reducing the state's role in healthcare provisioning, as India also opened up its health insurance sector to foreign direct investment (FDI), capped at 26 percent in 1999. The pharmaceutical sector was also liberalized from 1994 to 2002, and only 74 out of 500 commonly used bulk drugs were kept under statutory price control. The impact of such drug policy changes could be seen in the dramatic increase in drug prices during this period (Ghosh 2010).

This neoliberal agenda was further advanced by the Bank in its India-specific report: *India: Raising the Sights – Better Health Systems for India's Poor* (World Bank 2001). The report stressed that underfunding and privatization are defensible because the Indian economy has the potential to grow at a faster rate, leading to increased purchasing power among the population. Since public systems were assumed inefficient in meeting popular need, the obvious answer was marketization. Such neoliberal arguments continuously and publicly insist on the necessity of cuts in public investment that would, of course, open up investment opportunities for the private sector. Accordingly, underfunding provided a necessary first step in realizing a neoliberal strategy in healthcare: as this sector became a low political priority, inadequate public provisioning led to 'rational' user fees and, ultimately, private sector 'rationalization' (read: exploitation) of the healthcare market (Hooda 2020, 2021).

In this policy environment, India rolled out several liberalization policies to privatize the sector. One key policy move was to open up hospitals to foreign actors, approving 100 percent FDI in 2000. To further encourage domestic and foreign players, especially large corporations, additional measures included the relaxation of import duties on medical equipment and technology in 2000; long-term and cheap loans to private healthcare institutions; and redesignation of the hospital sector to industry status in the 2003–04 budget. Several tax benefits and other incentives were also granted for setting up private hospitals and clinics during this period. The state, thus, repositioned itself as a facilitator of private development, with an eye to investing in health but supporting the private sector through subsidies, credits and public-private partnerships (PPPs), and insurance

(Hooda 2021). In concrete terms, privatization then took various forms – ranging from disinvestment in hospitals, leasing contracts, and outsourcing of laundry, diet, diagnostic services, and pharmaceutical supplies, to private consulting facilities and, of course, the introduction of user fees in dispensaries and hospitals (JSA 2006).

Despite several shortcomings in market-based models, this pro-market phenomenon is spreading in many developing countries. In India, the liberalization and privatization reforms of the 1990s and 2000s have, ultimately, resulted in the very high presence of private healthcare providers. As of 2011, out of 106.7 million health enterprises, only 19.6 million were public entities. Presently, the private sector provides around three-quarters of all outpatient, and two-thirds of inpatient, care treatments – all at a very high cost (Hooda 2021). For instance, in 2018, the cost of hospitalization in a private facility was 6.37 times and 8.03 times higher than receiving care in a public facility in rural and urban areas, respectively (Hooda 2021). By 2018, the cost of hospitalization care in the private sector was 11 times higher than what it was in 1987. Costlier private care has resulted in high out-of-pocket health expenditure. This has made health services inaccessible, particularly to the poor, who cannot afford to pay in times of need; or, if they do pay, often face financial hardship and impoverishment as a result of selling their assets or borrowing money to meet their healthcare costs (Hooda 2021). In short, neoliberal reform has steepened inequality in relation to healthcare, diminishing access for the rural and poor, while leaving them financially squeezed or potentially ruined.

Health financing and policy paradigms: the recent phenomena

Achieving universal health coverage (UHC) has become an internationally accepted development goal. UHC demands that all people receive access to the healthcare they need without exposing users to financial hardship (WHO 2013). Thus, the paramount issue in health policy circles is which type of health financing mechanism can provide efficient financial risk protection to all people against the cost of healthcare. The WHO (2010, 2013) advocates for restructuring the financing of healthcare to achieve UHC, and suggests a road map for developing countries to achieve this goal. In particular, it recommends financing care through social health insurance (employer-based) as a tool to move toward universal coverage. However, this promotion of employer-based financing depends on pooling resources from employer and employee contributions, possibly supported by public funds. While many countries have done this, the Indian labor market is highly fragmented, where a large proportion (over 90 percent) of the workforce is engaged in the informal sector, leaving little room for organized employer contributions. Indeed, estimates of employer contributions in financing health declined from 5.7 percent in 2004–05 to 2.4 percent in 2013–14 (GOI 2018).

Nonetheless, since global practices have always had a discernible influence on Indian policy, India set up a High Level Expert Group (HLEG) on UHC in 2010. Its report suggested that India needs to increase its health spending to 2–3 percent of GDP. The planning commission's steering committee for the Twelfth Five-Year Plan appreciated the HLEG's recommendations. Yet, in its own assessment report, criticized the HLEG for ignoring the well-established private sector. The committee commented that given the major share of personnel, beds, and patients, 'the private sector has to be partnered with for health care' (Qadeer 2013: 229). India incorporated this notion in its third *National Health Policy, 2017* (GOI 2017). Here, there is a clearly specified role for comprehensive primary care provision in the public sector, supplemented by the strategic purchase of secondary and tertiary care services from private sectors, ensuring that universal healthcare and strategic purchasing will be promoted through publicly funded health insurance. Within this policy, the privatization agenda in healthcare has advanced, as the health sector is viewed as a 'service-providing' instrument of national economic growth (Bajpayee and Saraya 2018).

The government has launched a publicly funded health insurance scheme, PMJAY-2018, under the ambit of Ayushman Bharat, aimed at covering the 40 percent of Indian families who are poor and vulnerable. This has brought about a major shift in policy dialogue, oriented around the promotion of purchasing through a financial protection package (insurance), where the state appears to ensure access to, but not necessarily provide, services. That is, while public funds were previously directed toward bolstering provision capacity, they will now be redirected toward private providers. The strategic purchasing of services can only facilitate integration of qualified providers for in-patient care within the system. Thus, vigorous promotion of the private sector will result in large and corporate hospitals acquiring a dominant position in medical care provisioning, whereas a majority of outpatient care received by individuals (which the insurance-based system does not cover) remains scattered across individual practices and clinics in the informal sector. The significant emphasis on curative over preventative care, and use of high-end technologies in medical interventions, will result in high variations in service delivery across regions and boundaries. The success of such programs will be entirely reliant on the approach of the private sector in addressing geographical disparities in healthcare distribution. Experience suggests that private hospitals will, however, remain highly concentrated in metro areas, as private players are opportunistic in provision, rather than attuned to the equity issues of resource-poor regions. Insurance, in other words, does little to encourage and redirect private health providers toward filling critical gaps in the system – indeed, these gaps may be exacerbated. So far, it remains entirely unclear whether strategic purchasing can advance quality healthcare services in underserviced areas (Hooda 2021).

Ideally, 'coverage' as a strategy would focus on the establishment of a wide network of health providers and health institutions – extending access to health services for the majority of the population, rather than just broadening financing. Reducing financial barriers to care is certainly critical to reform, but the outcome of such reforms will be immensely more favorable in an equitably distributed system of provision and care (Hooda 2020).

Conclusion

This chapter has described the tensions and contradictions that have arisen with regard to the Indian healthcare sector in terms of equity, access, and quality. It explained how global neoliberalism has affected the role of the state in healthcare provisioning, and the extent to which this has led to a divergence away from historically and culturally entrenched institutions, in favor of a more neoliberal orientation. From the working conditions of Indian laborers, to the displacement of AYUSH health practices, to the promotion of private insurance and delivery, India has not witnessed the extension of healthcare provision for those who need it most. Instead, a highly tiered system that emphasizes curative over preventive medicine will service, most effectively, those with the ability to pay. The majority of the population, however, will be left with inadequate and uneven care.

Notes

1 Of course, it is pertinent to note that the process of hiring labor at low wage rates is not new, but rather started in the pre-liberalization period (Subrahmanian 1990).

2 Moreover, this profit has been relatively concentrated among firms in India. For instance, in 2018, 'business group-affiliated firms' – legally independent firms linked by formal and informal network ties – secured 55 percent of the total profit share, despite only comprising 25 percent of 48,916 registered companies (Saraswathy 2021).

References

Baer, H.A. 1982, 'On the political economy of health', *Medical Anthropology Newsletter*, 14(1), pp. 1–17.

Baeza, C.C., Peters, D., Pellathy, T., Javier, E. and Ramon, M. 2019, 'India health sector risk pooling: Challenges, opportunities, and options for improvement', in NITI Aayog (ed), *Health System for a New India: Building Blocks*, Government of India, New Dehli, pp. 19–80. <www.niti.gov.in/sites/default/files/2019-11/NitiAayogBook_compressed_1.pdf>.

Bajpayee, V. and Saraya, A. (eds) 2018, *Health Beyond Medicine: Reflections on the Policies and Sociology of India*, Aakar Book Publication, Delhi.

Choudhury, P.K. 2016, 'Role of private sector in medical education and human resource development for health in India', *Economic and Political Weekly*, 51(3), pp. 71–9.

Cylus, J., Papanicolas, I. and Smith, P.C. 2016, *Health System Efficiency: How to Make Measurement Matter for Policy and Management*, Health Policy Series No. 46, European Observatory on Health Systems and Policies and World Health Organization, accessed 1 May 2021, <https://www.ncbi.nlm.nih.gov/books/NBK436879/?report=reader>.

D'Silva, J. 2015, 'Corruption in India: India's private medical colleges and capitation fees', *British Medical Journal Clinical Research*, 350(8001).

DGFAS. n.d., *National Occupational Safety and Health (OSH) Profile (draft)*, Directorate General Factory Advice Service and Labour Institutes in collaboration with International Labor Organization, accessed 7 April 2022, <https://dgfasli.gov.in/sites/default/files/service_file/Nat-OSH-India-Draft%281%29.pdf >.

Duggal, R. 2005, *Financing Strategies for Universal Access to Healthcare*, Centre for Enquiry into Health and Allied Themes, Mumbai, accessed 7 April 2022, <http://www.cehat.org/cehat/uploads/files/A%20264%20Financingand%20budgetissues.pdf>.

Engels, F. 2009 [1845], *The Condition of the Working Class in England in 1844*, Oxford University Press, Oxford.

Ghosh, S 2010, 'Catastrophic payments and impoverishment due to out-of-pocket health spending: The effects of recent health sector reforms in India', *Asia Health Policy Program, Working Paper No. 15*, July, accessed 1 April 2021, <https://papers.ssrn.com/sol3/papers.cfm?abstract_id=1658573>.

GOI. 1969, *Report of the National Commission on Labour Government of India*, Ministry of Labour and Employment and Rehabilitation, Government of India, New Dehli, accessed 19 May 2022, <http://14.139.60.153/handle/123456789/4380>.

GOI. 2002, *The Second National Commission on Labour Report, Volume I: Main Report*, Ministry of Labour and Employment, Government of India, New Dehli, accessed 19 May 2022, <http://labour.nic.in/lcomm2/nlc_report.html>.

GOI. 2011a, *Report of the Working Group on Occupational Safety and Health*, prepared for The Twelfth Five Year Plan (2012 to 2017), Ministry of Labour and Employment, Government of India, New Dehli, accessed 27 March 2021, <https://www.ilo.org/wcmsp5/groups/public/---ed_protect/---protrav/---safework/documents/policy/wcms_211795.pdf>.

GOI. 2011b, *A Critical Assessment of the Existing Health Insurance Models in India*, Public Health Foundation of India, Report submitted to Planning Commission of India, Government of India, New Dehli, accessed 27 March 2021, <http://planningcommission.nic.in/reports/sereport/ser/ser_heal1305.pdf>.

GOI. 2015, *Report on Employment in Informal Sector and Conditions of Informal Employment (2013–14), Volume IV*, Ministry of Labour and Employment, Labour Bureau, Government of India, Chandigarh, accessed 30 March 2021, <https://labour.gov.in/sites/default/files/Report%20vol%204%20final.pdf>.

GOI. 2017, *Third National Health Policy*, Ministry of Health and Family Welfare, Government of India, New Dehli, accessed 27 March 2021, <https://mohfw.gov.in/sites/default/files/9147562941489753121.pdf>.

GOI. 2018, *National Health Accounts: Estimates for India 2015–16*, National Health Accounts Technical Secretariat, National Health Systems Resource Centre, Ministry of Health and Family Welfare, Government of India, New Delhi.

GOI. 2019a, *New Labour Code for New India: Biggest Labour Reform in Independent India*, Ministry of Labour, Government of India, New Dehli, accessed 1 May 2021, <https://labour.gov.in/sites/default/files/Labour_Code_Eng.pdf>.

GOI. 2019b, *The Key Indicators of Social Consumption in India: Health,* NSS 75th Round, National Sample Survey Office, Ministry of Statistics and Programme Implementation, Government of India, New Dehli, accessed 27 April 2021, <http://164.100.161.63/sites/default/files/publication_reports/KI_Health_75th_Final.pdf>.

GOI. 2019c, *Bulletin on Rural Health Statistics (RHS) in India*, Ministry of Health and Family Welfare, Government of India, New Delhi.

GRP. 2020, 'ESG INDEX 2020: Measure of risks for 176 countries', Global Risk Profile, accessed 7 March 2021, <https://risk-indexes.com/wp-content/uploads/2020/12/Brochure_ESG_EN_2020.pdf>.

Harvey, M. 2021, 'The political economy of health: Revisiting its Marxian origins to address 21st-century health inequalities', *American Journal of Public Health*, 111(2), pp. 293–300.

Hooda, S.K. 2015, 'Government spending on health in India: Some hopes and fears of policy changes', *Journal of Health Management*, 17(4), pp. 458–86.

Hooda, S.K. 2017, 'Growth of formal and informal private healthcare providers in India: Structural changes and implications', *Journal of Health Care Finance*, 44(2), pp. 1–29.

Hooda, S.K. 2020a, 'Penetration and coverage of government-funded health insurance schemes in India', *Clinical Epidemiology and Global Health*, 8(4), pp. 1017–33.

Hooda, S.K. 2020b, 'Health system in transition: Journey from state provisioning to privatisation', *World Review of Political Economy*, 11(4), pp. 506–32.

Hooda, S.K. 2020c, 'Decoding Ayushman Bharat: A political economy perspective', *Economic and Political Weekly*, 50(25), pp. 107–15.

Hooda, S.K. 2021, *Health Sector, State and Decentralized Institutions in India*, Routledge India, London.

Hsiao, W.C. 2003, 'What is a health system? Why should we care?' accessed 1 March 2021, <www.mediastudies.fpzg.hr/_download/repository/Hsiao2003.pdf>.

ILO. 2019, *Safety and Health at the Heart of the Future of Work: Building on 100 Years of Experience*, International Labour Office, International Labour Organization, accessed 7 April 2021, <www.ilo.org/wcmsp5/groups/public/---dgreports/---dcomm/documents/publication/wcms_686645.pdf>.

ITUC. 2020, *2020 ITUC GLOBAL RIGHTS INDEX: The World's Worst Countries for Workers*, International Trade Union Confederation, accessed 7 May 2021, <https://www.ituc-csi.org/IMG/pdf/ituc_globalrightsindex_2020_en.pdf>.

Jayaram, N. 1995, 'Political economy of medical education in India', *Higher Education Policy*, 8(2), pp. 29–32.

JSA. 2006, *Health System in India: Crisis and Alternatives, First Edition*, National Coordination Committee, Delhi, accessed 19 March 2021, <http://sanhati.com/wp-content/uploads/2009/09/health_system_in_india.pdf>.

Mahal, A., Singh, J., Afridi, F. and Lamba, V. 2001, *Who Benefits From Public Health Spending in India*, World Bank Group, Washington, DC, accessed 21 March 2021, <http://documents.worldbank.org/curated/en/930041468285004372/Who-benefits-from-public-health-spending-in-India>.

Mandal, A.K. 2009, 'Strategies and policies deteriorate occupational health situation in India: A review based on social determinant framework', *Indian Journal of Occupational and Environmental Medicine*, 13(3), pp. 113–20.

Navarro, V. 1985, 'US Marxist scholarship in the analysis of health and medicine', *International Journal of Health* Services, 15(4), pp. 525–45.

Pathak, K. 2014, 'Medical capitation fee zooms as seats go under knife', *Business Standard*, 28 June, accessed 27 May 2015, <https://www.business-standard.com/article/management/medical-capitation-fee-zooms-as-seats-go-under-knife-114062800094_1.html>.

Qadeer, I. 2013, 'Universal health care in India: Panacea for whom?', *Indian Journal of Public Health*, 57(4), pp. 225–30.

Roy, S. 2016, 'Faltering manufacturing growth and employment: Is 'making' the answer?' *Economic and Political Weekly*, 51(13), pp. 35–42.

Royal Commission on Labour in India. 1931, *Report of the Royal Commission on Labour in India*, June, Stationary Office, London, accessed 11 March 2022, <https://indianculture.gov.in/report-royal-commission-labour-india>.

Saraswathy, B. 2021, *Changing Business Group Strategies in India: An Inquiry from the Lens of Mergers and Acquisitions*, Report submitted to the Indian Council of Social Science Research (ICSSR), New Delhi.

Selvaraj, S., Abrol, D. and Gopakumar, K.M. 2014, *Access to Medicines in India*, Academic Foundation, New Delhi.

Selvaraj, S., Karan, A.K., Mao, W., Hasan, H., Bharali, I., Kumar, P., Ogbuoji, O. and Chaudhuri, C. 2021, 'Did the poor gain from India's health policy interventions? Evidence from benefit-incidence analysis, 2004–2018', *International Journal of Equity in Health*, 20(1), pp. 1–15.

Sood, A. 2020, 'The silent takeover of Labour Right', *The India Fourm*, 17 November, accessed 7 April 2021, https://www.theindiaforum.in/article/silent-takeover-labour-rights#:~:text=The%20three%20new%20labour%20codes,all%20in%20all%2C%20disempower%20labour.

Subrahmanian, K.K. 1990, 'Development paradox in Kerala: Analysis of industrial stagnation', *Economic and Political Weekly*, 25(37), pp. 2053–5.

Thirumal, P. 2021, 'Regurgitative violence: The sacred and the profane in higher education institutions in India', *Economic and Political Weekly*, 56(23), pp. 15–8.

WHO. 1978, *Report of the International Conference on Primary Health Care*, Alma Ata, USSR, 6–12 September, accessed 7 April 2022, <https://apps.who. int/iris/handle/10665/39228>.

WHO. 1980, *The Role of the Health Sector in Food and Nutrition*, Technical Report Series No. 667, World Health Organisation, Geneva.

WHO. 2002, *World Health Report 2002, Statistical Annex*, World Health Organisation, accessed 8 April 2022, <http://www.who.int/whr/2002/annex/en/index.html>.

WHO. 2010, *The World Health Report: Health System Financing – The Path to Universal Coverage*, World Health Organization, Geneva, accessed 8 April 2022, <https://apps.who.int/iris/handle/10665/44371>.

WHO. 2013, *World Health Report 2013: Research for Universal Health Coverage*, World Health Organisation, Luxembourg, accessed 7 April 2022, <https://www.who.int/publications/i/item/9789240690837>.

WHO-ILO. 2021, *WHO/ILO Joint Estimates of the Work-related Burden of Disease and Injury, 2000–2016, Global Monitoring Report*, World Health Organization and International Labour Organization, Geneva, accessed 19 May 2022, <https://www.ilo.org/wcmsp5/groups/public/@ed_dialogue/@lab_admin/documents/publication/wcms_819788.pdf>.

World Bank. 1993, *World Development Report: Investing in Health*, Oxford University Press, Oxford.

World Bank. 2001, *India: Raising the Sights - Better Health Systems for India's Poor*, HNP Unit-India, Report No. 22304, World Bank, Washington, DC.

Zodpey, S.P. and Negandhi, P.H. 2018, 'Tracking India's progress in health sector after 70 years of independence', *Indian Journal of Public Health*, 62(1), pp. 1–3.

29

THE POLITICAL ECONOMY OF THE POSTSOCIALIST MORTALITY CRISIS

Gabor Scheiring and Lawrence King

The declining life expectancy in deindustrialized, rustbelt areas of the core capitalist countries, and the accompanying deepening of health inequalities therein, signals the existential crisis of contemporary economic arrangements. Recent research by Ann Case and Angus Deaton (2020) has prompted wide attention to workers' declining health in the North American Rust Belt, igniting the 'deaths of despair' debate. Case and Deaton (2020: 183) argue that this mortality crisis has been driven by deindustrialization, highlighting that the 'faults of contemporary capitalism are widespread, and America is simply the leader of a more general disaster that is already taking root elsewhere'.

The US is, indeed, not alone. The postsocialist mortality crisis offers insightful parallels. Foreshadowing today's working-class epidemic of deaths of despair, an unprecedented mortality crisis hit Eastern Europe 30 years ago as ex-socialist countries transitioned to capitalism. As Case and Deaton (2020: 108) highlight, 'it is no exaggeration to compare the long-standing misery of these Eastern Europeans with the wave of despair that is driving suicides, alcohol, and drug abuse among less-educated white Americans'.

With some fluctuations, life expectancy stagnated in most socialist countries in the 1970s and 1980s. However, the transition from state socialism to capitalism was accompanied by increased mortality in postsocialist Europe, leading to an epidemic of premature deaths unprecedented in peace times. According to David Stuckler (2009), the number of excess deaths could have been around 7.3 million in Eastern Europe in 1991–99 – including five million in Russia. This estimate falls between UNICEF's (2001) smaller figure of 3.3 million for Eastern Europe, and much larger estimates that as many as 6.1 million excess deaths may have arisen in Russia alone (Rosefielde 2001).

Former members of the Soviet Union suffered the most, especially Russia, where life expectancy declined by five years between 1988 and 1994, and the Baltic states, where life expectancy fell by four years on average in the same period. In the first 15 years after the fall of Communism, Russia lost more than three times as many people as during World War One (Eberstadt 2010: 5). At the other end of the spectrum, in a few countries such as the Czech Republic, Slovakia, and Slovenia, life expectancy increased by one year between 1988 and 1994.

Even though life expectancy has improved after the tumultuous years of the early-1990s, the postsocialist mortality crisis has left lasting wounds on postsocialist countries, contributing to

 DOI: 10.4324/9781003017110-33

deep health inequalities that continue to exist until today. The postsocialist mortality crisis represents one of the largest demographic catastrophes seen outside famine or war in recent history (Eberstadt 2010).

This chapter[1] presents a concise overview of the literature on the causes of this population health crisis, paying particular attention to the political-economic factors rooted in the violent social dislocations wrought by rapid economic change and attendant public policies. We probe a collection of dominant, yet competing, explanatory frameworks, and highlight socioeconomic dislocations that shape health behavior such as drinking or drug abuse. The chapter shows that a political economy of health approach that moves beyond individualistic, biological, and psychological explanations is necessary to understand health crises such as the postsocialist mortality crisis properly.

What explains the postsocialist mortality crisis?

Though some see the postsocialist mortality crisis as a continuation of past demographic processes (Carlson and Hoffmann 2011; Bhattacharya *et al.* 2013), research shows that the wave of excess deaths in the 1990s went well beyond what could be explained by historical trends (Cornia *et al.* 1998; Shkolnikov *et al.* 1998a; Cornia 2000; Brainerd and Cutler 2005). High and growing health inequalities still plague most Eastern European countries. Mortality differences by education exploded in the 1990s (Shkolnikov *et al.* 1998b) and grew until the early-2000s (Murphy *et al.* 2006; Doniec *et al.* 2018; Mackenbach *et al.* 2018).

Like in the US, middle-aged men were hit harder than younger or older generations or women, suggesting that stress could have been an important factor behind these excess deaths. The trends of different cause-specific death rates also point toward the importance of despair and stress. Diseases sensitive to the quality of healthcare and the extent of extreme poverty – such as infant deaths and infectious diseases – declined (Brainerd and Cutler 2005). Health indicators related to pollution also improved following industrial decline from the end of the 1980s (Nell and Stewart 1994: 16–7). In contrast, deaths sensitive to psycho-social stress grew rapidly, including cardiovascular diseases, alcohol-related diseases (liver diseases, accidents, poisoning), mental health disorders, suicides, and homicides.

Hazardous drinking played a central role in most of these deaths (Leon *et al.* 1997; Leon *et al.* 2007). In a systematic review of medical studies published between 1967 and 1997, Britton and McKee (2000: 300) found that 'the association between binge drinking and sudden cardiovascular death appears to be causal, thus providing a mechanism for the observed association between alcohol consumption and cardiovascular disease in Eastern Europe'. Using administrative time-series data on suicides and alcohol consumption, Landberg (2008) found that in spirit-consuming countries of Eastern Europe (Russia, Belarus, and Poland), a 1-liter increase in per capita alcohol consumption was associated with an increase in overall suicide rates of 5.7 to 7.5 percent. Excessive drinking, especially hazardous binge drinking, is also directly linked to accidents and liver diseases.

Most scholars agree that psycho-social stress significantly contributed to binge drinking and ill-health during the postsocialist transformation (Ellman 1994; Shapiro 1995; Watson 1995; Shkolnikov *et al.* 1998a; Leon and Shkolnikov 1998; Gilmore *et al.* 2002; Kopp *et al.* 2007; Popov 2009). Stress and despair were also directly associated with cardiovascular diseases (Razvodovsky 2013) and suicides (Brainerd 2001). Drug abuse also exploded in Eastern Europe after the fall of state socialism, but its overall contribution to the mortality crisis is minor.

Fewer drug-related deaths, more alcohol-related deaths, and cardiovascular deaths also played a central role, but the age distribution and the upstream role of stress, inability to cope with stress, and despair are comparable to the North American deaths of despair epidemic. Case and Deaton (2020) also note that they consider cardiovascular deaths a potential fourth category of deaths of despair because of their close connection to psycho-social stress. They also note that cardiovascular deaths stopped declining among working-class Americans, contributing to the relative worsening of their health profile. Thus, the postsocialist mortality crisis was an epidemic of deaths of despair, albeit encompassing some different components.

The remainder of this chapter considers how this population health crisis may be accounted for, with particular emphasis accorded to identifying its political-economic roots.

Dislocation and stress

A large body of studies concentrated on identifying the empirical patterns and proximate causes of the postsocialist mortality crisis in detail. This literature led to a consensus that alcohol consumption and stress were the most critical proximal causes. Another body of literature investigated more distal causes – that is, the social determinants of these deaths of despair (for a review, see: Scheiring *et al.* 2019). These can be divided into two broad camps: those emphasizing economic stress associated with economic reforms (demand/despair approach) versus those emphasizing narrower policies concerning the availability of alcohol or the dysfunctional health habits of working-class people (supply/culture approach).

Followers of the demand/despair approach showed that labor market disintegration – measured by unemployment or labor market turnover – was associated with the wave of postsocialist excess deaths. Walberg *et al.* (1998) used data from the state statistics bureau in 52 regions in the European part of Russia to measure the impact of economic insecurity on mortality. Examining the change in life expectancy from 1990 to 1994, the most significant factor was labor market turnover (gains and losses per 1,000 employees in medium and large enterprises), which explained about 42 percent of the variance in a simple regression model.

Using a multistage sample of the Russian adult population, Bobak *et al.* (1998) found that perceived control over life was strongly related to poor self-rated health and low physical functioning, concluding that psycho-social factors rooted in labor market disintegration were crucial to the postsocialist mortality crisis. Comparing data from surveys of the adult population conducted in 1988 and 1995 in Hungary, Kopp *et al.* (2000) also found a significant decrease in perceived control at the workplace, significantly correlated with depressive symptoms and lower self-rated health. A subsequent survey using data on Hungarian adults robustly linked the lack of control, high weekend workloads, and job insecurity to premature cardiovascular mortality (Kopp *et al.* 2006). Using cross-national survey data collected in Poland, the Czech Republic, Lithuania, and Hungary, Pikhart *et al.* (2001) also found that lower perceived control and job stress, measured by the effort/reward ratio, were associated with worse self-reported health.

Perlman and Bobak (2009) exploited the Russian Longitudinal Monitoring Survey, which surveyed 4,000 households yearly from 1994 to 2003. They showed that the odds of dying increased by 104 percent for manual employees who became unemployed. Similar elevated odds of death (64 percent) were observed for the working-class when they were paid in non-monetary goods, a strategy widely employed by failing firms. Service sector and agricultural workers also displayed similar patterns of deaths, but not professional and managerial workers.

As also noted by Case and Deaton (2020), declining levels of social capital are another expression of social disintegration contributing to deaths of despair. Using nationally representative household survey data covering 40 regions of Russia, Kennedy *et al.* (1998) found significant associations between indicators of social capital and life expectancy, as well as mortality rates. In a nationwide representative sample of the adult Russian population, Rose (2000) confirmed that social capital accounts for a notable amount of variance in health. Using data from 20 counties of Hungary in 1995, Skrabski *et al.* (2003) also found a robust correlation between lower levels of social capital, mistrust, and mortality.

Privatization

Perhaps the most controversial analysis of the causes of the postsocialist mortality crisis was a cross-national time-series regression of 26 postsocialist countries, which identified large-scale and rapid privatization as a distal driver of these postsocialist deaths of despair (King and Stuckler 2007; King *et al.* 2009; Stuckler *et al.* 2009). These studies investigated whether one component of the 'shock therapy' policy package – namely, large-scale and rapid mass privatization (Irdam *et al.* 2015) – drove premature deaths among working-age men and, to a lesser extent, women.

The authors found that radical privatization policies were associated with the loss of almost two years of male life expectancy (and 0.7 years lost for women). They also found that privatization was associated with deaths primarily among working-age men and predicted alcohol consumption, suicide, unemployment, and ischemic heart disease (King *et al.* 2009). Stuckler *et al.* (2009) found that radical privatization was associated with a 12.8-percent increase in adult male mortality. These findings were consistent with an earlier study by Brainerd (1998), who found that the speed of such neoliberal economic reforms was positively correlated with rising death rates in 22 countries in Eastern Europe from 1989 to 1994.

The robust negative health effect of mass privatization is not surprising, since radical privatization is related to firm failure, state failure, and lower growth at the cross-national level (Hamm *et al.* 2012). Moreover, state socialist firms provided social rights, public services and benefits, and meaning and community for their employees. Even though the masses never had de facto control over state socialist companies, research showed a declining sense of control over workplace processes during the transition to capitalism: the share of workers who thought they had no influence in decision-making at the workplace increased from 14 percent in 1985 to 47 percent in 1991 in Hungary (Simon 1993: 234). Radical privatization was analogous to stripping workers of their social rights and services associated with being employed at socialist firms, which increased their stress and uncertainty.

A group of economists and political scientists attacked the studies on the mass privatization-mortality association on methodological grounds (Earle and Gehlbach 2010; Gerry 2012). However, a stream of studies emerging out of the Privatization and Mortality (PrivMort) research project (Irdam *et al.* 2016), the largest data-gathering effort so far on the upstream economic determinants of the postsocialist mortality crisis, provided further robust evidence for the association between rapid economic change and the postsocialist mortality crisis.

Most previous studies relied on either country-level or individual-level data, which leaves the potential for modeling error, as they cannot simultaneously assess distal (economic) and proximal (individual) causes of mortality. The PrivMort research project aimed to overcome these limitations and investigate the role of economic transitions and individual-level factors (*e.g.* alcohol consumption) in the mortality crises in postsocialist countries.

The project identified towns with different privatization strategies and collected administrative data on 539 municipalities in Russia, 96 towns in Belarus, and 52 towns in Hungary. The researchers identified the largest companies in these towns and collected data on their ownership structure. The researchers also conducted large-scale surveys using a retrospective cohort study approach. Respondents provided information on themselves and their relatives, including socioeconomic characteristics, health behavior, and the vital status of their relatives. In total, the research project collected data on 268,600 subjects in the three countries. Using this information, the researchers created a complex multilevel database linking towns' industrial characteristics and individual health outcomes covering three decades from 1980 to 2010.

Building on this project, Azarova *et al.* (2017) developed a study using a quasi-experimental design, based on surveys of individuals nested in a matched set of towns with and without mass privatization in Russia. This account found that rapid mass privatization was strongly associated with higher working-age male mortality rates of 13–21 percent – very close to the estimates from Stuckler *et al.* (2009).

Using the Hungarian leg of the PrivMort study, Scheiring *et al.* (2018) reported results from multilevel data related to Hungary between 1995 and 2004. Using population surveys conducted in 52 towns to collect data on vital status and other characteristics of survey respondents' relatives, they found that women living in towns with prolonged state ownership had significantly lower odds of dying than women living in towns dominated by privatized companies – either foreign-owned (8–31 percent lower odds of dying) or domestically owned (10–39 percent lower). Women were overrepresented in sectors with slow privatization compared to the general population, explaining this gendered effect of privatization.

Together, these studies provide strong evidence for the driving role of economic dislocation caused by neoliberal economic reforms, in particular rapid privatization. Based on evidence from Hungary, slow and gradual privatization was better for health, while the oft-hypothesized benefits of foreign-investment–driven privatization did not translate into better health. It is primarily the state that can intervene to offset the adverse health effects of privatization – either through direct ownership, or via social and industrial policies that mitigate the effects of rapid change. Notably, these analyses of privatization were not claiming that privatization was the only factor causing economic dislocation and, thus, deaths of despair. Instead, they merely maintained that privatization was the most easily measurable policy and that, among the big three components of shock therapy (stabilization/austerity, liberalization, and privatization), it varied the most cross-nationally.

Deindustrialization

Another study showed that deindustrialization could have been another crucial determinant to the mortality crisis. Scheiring *et al.* (2023) analyzed survival and two-way fixed-effects panel models covering 52 towns and 42,800 people from 1989 to 1995 in Hungary, as well as 514 medium-sized towns in the European part of Russia. The results showed that deindustrialization was significantly correlated with male mortality in both countries, and directly and indirectly mediated by adverse health behavior (alcohol abuse). Both countries experienced severe deindustrialization, but social policies seem to have offset the adverse health effect of Hungary's more immense industrial employment loss.

In addition to this quantitative analysis, a slew of qualitative research also revealed that deindustrialization in former socialist industrial towns led to social disintegration, status loss, the loss of communities, and a cascade of infrastructural, social, and health problems, prolonged stress, depression, and despair in Eastern Europe (for a review, see: Ghodsee and Orenstein 2021). Through interview narratives and ethnographic description, Kideckel (2008) analyzed the lived experience of the postsocialist transformation among coal miners in the Romanian Jiu Valley and chemical workers in Fagaras. Kideckel found that the collapse of working-class culture caused mental and physical harm. Relying on fieldwork in Moscow in the 1990s and 2000s – including participant observation, unstructured interviews, and 38 semi-structured life-history interviews – Parsons

(2014: 24) demonstrated the negative health consequences of social isolation and the disruption of work identity in Russia in the 1990s: noting that postsocialist workers 'died unconnected, unbound, unmoored'.

Based on 82 life-history interviews amounting to 2,000 pages of dialogue with workers in Hungary's rustbelt, conducted under the auspices of the PrivMort study, Scheiring and King (2023) explored how deindustrialization engenders individual and social processes that affect health by increasing stress and eroding coping resources. Based on this data, the authors developed a synthetic sociological framework to map the mechanisms that link upstream economic dislocation to the postsocialist deaths of despair, also highlighting the parallels between the health effects of deindustrialization in the US and Eastern Europe.

This study presented a novel neoclassical sociological synthesis theorizing the deindustrialization-health association. This account combined Durkheimian and Marxian concepts in order to demonstrate how deindustrialization created ruptures in economic production that spilled over to the field of social reproduction, and became embodied as ill-health or dysfunctional health behavior. Regarding the former, the collapse of industry as an institution has been a disintegrative process, creating ruptures in economic production that only a multidimensional analysis can capture. First, deindustrialization has been a prime source of *labor market dislocation (job/income loss)*. In Eastern Europe during the early-1990s, many lost their jobs and permanently exited the labor market. Some could retire, while others joined the ranks of the sub-proletariat (or underclass).

Second, deindustrialization also led to *increased exploitation (workload, precarity)*. Deindustrialization shifted the risks previously socialized through welfare arrangements back onto workers. For example, fewer workers have full-time jobs with an unlimited contract, and more work as freelance pizza delivery 'entrepreneurs', such that they individually take on all the risk this entails. This was even more pronounced in socialist Eastern Europe, where securing a modicum of stability and welfare for workers was crucial for the legitimacy of socialist regimes.

Third, deindustrialization *increased social inequality (income, race/ethnicity)*. The industrial sector typically offers higher wages than the service sector, where wages are lower and unequal. Deindustrialization, thus, has led to rising income inequality. The same is true for Eastern Europe, where inequalities have also grown, and upward mobility has stagnated. Deindustrialization disproportionately hit the Roma ethnicity in Hungary, contributing to racial discrimination and segregation.

Finally, deindustrialization *disrupted community services*. Industrial companies generally provided various fringe benefits and health insurance coverage. The jobs that emerged after deindustrialization provide fewer such benefits. The destruction of the industry has also placed local government budgets under pressure, which have been forced to downsize public services to maintain fiscal balance.

As deindustrialization transformed the field of economic production, its effects have spilled over to social reproduction, which has manifested in myriad forms. First, labor market dislocations and disruption of services caused *material deprivation and physical suffering*. Sudden loss of income created multiple new stresses, such as increased food insecurity, difficulties with paying the mortgage, rent, or utilities, and poor housing conditions, which negatively affected health.

Second, increased exploitation led to *job strain*. Several workers we interviewed talked about increased stress even though they could keep their jobs. Increased exploitation in the precarious jobs emerging after deindustrialization augmented job strain, leading to mental health problems. This implies that the effects of deindustrialization transcend income and job loss alone.

Third, labor market dislocations caused *fatalism and shame*. Work identity is central to workers' self-conception: they derive a positive sense of self from disciplined, hard industrial work. When individuals could not fulfill the roles prescribed by their identity, it has engendered fatalism, shame, and inferiority. Fatalism appears to be an essential factor in the deaths of the despair epidemic in the US. It was equally crucial among our interviewees in Eastern Europe.

Fourth, the disruption of public services also *increased domestic workload*. When companies closed, the decommodified public services they provided became untenable, shifting the cost of care work onto families. Unpaid care responsibilities and declining access to public or private care services intensified the domestic workload – an essential source of chronic stress, which subsequently led to lower self-reported health, as several interviewees described.

Fifth, social inequalities and the disruption of services have produced *anomie and anger*. Sudden economic change (crisis or rapid growth) propelled some individuals and groups to amass immense wealth, while others have fallen behind. In turn, many individuals have conceived of the distribution of social hierarchy as unjust, and that society's moral order has broken down – a situation labeled by Durkheim (2002 [1897]) as 'anomie'. Our interviewees reported widespread anger in response to the perceived injustices created by deindustrialization. Under these circumstances, people are more inclined to self-destruction.

Sixth, labor market dislocation, exploitation, and the disruption of communal services produced *community disintegration and hopelessness*. Such disintegration has negatively affected workplace communities, neighborhood communities, friendships, and families. According to Durkheim (2002 [1897]), individuals left on their own find it harder to find meaning in their lives and are more prone to hopelessness. Community disintegration is a crucial determinant of ill-health in the US and Eastern Europe. Our interviewees described in detail the emotional strain caused by the collapse of working-class communities.

Seventh, as Marx described, commodification, exploitation, and the disruption of services generate *alienation and powerlessness*. Capitalism in general causes alienation, but deindustrialization intensifies it. The corollary of alienation is the sense of powerlessness. Our interviews revealed that commodification of the labor process and the accompanying alienation and powerlessness have damaged their mental and physical health. Many workers reflected on a complete loss of control over their lives and a concomitant rise in hopelessness.

Deindustrialization, the upstream policies, and the global challenges driving it are not unique to Eastern Europe. The combination of severe deindustrialization and lack of effective regional and industrial policy created regionally locked-in, marginalized areas, with a cascade of social and economic problems in the East and West. In this sense, the neoclassical sociology of the lived experience of deindustrialization elucidates a great deal about the Eastern regions, but could also be a fruitful way to analyze the root causes of the deaths of despair in other countries.

Alcohol supply and dysfunctional culture

These findings on stress, labor market upheaval, privatization, and deindustrialization are consistent with the Case and Deaton hypothesis. However, proponents of the supply/culture approach question the association between socioeconomic dislocation, stress, despair, and mortality in Eastern Europe. One line of criticism comes from studies emphasizing the role of dysfunctional working-class culture inherited from the socialist past. Using data on 4,006 individuals from the Russian sample of the Living Conditions, Lifestyles, and Health project, Cockerham (2007: 459) concluded that 'there is a lack of evidence documenting a relationship between stress and health outcomes'. Cockerham proposed that the lack of a health-conscious middle-class is the main reason behind the postsocialist mortality crisis.

Regressing death rates on a measure of socialist over-industrialization in Europe's Eastern periphery between 1960 and 2005, Carlson (2001: 375) also concluded that state socialist development policies emphasizing industrial employment at the expense of the service sector 'created anomic conditions leading to unhealthy lifestyles and self-destructive behavior among men'. He argues that this explains the subsequent rise in working-age male mortality until the middle of the 1990s. While cultural differences in health behavior are likely important to explain long-running health inequalities between Western and Eastern European countries, it is much less plausible that they could explain a sudden spike in death rates.

Another line of criticism came from studies investigating the rebound effect after the Gorbachev anti-alcohol campaign. Using data on regional death rates and the number of liters of vodka that could be bought with the average regional monthly income (measured at the capital city of each region for high-quality alcohol), Treisman (2010) found that the decline in vodka price relative to those of other goods was the primary determinant of the postsocialist mortality crisis. He found that a 10-percent increase in the affordability of vodka translated into a rise of several percent in the male working-age death rate.

Using archival sources to build a new oblast-year dataset spanning 1978–2000, Bhattacharya *et al.* (2013) also found evidence suggesting that the end of the Gorbachev anti-alcohol campaign explains a large share of the postsocialist mortality crisis. They called this the 'rebound' hypothesis: Russians whose lives were saved by the reduced availability of alcohol during Gorbachev's campaign died once the transition occurred and alcohol became more affordable. Bhattacharya *et al.* (2013: 232) concluded that 'Russia's transition to capitalism [...] was not as lethal as commonly suggested'.

However, several studies questioned the centrality of the campaign's end in explaining excess postsocialist deaths. Shkolnikov *et al.* (1996: 144–5) demonstrated that the increase in life expectancy during the anti-alcohol campaign from 1985 to 1988 was achieved due to a decrease in violent deaths, while the reduction of life expectancy in the early-1990s included a substantial cardiovascular component. This mismatch in the types of deaths involved casts doubt on the validity of the alcohol campaign argument. Denisova (2010) utilized 12 rounds of the Russian Longitudinal Monitoring Survey spanning 14 years, and found no evidence supporting the positive correlation between low alcohol prices and high mortality rates. Furthermore, several countries in Eastern Europe, such as Bulgaria or Hungary, did not have an anti-alcohol campaign in the 1980s, but experienced a significant increase in middle-aged male death rates in the 1990s.

While we do not doubt that raising the cost of alcohol can lower drinking, it probably does not decrease drinking much for the addicted, who can simply substitute cheaper (and more dangerous) alcohol for more expensive alcohol. There is a long history of *samogon* (moonshine) in Russia, which can be very dangerous due to impurities. In Hungary, it is homemade *palinka* (brandy). This substitution was also achieved by 'alcohol substitutes' – industrially produced products that are ostensibly mouthwash or cologne, but are made to be consumed. They are taxed at far lower rates than beverages and, thus, are very cheap. The studies reviewed here suggest that factors related to alcohol supply could have played a role in the postsocialist mortality crisis – albeit, likely less central than often claimed – but should not be elevated above economic dislocation as the primary cause.

Conclusions

The postsocialist mortality crisis represents the most significant demographic catastrophe seen outside China since the Second World War (Eberstadt 2010). The extant research has identified crucial political-economic determinants behind this health disaster, such as privatization, deindustrialization, and general labor market dislocations. This research also offers vital lessons for the contemporary deaths of despair epidemic plaguing the North American Rust Belt.

The evidence suggests that deindustrialization and economic malaise, combined with the effects of broader public policies, jointly contributed to the mortality crisis and deaths of despair in the US. These mortality crises are not historically unique events that idiosyncrasies of the countries could explain. Dysfunctional health behavior in the form of alcohol and drug abuse is central to both deaths of despair epidemics. However, these are proximate and not ultimate causes and, in most cases, are on a shared causal pathway linking upstream economic dislocations to individual ill-health. Population health crises cannot be examined in isolation from the socially determined political-economic structures in which people operate.

The insight that abrupt socioeconomic change can harm health goes back to the roots of social science. Durkheim (2002 [1897]: 207) famously concluded that 'whenever serious readjustments take place in the social order, whether or not due to a sudden growth or an unexpected catastrophe, men [sic] are more inclined to self-destruction'. Engels (2009 [1845]: 106) captured another way in which economic change can lead to mortality:

> When society places hundreds of proletarians in such a position that they inevitably meet a too early and an unnatural death; when it deprives thousands of the necessaries of life, places them under conditions in which they cannot live, and yet permits these conditions to remain, its deed is murder.

The postsocialist mortality crisis of the 1990s and the contemporary working-class deaths of despair epidemic in the US prove these bold early insights. Only equally bold analyses and policies can prevent similar excess deaths in the future.

Note

1 The chapter builds on King *et al.* (2022); Scheiring and King (2023); and Scheiring *et al.* (2020).

References

Azarova, A., Irdam, D., Gugushvili, A., Fazekas, M., Scheiring, G., Horvat, P., Stefler, D., Kolesnikova, I., Popov, V., Szelényi, I., Stuckler, D., Marmot, M., Murphy, M., McKee, M., Bobak, M. and King, L. 2017, 'The effect of rapid privatisation on mortality in mono-industrial towns in post-Soviet Russia: A retrospective cohort study', *The Lancet Public Health*, 2(5), pp. e231–8.

Bhattacharya, J., Gathmann, C. and Miller, G. 2013, 'The Gorbachev anti-alcohol campaign and Russia's mortality crisis', *American Economic Journal: Applied Economics*, 5(2), pp. 232–60.

Bobak, M., Pikhart, H., Hertzman, C., Rose, R. and Marmot, M. 1998, 'Socioeconomic Factors, perceived control and self-reported health in Russia: A cross-sectional survey', *Social Science and Medicine*, 47(2), pp. 269–79.

Brainerd, E. 1998, 'Market reform and mortality in transition economies', *World Development*, 26(11), pp. 2013–27.

Brainerd, E. 2001, 'Economic reform and mortality in the former Soviet Union: A Study of the suicide epidemic in the 1990s', *European Economic Review*, 45(4–6), pp. 1007–19.

Brainerd, E. and Cutler, D.M. 2005, 'Autopsy on an empire: Understanding mortality in Russia and the former Soviet Union', *The Journal of Economic Perspectives*, 19(1), pp. 107–30.

Britton, A. and McKee, M. 2000, 'The relation between alcohol and cardiovascular disease in Eastern Europe: Explaining the paradox', *Journal of Epidemiology and Community Health*, 54(5), pp. 328–32.

Carlson, E. and Hoffmann, R. 2011, 'The state socialist mortality syndrome', *Population Research Policy Review*, 30(3), pp. 355–79.

Carlson, P. 2001, 'Risk behaviours and self rated health in Russia 1998', *Journal of Epidemiology and Community Health*, 55(11), pp. 806–17.

Case, A. and Deaton, A. 2020, *Deaths of Despair and the Future of Capitalism*, Princeton University Press, Princeton.

Cockerham, W.C. 2007, 'Health lifestyles and the absence of the Russian middle class', *Sociology of Health and Illness*, 29(3), pp. 457–73.

Cornia, G.A. 2000, 'Short-term, long-term, and hysteresis mortality models: A review', in Cornia, G.A. and Paniccia, R. (eds), *The Mortality Crisis in Transitional Economies*, Oxford University Press, Oxford, pp. 59–80.

Cornia, G.A., Honkkila, J., Paniccià, R., and Popov, V. 1998, 'Investment Behaviour, Population Structure and Long-Term Growth in Eastern Europe and Russia', *MOST: Economic Policy in Transitional Economies*, 8, pp. 1–5.

Denisova, I. 2010, 'Adult mortality in Russia', *Economics of Transition*, 18(2), pp. 333–63.

Doniec, K., Stefler, D., Murphy, M., Gugushvili, A., McKee, M., Marmot, M., Bobak, M. and King, L. 2018, 'Education and mortality in three Eastern European populations: Findings from the PrivMort retrospective cohort study', *European Journal of Public Health*, 29(3), pp. 549–54.

Durkheim, É. 2002 [1897], *Suicide: A Study in Sociology*, Routledge Classics, London.

Earle, J. S. and Gehlbach, S. 2010, 'Did mass privatisation *really* increase post-communist mortality?' *The Lancet*, 375(9712), p. 372.

Eberstadt, N. 2010, 'The enigma of Russian mortality', *Current History*, 109(729), pp. 288–94.

Ellman, M. 1994, 'The Increase in death and disease under "Katastroika"', *Cambridge Journal of Economics*, 18(4), pp. 329–55.

Engels, F. 2009 [1845], *The Condition of the Working-Class in England*, Oxford University Press, Oxford.

Gerry, C.J. 2012, 'The Journals are full of great studies but can we believe the statistics? Revisiting the mass privatisation-mortality debate', *Social Science and Medicine*, 75(1), pp. 14–22.

Ghodsee, K. and Orenstein, M. 2021, *Taking Stock of Shock: Social Consequences of the 1989 Revolutions*, Oxford University Press, Oxford.

Gilmore, A.B.C., McKee, M. and Rose, R. 2002, 'Determinants of and inequalities in self-perceived health in Ukraine', *Social Science and Medicine*, 55(12), pp. 2177–88.

Hamm, P., King, L. and Stuckler, D. 2012, 'Mass privatization, state capacity, and economic growth in post-communist countries', *American Sociological Review*, 77(2), pp. 295–324.

Irdam, D., King, L., Gugushvili, A., Azarova, A., Fazekas, M., Scheiring, G., Stefler, D., Doniec, K., Horvat, P., Kolesnikova, I., Popov, V., Szelenyi, I., Marmot, M., Murphy, M., McKee, M. and Bobak, M. 2016, 'Mortality in transition: Study protocol of the PrivMort Project, a multilevel convenience cohort study', *BMC Public Health*, 16(672), pp. 1–8.

Irdam, D., Scheiring, G. and King, L. 2015, 'Mass privatization', in Hölscher, J. and Tomann, H. (eds), *Palgrave Dictionary of Emerging Markets and Transition Economics*, Palgrave Macmillan, London, pp. 488–507.

Kennedy, B.P., Kawachi, I. and Brainerd, E. 1998, 'The role of social capital in the Russian mortality crisis', *World Development*, 26(11), pp. 2029–43.

Kideckel, D.A. 2008, *Getting By in Postsocialist Romania: Labor, the Body, and Working-Class Culture*, Indiana University Press, Bloomington.

King, L., Hamm, P. and Stuckler, D. 2009, 'Rapid large-scale privatization and death rates in ex-communist countries: An analysis of stress-related and health system mechanisms', *International Journal of Health Services*, 39(3), pp. 461–89.

King, L., Scheiring, G. and Nosrati, E. 2022, 'Deaths of despair in comparative perspective', *Annual Review of Sociology*, 48(July), pp. 299–317.

King, L. and Stuckler, D. 2007, 'Mass privatization and the post-communist mortality crisis', in Lane, D. (ed), *The Transformation of State Socialism: Studies in Economic Transition*, Palgrave Macmillan, London, pp. 197–218.

Kopp, M., Skrabski, Á. and Szedmák, S. 2000, 'Psychosocial Risk factors, inequality and self-rated morbidity in a changing society', *Social Science and Medicine*, 51(9), pp. 1351–61.

Kopp, M., Skrabski, Á., Szántó, Z. and Siegrist, J. 2006, 'Psychosocial determinants of premature cardiovascular mortality differences within Hungary', *Journal of Epidemiology and Community Health*, 60(9), pp. 782–8.

Kopp, M., Skrabski, Á., Székely, S., Stauder, A. and Williams, R. 2007, 'Chronic stress and social changes: Socioeconomic determination of chronic stress', *Annals of the New York Academy of Sciences*, 1113(1), pp. 325–38.

Landberg, J. 2008, 'Alcohol and suicide in Eastern Europe', *Drug and Alcohol Review*, 27(4), pp. 361–73.

Leon, D. and Shkolnikov, V. 1998, 'Social stress and the Russian mortality crisis', *Journal of the American Medical Association*, 279(10), pp. 790–1.

Leon, D.A., Chenet, L., Shkolnikov, V.M., Zakharov, S., Shapiro, J., Rakhmanova, G., Vassin, S. and McKee, M. 1997, 'Huge variation in Russian mortality rates 1984–94: Artefact, alcohol, or what?', *The Lancet*, 350(9075), pp. 383–8.

Leon, D.A., Saburova, L., Tomkins, S., Andreev, E., Kiryanov, N., McKee, M. and Shkolnikov, V.M. 2007, 'Hazardous alcohol drinking and premature mortality in Russia: A population based case-control study', *The Lancet*, 369(9578), pp. 2001–9.

Mackenbach, J.P., Valverde, J.R., Artnik, B., Bopp, M., Brønnum-Hansen, H., Deboosere, P., Kalediene, R., Kovács, K., Leinsalu, M., Martikainen, P., Menvielle, G., Regidor, E., Rychtaříková, J., Rodriguez-Sanz, M., Vineis, P., White, C., Wojtyniak, B., Hu, Y. and Nusselder, W.J. 2018, 'Trends in health Inequalities in 27 European countries', *Proceedings of the National Academy of Sciences*, 115(25), pp. 6440–5.

Murphy, M., Bobak, M., Nicholson, A., Rose, R. and Marmot, M. 2006, 'The widening gap in mortality by educational level in the Russian Federation, 1980–2001', *American Journal of Public Health*, 96(7), pp. 1293–9.

Nell, J. and Stewart, K. 1994, *Death in Transition: The Rise in the Death Rate in Russia Since 1992*, UNICEF, International Child Development Centre, Florence.

Parsons, M.A. 2014, *Dying Unneeded: The Cultural Context of the Russian Mortality Crisis*, Vanderbilt University Press, Nashville.

Perlman, F. and Bobak, M. 2009, 'Assessing the contribution of unstable employment to mortality in post-transition Russia: Prospective individual-level analyses from the Russian longitudinal monitoring survey', *American Journal of Public Health*, 99(10), pp. 1818–25.

Pikhart, H., Bobak, M., Siegrist, J., Pajak, A., Rywik, S., Kyshegyi, J., Gostautas, A., Skodova, Z. and Marmot, M. 2001, 'Psychosocial work characteristics and self rated health in four post-communist countries', *Journal of Epidemiology and Community Health*, 55(9), pp. 624–30.

Popov, V. 2009, *Mortality Crisis in Russia Revisited: Evidence from Cross-Regional Comparison*, University Library of Munich, Germany.

Razvodovsky, Y.E. 2013, 'Psychosocial distress as a risk factor of ischemic heart disease mortality', *Psychiatria Danubina*, 25(1), pp. 68–75.

Rose, R. 2000, 'How much does social capital add to individual health? A survey of Russians', *Social Science and Medicine*, 51(9), pp. 1421–35.

Rosefielde, S. 2001, 'Premature deaths: Russia's radical economic transition in Soviet perspective', *Europe-Asia Studies*, 53(8), pp. 1159–76.

Scheiring, G., Azarova, A. and Irdam, D. 2020, 'Analyzing the health impact of economic change: Insights from a multi-level retrospective cohort study', in *Sage Research Methods Cases: Medicine and Health*, SAGE, Thousand Oaks, pp. 1–19.

Scheiring, G., Azarova, A., Irdam, D., Doniec, K.J., McKee, M., Stuckler, D. and King, L. 2023, 'Deindustrialization and the postsocialist mortality crisis,' *Cambridge Journal of Economics*, 47(2), pp. 341–72.

Scheiring, G., Irdam, D. and King, L. 2019, 'Cross-country evidence on the social determinants of the post-is in Europe: A review and performance-based hierarchy of variables', *Sociology of Health and Illness*, 41(4), pp. 673–91.

Scheiring, G. and King, L. 2023, 'Deindustrialization, social disintegration, and health: A neoclassical sociological approach,' *Theory and Society*, 2023(52), pp. 145–78.

Scheiring, G., Stefler, D., Irdam, D., Fazekas, M., Azarova, A., Kolesnikova, I., Köllő, J., Popov, V., Szelényi, I., Marmot, M., Murphy, M., McKee, M., Bobak, M. and King, L. 2018, 'The gendered effects of foreign investment and prolonged state ownership on mortality in Hungary: An indirect demographic, retrospective cohort study', *The Lancet Global Health*, 6(1), pp. 95–102.

Shapiro, J. 1995, 'The Russian mortality crisis and its causes', in Aslund, A. (ed), *Russian Economic Reform at Risk*, Pinter Publishers, London, pp. 149–78.

Shkolnikov, V.M., Cornia, G.A., Leon, D.A. and Meslé, F. 1998a, 'Causes of the Russian mortality crisis: Evidence and interpretations', *World Development*, 26(11), pp. 1995–2011.

Shkolnikov, V., Mesle, F. and Vallin, J. 1996, 'Health crisis in Russia: Recent trends in life expectancy and causes of death from 1970 to 1993', *Population: An English Selection*, 8, pp. 123–54.

Shkolnikov, V.M., Leon, D.A., Adamets, S., Eugeniy, A. and Deev, A. 1998b, 'Educational level and adult mortality in Russia: An analysis of routine data 1979 to 1994', *Social Science and Medicine*, 47(3), pp. 357–69.

Simon, J. 1993, 'Post-paternalist political culture in Hungary: Relationship between citizens and politics during and after the "melancholic revolution" [1989–1991]', *Communist and Post-Communist Studies*, 26(2), pp. 226–38.

Skrabski, Á., Kopp, M. and Kawachi, I. 2003, 'Social capital in a changing society: Cross sectional associations with middle aged female and male mortality rates', *Journal of Epidemiology and Community Health*, 57(2), pp. 114–9.

Stuckler, D. 2009, 'Social causes of post-communist mortality: A macro-sociological analysis', Ph.D. thesis, University of Cambridge.

Stuckler, D., King, L. and McKee, M. 2009, 'Mass privatisation and the post-communist mortality crisis: A cross-national analysis', *The Lancet*, 373(9661), pp. 399–407.

Treisman, D. 2010, 'Death and prices: The political economy of Russia's alcohol crisis', *Economics of Transition*, 18(2), pp. 281–331.

UNICEF. 2001, *A Decade of Transition: Regional Monitoring Report 8*, UNICEF International Child Development Centre, Florence.

Walberg, P., McKee, M., Shkolnikov, V., Chenet, L. and Leon, D. 1998, 'Economic change, crime, and mortality crisis in Russia: Regional analysis', *British Medical Journal*, 317(7154), pp. 312–8.

Watson, P. 1995, 'Explaining rising mortality among men in Eastern Europe', *Social Science and Medicine*, 41(7), pp. 923–34.

30

HEALTHCARE IN AUSTRALIA

Contesting marketized provision

Ben Spies-Butcher

Australia's experience of healthcare appears full of contradictions. It is usually considered typical of OECD norms, providing universal public healthcare through the popular public insurance scheme, Medicare. Yet, public healthcare arrived relatively late. Efforts to nationalize health in the immediate post-War years were frustrated by constitutional barriers and partisan opposition. Only in the 1970s was public insurance legislated following a fierce political and parliamentary battle against an organized and aggressive medical profession and conservative parties. Opposition continued under a subsequent conservative government, and Australia became relatively unique when it stepped back from a functioning public health scheme. Ironically, the scheme was reintroduced and entrenched, as Medicare, from the 1980s, just as neoliberalism was eroding universalism in welfare states globally.

The tumultuous history of health reform shaped a hybrid model of public provision. While Medicare is a universal public insurance scheme, it sits alongside existing systems of private hospitals, private health insurance, and fee-for-service medicine. Despite bipartisan commitment to, and strong public support for, public insurance, governments have continued to provide substantial subsidies to the private sector. The private sector has undergone its own transformation. Regulation has shifted from ensuring cross-subsidies for poorer and sicker members to penalizing non-members, and from non-profit ownership to corporatization. These transformations reflect a politics of liberalization alongside the overt and ongoing commitments to universalism.

The combination of public and private provision within Australian healthcare, where universalism and liberalization advanced together, can make it more difficult to assess and to identify significant changes over time. As institutionalist scholars have noted, democratic opposition to privatization often leads to less visible 'market' strategies of welfare state retrenchment, or, as in the case of the USA, 'adaptive accumulation' (see: Loeppky, this volume). Medicare's hybrid configuration not only facilitates these privatized arrangements, but it also facilitated the expansion of public provision using surprisingly similar strategies, suggesting new forms of contestation. Medicare was designed by neoclassical economists, as much to address inefficiencies and promote competition as to address need (Scotton and Deeble 1968). Thus, it provides a useful example for understanding how liberalization changes the nature of policy contestation: not only to erode social provision but also to reconfigure the axes of politics (Spies-Butcher 2023).

 DOI: 10.4324/9781003017110-34

This chapter examines the mixed political economy of Australian healthcare and reflects on how it might inform broader understandings of liberalized welfare, in terms of both threats and opportunities for egalitarian provision. It begins with an historical overview, from early attempts to nationalize healthcare at the state level, through to more recent contests over fiscal support offered to public and private healthcare. It then provides an analytic account of Medicare as a quasi-market model of universal provision, which I examine through the lens of hybridity. Next, it applies this model to an analysis of policy contestation over the boundaries of public and private health, drawing on historical institutionalist accounts of liberalization. Finally, the chapter reflects on what lessons such an analysis provides – both for Australian health policy scholars and for welfare state scholars more broadly.

Australian healthcare: from private market to universalism

Health policy has an unusually contentious history in Australia. While bipartisanship was entrenched by the end of the Twentieth Century, fierce opposition to universalism played an important role in shaping the marketized system that emerged. Twice Labor Governments successfully passed legislation to establish a public health system, only to have it subsequently rescinded. Opposition was led by a well-organized and conservative medical profession with close ties to Australia's conservative political parties. In this context, marketization partly facilitated universalism, helping to overcome legal and ideological barriers, and mobilized competition to undermine producer power. Once entrenched, Medicare has become a totemic political issue, making its overt disassembly difficult, although its marketized structure has facilitated ongoing forms of less visible contestation.

Boxall and Gillespie (2013) provide a comprehensive account of the development of Australia's healthcare system. During the early-Twentieth Century, healthcare was dominated by private practice and a form of working-class insurance via friendly societies, called the lodge system (Boxall and Gillespie 2013: 19). Under this system, doctors would accept regular capitation payments for each of the members in return for a range of free services, while middle-class patients received fee-for-service medicine in more exclusive private rooms. In the wealthier states, charitable hospitals had been established, while in the poorer ones, and Labor-dominated Queensland, state hospitals were the norm. The first serious attempt at a national health policy came from the conservatives, who included health alongside proposals for a range of social insurance schemes in the 1930s. A social insurance model was legislated, but remained unimplemented largely due to doctor opposition, expressed via the Country Party, Australia's smaller, rural conservative party. Doctors opposed capitation payments, in part because of their experience with the lodge system, while bureaucrats balked at the fiscal implications of fee-for-service medicine (Boxall and Gillespie 2013: 15–18).

Both the Labor Party and the federal public service supported a more strongly nationalized model. Labor won office during the War and then assumed powers over income tax from the states, which the courts confirmed could remain post-War. Access to fiscal resources led Labor to begin implementing a welfare state in the later years of the War. The first element of a national health plan came via a Pharmaceutical Benefits Scheme. This was subsequently struck down by the courts as beyond federal powers, leading Labor to leverage its wartime popularity to propose a successful referendum. However, to reduce conservative opposition, Labor agreed to qualify new constitutional health powers to limit any form of 'civil conscription', that is, compulsion on the part of doctors, a key demand of the medical profession, again conveyed via conservative opposition parties (see: Gillespie 1991: 223). After the War, doctors launched an extraordinary campaign against 'nationalized medicine': fundraising, advertising, and mobilizing a significant grassroots campaign, including a boycott of the new public system (Mackay 1995). When Labor introduced penalties for non-compliance, the courts struck down the scheme, or at least elements of it, as 'civil conscription', while the doctors' campaign contributed to a change in government (Mendelson 1999).

It took some time for the conservatives to fill the void left by Labor's attempt at nationalization. Public expectations had risen, and some form of the public scheme was clearly required, while doctor insistence on fee-for-service had also proven politically powerful. The result was the Page Scheme, named after the Health Minister and rural specialist Earl Page, which unwound free hospital access through means-tests, while subsidies supported private insurance through non-profit, doctor-controlled funds. Over time, means-testing strengthened, while fee-for-service medicine increased premiums and out-of-pocket costs. Insurance coverage declined, while public subsidies – structured through concessional tax arrangements – reinforced inequalities (Scotton 1969).

Across the 1950s and 1960s, Labor remained committed to nationalization, but also spent an extended period in opposition. By 1969, Labor's leadership determined to change course: embracing a scheme for universal public insurance modeled on the Canadian system, which shared a similar division of powers between federal and provincial governments. The scheme, which became Medicare, was developed by health economists critical of the poor price control and uncompetitive dynamics of the doctor-run health funds (Scotton and Macdonald 1993: 16–7). The insurance model sought to solve the problems of healthcare, not through nationalization, but a single-payer model of finance.

Medicare is effectively two schemes. A hospital scheme ensures free access to a public hospital as a public patient. States guarantee free hospital access in exchange for federal funding through regularly negotiated funding agreements. Private hospitals remain, as does access to a public hospital as a private patient. Private patients gain more timely access (jumping waiting lists), choice of doctor, and more comfortable accommodation. Medicare also funds private hospital treatment, through subsidies for medical procedures, but in most cases, co-payments are required in addition to private insurance coverage.

The medical scheme provides universal insurance for medical services from general practitioners and specialists, who are licensed to receive public funds through Medicare provider numbers on a fee-for-service basis. Doctors retain the right to set their own fees, with Medicare providing the patient with a rebate based on a government fee schedule, rather than the actual fee. Alternatively, doctors can agree to 'bulk bill', an arrangement in which doctors agree not to charge the patient, and in return, the government provides a bulk payment for all services, reducing administrative costs and bad debts (see: Gray 1991). The medical scheme does not generally cover dental or optical services, and has only recently begun to cover some mental health services (see: Cook 2019).

Labor finally returned to office in 1972 and sought to introduce its new health policy under the name Medibank. The legislation faced fierce opposition, again led by the medical profession, and was blocked in Australia's powerful Senate. Labor used the rejection as a trigger to call an election and dissolve the Senate. While retaining government in the House, the Senate again blocked passage, leading to Australia's only Joint Sitting – a special constitutional mechanism to resolve parliamentary deadlock – to finally pass the scheme (Parliament of Australia 2018: Chapter 13). However, by the time Medibank began operation, a new Senate standoff had developed, which eventually saw the Labor Government controversially sacked by the Governor General and a return to conservative rule. The incoming Coalition Government gradually unwound Medibank, effectively dismantling it by the early-1980s, and returning to a version of the Page Scheme.

The current Medicare scheme was reintroduced by the next Labor Government in 1984, as part of a formal Accord with the union movement. The additional costs were funded by an income tax levy, the Medicare Levy, which is not formally hypothecated, but notionally supports health provision (Briggs 2013). Conservative opposition remained until the mid-1990s, when an unexpected election win, partly driven by Medicare's popularity (Bean 1994), extended Labor's longest period in office, leading conservatives to explicitly commit to retaining public insurance. While leaving Medicare in place, conservative governments provided growing support to the remaining elements of private medicine, through new subsidies and regulatory interventions in favor of private health insurance. Ongoing contestation over support for private insurance, levels of bulk billing, out-of-pocket fees, and waiting lists belie formal bipartisan support for Medicare.

Marketization, dual welfare, and hybrid politics

Understanding ongoing contestation within Medicare requires an analysis of marketization. Marketization has generally been framed as part of liberalization, where previously public services are reorganized to incorporate aspects of market competition (Whitefield 2006). This positions marketization as a shift in service provision from public to private. More recently, institutionalist scholars have highlighted diversity among models of marketization. Social service markets can prioritize different interests and produce different outcomes, reflecting different welfare state histories and partisan orientations (Gingrich 2011; Meagher and Goodwin 2015). This complicates a simple 'marketization as privatization' reading, but often emphasizes continuity rather than situating marketization itself as a site of ongoing contestation. Drawing on both these accounts, and more general accounts of 'actually existing neoliberalism' (Peck *et al.* 2018), I suggest that Australia's healthcare points to the possibility of 'hybrid' forms of marketization, which facilitate ongoing contestation over universalism.

The welfare state was a target of neoliberal politics as it emerged in the 1970s and 1980s (Pierson 1994). New Right politicians, public choice theorists, and international organizations identified what they claimed was an overreach of democracy. Politicians, they claimed, overcommitted fiscal resources as they appealed to voters. The resulting welfare states then eroded competitive incentives, taxing enterprise, and rewarding sloth. The solution was to cut social spending, forcing citizens to become financially 'independent' or rely on family and mutual aid. Tax revolts and independent monetary policy placed explicit limits on state finances, creating what James O'Connor called a 'fiscal crisis of the state' (1973), in which the neoliberal mantra that 'there is no alternative' seemed increasingly real. However, over time, it became clear that neoliberalism did not straightforwardly lead to the end of welfare. While privatization significantly eroded state ownership, there was a little decline in social spending and few explicit examples of existing social programs were being formally dismantled (Pierson 2001) – Medibank being an international exception. Instead, within the welfare state, liberalization advanced through marketization and workfare.

Marketization gained traction as a policy approach through economic ideas linked to Third Way politics. In the UK, Julian Le Grand (1991, 1997) used the National Health Service as the focus of his analysis. Nationalization, he claimed, placed too much power in the hands of medical professionals, who were understood by policy-makers as 'knights', but which positioned patients as docile 'pawns'. Alternatively, policy-makers avoided competition because of a fear it would breed profit-hungry 'knaves'. The health system could be improved, Le Grand (1997) argued, by combining elements of public and private provision. This would give patients power and choice as consumers while ensuring equity in access through public financing. Le Grand's ideas proved influential within the UK Labor Party, as did Nicholas Barr's (2001) similarly constructed welfare economics. Marketization was, thus, conceived as a Third Way response to the extremes of market competition and socialization, with technocratic expertise, rather than partisan conflict, used to 'manage markets' according to both equity and efficiency.

Marketization became far more common internationally across the 1990s and 2000s. Framed as a shift from the public sector toward the market, even if not as dramatic as full privatization or state retrenchment, this global trend seemed to suggest convergence toward a liberalized policy model. Alternatively, the inability of even committed market-reforming governments to reduce social spending suggested limits to liberalization. Against this background, institutionalist scholars began to develop a more nuanced account of liberalization. Wolfgang Streeck and Katheleen Thelen (2005) suggested liberalization had gone further than many thought, but had advanced more incrementally through a process they dubbed 'gradual transformation'. Less overt, gradual changes reduced political resistance from publics defending social programs. Layering, for example, keeps in place the existing policy institutions, while establishing a new set of institutions alongside them. Similarly, the USA's highly privatized model increasingly relies on growing public support to create stable revenues through 'adaptive accumulation' (Loeppky, this volume). Over time, policy logics are reoriented to new ends, contributing to a 'risk shift' (Hacker 2019) from governments and corporations toward households.

Drawing on similar conceptual tools, other policy scholars noted differences in national trajectories, despite what appeared a common marketized policy model. Jane Gingrich (2011) showed 'variety' within marketization. She focused particular attention on where power is located within social markets and whether access is understood as universal. Her framework identifies a number of ideal types, where the state, producers, or consumers, respectively, hold power. Where Streeck and Thelen mapped change within apparent continuity, Gingrich used her typology to demonstrate continuity within change. Rather than converging on a liberal norm, marketization occurred differently in social democracies, where consumers gained power and states ensured access, compared to liberal welfare states, where producers often gained power or services were residualized.

Two of Gingrich's ideal types are particularly useful for understanding Australian health policy. Two-tier markets closely resemble Australia's broader dual welfare model (Stebbing and Spies-Butcher 2010), in which governments subsidize consumers to access services in a market. These models typically create significant producer power, as was the case in the Page Scheme, increasing prices and leading to stratification as better off consumers top up their public subsidy – hence, 'two-tiers'. Most people can access some health services, but there are clear differences between 'private/elite' and 'public/basic' versions. Alternatively, state-managed markets use monopsony power, or leverage, to discipline producer interests, concentrating power in the state. This constrains costs and facilitates universal access, a situation analogous to Medicare's single-insurer model.

These two models, I argue, provide a useful lens to understand Australia's health system, but are best understood through a model of hybridity developed through work on 'actually existing neoliberalism'. Drawing on Polanyi, Jamie Peck sees liberalization as an uneven and contested process, where 'actually existing neoliberalism' transforms to accommodate existing institutions and local interests, creating 'hybrid combinations' (Peck 2013: 1555) that integrate elements of state distribution and market exchange. Hybridity reflects the possibility of 'collibration' (Jessop 2016: 171–8), where states coordinate via both exchange-based tools and centralized distribution, opening possibilities for ongoing political contestation in what appears market forms (Bryant and Spies-Butcher 2020). On this account, we might see different models of marketization (such as two-tier and state-managed markets), reflecting different hybrid combinations, which are contested through 'gradual transformations' – that is, less explicit and direct partisan politics than is typical of Twentieth Century welfare state politics.

Conceptualizing marketization as hybridity focuses attention on how state power and market forms are combined and contested. This not only highlights politically distinct models of marketization and incremental modes of liberalization. In the Australian case, it can also explain how competition can advance universalism. It is Medicare's marketized form, I argue, that facilitated a process of layering: allowing public insurance to overcome institutional and political resistance to universalism, and establishing tools to slowly transform a two-tier market into a state-managed market. At the same time, its hybrid configuration potentially limits its transformative capacity and leaves it susceptible to erosion through more conventional liberalization.

Contesting universalism and liberalization

The partisan history of Australian health policy seems to accord with traditional accounts of welfare state contestation. In this reading, the depoliticization of health policy since Medicare reflects universalism becoming entrenched. This echoes the liberalization thesis, in which overt political contestation is replaced by technocratic rule, leading to forms of fiscal austerity and forms of gradual transformation (Mair 2013; Streeck 2014). Yet, on key measures of access and equity, Medicare did not mark healthcare's 'end of history'. Levels of bulk billing increased consistently from Medicare's introduction until the mid-1990s (Elliot 2002: Graph 1). Private hospital insurance coverage also remained high for some time, only gradually falling to under one-third of households, before surging back more recently (Briggs 2017). Despite rising bulk billing rates and the option of free hospital care, out-of-pocket costs are among the highest in the OECD, and total voluntary health expenditure per person is similar to that found in the USA (OECD 2021).

Ongoing changes in the lived experience of accessing healthcare suggest the ongoing importance of partisanship. Drawing on the previous section, I argue hybridity can help us understand the nature of this contest. First, Labor's embrace and entrenchment of Medicare reflect its marketized structure. Traditional forms of politics remained important – the scheme's reintroduction was part of a formal Accord with the trade union movement and followed a rare general strike. However, its market form proved significant in both reducing opposition and facilitating a form of gradual transformation away from private medicine and toward universal access. Second, the new marketized landscape reshaped conservative strategies away from overt retrenchment. Instead, conservatives expanded fiscal and regulatory support for private healthcare to foster a two-tier market. Thus, a partisan politics remained, but it has been increasingly decoupled from strict understandings of nationalization and liberalization.

Public insurance was initially controversial within the Labor Party. The party's left-wing saw the shift in policy from nationalization to universal insurance as a clear step back from Labor's socialist ambitions (Boxall and Gillespie 2013: 43–5). However, it offered Labor's leadership a model that was less constitutionally risky. An insurance model also reflected a shift away from traditional socialization, toward what would become 'Third Way' alternatives. However, this suggests that universalism is achieved by the more statist elements of regulation and social spending, with marketization facilitating the partial continuation of private medicine. That is only partly true. Competition was also at the heart of advancing universalism.

Competition proved useful to advancing universalism in three ways (Spies-Butcher 2014). First, the scheme framed public insurance as pro-competition. It was not simply an alternative to nationalization, but a strengthening of competition within the existing (private) health system. The scheme's architects, Richard Scotton and John Deeble, were health economists. They framed the policy problem in terms of market failure, identifying oligopolistic and anti-competitive practices among private insurers that led to price inflation. That framing appealed to the financial press, which proved an influential advocate of public insurance, and fragmented parliamentary and medical opposition that had been built around anti-communism. Framing universalism through the lens of competition also facilitated an alliance with the emerging consumer rights movement, which advocated for public insurance on much the same grounds as Scotton and Deeble (Browning 1992).

Second, the scheme expanded access by creating public competitors to private provision. This reflects a process of 'layering', usually identified with liberalization, in which social provision is reorganized by adding a new layer onto an existing system, rather than replacing one system with another. Medicare left the existing institutions of private healthcare in place. Private hospitals, private health insurance, and fee-for-service medicine all remain, however, layering facilitated competition. Free hospital care required increased public funding, which largely came from removing tax concessions for private health insurance. Even with longer wait times, shared rooms, and an allocated surgeon, free hospital care is clearly a powerful competitor to private provision, especially when private insurance became more expensive as subsidies were reduced. The continuation of private systems also made it more difficult for doctors to boycott or challenge constitutionally.

Alternatively, the continuation of fee-for-service medicine delayed equitable access to medical services. The retention of private insurance and hospitals meant most people remained in the private system, at least notionally, for some time. Doctor resistance saw relatively low rates of bulk billing. However, over time, competition also expanded access, at first through the minority of doctors sympathetic to public medicine, then as more doctors began to selectively bulk bill poorer patients (Gray 1991) and, finally, through the competition effect that comes from having some doctors provide services for free. Doctors in working-class areas became dependent on bulk billing (Scotton 1980: 208–9), and later, analysis suggests higher rates not only where incomes are lower, but also where there are more doctors competing for patients (Spies-Butcher 2014: 29). Bulk billing rates rose from approximately 45 percent when Medicare was introduced, to over 70 percent by the mid-1990s (Elliot 2002), and over 80 percent today (Hunt 2021). Conversely, private hospital cover fell from 50 percent after Medicare's introduction, to 30 percent by the late-1990s (Briggs 2017), reflecting the use of competition to gradually advance universalism.

Finally, public insurance facilitated a model of governing medicine via prices. Cost containment was an important part of the economic case for Medicare. Not only would a public insurer challenge the oligopolistic tendencies of private insurers, but it would also grant the state a degree of monopsony power. That argument helped persuade a fiscally cautious Labor Party to retain Medicare when it returned to office in the 1980s, after economists persuaded the party leadership that a single insurer would prove more effective at reining-in medical price inflation (Scotton and Macdonald 1993: 268–9). The hybrid model of insurance, where premiums are organized through a tax levy, further aided the fiscal case. This meant that the reduction in private health spending contributed to curbing inflation, while the new levy did not add to it (see: Sax 1984: 241).

The mobilization of monopsony reflects a combination of market and state power. As a single buyer, Medicare can moderate medical prices. Doctors feared exactly this outcome, leading to fierce resistance. Australia's public health spending now sits around the middle of the OECD as a proportion of GDP (OECD 2021). Indeed, general practice has undergone something of a 'proletarianization', as high administrative costs and price discipline have forced many into medical centers (Collyer and White 2001). These centers do not create a public salaried workforce, but they produce a similar effect in the private sector, and potentially create a model for integrated public provision (see: Spies-Butcher 2014: 32).

While monopsony expresses a form of market power, the mechanisms for doing this often reflect forms of state distribution. The Medicare schedule of fees is determined through bureaucratic processes that integrate medical, actuarial, and economic expertise, and that are grounded in normative commitments to deliver health outcomes as a 'need', rather than simply reflecting consumer/patient demands. The immense data produced by Medicare also allows policing of over-servicing and price dynamics, much in the vein of a regulator. Even greater discipline is exerted by the Pharmaceutical Benefits Scheme, which can either create or withhold a market for many drugs through listing them for subsidy (see: Harvey *et al.* 2004).

Medicare not only reflects a reorientation of center-left politics away from nationalization and toward marketization, but it has also reoriented conservative responses, such that it has changed the dynamics of contestation. The electoral popularity of Medicare saw the conservative parties relinquish any explicit opposition to the scheme, even claiming to be the 'best friend Medicare ever had' (Elliot 2006). However, this has not meant an end to support for private provision. Conservative reforms explicitly aimed to support the expansion of private health insurance coverage, while rates of bulk billing simultaneously stalled and then began to decline. There has also been a steady drift toward for-profit insurance since changes to private insurance allowed their entry alongside the introduction of Medicare (Collyer *et al.* 2015). These changes, however, reflect contestation within the marketized Medicare framework.

In the late-1990s, the conservatives introduced three significant changes that have remained in modified form through to the present (see: Briggs 2013). First, new public subsidies support private hospital insurance, initially targeting those on low incomes, and then extending to all. Second, the conservatives introduced a new tax penalty for high-income earners without private hospital insurance. This mirrors tax concessions within the Page Scheme, but in reverse. For many high-income earners, the tax penalty is larger than the cost of basic insurance products, meaning insurance has a negative price (McAuley 2005). Finally, community rating was restructured so that premiums can vary based on the age at which a person first takes out insurance, thereby penalizing those who only take out insurance later in life.

Following these changes, health insurance coverage surged – from roughly 30 to 40 percent of households. The timing of coverage increases suggests the changes to community rating were the primary contributor to this trend (Palangkaraya and Yong 2005). Labor has broadly accepted the rationale for the changes – ensuring private health insurance coverage is maintained. From the mid-1990s, both Labor and conservative governments began to express concern that coverage – then nearing 30 percent – was too low. Neither side of politics was eager for the competitive dynamics Medicare fostered to collapse the private sector, fearing this would increase the fiscal cost of public healthcare.

Political contestation of healthcare, thus, reflects two apparently bipartisan commitments: (i) to retain Medicare as a universal public system, and (ii) to ensure a dual welfare state where a significant minority are privately insured. Rather than removing support for private health, Labor instead sought to modify its fiscal incidence. By the 2000s, the private health insurance rebate, as it is known, was the fastest-growing component of federal health spending, leading a then-Labor Government to means-test access for high-income earners (Spies-Butcher and Stebbing 2019: 1425). Likewise, it extended the tax penalty by implementing higher rates for (very) high-income earners.

Limits have also emerged to the erosion of Medicare's universalism. In the 2000s, as private insurance coverage stayed high, bulk billing rates began to decline, and out-of-pocket costs rose. The changes potentially reflected failure to increase the public schedule of fees in line with medical inflation, leading to opposition charges of conservative hostility to universalism. The conservative Coalition Government's response suggests the campaign was effective. They sought to defend bulk billing without reinforcing universalism. Doctors were provided with new incentives to bulk bill low-income and older patients, while new tax concessions were introduced for those with very high out-of-pocket costs. The incentives saw a bifurcation of costs, with out-of-pocket costs falling for low-income patients, but increasing for higher-income patients (Wong *et al.* 2017). Labor has continued the pattern of targeting incentives to increase bulk billing rates (Treasury 2023).

The politics of healthcare is shaped by broader changes in political alignment, consistent with experience elsewhere. A long-term reorganization of political allegiances has seen educated voters move from more conservative to more progressive parties, while many older, blue-collar voters have become more conservative. These dynamics foster age (and potentially generational) cleavages, making conservative parties more responsive to the welfare state demands of older voters (Mair 2013). Coalition Government changes have particularly targeted older voters, providing larger subsidies for private insurance and larger incentives for bulk billing. Alternatively, health retains its ability to swing votes, with evidence in 2016 that any suggestion of 'privatization' significantly aids Labor's electoral prospects (Carson *et al.* 2020).

The outcome is a model that increasingly combines state and market forms to both promote competition and reflect equity concerns. Efforts to expand private provision depend on large fiscal expenditures and penalties. Both the defense of private insurance and bulk billing reflect the equity principles of the tax system – with fiscal support/penalties falling/rising with income, and access to bulk billing explicitly linked to ability to pay. Competition remains an important driver of universalism, evidenced both in monopsony power and in the lack of price (and fiscal) discipline within private insurance. Concomitantly, the most effective policy to expand private healthcare – changes to community rating – reflects an attempt to limit adverse selection and, thus, negate the public sector's competitive edge.

These dynamics are not well captured by traditional understandings of social policy. The alignment between state regulation aiding universalism and market exchange driving competition is hard to sustain. Private medicine expands with state finance, while competition fosters universalism. At the same time, Medicare has entrenched a normative commitment to universalism far more successfully than universal access or public control. A two-tiered market remains, although the more explicit fiscal support it now receives ensures a more equitable structure to subsidies and taxation than under the old Page Scheme.

Conclusion

Australia's health system reflects the twin dynamics of popular support for universalism and liberalization of welfare. Its expansion of public healthcare came later than most in the OECD. The public insurance model that emerged left in place much of the private system that preceded it. This partly reflects the influence of liberalization on global politics, and especially within the Anglosphere. However, unlike the UK, marketization was not a step toward private provision. Instead, public insurance mobilized competition to challenge producer power and universalize access. In response, conservative parties have used more explicit forms of state power – both fiscal and regulatory – to maintain a two-tier system. Ongoing contestation has shaped a system where support for private health expands, but is increasingly disciplined by a distributive logic of targeting. Targeting is not focused on the poor, but rather on limiting benefits provided to high-income earners. Australia's experience complicates our understanding of marketization as purely liberalizing, yet it also demonstrates its limits as an egalitarian strategy. High out-of-pocket costs and growing private subsidies suggest universalism is less entrenched than it appears, while the popular conception of Medicare as universal similarly limits efforts for more expansive public provision.

References

Barr, N. 2001, *The Welfare State as Piggy Bank: Information, Risk, Uncertainty, and the Role of the State*, Oxford University Press, Oxford.

Bean, C. 1994, 'Issues in the 1993 election', *Australian Journal of Political Science*, 29, pp. 134–57.

Boxall, A. and Gillespie, J. 2013, *Making Medicare: The Politics of Universal Healthcare in Australia*, University of New South Wales Press, Sydney.

Briggs, A. 2013, 'A short history of increases to the medicare levy', *Australian Parliamentary Library*, 3 May, accessed 14 June 2021, <https://parlinfo.aph.gov.au/parlInfo/download/library/prspub/2422887/upload_binary/2422887.pdf;fileType=application%2Fpdf#search=%22library/prspub/2422887%22>.

Briggs, A. 2017, 'Private health insurance: A quick guide', *Australian Parliamentary Library*, 4 August, accessed 10 October 2022, <https://www.aph.gov.au/About_Parliament/Parliamentary_Departments/Parliamentary_Library/pubs/rp/rp1718/Quick_Guides/PrivateHealthInsurance>.Browning, B. 1992, *Exploiting Health: Activists and Government v. The People*, Canonbury Press, Kew.

Bryant, G. and Spies-Butcher, B. 2020, 'Bringing finance inside the state: How income-contingent loans blur the boundaries between debt and tax', *Environment and Planning A: Economy and Space*, 52(1), pp. 111–29.

Carson, A., Martin, A.J. and Ratcliff, S. 2020, 'Negative campaigning, issue salience and vote choice: Assessing the effects of the Australian Labor Party's 2016 "Mediscare" campaign', *Journal of Elections, Public Opinion and Parties*, 30(1), pp. 83–104.

Collyer, F., Harley, K. & Short, S. 2015, 'Money and markets in Australia's healthcare system'. In Meagher, G. & Goodwin, S., *Markets, rights and power in Australian social policy*, Sydney University Press. Sydney, pp. 257–292.

Collyer, F. and White, K. 2001, 'Corporate control of healthcare in Australia', *Discussion paper no. 42*, The Australia Institute, Canberra.

Cook, L. 2019, 'Mental health in Australia: A quick guide', *Research Paper Series, 2018–19*, Australian Parliamentary Library, Canberra, accessed 14 June 2021, <https://parlinfo.aph.gov.au/parlInfo/download/library/prspub/6497249/upload_binary/6497249.pdf>.

Elliot, A. 2002, 'The decline in bulk billing: Explanations and implications', *Current Issues Brief no.3 2002–2003*, Australia Parliamentary Library, Canberra.

Elliot, A. 2006, '"The best friend Medicare ever had"?: Policy narratives and the changes in Coalition health policy', *Health Sociology Review*, 15(2), pp. 132–43.

Gillespie, J. 1991, *The Price of Health: Australian Governments and Medical Politics, 1910–1960*, Cambridge University Press, Melbourne.

Gingrich, J. 2011, *Making Markets in the Welfare State: The Politics of Varying Market Reforms*, Cambridge University Press, New York.

Gray, G. 1991, *Federalism and Health Policy: The Development of Health Systems in Canada and Australia*, University of Toronto Press, Toronto.

Harvey, K., Lokuge, B., Drahos, P. and Faunce, T. 2004, 'Will the Australia-United States free trade agreement undermine the pharmaceutical benefits scheme?' *Medical Journal of Australia*, 181(5), pp. 256–9.

Hunt, G. 2021, 'Medicare bulk billing rates continue to grow', Department of Health, Canberra, accessed 15 June 2021, <https://www.health.gov.au/ministers/the-hon-greg-hunt-mp/media/medicare-bulk-billing-rates-continue-to-grow>.

Jessop, B. 2016, *The State: Past, Present, Future,* Polity Press, Cambridge.

Le Grand, J. 1991, 'Quasi-markets and social policy', *The Economic Journal*, 101(408), pp. 1256–67.

Le Grand, J. 1997, 'Knights, knaves or pawns? Human behaviour and social policy', *Journal of Social Policy*, 26(2), pp. 149–69.

MacKay, D. 1995, 'The politics of reaction', in Gardner, H. (ed), *The Politics of Health: The Australian Experience*, 2nd ed., Churchill Livingstone, Melbourne.

Mair, P. 2013, *Ruling the Void*, Verso, London.

McAuley, I. 2005, 'Private health insurance: Still muddling through', *Agenda*, 12(2), pp. 159–78.

Meagher, G. and Goodwin, S. 2015, 'Introduction: Capturing marketisation in Australian social policy', in Meagher, G. and Goodwin, S. (eds), *Markets, Rights and Power in Australian Social Policy*, Sydney University Press, Sydney, pp. 1–28.

Mendelson, D 1999, 'Devaluation of a constitutional guarantee: The history of Section 51(xxiiiA) of the Commonwealth Constitution', *Melbourne University Law Review*, 23, pp. 308–44.

O'Connor, J. 1973, *The Fiscal Crisis of the State*, St. Martin's Press, New York.
OECD. 2021, 'Health spending (indicator)', accessed 11 June 2021, https://www.oecd-ilibrary.org/social-issues-migration-health/health-spending/indicator/english_8643de7e-en
Palangkaraya, A. and Yong, J. 2005, 'Effects of recent carrot-and-stick policy initiatives on private health insurance coverage in Australia', *Economic Record*, 81(254), pp. 262–272.
Parliament of Australia. 2018, *House of Representatives Practice*, 7th ed, June, Parliament of Australia, Canberra.
Peck, J. 2013, 'For Polanyian economic geographies', *Environment and Planning A*, 45(7), pp. 1545–68.
Peck, J., Brenner, N. and Theodore, N. 2018, 'Actually existing neoliberalism', in Cahill, D., Cooper, M., Konings, M. and Primrose, D. (eds), *The Sage Handbook of Neoliberalism*, Sage, London, pp. 3–15.
Pierson, P. 1994, *Dismantling the Welfare State? Reagan, Thatcher, and the Politics of Retrenchment*, Cambridge University Press, Cambridge.
Pierson, P. 2001, 'Coping with permanent austerity welfare state restructuring in affluent democracies', in Pierson, P. (ed), *The New Politics of the Welfare State*, Oxford University Press, Oxford, pp. 410–56.
Sax, S. 1984, *A Strife of Interests*, Allen and Unwin, Sydney.
Scotton, R.B. 1969, 'Membership of voluntary health insurance', in Butler, J.R. and Doessel, D.P. (eds), *Health Economics: Australian Readings*, Australian Professional Publications, Sydney.
Scotton, R.B. 1980, 'Health insurance: Medibank and after', in Cotton, R.B. and Ferber, H. (eds), *Public Expenditure and Social Policy in Australia: The First Fraser Years, 1976–8*, Vol. 2, Longman Chesire, Melbourne.
Scotton, R.B. and Macdonald, C. 1993, *The Making of Medibank*, University of New South Wales Press, Kensington.
Scotton, R.N. and Deeble, J. 1968, 'Compulsory health insurance in Australia', *The Australian Economic Review*, 1, pp. 9–16.
Spies-Butcher, B. 2014, 'Markets, universalism and equity: Medicare's dual role in the Australian welfare state', *Journal of Australian Political Economy*, 73, pp. 18–40.
Spies-Butcher, B. 2023, *Politics, Inequality and the Australian Welfare State After Liberalisation*, Anthem Press, London.
Spies-Butcher, B. and Stebbing, A. 2019, 'Mobilising alternative futures: Generational accounting and the fiscal politics of ageing in Australia', *Ageing and Society*, 39(7), pp. 1409–35.
Stebbing, A. and Spies-Butcher, B. 2010, 'Universal welfare by "other means"? Social tax expenditures and the Australian dual welfare state', *Journal of Social Policy*, 39(4), pp. 585–606,
Streeck, W. 2014, *Buying Time: The Delayed Crisis of Democratic Capitalism*, Verso, London.
Streeck, W. and Thelen, K. 2005, 'Introduction: Institutional change in advanced political economies', in Streeck, W. and Thelen, K. (eds), *Beyond Continuity: Institutional Change in Advanced Political Economies*, Oxford University Press, New York, pp. 1–39.
Treasury 2023, 'Historic investment in Medicare, Budget 2023-24', accessed 14 July 2023, <https://budget.gov.au/content/02-medicare.htm>.
Whitfield, D. 2006, 'A typology of privatisation and marketisation', *European Services Strategy Unit*, pp. 1–12.
Wong, C.Y., Greene, J., Dolja-Gore, X. and van Gool, K. 2017, 'The rise and fall in out-of-pocket costs in Australia: An analysis of the strengthening Medicare reforms', *Health Economics*, 26(8), pp. 962–79.

31

THE POLITICAL ECONOMY OF THE NATIONAL HEALTH SERVICE IN THE UNITED KINGDOM

Jonathan Filippon

The British National Health Service (NHS) has been regarded as an international role model of how to plan and organize a universal national healthcare system, at least until the influence of neoliberalism and New Public Management on health policy-making during the 1980s (Hart 2010). Part of a wider state-led welfare structure, the NHS is publicly funded through taxation and free at the point of delivery (financed by general taxation), providing comprehensive healthcare through universal access to services. From the citizen's perspective, despite numerous market-based health policy reforms since the Thatcher era (1979–90), the system has remained largely unchanged: still based on universal access, hierarchically structured over a large primary care basis of General Practitioner Practices acting as 'gate keepers' and, therefore, rationalizing use based on clinical needs. Moreover, other 'walk-in' and preventive services have been expanded over the last three decades.

Yet, the organization of the system and its policy reforms have been a constant and contentious subject of political deliberation during and after election campaigns, when all sides of the political spectrum seem to defend 'no change to our NHS'. The reality is that the NHS, founded in the context of post–World War Two optimism, has thoroughly changed in the ensuing seven decades – heavily influenced by market reforms and, since the process of devolution across the UK, nudged toward more diverse national policy choices by each member of the Union (Woods 2004). The foundational principles of the NHS embodied what was then a solid welfare state ethos of universal access to basic life conditions (minimum life standards), guaranteed by the state, and buttressed by popular support during every election. In relation to the triad of housing, education, and health, the welfare state pointed a way forward from the scant picture of social deprivation experienced in Britain during the 1940s (Fraser 1992). Most recognizably, the *Beveridge Report* (Beveridge 1942) postulated a foundational set of minimum life conditions that should be guaranteed by the state. Over time, however, health and social care in the UK have gradually changed from comprising a social system based on solidarity and cooperation, to a set of services arranged through mutual competition under contractual market rules (Barr 2020). When it comes to healthcare, English citizens have effectively been converted into clients, at least from an organizational perspective, based on performance and competition – as consolidated under the *Health and Social Care Act* (HSCA) of 2012. Regrettably, despite its rhetorical emphasis on 'cooperation', an even

DOI: 10.4324/9781003017110-35

more marketized approach has recently been codified in the recently legislated *Health and Care Act* (HCA) of 2022 (Alderwick *et al.* 2021; Roderick and Pollock 2022).

The purpose of this chapter is to explore the different NHS policy reforms since its inception, with an explicit focus on NHS England and its previous three decades of change. In particular, the chapter seeks to grasp the comprehensive nature of the HSCA of 2012 by examining its motivation and purpose in the context of the different stages of institutional reform that preceded it. Prior to the introduction of the HCA in 2022, the HSCA was the most expansive health policy reform introduced in the UK since the creation of the NHS in 1948, though it concerns only the English NHS. For some, it brought NHS England to its end as a truly 'public' health system (Pollock *et al.* 2012). Even though the HSCA did not alter the system from the user's perspective (services remained comprehensive and financed through general taxation), the chapter demonstrates that the changes it engendered at the level of service provision were remarkable and poorly corresponded to a public health rationale.

This critical historical review also helps reveal the rationale for the more recent HCA as a reform intended to address the shortcomings of the HSCA. Note, however, that at the time of completing this chapter in mid-2022, the HCA had only just received Royal Assent. Accordingly, the following discussion will primarily focus on examining the reform processes undertaken prior to this latest development, while offering some reflections on its form and likely future political-economic implications.

The NHS and devolution

From an international perspective, a common misconception is that the NHS is the same system all over the UK. This is largely a historical representation of the system that no longer corresponds to its current form, as much has changed over the last 30 years through the process of political devolution – as discussed in detail below. Indeed, since devolution in 1997–98 gradually implemented semi-independent, locally elected governments and national assemblies in Wales, Scotland, and Northern Ireland, there have been four independent NHS systems (McCartney 2018), with decision-making powers also devolved from the national level. This is no small detail for the health system, as it profoundly affects its arrangement of services, financing, and comprehensiveness. With the 'devolution', a fundamental change emerged at an early stage in Wales and Scotland: the reversal of the split between service provision and purchasers of healthcare services, which had initially introduced market competition in the NHS – the so-called 'internal market' reforms started by Thatcher; continued by the Labour governments of Tony Blair and Gordon Brown (1997–2010); and finally opened to the for-profit private sector, with the HSCA 2012 under the Conservative Prime Minister, David Cameron. The system has fundamentally changed again in light of the 2022 HCA introduced under the premiership of Boris Johnson, which aims to end the purchaser/provider split in England, invest in regional 'cooperation' through Integrated Care Services, and return powers to the central government (Cowper 2021; Bayliss 2022; Roderick and Pollock 2022).

Health systems are social systems and, therefore, a reflection of sociopolitical arrangements, values, agreements (and disagreements) of the populations in which they are generated (Donaldson and Rutter 2017). Accordingly, each NHS in the UK reflects the historical values and political consensus in which it is embedded. From a healthcare policy perspective, each system has, since devolution, been gradually reformed in varying directions. From the four cases, the most distinct contrast has been between NHS England and NHS Scotland. In England, as outlined below, policy-makers have focused on increasing competitive mechanisms between independent agents, mediated by commercial contracts, and multiplying regulatory organizations outside the government apparatus. Scotland, however, has endeavored to reduce layers of management while increasing reliance on clinical networks and professional expertise organized into geographically defined health boards. The latter remains closer to a classic public health approach based on territory, rooted in an understanding of local needs and public health knowledge (Filippon *et al.* 2020).

As in the past, all four countries offer comprehensive protection from financial catastrophe in the face of unavoidable medical expenses. This shared characteristic is fundamental when compared to other health system financing models, protecting the population from out-of-pocket (OOP) payments and avoiding catastrophic medical expenditure. When compared to its European counterparts, the UK has a slightly lower GDP/health expenditure ratio, likely linked to the use of primary care professionals as systemic 'gatekeepers'. Such models can be very efficient if primary care is truly prioritized and properly financed (Starfield 1998). Finally, financing for all four systems is based on general taxation, with block grants transferred to Scotland, Wales, and Northern Ireland under political devolution arrangements.

The remainder of this chapter examines the multitude of institutional reform processes that have profoundly affected the operation of NHS England since the mid-1970s, and considers their political-economic implications for the effective delivery of comprehensive public health objectives.

Post-War origins, the winter of discontent, and the seeds of change

After a tumultuous post-War start, with the nationalization of all UK hospitals through a 'pen stroke' reform, a hierarchical 'tripartite' division was eventually applied across the NHS between primary (and preventative), secondary, and tertiary care. Such division has been used as an organizational base for most national health services established in late-industrialized countries that attempted the 'NHS model'. Health and Social Security departments were reunited in 1968, leading to the formation of the UK Department of Health and Social Security. While a comprehensive view of health should involve both arenas, NHS budget practices have kept health and social care fragmented. A major administrative reorganization occurred in 1974 when Local Health Authorities were established under the *National Health Service Reorganization Act*, aimed at increasing cooperation, reducing service fragmentation, and increasing funding availability for local services. Territorial authorities were established and financed using a needs-based resource allocation formula, which replaced block transfers calculated using historical averages. Despite some improvement in resource allocation, the end of Labour rule in the late-1970s was marked by various healthcare workforce industrial actions, chronic underfunding, and a system deemed to be excessively bureaucratic (Crinson 2008).

Conservatives won the election following the Winter of Discontent (1978–79),[1] ending Labour rule over the NHS, and initiating the 'market reforms' cycle. When Margaret Thatcher took office, the NHS was politically and administratively centralized: hospitals were owned, financed, and managed by the state. In England, Regional Health Authorities led, planned, and managed services within their territories, providing community and hospital care. These characteristics would soon give away to a rationalized approach focused on cost-containment, 'rewards' for efficiency, and managerialism through New Public Management approaches.

Organizational change began with the publication of the *Griffiths Report* (1983), which placed emphasis on managerial roles within the system, thereby increasing hierarchical relations. The establishment of directors' boards, subject to shareholders' scrutiny, mimicked private companies. Gradually, systematic control was handed to administrators, favoring a technocratic approach focused on individual and institutional performance (Verzulli *et al.* 2018). Furthermore, the late-Thatcher period (early-1990s) brought significant change: outsourcing and the purchaser-provider split, which would allow for the creation of the so-called internal market.

Outsourcing began outside clinical practices, primarily in cleaning, laundry, nutrition, and general maintenance of hospital services – all previously internally managed by the NHS. Since then, outsourcing has become one of the most common practices for reducing state costs in service provision, and it is frequently part of the privatization process in public healthcare provision across Western economies (Fine 2009).

The imposition of the purchaser-provider split is historically recognized as a critical privatization turning-point within the NHS. To place such a large system within a market framework that privileged competition and efficient performance required a corresponding legal and administrative framework. Despite some reorganizational changes throughout the 1980s, it was the Internal Market Reform that fundamentally changed the rationale of healthcare service provision in the UK. Importantly, some of these reforms were 'undone' by the Scottish and Welsh governments after political devolution. Under this reform, Department of Health funds could be allocated to purchasers, who would then pay providers based on competitive contracts. The rationale was that such a mechanism would work as the main driver for cost-efficiency across the system – from GP practices to specialized hospital care.

These changes were promoted in stages, and decision-making was gradually decentralized. Initially, the purchasers were the General Practitioners-Fundholders (GP-FH) and District Health Authorities (DHAs), who were responsible for acquiring primary and secondary services. GP-FH covered some secondary services for their population, and DHAs would contract services based on local needs for the population otherwise not covered. Each would cover populations up to 200,000 people, based on a needs-adjusted budget *per capita* (capitation). The internal market was a sweeping health policy reform that reverberated in the policy literature of other high- and middle-income economies, whereby the British approach was modeled as a way to maintain universal healthcare systems under the internationally shared pressure of increasing healthcare spending (Akerman 1993).

1991–2007: advancing the internal market

Market relations of buying and selling services can only occur if a certain legal framework exists, even if buyers and sellers are part of the same hierarchical system composed of primary and secondary public healthcare. For the newly established internal market, a whole set of administrative layers and legal tools had to be instituted. These were heavily influenced by New Public Management (NPM) principles, such as decentralization and competition via contractual relationships, contained within the Conservative Party's 1990 *National Health Service and Community Care Act*. Having already introduced management layers and boards of directors during the 1980s, this Act facilitated the move toward reshaping public healthcare services in England into business-like entities during the 1990s. Hospitals turned into 'trusts' and adopted yearly budgets that could be 'balanced' by selling assets (goods divestiture), establishing cash flow statements, and maintaining accounting records similar to private companies.

John Major (1992–97) succeeded Thatcher and used the internal market reform as a flagship policy aimed at reducing state bureaucracy (Ham 1999). Health Authorities' and the GP Fundholders' model was adopted, while salaried payments for GPs were introduced. By 1996, around 50 percent of GPs were financed through some kind of the fundholding model, and those who remained 'independent' adhered to cost-containment, mostly linked to prescriptions. In the same year, there were 350 NHS Trusts structuring service packages, workforce pay, and composition.

These operated as not-for-profit social organizations – an archetype that subsequently influenced the 'social enterprise' model undertaken by different middle-income countries around the world, manifest in increased third sector participation in healthcare services provision.

There were structural issues, which affected the model based on competition and market rules: purchasers were limited in their bargaining scope, weakening price competition; Health Authorities lacked information (market asymmetry); and local service providers manipulated monopolies. Further, issues around the fundamental definition of core services, and the dividing line between 'social care' and 'extra care', remained a constant matter of debate. While decentralized decisions increased inequalities of access based on geographic location, local services were reluctant to compete with each other (Russell *et al.* 2013). The assumption of the reform was that competition would 'naturally' lead to gains in efficiency and service quality by (i) keeping the purchaser-provider split, (ii) stimulating private providers' participation, and (iii) decentralizing administration. These characteristics formed the basis of a 'quasi-market' arrangement, while their weak realization as 'reforms' has occasioned political and social criticism in most Western democratic states (Crinson 2008), including the UK. The quasi-market arrangement, however, continued to hold sway in the political arena as a general 'modernization of the state apparatus' (Turino *et al.* 2021). Sectors other than healthcare were reformed during the same period, whereby the state could control demand through selected agents (purchasers), with provision by either public companies or not-for-profit entities. The unifying thread throughout was competition as a means to 'service improvement' and cost-efficiency (Gaynor *et al.* 2017).

The final stage of these reforms, under the auspices of 'New Labour' (1997–2010), consolidated the corporate culture within UK public services, including the NHS. Despite publicly condemning the health policy reforms of its predecessors, the Labour government entrenched the purchaser-provider split by creating Primary Care Groups (PCGs), which were later arranged as Primary Care Trusts (PCTs), and increased reliance on the decentralized Fundholders' model. By 1999, all GPs were asked to join one of the 481 PCGs under the *New NHS Act* (1997): an effort to budget specifically primary care, with a partial return to territorial responsibility. After 2000, PCTs were established as legal entities in primary care, accompanied by the creation of Foundation Trusts (FTs), which were even more independent from government, closer to commercial and corporate arrangements from a legal, financial, and governance perspective (Allen 2009).

Ultimately, PCTs came to be organized in a territorial way (with constituencies of up to 200,000 people) and were focused on: (i) territorial health improvement (public health), (ii) commissioning of services (purchasing), and (iii) enhancement of local primary care procedures (Oliver 2005). By 2003, there were 211 PCTs, and larger Health Authorities were rearranged into 28 Strategic Health Authorities (SHAs). SHAs, then, were responsible for planning and management, while PCTs retained responsibility to commission actual services (Peckham 2007). Over the years, the Department of Health (DH) gradually transferred other responsibilities to semi-independent institutions. For instance, the National Institute for Health and Care Excellence (NICE), initially only responsible for health technology assessments, was tasked with the organization of university research and the setting up of clinical guidelines. Additionally, the Care Quality Commission (CQC) came to regulate licensing, quality, and performance among healthcare services (NHS or independent).

We see, then, a transition toward regulatory services that act independently but on behalf of the state, with the latter remaining responsible for financing the system (taxation/collection and pooling) and 'stewardship' (WHO 2000; Navarro 2020). During this time, despite an apparent move from competition to regulation under centralized performance management, there is also a greater distance from a 'needs-based' public health system, relying more overtly on individualized behavior change and 'self-accountability' (Williams and Dickinson 2016).

This move toward a regulatory state in the English NHS was consolidated during Tony Blair's second term in office (2001–04), concomitant with further political devolution to Wales, Scotland, and Northern Ireland. From this period onward, the path toward a more 'liberalized' NHS was followed only within England, while Scottish and Welsh policies focused on rebooting key aspects of the purchaser-provider split and prescription charges. In England, targets and performance remained as the central focus, triggering a second wave of reforms, with incentives to private sector participation (to compete with public providers) being characteristic of this wave. This signals the clear opening of the NHS to the participation of private providers via market competition (Smith *et al.* 2010). The general belief was that private providers could also encourage efficiency among public actors if all actors were subject to similar targets and regulation rules (McDonald 2009). The introduction of Payment by Results (PbR) was an attempt to make 'the money to follow the patient', providing both larger scale programs and barriers to care for complex cases, such as those with chronic conditions and comorbidities (Sussex and Farrar 2009). 'Choice Initiative' was yet another way of inciting competition, by expanding choice in users' preferred location for treatments or specialized care referrals. Ultimately, neither PbR nor the 'Choice Initiative' led to the system delivering quality improvement or greater cost-efficiency.

Labour's consolidation of market reforms started by the Thatcher government can be considered a political betrayal of its center-left supporters. Yet, beyond choosing not to abolish the internal market (despite being elected under the promise of doing so), its implementation of Private Finance Initiatives (PFIs) may be more consequential. PFIs are not the creation of the Labour Party, instead coming of age during the 1990s as a way of capitalizing investment in 'public' infrastructure (Pollock *et al.* 2005). In a nutshell, under such initiatives, private companies (construction sector, banks, and service providers) are allowed to raise funds through the financial market (for large borrowing of funds) to build infrastructure for 'public' use. In the case of healthcare and the NHS, this has usually applied to hospitals and clinical settings. The return on investment occurs through long-term contracts (20 to 30 years, or even more when these are reviewed), where the government assures lease of the structure for the duration of the contract. In theory, the government (society) benefits through new capital projects for prompt public use, without the need to increase taxes or public spending. However, as with other reform 'efficiencies', mid- to long-term calculations indicated that the system was highly onerous to the state and would likely necessitate the reduction of services and/or eventual closures to remain an economically 'sustainable' model (Pollock *et al.* 2011).

The road to the HSCA 2012 and beyond

Competition in healthcare services provision was subsequently taken a step further in England. Already in 2005, a policy known as Practice Based Commissioning (PCB) was used to aid GPs with budget management through standardized care plans. These were considered part of decentralization, through changing cooperative ties between secondary and tertiary care to competitive and contractual relationships (Roland and Rosen 2011). As such, this constituted the first stage toward the establishment of Clinical Commissioning Groups (CCGs). Through the HSCA 2012 (termed the 'Lansley Reforms'), CCGs replaced the previous territorial health models (PCTs), allowing private providers to sell services within NHS England – a fully liberalized, yet publicly financed arrangement (Filippon *et al.* 2016).

Certainly, many developments led the English NHS toward the HSCA in 2012, one of which was the gradual use of private entities to manage 'soft services': routine data management, administrative services, diagnostic services (pathology and radiology), and scientific research commissioning (Reynolds and McKee 2012). However, it was the creation of CCGs that limited the scope of procedures to be purchased – restricting supply and undermining system comprehensiveness. CCGs inaugurated a new mechanism of resource allocation for NHS England: rather than being based on territory, these entities were guided by risk profile (particularly by age), based on their 'clientele' population. Under such a format, resource allocation was especially challenging when concerned with the reduction of known and unknown health inequalities. In other countries, similar models are used for 'sickness funds' and can lead to risk selection, introduction of co-payments, and the use of extra services (dental care and prescription charges) to compensate for the lack of comprehensive care.

Moreover, services could be purchased by CCGs from NHS Foundation Trusts or 'any qualified provider' (AQP Contracts), which left the door open for private provisioning. Under this arrangement, equity of access would become problematic if not planned at the national level, and tellingly, public health experts were integrated into local councils rather than being members of CCGs. The danger, in turn, lay in NHS England moving away from a public, risk-sharing culture, toward a model in which non-state institutions assumed social risk and accountability similar to the private health insurance system. Under this arrangement, Foundation Trust Hospitals could generate up to 49 percent of their budget through the provision of private healthcare. Such realities threatened the comprehensiveness of care, with quasi-private health insurance models portending to stand in for NHS purchasing. The temptation of citizens/patients to 'jump the queue' via payment for private insurance, in turn, appeared to lay the groundwork for the next logical step: full for-profit privatization.

These fundamental changes, which put the universal character of the system in jeopardy, were largely invisible to the population, as care remained free at the point of delivery. Since the HSCA 2012, NHS England moved further away from state control and has been decisively influenced by the American model of medical insurance, notably with the implementation of Integrated Care Models similar to *Kaiser Permanente* and the *Veterans Health Administration* (Ham and Curry 2011). CCGs were open to Any Qualified Provider (AQP) (Regan and Ball 2016), and the process of tendering contracts has been based on principles (and legislation) that govern commercial relationships. Oddly, however, five years after the HSCA 2012 made this possible, NHS England's Chief Executive stated that 'accountable care organizations or systems [...] will [...] effectively end the purchaser-provider split, bringing about integrated funding and delivery for a given geographical population' (House of Commons Public Accounts Committee 2017: n.p.). So, what has happened since 2012 that allowed Conservatives to apparently turn away from the central organizing principle of their own internal market, toward a new 'collaboration and cooperation' at the local level?

Importantly, the constant search for providing incentives that 'reward' higher efficiency (McDonald 2009) remains a consistent rationale across Health Management Organizations (HMOs), Accountable Care Organizations (ACOs), but also Integrated Care Systems (ICS). In this sense, the Conservative move away from the HSCA 2012 was undertaken to import *corporate reform* inside NHS England that could further the implementation of ICS (Bayliss and Gideon 2020). After all, the NHS reforms prevailing prior to the introduction of HCA in 2022 were originally justified on the assumption that by 2020/21, the ballooning deficit (£30 billion) would restrict government provision of supplementary funding, leaving only the need for higher efficiency mechanisms. Thus, the 2014 *NHS Five-Year Forward View* involved a major system overhaul, which would be undertaken through local Sustainability and Transformation Plans (STPs). The government guaranteed financing increases between 2015 and 2020, coupled with efficiency savings of 2–3 percent per year that were to be generated by STPs. The generic rhetoric of STPs favoring cooperation, better quality, and value-for-money was, in principle, met without opposition among NHS actors. In practice, however, STPs brought about service reduction and budget cuts, with a 'difficult-to-trace' accountability at the national level. The pandemic years of 2020–22 are exceptions to this process, as systemic reforms were temporarily put on hold. Not surprisingly, in 2022, the HCA was introduced as a means to 'legislate' changes already implemented via STPs, without parliamentary deliberation.

Ultimately, between 2012 and 2022, the private sector was further embedded within NHS England. International healthcare provider companies now own large groups of GP practices across England, and under their recent abolition under the HCA, CCGs spent around one-sixth to one-fifth of their budget on private providers (Rowland 2021). STPs were always supposed to be a temporary solution for the full implementation of ICS boards. These 'boards' function to 'integrate' care services at the level of delivery by extinguishing the CCG model, receiving block grants at the local level, and redesigning service provision. Boards are to be comprised of different NHS officials, local authorities, and private providers, who can then plan services for a given geographic region within their allocated budget, using a loose 'cooperative' framework. The sudden substitution of the current regulated market mechanism with an abstract idea of 'collaboration' between providers offers considerable space for conflicts of interest and lower integrity of service provision. In the end, despite these obvious pitfalls, the (undoubtedly problematic) outcomes of the HCA will likely be praised as delivering 'comprehensiveness and universality', and they will be heralded as proof of the efficacy of reform by British Conservatives.

Conclusion

The history of NHS reform has always been embedded within major processes of globalization, an overall rise in social inequalities, and the increased influence of private corporations in public affairs. In the move to accommodate commercial growth and the 'sustainability of the sector', the latter influence directly affects and threatens universal health and healthcare entitlement. Within NHS England, there is a clear trend of state retrenchment when it comes to not only safeguarding health systems as comprehensive, but also addressing issues of existing socioeconomic inequality. As the former has advanced, the latter has become an increasingly pressing contemporary concern.

From the introduction of the system according to the principles of solidarity and cross-subsidization, to the 'market reverence' promoted by Thatcher and ushered in by 'new Labour', to the post-Brexit scenario of integration with no framework, NHS England has remained in a state of constant policy reform. The most recent round of reforms, manifest in the HCA, will add to a system already under considerable influence from American insurance and service providers. There is an overarching intention to transfer decision-making and risk from the national level under a common pool of resources to provider-based networks (either public, for-profit, not-for-profit, or social enterprises). Providers will bear responsibility for decisions around comprehensiveness, which will have unpredictable medium- and long-term consequences. Importantly, the main incentive of the ICS board model is to promote 'savings' that can be shared between providers – akin to Thatcherism's 'rewards for efficiency' (see: Bayliss 2022; Roderick and Pollock 2022). How to regulate against the reduction of service delivery in the face of 'cost-efficiency' and 'sustainability' imperatives will remain the system's biggest challenge. It is a rather puzzling and confounding problem, given that the initial intention of reforms was putatively to maintain comprehensive and universal care for all.

Note

1 The UK winter of 1978/79 was marked by strong storms and the coldest weather in 16 years, which isolated parts of the country, coupled with generalized strike action across the private and public sectors. The Labour Party was also under internal and external scrutiny over its macroeconomic strategy during the 1960s and 1970s. Margaret Thatcher was elected four months after Labour Prime Minister James Callaghan suffered a no-confidence vote, triggering the 1979 general election.

References

Akerman, M. 1993, 'The British healthcare system after the 1991 reforms: Preliminary considerations', *Saúde e Sociedade*, 2, pp. 85–99.

Alderwick, H., Gardner, T. and Mays, N. 2021, 'England's new health and care bill', *British Medical Journal*, 374(1767), p. 1.

Allen, P. 2009, 'Restructuring the NHS again: Supply side reform in recent English health care policy', *Financial Accountability and Management*, 25(4), pp. 373–89.

Barr, N. 2020, *Economics of the Welfare State*, Oxford University Press, Oxford.

Bayliss, K. 2022, 'Can England's national health system reforms overcome the neoliberal legacy?' *International Journal of Health Services*, 52(4), pp. 480–91.

Bayliss, K. and Gideon, J. 2020, 'The privatization and financialization of social care in the UK', *Working Papers 238*, Department of Economics, SOAS, University of London.

Beveridge, W.H. 1942, *Social Insurance and Allied Services*, H.M. Stationary Office, London.

Cowper, A. 2021, 'Leaked government white paper ends England's NHS internal market and returns power to health secretary', *British Medical Journal*, 372(384).

Crinson, I. 2008, *Health Policy: A Critical Perspective*, Sage, London.

Donaldson, L.J. and Rutter, P. 2017, *Donaldsons' Essential Public Health*, CRC Press, Boca Raton.

Filippon, J., Bremner, S., Giovanella, L. and Pollock, A.M. 2020, 'An ecological study of publicly funded elective hip arthroplasties in Brazil and Scotland: Do access inequalities reinforce the inverse care law?' *JRSM Open*, 11(5), pp. 1–7.

Filippon, J., Giovanella, L., Konder, M. and Pollock, A.M. 2016, '"Liberalizing" the English national health service: Background and risks to healthcare entitlement', *Cadernos de Saúde Pública*, 32(8), p. e00034716.

Fine, B. 2009, 'Neoliberalism as financialisation', in Saad-Filho, A. and Yalman, G.L. (eds), *Economic Transitions to Neoliberalism in Middle-Income Countries*, Routledge, London, pp. 11–23.

Fraser, D. 1992, *The Evolution of the British Welfare State: A History of Social Policy Since the Industrial Revolution*, Macmillan International Higher Education, London.

Gaynor, M., Mostashari, F. and Ginsburg, P.B. 2017, 'Making health care markets work: Competition policy for health care', *Journal of the American Medical Association*, 317(13), pp. 1313–4.

Ham, C. 1999, 'Learning from the NHS internal market: A review of the evidence', *British Medical Journal*, 318(7182), p. 543.

Ham, C. and Curry, N. 2011, *Integrated Care*, The Kings Fund, accessed 19 September 2020, <https://www.kingsfund.org.uk/sites/default/files/field/field_publication_file/integrated-care-summary-chris-ham-sep11.pdf>.

Hart, J.T. 2010, *The Political Economy of Health Care: Where the NHS Came From and Where It Could Lead*, Policy Press, Bristol.

House of Commons Public Accounts Committee. 2017, 'Oral evidence: Integrated health and social care', HC 959, Q93, 27 February, accessed 19 October 2021, <http://data.parliament.uk/writtenevidence/committeeevidence.svc/evidencedocument/public-accounts-committee/integrated-healthand-social-care/oral/48009.html>.

McCartney, M. 2018, 'The NHS's slow decline is a preventable disease', *British Medical Journal*, 361, p. k2740.

McDonald, R. 2009, 'Market reforms in English primary medical care: Medicine, habitus and the public sphere', *Sociology of Health and Illness*, 31(5), pp. 659–72.

Navarro, V. 2020, 'Assessment of the World Health Report 2000', in Navarro, V. (ed), *Neoliberalism, Globalization, and Inequalities*, Routledge, London, pp. 441–50.

Oliver, A. 2005, 'The English national health service: 1979–2005', *Health Economics*, 14 (Suppl. 1), pp. S75–S99.

Peckham, S. 2007, 'The new general practice contract and reform of primary care in the United Kingdom', *Healthcare Policy*, 2(4), pp. 34–48.

Pollock, A.M., Player, S. and Price, D. 2005, *The Private Finance Initiative: A Policy Built on Sand,* UNISON Report, accessed 8 October 2021, <https://allysonpollock.com/wp-content/uploads/2013/04/UNISON_2005_Pollock_PFIPolicyBuiltOnSand.pdf>.

Pollock, A.M., Price, D. and Liebe, M. 2011, 'Private finance initiatives during NHS austerity', *British Medical Journal*, 342(7794), p. d324.

Pollock, A.M., Price, D., Roderick, P., Treuherz, T., McCoy, D., McKee, M. and Reynolds, L. 2012, 'How the Health and Social Care Bill 2011 would end entitlement to comprehensive health care in England', *The Lancet*, 379(9814), pp. 387–9.

Regan, P. and Ball, E. 2016, 'NHS market liberalisation and the TTIP agreement', *British Journal of Community Nursing*, 21(7), pp. 356–8.

Reynolds, L. and McKee, M. 2012, 'Opening the Oyster: The 2010–11 NHS reforms in England', *Clinical Medicine*, 12(2), pp. 128–32.

Roderick, P. and Pollock, A.M. 2022, 'Dismantling the National Health Service in England', *International Journal of Health Services*, 52(4), pp. 470–9.

Roland, M. and Rosen, R. 2011, 'English NHS embarks on controversial and risky market-style reforms in health care,' *New England Journal of Medicine,* 364(14), pp. 1360–6.

Rowland, D. 2021, 'Conflicts of interest in the post Lansley NHS – From a regulated to an unregulated healthcare market?', *Thebmjopinion*, 28 May, accessed 19 October 2021, <https://blogs.bmj.com/bmj/2021/05/28/conflicts-of-interest-in-the-post-lansley-nhs-from-a-regulated-to-an-unregulated-healthcare-market/>.

Russell, J., Greenhalgh, T., Lewis, H., Mackenzie, I., Maskrey, N., Montgomery, J. and O'Donnel, C. 2013, 'Addressing the "postcode lottery" in local resource allocation decisions: A framework for clinical commissioning groups', *Journal of the Royal Society of Medicine*, 106(4), pp. 120–3.

Smith, J., Curry, N., Mays, N. and Dixon, J. 2010, 'Where next for commissioning in the English NHS?', Research Report, Nuffield Trust and King's Fund, accessed 7 April 2022, <www.nuffieldtrust.org.uk/research/where-next-for-commissioning-in-the-english-nhs>.

Starfield, B. 1998. *Primary Care: Balancing Health Needs, Services, and Technology*, Oxford University Press, New York.

Sussex, J. and Farrar, S. 2009, 'Activity-based funding for National Health Service hospitals in England: Managers' experience and expectations', *The European Journal of Health Economics*, 10(2), pp. 197–206.

Turino, F., Filippon, J., Sodré, F. and Siqueira, C.E. 2021, 'Reinventing privatization: A political economic analysis of the social health organizations in Brazil', *International Journal of Health Services,* 51(15), pp. 90–100.

Verzulli, R., Jacobs, R. and Goddard, M. 2018, 'Autonomy and performance in the public sector: The experience of English NHS hospitals', *The European Journal of Health Economics*, 19(4), pp. 607–26.

Williams, I. and Dickinson, H. 2016, 'Going it alone or playing to the crowd? A critique of individual budgets and the personalisation of health care in the English National Health Service', *Australian Journal of Public Administration*, 75(2), pp. 149–58.

Woods, K.J. 2004, 'Political devolution and the health services in Great Britain', *International Journal of Health Services*, 34(2), pp. 323–39.

World Health Organisation. 2000, *The World Health Report 2000: Health Systems: Improving Performance*, WHO, Geneva.

32
HEALTH AND HEALTHCARE IN THE UNITED STATES

Rodney Loeppky[*]

The story of health and healthcare in the United States has always been – and continues to be – controversial and contradictory. It is surely a story of expanding profitability in healthcare delivery, and the growth of the largest healthcare market in the world – estimated to reach 20 percent of the country's GDP by 2026 (Himmelstein *et al.* 2018: 9). However, at the center of this story, cutting-edge biomedical research and world-class care sit uncomfortably with grossly unequal healthcare access and, at best, mediocre societal health indicators. Indeed, tens of millions of US citizens remain excluded from healthcare coverage altogether.

The prime movers of US healthcare are corporate actors, while to the extent that government has become more heavily involved, it fails to form an effective counterweight to such corporate agency. At least in relation to health, this is not true across comparable advanced industrial countries that have experienced similar corporate pressure (Giaimo and Manow 1999; Loeppky 2014). The US is generally taken as the ongoing neoliberal baseline, against which other health systems are compared. However, taking the notion of 'varieties of neoliberalism' seriously (Albo 2005), this chapter suggests that the US state has, indeed, gone further than other countries to foster market-led health. More recently, though, neoliberal growth has a paradoxically involved government intervention that enables corporations as quasi-public actors. Corporate actors engage in 'adaptive accumulation': securing private revenue at the crossroads between public policy objectives, a disjointed health system, and government funding. Indeed, at the height of neoliberalism, corporate health actors have latched onto a perverse interpretation of the Keynesian notion that 'what we want is not no planning, or even less planning, indeed [...] we almost certainly want more' (Christainsen 1993: 52).

The chapter begins by mapping out landmark evolutionary moments that have laid the groundwork for the explosion of public-private interactions in the contemporary era. Following this, it explores component parts of US health delivery that exhibit attributes of adaptive accumulation, including the growing Medicare Advantage program; Medicare's prescription drug program; and select attributes of the *Affordable Care Act* (ACA), particularly its expansion and subsidization of the commercial insurance market. Finally, the chapter closes with a discussion of ACA-centered healthcare in post-Trump America.

[*] This chapter is a modified and adapted version of Loeppky (2019).

DOI: 10.4324/9781003017110-36

Whence the mess? The growth of a neoliberal market in US health

Healthcare in the US constitutes one of the more blatant examples of neoliberal contradiction, wherein the country that leads the advanced industrial world in biomedical advances also tends toward a health delivery system that is grossly inefficient and fails vast swaths of its population. Viewed from a comparative public policy standpoint, US healthcare is not the 'envy of the world'. It costs more than any other health system, with 2019 (pre-COVID) *per capita* spending at US$11,072 – amounting to a whopping 17 percent of GDP, roughly twice as much spending as found in most other OECD countries (OECD 2021). Despite this spending, the system does not bring about the health outcomes purported by its advocates. Prior to the implementation of the ACA, some 52 million were without healthcare, with another 34 million understood as underinsured (with out-of-pocket costs acting as an impediment to care) (Rao and Hellander 2014: 216). Even following the rollout of the ACA, some 29 million remained uninsured, with another 50 million-plus experiencing underinsured status. Even more damning is that multiple outcome indicators (such as mortality, life expectancy, infant mortality, and mental health) place US healthcare definitively low on the list among its peer countries (OECD 2019).

Ultimately, market-based organization does not make healthcare systems more efficient or lower their costs. The singular most important reason for this is weak price leverage in a free-ranging, largely unregulated myriad of healthcare actors (Loeppky 2014: 69). Payment and provision remain extensively divided, where no payer (even large private insurers) possesses the systemic leverage to affect prices charged by providers. The US government proves singularly unwilling to regulate in this regard, leaving health providers to charge what the 'market will bear' for goods and services. This, combined with the reality that health and healthcare are handled as a form of industrial and economic development, has rendered costs that continue to climb faster than anywhere else. Yet, how did it come to this? Why has the US continued to encourage market-led healthcare, even as its peer countries moved in the opposite direction?

Early in the Twentieth Century, healthcare was largely administered by hospitals, run for the poor by charitable organizations, and medical costs were often out-of-pocket (Berkowitz 2010: 3). Efforts to create medical coverage for workers in moments of disability, led by the American Association for Labour Legislation (AALL), managed grassroots support in key states – the most prominent of which was New York. In that state, a 1919 bill supporting health insurance passed the state Senate, but was shut down in the House by the Speaker and a host of lobbying interests, including physicians, hospitals, and insurance companies (Hoffman 2010: 1541).

Even in the wake of the depression, the American Medical Association (AMA) recoiled at the prospect of New Deal legislation that might orchestrate change in healthcare, fearing regulation of fees and lowered income for physicians. The proposed inclusion of health reform within the *Social Security Act* of 1935 was abandoned, after it became clear that physicians' opposition would likely derail the entire bill. Even after Franklin Delano Roosevelt's re-election in 1936, the administration was not able to find political currency for such reform, and Congressional figures, lobbied by the AMA, indicated that they would shut down any attempts at legislation (Starr 2013: 46–8). Similarly, the Truman administration's support for national insurance was blocked by a Congress heavily influenced by providers' lobbying efforts. Public debate was steered toward a fear of 'socialized medicine', and the possibilities for change were pre-emptively foreclosed.

Only in the 1960s did meaningful policy reform emerge, with the advent of Medicare and Medicaid in 1965. These measures established almost universal purchasing of healthcare for US citizens over the age of 65, covering hospital care (Medicare Part A), physician and home care (Medicare Part B), and a federally backed but state-administered program for the poor (Medicaid).

Arguably, these programs were just as much a victory for the private healthcare market, providing care to vulnerable segments of the population, who were also viewed as unprofitable by market actors (Hacker 2008: 290). Tellingly, while the long-term goal of Medicare advocates had been its extension to the entire US population, this would prove unattainable in a US health landscape dominated by the AMA, the health insurance industry, myriad providers, and many Republican critics (Berkowitz 2017: 522–6).

As the strength and complexity of private coverage and provision in the US grew through the Reagan-Bush years, the failed health reform of the Clinton administration in the early-1990s stands as a watershed moment. It formed the political experience from which subsequent reforms would be shaped: clearly demonstrating both the dominance of market actors and power of political figures resistant to equitable healthcare coverage. By the early-1990s, healthcare costs had long since become unmanageable in the country, with the rising costs of coverage now felt by large corporations supplying health benefits, and the dilemma of uninsured Americans reaching catastrophic proportions (Béland and Waddan 2010: 219). The administration's strategy to get large corporations (with health plans) onside was intended as a means to create political momentum toward reform. This strategic move, while successful at first, proved to be the Achilles heel of the administration's efforts.

Large corporations' support did not signal any changing political culture, but rather a corporate desire to cut costs (Swenson and Greer 2002). The health industry quickly understood the 'harmful' political situation, wherein any call for greater government involvement could usher in price controls and disrupt revenue streams. As such, pharmaceutical and health maintenance organizations (HMOs) worked individually with major corporate actors to reduce, or at least stabilize, prices for the time being. Along with a concerted media campaign, this immediately undermined the publicly stated basis for reforms – making US corporations competitive – and brought a wave of resistance from foes and, eventually, existing corporate allies. The *Health Security Act*, the legislative expression of Clinton's 'managed competition' (mandating expanded employer-based health insurance), was intensely resisted by Republicans, while the insurance, pharmaceutical, and small business lobbies also forcefully denounced it (Béland and Waddan 2010: 220). In this field of hostility, hitherto corporate allies failed to back the administration – instead, perceiving greater opportunities to successfully negotiate better terms for their healthcare coverage on the open market (Giaimo and Manow 1999: 989). Politically, the effects of this failure cannot be understated: the space for broad healthcare reform disintegrated, and it would remain extremely limited for almost two decades.

When competition prevails: adapting neoliberal healthcare

Following the downfall of the Clinton reform, the political message was clear in US health: policy reform that interfered with, rather than bolstered, market presence in purchasing and delivery would be viewed unfavorably. The result was stepped-up competition between insurance companies and HMOs to tap into the extant, but still lucrative, health domains. In this neoliberal marketplace, the insurance industry opted to extend high-cost coverage to those who could pay (either individually or, more frequently, through their employer), rather than extend coverage more broadly. Moreover, it relied on actuarial risk and back-end rationing to enhance profit. Policy exclusion for 'high-risk' populations, denial of coverage, high deductibles and, if all else failed, insurance rescission were combined strategies that had accompanied the growth of a highly profitable market.

All markets, however, have their limits, and as the growing ranks of the uninsured meant relatively fewer paying beneficiaries, stepped-up premium prices could not compensate for this finite consumer base. In this competitive sphere, then, health industry actors necessarily sought alternative growth strategies. To do this, they have capitalized on healthcare reform in a manner that not only elevates their own public prominence, but also optimizes their potential for politically secured profit streams. Health, in this sense, follows a model that modifies neoliberal practice through adaptive accumulation. Adaptive accumulation distances us from the neoliberal archetype of lean regulation, state sell-offs, and a general state retrenchment from the public arena. Instead, the structures of public institutions can and do provide important platforms from which to enter or expand new avenues of private accumulation. Public objectives can be harnessed, such that a stable stream of revenue flows are secured for private actors undertaking public tasks, ostensibly with new integrity or effectiveness. The goal is not to remove the specter of government involvement or organization, but rather to subject its operationalization to private actors. In this sense, adaptive accumulation often involves advocacy for stronger government involvement, not less. It highlights the attention paid by corporate agents to read signals arising from both the market *and* legislative and regulatory fields. The total effect of this – in health, military, education, prisons – presents an image of American capitalism that, alongside being lean and anti-interventionist, contains a strong and contradictory dose of state largesse and corporate dependence.

The presence of adaptive accumulation within US neoliberalism brings with it select advantages for its protagonists – in the health sector and elsewhere. There are, first, amplified opportunities for private revenue, rooted in an expanding field of operations and stable, government-issued payments. In this way, market activity and profitability are augmented with a far more predictable field of public revenues redirected into private channels. To the extent that corporate actors within the US health sector have certainly experienced profitability pressures (Kelly 2016), adaptive accumulation offers an obvious (countertendential) release valve. Second, from a public imaging standpoint, private actors are slotted into a role that appears to be fulfilling social needs, shaped and expanded through public action. These needs can quickly transform into political necessity, even widespread public entitlement. This not only ensures market demand, but also crafts a kind of social legitimacy, as corporations 'selflessly' meet public needs. Finally, adaptive accumulation taps into a strain of American political culture that disparages the role of the state, taxation, and those 'undeserving' of public care. It captures both a long-term neoliberal ethic, and capitalizes on a more recent right-wing political theme: directing blame at 'lazy' sections of society while reinvigorating a call to 'save' the republic – and its misdirected public programs – through the moral discipline and efficiency of market imperatives.

What follows is an exploration of this dynamic through various components of US healthcare delivery, investigating both their origins and contemporary features, in order to shed light on the adaptive arrangements secured by market players. This is not an exhaustive survey of US healthcare delivery, but it does point to the highly profitable public-private dynamic upon which market actors depend for expansion. Further, while the US is hardly the only country to utilize such relationships in the health sector, its governmental actors demonstrate a particular willingness to reproduce conditions that render extraordinary market returns.

Medicare Advantage

While the move to profit from public, single-payer Medicare was initiated in the 1980s, it was in the late-1990s that insurers 'turned to Medicare for new sources of revenue. In the fight for beneficiaries, insurers offered richer and richer benefit packages, as well as lower cost sharing [...] even if that meant incurring short-run losses' (Kelly 2016: 331). The basis for this had been laid in 1982, with the passage of the *Tax Equity and Fiscal Responsibility Act* (TEFRA), which allowed private plans to offer Medicare coverage outside of the boundaries set by traditional Medicare (TM) fee-for-service (FFS) coverage (Hacker 2004: 253). Formalized as a Medicare option under the Clinton administration, it was the passage of the *Medicare Modernization Act* (MMA) in 2003 under George W. Bush that cemented this program, renaming it 'Medicare Advantage' (MA). Aimed at enhancing the attractiveness of seniors' coverage to the health industry, MA afforded more generous payment structures for those beneficiaries willing to convert to such arrangements. Major insurers have carved out a substantial portion of this market, and industry lobbyists devote time and resources to defend it (Kelly 2016: 336). The political leverage of industry actors has also grown with these beneficiary markets. Their power is substantial, as they can withdraw from participating in MA, retreat from certain counties, or charge higher premiums or extend modified benefits to the millions of seniors enrolled in their plans, 'the potential effect of which is to throw a growing portion of the Medicare market into turmoil' (Kelly 2016: 337). In other words, once private provision reaches a critical mass of participation, regulatory modifications around corporate participation present the strong possibility for political pain through disruption of care. From this advantageous position, corporate actors fend off regulatory constraints that might otherwise temper their profit expectations.

The Center for Medicare and Medicaid Services (CMS) has long attempted to reduce overly lucrative payment structures, utilizing a risk-adjustment scheme to modify FFS payments to insurers. A singular risk score is assigned to each insurance pool (usually by county), based on coded data submitted on each beneficiary. From this data, only higher risk pools receive enhanced FFS payments. How can the insurance industry adapt and still profit in such a carefully regulated payment structure? First, industry actors are selective about where they offer coverage, chosen on a county-by-county basis, as well as the structure of that coverage. With this, they maintain a pre-emptive, group-based adverse selection process (Brown *et al.* 2014; Newhouse *et al.* 2015). Moreover, beneficiaries with chronic conditions, or in need of acute care, tend to self-select back into traditional Medicare, avoiding the often-brutal limitations of 'care networks' (Rahman *et al.* 2015). Additionally, the industry engages in risk 'upcoding', where beneficiaries' health data is recorded within increased risk scores – a 5.3-percent climb among those who switched from TM to MA in 2008, increasing to a figure of 8 percent by 2012, and subsequently rising by an annual rate of 1.2 percent (Burns and Hayford 2017; Kronick 2017). Corporate players deftly navigate 'risk' as a regulatory structure, delivering quasi-public insurance plans that enhance structured revenue. By the end of the Bush administration, the average federal overpayment to MA already amounted to somewhere between 12 percent and 14 percent, totaling US$12 billion in yearly additional costs for the Medicare program (McGuire *et al.* 2011: 319).

The Obama administration recognized this problem as a drain on government resources, and signaled its intention to 'eliminate billions in unwarranted subsidies to insurance companies in the Medicare Advantage program – giveaways that boost insurance company profits but don't make you any healthier' (quoted in Volsky 2014). Yet, the industry's entrenched political leverage in this arena said otherwise. Its central lobbying body, America's Health Insurance Plans (AHIP), threatened that 'reimbursement reductions could drastically reduce enrollment in Medicare Advantage and disrupt plan offerings' (Jennings 2015). Under pressure, the administration compensated with the US$8 billion Quality-Based Bonus Payments Program (QBP), awarding increases in benchmark payments to a deeper range of recognized county plans over the ACA's first three years. In early 2013, when CMS finally gave notice of a 2014 MA payment *reduction* of 2.3 percent, the final payment rates, issued months later, nonetheless registered a payment rate *increase* of 3.3 percent (Haberkorn and Norman 2013). These upward adjustments would continue over the next six years, as AHIP advertising campaigns (highlighting the 'threat' to seniors' healthcare) and stepped-up Congressional lobbying consistently and pre-emptively derailed benchmark reductions (Norman 2014). Industrial players have harnessed the leverage associated with some 20 million beneficiaries (and voting citizens), thereby frustrating cost control aspirations of CMS officials. The utilization of market choice in Medicare – originally intended to infuse 'efficiency' – has been largely successful in converting public use into private gain.

Medicare Part D

The actual centerpiece of the MMA was a Republican-led effort to create Medicare drug coverage, a program since known as Medicare Part D (MpD). By 2000, political pressure was mounting to do something about spiraling drug costs, the most profound and visible effects from which were exerted on vulnerable US seniors. The industry, represented by the Pharmaceutical and Research Manufacturers of America (PhRMA), recognized the poor optics and lobbied to 'optimize' any potential regulatory result. In fact, Medicare had always existed in a tense peace with pharmaceutical providers. As the largest payer for healthcare in the US (44 million enrollees in 2017), it certainly retains the potential to utilize its position for price leverage against drug manufacturers. Typically, in the US system – especially in relation to the drug industry – purchasers are divided up between multiple parties, and no one party possesses enough leverage to exert strong downward pressure on drug prices. This has meant that pharmaceutical prices are, by a considerable margin, the most expensive in the advanced industrial world.

For the drug industry, then, the MMA became a vehicle not only to defend existing market practices, but also grow them in ways that would boost rather than detract from profitability. It became deeply involved in the drafting of legislation, which ultimately offered 'an extraordinary opportunity to pursue their aims with $400 billion on the table – a pursuit made easier by the desire of both the Bush administration and Congress to expand the private sector in Medicare' (Oberlander 2007: 198). Its design included a gap in coverage, known as the 'doughnut hole', wherein the federal government would cover 75 percent of beneficiaries' drug costs up to a set amount (US$2250 in 2006) and only pick up costs again once 'catastrophic coverage' levels were exceeded (US$5100 in 2006) (Henry J. Kaiser Family Foundation 2017b). MpD put the insurance industry in charge of plan administration and made the likelihood of serious cost control effectively disappear, as it includes a clause prohibiting the Department of Human Health and Services (DHHS) from leveraging drug prices (*Medicare Prescription Drug, Improvement, and Modernization Act 2003*: 2099). With a legal prohibition on price negotiation, spending in MpD increased from US$44.3 billion in 2006 to US$92 billion in 2018, thereby growing from 10.8 percent to 15.9 percent of Medicare totals, with a 4.7 percent projected annual growth rate through 2026 (Hoadley *et al.* 2015: 1682–3). Accordingly, the role of MpD in total US prescription drug spending has increased substantially, growing from 18 percent of the market in 2006 to 29 percent in 2015, with growth projected to reach 35 percent in 2025 (Henry J. Kaiser Family Foundation 2016, 2017a). In all, MpD spending has robustly enhanced the bottom line of firms – both payers and providers alike.

As with Medicare Advantage, the ACA was supposed to reduce the severity of drug spending in MpD. It aimed to close the 'doughnut hole' by subsidizing out-of-pocket balance. While surely helpful to seniors, this did nothing to address the issue of price escalation. Tellingly, political negotiations revolved around *how much*, not whether or not, government should subsidize a market-administered system of drug purchasing (Roy 2012; Osborn 2017). Reintroducing government price leverage, as exists in the profound majority of OECD countries, was certainly not on the table. As we will see, the ACA generally works to reinforce the status quo, while softening the impact of market prices on beneficiaries. MpD, in this regard, continues to furnish adaptive accumulation: channeling public revenues into insurance, pharmaceutical, and biopharmaceutical coffers.

The Affordable Care Act

Nowhere has the adaptation of the health industry been more obvious than in the largest instance of healthcare reform since the passage of Medicare and Medicaid in 1965. Democratic victories in 2008 opened a unique political window, but the desire for an Obama administration 'achievement' arguably outpaced the substantive outcomes of reform. In this sense, the administration retained 'the prime directive of [post-Clinton] health reform: do not disturb the existing insurance system and the already insured', and ensured 'various formidable interests –insurers, employers, the medical care industry, and states – were invested in the prevailing order' (Oberlander 2016: 804–5). The administration was able to bring onside all major players in the health industry, but its 'surrender-in-advance' strategy would certainly come with costs (Geyman 2017: 8). During this process, industrial actors were able to build their interests directly into the makeup of the ACA, ensuring that the systemic features of US healthcare would not only be preserved, but new markets and regulatory protections could also be created.

This began with the pharmaceutical and hospital industries, from which political support and some resources were extended, at a price. The MMA's prohibition on government involvement in price leveraging or formularies was extended into the legislation. Well aware that a government-driven, enlarged healthcare market would translate into more patients/customers, these industries 'limited the law's ability to deliver tangible benefits to the middle-class and largely took off the table tools of cost control used in other nations, such as provider rate-setting and government negotiation of drug prices' (Hacker 2010: 865). Once again, drug prices have accelerated under the ACA, particularly in recent years, and this is especially true in the most utilized prescription drug classes (Norman and Karli-Smith 2016).

The most important impact of the ACA, however, was on the insurance industry. The Act was designed for minimal disruption of the existing insurance system, but it then created a mechanism to extend private coverage to a substantial portion of the population that would otherwise not have access. In part, this came about through more generous Medicaid qualifications, but it also expanded the individual insurance market and employment-based (private) insurance requirements for companies of 50 employees or more. The *quid-pro-quo* was straightforward: coverage for 'riskier' beneficiaries, with less purchasing power, required an 'individual mandate' that would make health insurance legally compulsive, thereby expanding the pool of paying customers. Indeed, the prospect of any real free market 'worried private insurers who [...] feared that millions of young, healthy and/or low-income people would pay [any weak] penalty and skip coverage. They wanted *more government regulation*, and a *stronger mandate*, not less' (Lichtenstein 2017: 127, emphasis added). To foster this scenario, AHIP rejected a potential public insurance option, instead securing government subsidies on private insurance premiums, in order to fulfill the individual mandate, as well as cost-sharing reduction payments for insurance companies participating in the insurance exchanges (Levitt *et al.* 2017).

There is no getting around the reality that the ACA was structured to maintain the complexity and fragmentation of US healthcare that preserves and expands its profoundly accumulative nature (Waitzkin and Hellander 2016). There is, then, little surprise that all industrial parties sought to defend ACA in the face of post-2016 Republican attempts to dismantle it. AHIP made clear that such attempts would, 'destabilize the individual market; cut Medicaid; pull back on protections for pre-existing conditions; not end taxes on health insurance premiums and benefits; and potentially allow government-controlled, single-payer healthcare to grow' (Hellman 2017; Pear 2017). This, of course, not only turns actual Republican wishes on their head, but it also demonstrates the ferocity with which industry defended expanded government-subsidized coverage. When repeal attempts ultimately failed, Republicans turned toward the elimination of the individual mandate. Once again, AHIP invoked the potential for crisis, warning of 'serious consequences if Congress simply repeals the mandate while leaving the insurance reforms in place: millions more will be uninsured or face higher premiums, challenging their ability to access the care they need' (AHIP, AAFP and AHA 2017). In the end, even the powerful healthcare lobby could not forestall Republicans' political urge to somehow make good on nine years of ACA repeal pledges, as the individual mandate fell victim to the very legislative instrument that gave it life: budget reconciliation. The insurance exchanges, however, had taken root, and there has been only a modest drop in participation, with 11.5 million beneficiaries in 2020, even without any compulsive tax enforcement (Henry J. Kaiser Family Foundation 2020).

With its subsidization of the status quo in health coverage, open to price increases and high deductibles, the ACA has turned into a productive terrain for the health industry. Further, while each industrial group within the sector cannot and does not retain fully optimized profitability in the face of the law's volatile political course, there has been a concerted effort across these groups to capitalize on government spending while minimizing their own revenue contributions (such as industrial taxes or forced discounts) and market risk. The ACA is not so much government 'meddling', as its loudest critics suggest, but rather a government reassurance to many sectors benefitting from, and seeking to expand, market-oriented health in the US.

Adaptive accumulation and the future of US health

At writing, US political culture has persevered through the Trump administration and its contempt for 'Obamacare', including the rejection of the latest (and probably last) Supreme Court challenge, *California v. Texas* (Luthi 2021). Moreover, 2020–22 has witnessed the worst US health crisis on record, with COVID-19 leading to the death of over one million of its citizens, a health system in disarray, and a politico-economic situation that has grossly divided the nation. In a telescoped manner, COVID demonstrated the harm done to impoverished and racialized communities in an unequal and uneven health and social system (Krutika and Cox 2021). As the virus ebbed and flowed across different US states, the repeated declaration that low-income and racialized groups were bearing the brunt of both morbidity and mortality has provoked a new political debate around the possibilities of social and political reform – in healthcare, if in nothing else.

This new reality has breathed new life into calls for 'Medicare for All', a proposal to expand the domain of Medicare to include larger and larger portions of the population. The benefits of this are undeniable. On the one hand, access to healthcare would increase. On the other hand, its cost – from an overall social perspective – would decline, as a function of massively broadened risk pools; lowered administrative costs; and public leverage over the upward march of provision costs. Indeed, its current legislative form has been 'scored' with an overall drop in healthcare costs of US$650 billion (Gaffney *et al.* 2021). On the issue of inequalities, so clearly revealed during the COVID pandemic, universal and equitable healthcare access will not solve every social ill, but it will go some distance toward mitigating one of the most trenchant stress points traversing racial, gender, and class inequalities in America. In the immediate wake of COVID-19, frequently conducted polling places support for a publicly funded healthcare system above 70 percent (Michels 2021). Critically, however, the devil is in the details: more than half of those polled feel that such a system would not require them to relinquish their private insurance plans (Altman 2021). This inconsistency reflects overall confusion in a healthcare system that is unnecessarily, but strategically, complicated. Industrial actors, of course, prey on this inconsistency to resist any potential changes toward a universally-funded, public system.

In this regard, the difficulty of the path to be forged ahead in American health delivery could not be more apparent. Industry, having pushed the limits of profit accumulation through MA, MpD, and the ACA, will forcefully advocate for a system in which the competitive market mechanisms within these programs are validated, while government subsidization expands progressively, always avoiding markets deemed of little value. In this, there is perfect consistency in the industrial call for *both* an expansion of the healthcare exchange markets *and* enhanced Medicaid funding, because the latter 'cleans up' the inevitable adverse selection in healthcare purchasing, and thereby mitigating negative associations with industry. In the end, of course, this is far more expensive for society. A recent study of private coverage *versus* Medicaid costs concluded that, 'overall healthcare spending was more than 80 percent higher among Marketplace-eligible adults than among Medicaid-eligible adults' (Allen *et al.* 2021: 9). This included '10-fold higher out-of-pocket costs for low-income enrollees', despite the fact that claims of higher quality care in private plans found little-to-no evidentiary corroboration.

Political momentum toward Medicare for All has certainly built beyond previous expectations. However, arrangements under adaptive accumulation will not be relinquished without a colossal fight from the health industry, which deployed record lobbying of $615 million in 2020 (Evers-Hillstrom 2021). In the context of COVID-19, the insurance industry has already demanded and won increased subsidies to both COBRA premiums (allowing people to keep private, employer-based plans after termination) and individual market premiums, while it has further insisted on stabilization of funding for Medicare Advantage plans, with an extra emphasis on MpD (AHIP 2020). There can be no doubt that industry – from insurance to hospitals to pharmaceuticals – seeks to avoid the potential demonstration effect of government-run programs (except for the extremely impoverished). From this perspective, Medicare for All constitutes the worst of all outcomes, as the industry's fights against state-based public payer models in Michigan, Washington, Colorado, and California make abundantly clear (Michels 2021; Rock 2021; Wilkins 2021).

Scaled-down proposals also draw fire from industry and its supporters, such as dropping the eligibility age of Medicare to 60 or 55, even though the effects on market provision remain unclear. Will new enrollees have access to Medicare Advantage, or will they be limited to traditional Medicare? How would either differential access or complete reversion to TM be sold politically? Both of these questions offer obvious points of vulnerability for AHIP, PhRMA, and the AHA to exploit during any future politico-legislative process. Additionally, the seemingly endless quest for the so-called 'public option' is likely to fare no better. Were such an option to emerge within ACA coverage, surrounded by market provision, it would possess no particular purchasing leverage, and its inevitable orientation toward higher risk pools would render its appearance costly and bloated. It will, in other words, be low-hanging fruit for conservatives and the health industry, who will use it as an example of why government should not be allowed to 'take away your healthcare choices'. Perhaps the only bright spot in the current state of affairs is the inclusion of very limited MpD price negotiation for select pharmaceuticals in the *Inflation Reduction Act of 2022* (Bunis 2022). While this Act presents a progressive timetable for expanded negotiations from 2026, the PhRMA is very unlikely to accept this implementation process without political struggle, and much will hinge on congressional and presidential electoral outcomes.

Ultimately, any realistic assessment of healthcare reform in the US steers us toward an all-or-nothing conclusion. Either there is a sea-change in at least purchasing (a single-payer system), where either government or regulated non-profit associations take the helm, or market provision and adaptive accumulation will continue to rule the day. Corporate actors, along with policymakers of all stripes, have proven adept at creating a complicated labyrinth of purchasers and providers, where the possibilities for commercial intervention abound. Moreover, once in place, the notion of selectively 'taking away' citizens' existing commercial healthcare plans, whatever their actual efficacy, will prove to be a political dead-end.

References

AHIP. 2020, 'Letter to Mitch McConnel, Nancy Pelosi, Chuck Shumer, and Kevin McCarthy', 3 December, accessed 31 August 2021, <ahip.org/wp-content/uploads/AHIP-BCBSA-Leg-Rec-12.3.20.pdf>.

AHIP, AAFP and AHA. 2017, 'Letter to congressional leadership', 14 November, accessed 20 March 2020, <ahip.org/wp-content/uploads/2017/11/IM-Coalition-Letter-11_14_2017.pdf>.

Albo, G. 2005, 'Contesting the "new capitalism"', in Coates, D. (ed), *Varieties of Capitalism, Varieties of Approaches*, Palgrave Macmillan, London, pp. 63–82.

Allen, H., Gordon, S.H., Lee, D., Bhanja, A. and Sommers, B.D. 2021, 'Comparison of utilization, costs, and quality of medicaid vs subsidized private health insurance for low-income adults', *Journal of the American Medical Association Network Open*, 4(1), pp. 1–13.

Altman, D. 2021, 'Even supporters may not understand medicare for all', *Axios*, 2 March, accessed 9 January 2022, <axios.com/bernie-sanders-supporters-medicare-for-all-44b8e5bd-45b6-4a91-bcb9-856265b48706.html?utm_source=newsletter&utm_medium=email&utm_campaign=newsletter_axiosvitals&stream=top>.

Béland, D. and Waddan, A. 2010, 'The politics of social policy change: Lessons of the Clinton and Bush presidencies', *Policy and Politics*, 38(2), pp. 217–33.

Berkowitz, E.D. 2010, 'The scenic road to nowhere: Reflections on the history of national health insurance in the United States', *The Forum*, 8(1), pp. 1–20.

Berkowitz, E.D. 2017, 'Getting to the affordable care act,' *Journal of Policy History*, 29(4), pp. 519–42.

Bunis, D. 2022, *How Medicare Price Negotiations Work Under New Law*, AARP, accessed 20 October 2022, <https://www.aarp.org/politics-society/advocacy/info-2022/medicare-drug-price-negotiations.html>.

Burns, A. and Hayford, T. 2017, *Effects of Medicare Advantage Enrollment on Beneficiary Risk Scores*, Congressional Budget Office, Washington, accessed 19 September 2021, <https://www.cbo.gov/system/files/115th-congress-2017-2018/workingpaper/53270-workingpaper.pdf>.

Brown, J., Duggan, M., Kuziemko, I. and Woolston, W. 2014, 'How does risk selection respond to risk adjustment? New evidence from the Medicare advantage program', *American Economic Review*, 104(10), pp. 3335–64.

Christainsen, G.B. 1993, 'What Keynes really said to Hayek about planning', *Challenge*, 36(4), pp. 50–3.

Evers-Hillstrom, K. 2021, 'Healthcare interests, restaurants among COVID relief bill winners', Center for Responsive Ethics, 11 March, accessed 10 April 2021, <opensecrets.org/news/2021/03/covid-relief-bill-winners/>.

Gaffney, A., Himmelstein, D. and Woolhander, S. 2021, 'Congressional budget office scores medicare-for-all: Universal coverage for less spending', *Health Affairs Blog*, 16 February, accessed 10 April 2021, <healthaffairs.org/do/10.1377/hblog20210210.190243/full/>.

Geyman, J. 2017, 'Crisis in U.S. healthcare: Corporate power still blocks reform', *International Journal of Health* Services, 48(1), pp. 5–27.

Giaimo, S. and Manow, P. 1999, 'Adapting the welfare state', *Comparative Political Studies* 32(8), pp. 967–1000.

Haberkorn, J. and Norman, B. 2013, 'CMS reverses course on cuts', *Politico*, 3 April, accessed 1 March 2021, <https://politico.com/story/2013/04/insurance-medicare-advantage-cuts-health-care-089569>.

Hacker, J. 2004 'Privatizing risk without privatizing the welfare state: The hidden politics of social policy retrenchment in the United States', *American Political Science Review*, 98(2), pp. 243–60.

Hacker, J. 2008, *The Divided Welfare State: The Battle Over Public and Private Social Benefits in the United States*, Cambridge University Press, Cambridge.

Hacker, J. 2010, 'The road to somewhere: Why health reform happened', *Perspectives on Politics*, 8(3), pp. 861–76.

Hellman, J. 2017, 'Insurer trade group blasts latest ObamaCare repeal bill,' *The Hill*, 20 September, accessed 7 April 2021, <thehill.com/policy/healthcare/351592-insurer-trade-group-opposes-latest-obamacare-repeal-bill>.

Henry J. Kaiser Family Foundation. 2016, 'Medicare Part D in 2016 and trends over time', 16 September, accessed 9 March 2019, <kff.org/medicare/report/medicare-part-d-in-2016-and-trends-over-time/>.

Henry J. Kaiser Family Foundation. 2017a, '10 essential facts about Medicare and prescription drug spending', 20 November, accessed 9 March 2019, <kff.org/infographic/10-essential-facts-about-medicare-and-prescription-drug-spending/>.

Henry J. Kaiser Family Foundation. 2017b, 'The medicare Part D prescription drug benefit', 2 October, accessed 9 March 2019, <kff.org/medicare/fact-sheet/the-medicare-prescription-drug-benefit-fact-sheet/>.

Henry J. Kaiser Family Foundation. 2020, 'Marketplace enrollment, 2014-2020, state health facts', accessed 20 March 2020, <kff.org/health-reform/state-indicator/marketplace-enrollment/?currentTimeframe=0&so rtModel={"colId": "Location", "sort": "asc"}>.

Himmelstein, D.U., Woolhander, S., Almberg, M. and Fauke, C. 2018, 'The US healthcare crisis continues: A data snapshot', *International Journal of Health Services*, 48(1), pp. 28–41.

Hoadley, J.F., Cubanski, J. and Neuman, P. 2015, 'Medicare's Part D drug benefit at 10 Years: Firmly established but still evolving', *Health Affairs*, 34(10), pp. 1682–7.

Hoffman, B. 2010, 'The challenge of universal healthcare', in Banaszak, H.J., Levitsky, S. and Zald, M. (eds), *Social Movements and the Transformation of American Healthcare*, Oxford Scholarship Online, Oxford, pp. 39–49.

Jennings, K. 2015, 'Nonprofit insurers lose on medicare under new Obamacare rules', *Politico*, 19 August, accessed 21 November 2021, <https://politico.com/states/new-york/albany/story/2015/08/nonprofit-insurers-lose-on-medicare-under-new-obamacare-rules-000000>.

Kelly, A.S. 2016, 'Boutique to booming: Medicare managed care and the private path to policy change', *Journal of Health Politics, Policy and Law*, 41(3), pp. 315–54.

Kronick, R. 2017, 'Projected coding intensity in medicare advantage could increase medicare spending by $200 billion over ten years', *Health Affairs*, 36(2), pp. 320–7.

Krutika, A. and Cox, C. 2021, 'COVID-19 pandemic-related excess mortality and potential years of life lost in the U.S. and peer countries', *Kaiser Family Foundation*, Health Tracker Brief, 7 April, accessed 10 May 2021, <healthsystemtracker.org/brief/covid-19-pandemic-related-ex...1of102021-04-27>.

Levitt, L., Cox, C. and Claxton, G. 2017, 'The effects of ending the Affordable Care Act's cost-sharing reduction payments', *The Henry J. Kaiser Family Foundation*, 25 April, accessed 9 March 2019, <kff.org/health-reform/issue-brief/the-effects-of-ending-the-affordable-care-acts-cost-sharing- reduction-payments/>.

Lichtenstein, N. 2017, 'Who killed Obamacare?' *Dissent*, 64(2), pp. 121–9.

Luhti, S. 2021, 'The Supreme Court saved Obamacare. Now supporters want Biden to fix the law', *Politico*, 24 June, accessed 27 March 2022, <https://www.politico.com/news/2021/06/24/supreme-court-obamacare-law-495755>.

Loeppky, R. 2014, *Accumulation and Constraint: Biomedical Development and Advanced Industrial Health*, Fernwood, Halifax.

Loeppky, R. 2019, 'The real meaning of "managed care": Adaptive accumulation and U.S. health care', *International Journal of Health Services*, 49(4), pp. 733–53.

McGuire, T.G., Newhouse, J.P. and Sinaiko, A.D. 2011, 'An economic history of medicare Part C', *Milbank Quarterly*, 89(2), pp. 289–332.

Medicare Prescription Drug, Improvement, and Modernization Act of 2003, Public Law 108–173, US Statutes At Large 117.

Michels, J. 2021, 'Winning Medicare for all would have massive implications beyond healthcare', *Jacobin Magazine*, 31 March, accessed 19 September 2022, <jacobinmag.com/2021/03/medicare-for-all-citizens-guide-health-care>.

Newhouse, J.P., Price, M., McWilliams, J.M., Hsu, J. and McGuire, T.G. 2015, 'How much favorable selection is left in medicare advantage?' *American Journal of Health Economics*, 1(1), pp. 1–26.

Norman, B. 2014, 'Ad blitz to preempt medicare cuts', *Politico*, 14 January, accessed 21 December 2021, <https://politico.com/story/2014/01/insurance-industry-ads-medicare-cuts-102158>.

Norman, B. and Karli-Smith, S. 2016, 'The one that got away: Obamacare and the drug industry', *Politico*, 13 July, accessed 21 December 2021, <politico.com/story/2016/07/obamacare-prescription-drugs-pharma-225444>.

Oberlander, J. 2007, 'Through the looking glass: The politics of the medicare prescription drug, improvement, and modernization act', *Journal of Health Politics, Policy and Law*, 32(2), pp. 187–219.

Oberlander, J. 2016, 'Implementing the affordable care act: The promise and limits of healthcare reform', *Journal of Health Politics, Policy and Law*, 41(4), pp. 803–26.

OECD. 2019, *Health at a Glance 2019: OECD Indicators*, accessed 1 April 2021, <https://www.oecd-ilibrary.org/social-issues-migration-health/health-at-a-glance-2019_4dd50c09-en>.

OECD. 2021, *Health Spending (Indicator)*, OECD Data Online, accessed 11 June 2021, <https://www.oecd-ilibrary.org/social-issues-migration-health/health-spending/indicator/english_8643de7e-en>.

Osborn, J. 2017, 'Repealing and replacing' Obamacare: Whatever you do, preserve medicare Part D and fill the donut hole', *Forbes*, 17 January, accessed 9 April 2021, <forbes.com/sites/johnosborn/2017/01/13/repealing-replacing-obamacare-whatever-you-do-preserve-medicare-part-d-and-fill-the-donut-hole/3/#3792b83c4d53>.

Pear, R. 2017, 'Insurers come out swinging against new republican healthcare bill', *New York Times*, 20 September, accessed 21 March 2021, <nytimes.com/2017/09/20/us/politics/insurers-oppose- obamacare-repeal.html>.

Rahman, M., Keohane, L., Trivedi, A.N. and Mor, V. 2015, 'High-cost patients had substantial rates of leaving medicare advantage and joining traditional medicare', *Health Affairs*, 34(10), pp. 1675–81.

Rao, B. and Hellander, I. 2014, 'The widening U.S. healthcare crisis three years after the passage of 'Obamacare', *International Journal of Health Services,* 44(2), pp. 215–32.

Rock, J. 2021, 'The fight for healthcare for all is opening up in the States', *Jacobin Magazine*, 19 April, accessed 7 April 2022, <jacobinmag.com/2021/04/public-option-health-care-biden-washington-colorado>.

Roy, A. 2012, 'Why closing Medicare's 'donut hole' is a terrible idea', *Forbes*, 23 May, accessed 7 April 2022, <forbes.com/sites/theapothecary/2012/05/23/why-closing-medicares-donut-hole-is-a-terrible-idea/#506b87a0563>.

Starr, P. 2013, *Remedy and Reaction: The Peculiar American Struggle Over Health Care Reform*, Yale University Press, New Haven.

Swenson, P. and Greer, S. 2002, 'Foul weather friends: Big business and healthcare reform in the 1990s in historical perspective', *Journal of Health Politics, Policy and Law*, 27(4), pp. 605–38.

Volsky, I. 2014, 'Obama makes surprise reversal on Obamacare', *Think Progress*, accessed 8 April 2021, <https://thinkprogress.org/obama-makes-surprise-reversal-on-obamacare-f8214392f8d2/>.

Waitzkin, H. and Hellander, I. 2016, 'Obamacare: The neoliberal model comes home to roost in the United States – If we let it', *Monthly Review*, 68(1), pp. 1–18.

Wilkins, B. 2021, 'With California single-payer bill shelved, advocates call on Newsom to take lead on Medicare for all', *Common Dreams*, 23 April, accessed 10 May 2021, <commondreams.org/news/2021/04/23/california-single-payer-bill-shelved-advocates-call-newsom-take-lead-medicare-all>.

33

THE NEW HEALTH POLITICS OF AUSTERITY IN EUROPE

Scott L. Greer and Margitta Mätzke

Citizens of the European Union are mostly proud of their countries' commitment to universal healthcare access, and Europe has most of the world's most effective and globally admired health systems. European healthcare systems are also often integrated with extensive and generous welfare state and labor market systems. This, in turn, attenuates the link between healthcare and personal assets or labor market income that shapes health and social prospects in much of the rest of the world. Conversely, while the proliferation of austerity in Europe has often been presented as an agenda of realizing efficiency gains, we know after a generation of such policies that it is, at its core, a challenge to universalism and integrated social protection. This chapter explains the effects of austerity on governance and social cohesion as institutionalized in European health systems.

First, we discuss the organizational form. The names of two European leaders – Bismarck and Beveridge – were appropriated by social scientists as ideal types for health system design: specifically, Social Health Insurance and National Health Service systems. These two organizational forms are interesting dependent variables, reflecting different health and welfare politics. In particular, they reflect the interaction between parties, interest group politics, and state structures during the latter half of the Twentieth Century, when modern welfare states took on their basic shapes. They are also independent variables, shaping interest groups, healthcare practice, policy tools, and the interactions of health with other political institutions such as federalism or social partnership.

In turn, contrary to claims of decentralization or markets and New Public Management, we argue that systems across Europe are actually converging on increased state claims of authority at the expense of power-sharing arrangements and intermediate organizational layers, such as regional offices, social insurance funds, or professional associations. State intervention in health systems is shifting from constitutive to directive – that is, from setting rules of the game, formally or informally, to directing health systems to do particular things.

We then trace policy developments and the evolution of health system governance during the 'age of permanent austerity' (Pierson 2001; Streeck and Schäfer 2013). Since the 1990s, we have seen convergence of health system governance, and discussion about what kind of convergence is happening and how it relates to the distributional struggles about and within health systems. One of the victims of austerity is diversity in health system governance. The great variety of power-sharing arrangements and dispersed authority in regulating and administering healthcare has given way to a more important role of central governments. We find central governments,

DOI: 10.4324/9781003017110-37

claiming authority, assuming control and responsibility in healthcare delivery, notwithstanding public pronouncements of autonomy and diversity, and idiosyncratic manifestations of the shared trend. Finally, we discuss the unusual and changing EU role in public health policies and politics.

Taxonomies and ideal types

We distinguish between healthcare and public health systems. Healthcare is related to curative medical attention in all its complexity, including finance, payment systems, management, professional organization, and workforce. Public health, in contrast, is a broader and more cross-nationally varied field that deploys public power and expertise to manage risks to health, whether through health education, surveillance, or microbiology. The two systems will constantly intersect, with border conflicts and cooperation of all sorts, but they will also ebb and flow with threats to health, interest groups, and state finances.

There is an established and internationally influential pair of archetypes for healthcare financing: the National Health Service (NHS) and Social Health Insurance (SHI) models (Evans and Stoddart 1990; Freeman 2000; Evans 2002). In the first, healthcare is provided or contracted by the state, and funded primarily out of general taxation and through the budget. In the second, the key healthcare financing mechanism is a social insurance fund that charges payroll taxes as the main form of healthcare, and then sets fixed prices in negotiations with providers.

For many purposes, ownership is a distinction without a difference. The actual ownership of healthcare facilities and provision of healthcare does not follow from either funding model. Neither does the universality, equity, or efficiency of the system. What matters is that each system has the essential requirements for a functional healthcare system: universality, price controls, and effective monopsony (White 2013). To the extent that any one of these characteristics is weakened, the result tends to be a worse value or lower-performing health system; if they are too weak, the result is a wasteful and inequitable situation rife with cost- and blame-shifting, such as that which prevails in the US.

However, below that level, the type of the healthcare system is a dependent variable for many other things. The development of universal healthcare systems is often a fascinating political story, involving a mixture of path dependency, party ideology, critical junctures such as war and democratization, diffusion of the models in international policy conversations and, above all, intricate interest group politics (Mätzke 2011). Thus, for example, it is plausible that the SHI systems were often the ones in which doctors won the most complete victory, while NHS systems were found in less consensual or new democracies that could make more drastic policy decisions at the expense of powerful medical lobbies (Baldwin 1992; Immergut 1992).

The type of health system, as well as the particular health system in all its complexity, is also an independent variable in many ways. The type of system encodes particular actors, such as unions, professional associations, and governments in different positions of power and structural relationships. To illustrate how system types can be an independent variable in policy research, consider federalism (Greer 2017; Greer and Elliott 2019). The study of health policy and federalism looks quite different in Bismarckian and Beveridgean systems. In Bismarckian systems, the logic of social insurance and its norms of redistribution and broad solidarity are held to be separate from the financial constitutions of federal systems – that is, the logic of fiscal federalism. Social insurance is often tied to the development and the fate of the nation-state and the consolidation of federal policy capacity. This is so even when much of the organizational structure and informal networks that govern the healthcare and, especially, hospital sectors is organized territorially, as in Austria (Mätzke and Stöger 2015), or where there is a substantial private or regional government role in organizing and even owning healthcare provision, as in Germany (Mätzke 2013; Pamphilis *et al.* 2019). The result is that Bismarckian systems, from the perspective of federalism, provide almost no territorially useful data and only sporadic interactions with the federal structure of public finances. Emblematically, a study of all OECD federations found no social insurance model countries that supplied useful data at a territorial level (Greer and Elliott 2019).

Indeed, it is easy to see why people invested in a social insurance system rooted in individual or occupational logics would prefer that its territorial dimensions be invisible. We all know that the German social insurance system redistributes from the richer and healthier south to the sicker and poorer east. Yet, given the polemics around that redistributive pattern in the policy sectors where it is visible, why would anybody involved in the social insurance system care to make it clear just how much money is moving (Pamphilis *et al.* 2019)? This was confirmed by the German Federal Constitutional Court in 2005, when southern German *Bundesländer* complained about solidaristic health legislation that unduly (from their perspective) impaired their finances by systematically redistributing from the south to the east of Germany within the social insurance system (Mätzke 2013: 202). In contrast, in Beveridgean systems – be they Canada, the UK, Spain, or Italy – subnational governments are largely responsible for the organization and finance of healthcare. Much of intergovernmental politics and policy revolves around these issues. It is hard to hide revenues, expenditures, and intergovernmental transfers in decentralized NHS systems, which is why health policies and expenditures are constantly on the agenda in their intergovernmental debates (Greer *et al.* 2022).

Finally, the type of health system shapes the kind of analysis scholars must perform. For example, it is very easy to have a communication breakdown in conversations across systems, because the set of policy instruments in NHS and SHI systems is quite different. In the latter, the state traditionally plays a *constitutive* role: setting the rules of the game through statutes and, perhaps, subsidies (Feeley 2012). The result is that the policy instruments tend to be laws and sometimes budgets. If, for example, a government in a social insurance system wishes to introduce Health Technology Assessment, it must not simply create the institution, but then also either persuade social partners to use its findings or legislate that they must (Löblová 2016). In contrast, in an NHS model system, it is possible to create an agency and then inform managers that they must respond to it; the obstacles will be practical and organizational rather than legal or legislative (Williams 2013). Much public policy in NHS systems looks like management reorganizations or interventions to those used to the legislative focus of a SHI system, primarily because there are few obstacles to reorganization within the structure of the healthcare system (Hacker 2004). This is why work that tries to track health policy changes by focusing on legislation faces fewer methodological challenges in SHI systems than in NHS systems (*e.g.* Immergut *et al.* 2021)

Even if the outcomes were identical, the different institutional structures and legacies mean that the systems look and work differently, and have different politics. Health systems analysts often focus on big issues such as the provision of money and workforce, cost as a proportion of GDP, or access. These are important, but if we are to understand the workings of systems, we should still understand these types and their evolution.

Health system convergence on what?

There are many authors who have argued that distinguishing health system types is becoming less useful as health systems evolve and converge (*e.g.* Schmid *et al.* 2010), such that analysts should instead focus on conceptual issues such as risk pooling and access (Kutzin *et al.* 2016). Yet, what are they converging on? There are a variety of answers – from diversity in funding sources, to increased focus on primary care, to a blurring of NHS and SHI models, to broader claims about marketization and neoliberalism. Such accounts tend to be not entirely compelling – in part, because established health systems only change slowly and, in part, because it is easy to confuse rhetoric and action in health reforms (evidence for a shift toward primary care dominance or focus on reducing health inequalities is especially hard to find) (Lynch 2020).

The thread that ties together contemporary trends of convergence in Europe is not so much attitudes toward markets or healthcare models. Instead, it is state power, claimed at the expense of intermediate bodies such as professions or local governments, and exercised through a variety of technocratic, market, or other mechanisms. In particular, it is important to note that 'market' reforms in healthcare often involve highly artificial markets designed and constantly manipulated by governments (*e.g.* through setting tariffs or changing regulatory priorities).

The driving force of these convergent trends is austerity. Broadly, the mechanism that we identify pictures governments, once they have extended universal coverage to a population, immediately becoming the target of extensive interest group lobbying and public interest, while also having to trade-off healthcare expenditures against everything else, from defense to tax cuts to schools. At its core, distributional politics drive central governments deeper into the micro-management of healthcare systems. As healthcare budgets show inflationary propensities, governments are recurrently faced with a choice: contain costs and risk (often justified) accusations that they are diminishing the quality and accessibility of healthcare, or increase expenditure, which might reduce health sector complaints, but involves trading-off some other interest. Wishing to escape this trap, health and finance ministers alike are a perfect audience for policy advocates, management thinkers, technologists, consultants, and others, who offer a way out of the cost-quality tradeoff by reorganizing some aspect of healthcare delivery.

The list of policies that promise to ease or change the cost-quality tradeoff is endless. Some of the most salient include the following: co-payments (reducing putatively needless patient demand); health informatics (increasing the legibility of the system to policymakers while avoiding duplication); managerial approaches of shifting control from professionals to paid expert managers; internal markets (purchaser-provider splits and strategic purchasing); tariff or diagnosis-related group (DRG) fixed-price systems, or more complex value-based purchasing models (which promise to use economic incentives to improve efficiency); privatization; use of contracts; health technology assessment; and complex workforce or skill mix policies. The rhetoric around these can be quite different, but the basic argument they share is that they will allow policy-makers to change the way health systems operate to increase efficiency without being blamed for worsened quality and access.

Each of these policies entails centralization in that it diminishes the role of intermediate institutional layers between the central government and the organizations that had been important in managing health systems, including organized professions, social insurance funds, and territorial management units such as NHS regions. These policies amount to government claims of authority over healthcare at the expense of intermediate bodies. This is more widely recognized in comparative politics with regard to the SHI systems, which to many scholars seemed self-evidently wasteful, overly complex, and ready for reform (Levy 1999; Wendt *et al.* 2004; Hassenteufel and Palier 2007; Gerlinger and Schmucker 2009). The informal and changing role of intermediate bodies in, for example, the UK NHS systems (Moran 2003; Harrison 2004; Klein 2010) was less widely recognized in the comparative politics literature, which obscured the similarity of the state's increasing claims of authority in both health system types.

These policies claim authority to micro-manage medical practice. Information technology investments create abundant data about what is being done in healthcare systems. Payment system changes, most of which try to add details about exact procedures and diagnoses, create new bureaucracies and shape healthcare in response to government incentives. Health technology assessment competes with doctors in choosing treatments. Reorganizations allow the center to design organizations from scratch, with new lines of accountability and roles. These constant policy initiatives mean that more and more of the healthcare system procedures and outputs become a creature of the government, while the government invests effort in developing more understanding of the system and more intrusive mechanisms of rule.

In particular, both payment systems and health informatics (or other data-gathering enterprises) are important because they purport to make the system more 'legible'. This concept, associated with James C. Scott (1998), emphasizes the importance to states of being able to understand and read their populations – in this case, healthcare systems and their activities. Making social life legible to government, Scott (1998) posits, is almost an innate drive of states, while resisting legibility constitutes a key modality of retaining autonomy (Scott 2009). The most developed area of scholarship that focuses on the role of health IT and payment systems largely confirms that, while their effects are often unexpected, they are serious and sometimes successful investments in making clinical decisions accessible to, and therefore manipulable by, management. The incentives of the latter are, in turn, more easily controlled by policy-makers and researchers, who can enable the state to formulate new policies for the management of healthcare (Timmermans and Berg 2003).

One example of policies that bring together all these strands is the concept of strategic purchasing. In it, we find state claims of authority, ostensible reliance on market and neoliberal thinking, mechanisms that increase central information and ambition and, in most cases, failure. Strategic purchasing is currently being advocated by a variety of international organizations again after a wave of popularity in the 1980s and 1990s (Klasa *et al.* 2018). It was originally developed by Margaret Thatcher's government in England as part of an NHS reform intended to introduce the discipline of competition. It turned primary care doctors into purchasers for their patients, and hospitals into competitive firm-like trusts. The economist who claimed to have originated the idea (and who would later disown most implementations of his idea) argued at different times that the introduction of market mechanisms would lead to both better data and less need for data (Enthoven 1979; Enthoven 1989). In practice, it led to a massive reorganization, which reduced local idiosyncrasy and created a standardized set of contracting mechanisms and organizations that were legible to the center, even if the actual benefits to healthcare efficiency or quality did not impress (Robinson and Le Grand 1993; Powell 1997). Nonetheless, the concept of strategic purchasing spread widely, trailing state claims of authority in its wake. On the one hand, implementing strategic purchasing creates a new and standardized set of data – prices and quantities – organized by the state in DRGs or other tariff schemes, and perhaps crude quality measures, while the legal and organizational work entrenched managers who were at least presumptively responsive to the state. On the other hand, its effects on any identifiable health outcome were, as the English data would have led us to expect, trivial (Klasa *et al.* 2018). The state's claim to be able to structure a market that would undo basic structural features of health system, such as professional power and localism, was largely defeated (Greer *et al.* 2020). Nonetheless, the idea spread widely, adopted in systems as different as the English, Dutch, German, Swedish, and even extending as far as parts of the US.

Strikingly, during the COVID-19 pandemic, most governments in Europe simply muscled their strategic purchasers aside. It turns out that 'strategic purchasing' systems were, for example, unable to cope with the prospect of canceled elective procedures and unusually high ICU utilization. The systems had been set up by governments within a narrow range of assumptions, and governments barely considered using them to respond to a serious crisis. In general, this COVID-19 response showed us how little resilience was built into any system designed on the principles of New Public Management (Sagan *et al.* 2021). In the Coasian sense of 'make versus buy' (Coase 1937), it turned out that systems premised on buying what they needed were often more vulnerable because, in a crisis, they had driven slack out of the system and nobody could or would sell what they wanted.

This analysis stands in contrast to many that see marketization, New Public Management, privatization, or any other neoliberal idea, as being primarily about the relative role of the market and the state, or the public and the private. Without trying to adjudicate definitions of neoliberalism – which is often just a pejorative term – we can argue that the core of neoliberalism is an approach to policy that preferentially supports the use of market mechanisms, and that shows up in public administration as 'New Public Management' (Ban 2016; Offer and Söderberg 2016). The problem with the idea that neoliberalism is predominantly about markets is that it obscures the extent to which markets are creations of state power. There is scarcely a more obvious example of this point than strategic purchasing models in which buyers, sellers, prices, and the product are all constituted by public policy. It is about as far from a Hayekian spontaneous order as we can get.

We can view, in particular, most research in health economics as constitutive of this fallacy. It is popular and well funded, like management consultancy, precisely because it serves the desire of policy-makers for technical and market solutions to distributional problems between sectors (Fourcade 2010). By increasing the legibility of the system and creating new opportunities for policy to intervene, as well as more or less coherent rationales for intervention, health economics could appear to serve this objective, even while its practitioners could personally adhere to egalitarian or libertarian agendas.

Bismarck, Beveridge, and convergence

State claims of authority manifest differently in different health system types, which is testimony to our point that 'type' is an independent variable. That is why illustrative cases can be valuable. NHS and SHI models are also known in the social policy literature as 'Beveridgean' and 'Bismarckian' after leaders involved in their creation. They have long been, effectively, ideal types of the two kinds of welfare states.

England

The UK has four health systems, each of them an NHS model. England makes up around 85 percent of the population, is directly run by the UK government (there is no English government *per se*), and has by far the largest and most politically contentious health system. The other three, in Northern Ireland, Scotland, and Wales, are much stable, and the UK government has shown relatively little interest in their decisions since 1998 (Greer 2016).

To say that English health policy is centralizing might seem puzzling, given that on paper it is extremely centralized, and because UK governments engaged in endless reforms from 1988 onward that tried to make it more like a regulated market and less of a centralized organization. Understanding this paradox requires starting with the baseline of the NHS in the late-1970s. It was a substantially unmanaged organization, with limited information of any kind flowing to the center, and limited central tools to control or plan the activities of the system. Formal centralization was of little use to a government that knew very little of what was happening across the vast and complex NHS. Frustrated with this situation, Margaret Thatcher first introduced a Management Executive that she hoped would make the NHS more closely resemble a big firm – indeed, she took the advice of a supermarket executive on this plan (Greer *et al.* 2016)!

The Management Executive and general management were scarcely implemented when Thatcher pushed ahead to introduce the 'purchaser-provider divide' that would eventually become the globally influential internal market and strategic purchasing model, and that all subsequent governments maintained for England (discussed above). Depending on how we count, after 1989 the English NHS was reorganized at least four times, with another under debate as we write in 2022. That count does not count the creation, reorganization, and abolition of multiple public health, regulatory, quality improvement, inspection, and other agencies, target regimes, and revised payment systems and schemes for integrated care (Ham 2009). All the while, the NHS enjoyed unusual funding under Labour (2000–10), and then one of the biggest periods of austerity in its history under the Conservatives, which is why England faced COVID-19 with among the fewest hospital beds, doctors, and nurses in the OECD (Williams *et al.* 2021). Perhaps all the reorganization meant that the NHS was more efficient than it otherwise would have been, but there are limits to the ability of any system, no matter how reorganized, to do more with less.

England has been one of the world's premier sites for experimentation in healthcare policy for decades now. Almost every policy – from targets to clinical governance, from health technology assessment to tariffs, and from integrated care to skill mix changes – has been adopted and sometimes implemented. This can happen because of the English institutional environment, with a parliamentary system that affords the executive great power and a centralized health service under formal government control. This plethora of policies, many of them announced under the rhetoric of decentralization, shares the common attribute that their implementation and operation increase the claims of the center of authority over others in the healthcare system.

Germany

Bismarckian SHI systems underwent major changes in the two decades around the turn of the millennium, and German healthcare policy development is the cardinal example (Palier 2010). Here, too, while centralization of authority was paramount, this is not the first thing that comes to mind when looking at the country's policy history of the last half-century. Health, after all, is a major part of the public sector, regardless of whether it is marked by corporatist governance (Döhler 1995). Moreover, the principal institutions of social insurance and professional self-government of medical practice have remained fairly stable, while the rhetoric surrounding health reform, if anything, has stressed the benefits of market competition and decentralized decision-making autonomy by individual patients and healthcare providers. That rhetoric emphasized the lineages of the SHI model, which have long been portrayed as institutional 'nodes' (Katzenstein 1987) that put a question mark behind central governments' authority to determine healthcare policies and institutions unilaterally (Mayntz 1990).

Although cost pressures mounted as early as the 1970s, it took roughly two decades of experimentation within the established corporatist model until healthcare cost containment policies substantially altered governance structures and constellations of interests and power in the health system. Starting in 1992, this took the form of experiments with competition and market mechanisms as a means of encouraging cost-conscious behavior in the health system. Accompanied by a rhetoric of micro-regulatory price mechanisms and decentralized decision-making autonomy, most of the reforms of the 1990s relied on centralized organizational structures for securing quality and guaranteeing the population's access to medical care, while simultaneously subjecting self-government institutions and individual health service providers to increasingly detailed rules about the range and quality of medical services (Burau 2007; Gerlinger and Schmucker 2009).

By the 2000s, however, it had become obvious that the simulated market needed hard budget constraints, so quasi-markets as governance tools were complemented by an institutional macro-structure of much tighter central government control over the country's healthcare finances. Public rhetoric about a 'preference for self-government' notwithstanding, this reform trajectory was characterized by a rapidly growing scheme of state-mandated resource transfers between wealthier and poorer public health insurance organizations, and an ever-tightening web of rules and instructions about physicians' practices in treating patients and prescribing drugs. Attempts to gain control of the health budget peaked in 2009 (in a reform enacted in 2007), when social health insurance funds lost their financial autonomy, contribution rates were set by the central government, and the finances of the public health insurance system were consolidated into a system of centralized resource allocation on a risk-adjusted per capita basis (Schroeder and Paquet 2009).

Shortly after this reform came into force in 2009, the Global Financial Crisis became the focus of public interest and captured all political attention. For health insurance, however, this eased cost containment pressures in the short-term, with stimulus packages allowing for reductions in contribution rates. Smaller changes involved increasingly elaborate modalities for setting health insurance contributions, capitation fees, or social compensation for low-income members. A series of reforms during the 2010s consisted of this kind of fine-tuning of money flows into and out of the health fund. Complementing this, the decade saw a number of reforms to improve healthcare delivery and access to healthcare. This legislation often included very specific instructions for the behavior of health system micro-actors, with less austerity in the overall environment. From our perspective, this development is not surprising: to the extent that health policy has changed from a constituent to a directive policy, this is unlikely to change as fiscal pressures ease. This has, indeed, been the situation of Germany's public finances: one of fiscal permissiveness, public perceptions to the contrary notwithstanding. Under these conditions, a weakening of the centralist reform zeal is exactly what we would expect.

The European Union: an ever-closer Union?

In the two countries that epitomize NHS and SHI models examined above, and whose health reformers personified the two models, we see extensive reforms since the 1970s. They were undertaken to contain costs and achieve efficiency gains – that is, they were driven by austerity. Yet, they have not led to a converging trend toward marketization. Contrary to that neoliberal scenario, austerity has enhanced the role of the state. It has boosted the centralization of decision-making, and this amounted to an increasing presence of state claims of authority in the health sector. The logic of distributional decisions within and between sectors has dragged politicians in very different healthcare systems into increasingly elaborate policy designs, increasing demands for legibility in the system, and increasing impatience with the competence of intermediate bodies at every level. The result has been greater state involvement in health system governance. This cuts both ways: healthcare is becoming a central pawn in the pursuits of nation-states, and conversely, the fate of states – their ambitions, the challenges they face, and the resources at their disposal – fully affects the situation, prospects, and institutional development of healthcare systems. Does this development stop at the level of the nation-state, or does the centralizing thrust extend to the supranational level and affect EU health politics as well?

There are many reasons to expect that the EU should not have much of a health policy. One reason is the diversity of healthcare systems: how many problems do health ministers, typically junior members of labor ministries, really have in common? Another is the limited legal basis for explicit health policy in the EU treaties. The latter enumerates the powers of the Union and ties them to specific tasks, such that it is difficult to make policy without a treaty base. The key obstacle has simply been the unwillingness of most member-states to accept serious fiscal redistribution. The reasons are not hard to understand, given that the gap between the GDP of the richest and the poorest member-states makes the EU one of the most internally unequal federations in the world. In most federations, class or other cleavages cross-cut territory, so it is possible to redistribute on grounds of shared nationhood (*e.g.* Germany) or, at least, direct distributional conflict away from the territory (Greer *et al.* 2022). In the EU, distributional conflicts about rich and poor map onto international differences that make appeals to solidarity difficult to sustain, as we saw in the carnival of national stereotyping that accompanied the 2008–12 debt crisis. When the massive internal economic divergences in the EU led to catastrophe, the first reaction of Europe's creditor governments was the construction of an elaborate and largely ineffective 'fiscal governance' system designed to keep countries from running deficits. Only the shock of COVID-19 helped to move them toward an effective, rather than reactive, form of debt mutualization (Greer and Brooks 2020; Greer *et al.* 2022).

Why, then, has *any* European integration in health become a reality? European integration proceeds by a process (known to scholars of integration as 'neofunctionalism') in which integration of one kind – whether it is a policy area or law – creates pressures for integration of another kind (Haas 2004). It also creates opportunities – whether it is to use EU law to deregulate professions, or to share in EU joint purchasing for pharmaceuticals. This is not just a mechanical process; it also depends on European heads of government, ministers, and civil servants becoming increasingly embedded in the EU as a reference point and way of working (Van Middelaar 2013). EU policy tools and constraints come to be second nature for many of them, a feature that was probably reinforced by watching the experience of Brexit (Greer and Laible 2020).

In 2019, therefore, the EU had a limited and largely indirect healthcare policy, which was driven by internal market rules and policies designed to contain deficits in member-states with weaker economies. The EU's powerful court had decided that EU internal market law applied to healthcare, sparking off legal and policy debates that culminated in legislation, intended to prevent disruptive extension of internal market rules to healthcare systems. EU law produced more of a political response than actual market openings in healthcare (Greer and Rauscher 2011a, b). Its public health policies could be thought of as more ambitious, except they were mostly made under other enumerated powers such as consumer protection, agriculture, labor law, and environmental protection. There were some fairly minor public health initiatives built around Article 168 – notably, a European Center for Disease Control and Prevention that would perform well in 2020–22 – but they were not large-scale policies by any standards (Mätzke 2012; Greer and Kurzer 2013).

During the COVID-19 pandemic, member-states – which had mostly restricted the EU to a very basic and contested constitutive role in setting regulations for healthcare markets – instead decided to use the institution as an active agent of intervention in health policy (Brooks *et al.* 2020; Brooks *et al.* 2021; Deruelle and Engeli 2021; Greer *et al.* 2021; Greer *et al.* 2022). Such initiatives expanded both public health and civil protection budgets enormously, and focused on joint purchasing of vaccines and pharmaceuticals as a single bloc. In other words, the EU member-states focused on areas where the logic of insurance (civil protection stockpiles) and size (*e.g.* joint purchasing agreements for vaccines, shared technical capacity, or investment in pharmaceutical production) worked for the larger unit. What is, at the time of writing, less clear is whether the EU can or will start to invest much money in healthcare systems.

A big surprise arising from the COVID-19 pandemic in most contexts around the world is just how little political and policy change it created. The EU stands out for being a case of real change, directly and quickly engendered by the pandemic. The reason might be fairly simple: European integration had outpaced European public health capacity. Faced with a choice of decoupling their tightly integrated economies or further integrating their health policies, member-states agreed on the latter.

Conclusion

This chapter has argued that health, as an expensive good, has been a preoccupation of governments as long as they have been accountable for healthcare access and public health. Delivering accessible healthcare to the population is expensive, but has become an entrenched norm, and it is difficult to take benefits away from populations once they are used to them. Governments, trapped by the tradeoff between good quality universal healthcare and every other potential expenditure or tax cut, become amenable to ideas that might seem managerial, neoliberal, or a top-down directive, but that are basically all about schemes to enlarge the role of the state in healthcare at the expense of intermediate bodies. Do such schemes work? The evidence is, at best, unclear, in part because the objectives are unclear. Do they spill over into 'public health' campaigns that are fundamentally primary prevention? Yes. Do they show the pressure to manage distributional tradeoffs across government by managing the healthcare system more intensively? Yes. Does this political economy lead to greater efficiency, quality, or access to healthcare? That, we cannot say.

References

Baldwin, P. 1992, *The Politics of Social Solidarity: Class Bases of the European Welfare State, 1975–1975*, Cambridge University Press, Cambridge.

Ban, C. 2016, *Ruling Ideas: How Global Neoliberalism Goes Local*, Oxford University Press, Oxford.

Brooks, E., de Ruijter, A. and Greer, S.L. 2020, 'COVID-19 and European Union health policy: From crisis to collective action', in Vanhercke, B., Spasova, S. and Fronteddu, B. (eds), *Social Policy in the European Union: State of Play 2020*, European Social Observatory and European Trades Union Institute, Brussels, pp. 33–52.

Brooks, E., de Ruijter, A. and Greer, S.L. 2021, 'The European Union confronts COVID-19: Another European rescue of the nation-state?', in Greer, S.L., King, E., Peralta, A. and Massard, E. (eds), *Coronavirus Politics: The Politics and Policy of COVID-19*, University of Michigan Press, Ann Arbor, pp. 235–48.

Burau, V. 2007, 'The complexity of governance change: Reforming the governance of medical performance in Germany', *Health Economics, Policy and Law*, 2(4), pp. 391–407.

Coase, R.H. 1937, 'The nature of the firm', *Economica*, 4(16), pp. 386–405.

Deruelle, T. and Engeli, I. 2021, 'The COVID-19 crisis and the rise of the European centre for disease prevention and control (ECDC)', *West European Politics*, 44(5–6), pp. 1376–400.

Döhler, M. 1995, 'The state as architect of political order: Policy dynamics in German health care', *Governance*, 8(3), pp. 380–40.

Enthoven, A.C. 1979, 'Consumer-centred vs. job-centred health insurance', *Harvard Business Review*, 57(1), pp. 141–52.

Enthoven, A.C. 1989, 'What Europeans can learn from Americans', *Health Care Financing Review Annual Supplement*, 1989(suppl), pp. 49–77.

Evans, R.G. 2002, 'Financing health care: Taxation and the alternatives', in Mossialos, E., Dixon, A., Figueras, J. and Kutzin, J. (eds), *Funding Health Care: Options for Europe*, Open University Press, Buckingham, pp. 31–58.

Evans, R.G. and Stoddart, G.L. 1990, 'Producing health, consuming health care', *Social Science and Medicine*, 31(12), pp. 1347–63.

Feeley, M.M. 2012, 'Scheingold's failure: His finest book', in Sarat, A. (ed), *Special Issue: The Legacy of Stuart Scheingold* (*Studies in Law, Politics, and Society*), 59, Emerald Group Publishing Limited, Bingley, pp. 179–98.

Fourcade, M. 2010, *Economists and Societies: Discipline and Profession in the United States, Great Britain and Finance*, Princeton University Press, Princeton.

Freeman, R. 2000, *The Politics of Health in Europe*, Manchester University Press, Manchester.
Gerlinger, T. and Schmucker, R. 2009, 'A long farewell to the Bismarck system: Incremental change in the German health insurance system', *German Policy Studies/Politikfeldanalyse*, 5(1), pp. 3–20.
Greer, S.L. 2016, 'Devolution and health in the UK: Policy and its lessons since 1998', *British Medical Bulletin*, 118(1), pp. 16–24.
Greer, S.L. 2017, 'Health policy and territorial politics: Disciplinary misunderstandings and directions for research', in Detterbeck, K. and Hepburn, E. (eds), *Edward Elgar Handbook of Territorial Politics*, Edward Elgar, Cheltenham, pp. 232–45.
Greer, S.L., Béland, D., Lecours, A. and Dubin, K.A. 2022, *Putting Federalism in its Place: The Territorial Politics of Social Policy Revisited*, University of Michigan Press, Ann Arbor.
Greer, S.L. and Brooks, E. 2020, 'Termites of solidarity in the house of austerity: Undermining fiscal governance in the European Union', *Journal of Health Politics, Policy and Law*, 46(1), pp. 71–92.
Greer, S.L., de Ruijter, A. and Brooks, E. 2021, 'The COVID-19 pandemic: Failing forward in public health', in Riddervold, M., Trondal, J. and Newsome, A. (eds), *Palgrave Handbook of EU Crises*, Palgrave Macmillan, Basingstoke, pp. 747–64.
Greer, S.L. and Elliott, H. (eds) 2019, *Federalism and Social policy: Patterns of Redistribution in Eleven Democracies*, University of Michigan Press, Ann Arbor.
Greer, S.L., Klasa, K. and Van Ginneken, E. 2020, 'Power and purchasing: Why strategic purchasing fails', *The Milbank Quarterly*, 98(3), pp. 975–1020.
Greer, S.L. and Kurzer, P. (eds) 2013, *European Union Public Health Policies: Regional and Global Perspectives*, Routledge, Abingdon.
Greer, S.L. and Laible, J. (eds) 2020, *The European Union After Brexit*, Manchester University Press, Manchester.
Greer, S.L. and Rauscher, S. 2011a, 'Destabilization rights and restabilization politics: Policy and political reactions to European Union health care services law', *Journal of European Public Policy*, 18(2), pp. 220–40.
Greer, S.L. and Rauscher, S. 2011b, 'When does market-marking make markets? EU Health services policy at work in the UK and Germany', *Journal of Common Market Studies*, 49(4), pp. 797–822.
Greer, S.L., Rowland, D. and Jarman, H. 2016, 'The central management of the English NHS', in Exworthy, M., Mannion, R. and Powell, M. (eds), *Dismantling the NHS?: Evaluating the Impact of Health Reforms*, Policy Press, Bristol, pp. 87–104.
Greer, S.L., Rozenblum, S., Fahy, N., Brooks, E., de Ruijter, A., Palm, W.I. and Wismar, M. 2022, *Everything You Always Wanted to Know About European Union Health Policy But Were Afraid to Ask* (3rd ed.), WHO/European Observatory on Health Systems and Policies, Brussels.
Haas, E.B. 2004, *The Uniting of Europe: Political, Social, and Economic Forces, 1950–1957* (3rd ed.), University of Notre Dame Press, Notre Dame.
Hacker, J.S. 2004, 'Reform without change, change without reform: The politics of U.S. health policy reform in cross-national perspective', in Levin, M.A. and Shapiro, M. (eds), *Transatlantic Policymaking in an Age of Austerity: Diversity and Drift*, Georgetown University Press, Washington, DC, pp. 13–63.
Ham, C. 2009, *Health Policy in Britain* (6th ed.), Palgrave Macmillan, Basingstoke.
Harrison, S. 2004, 'Medicine and management: Autonomy and authority in the national health service', in Gray, A. and Harrison, S. (eds), *Governing Medicine: Theory and Practice*, Open University Press, Maidenhead, pp. 51–60.
Hassenteufel, P. and Palier, B. 2007, 'Towards neo-Bismarckian health care states? Comparing health insurance reforms in Bismarckian welfare systems', *Social Policy and Administration*, 41(6), pp. 574–96.
Immergut, E.M. 1992, *Health Politics: Interests and Institutions in Western Europe*, Cambridge University Press, Cambridge.
Immergut, E.M., Anderson, K.M., Devitt, C. and Popic, T. 2021, *Health Politics in Europe: A Handbook*, Oxford University Press, Oxford.
Katzenstein, P. 1987, *Policy and Politics in West Germany: The Growth of a Semisovereign State*, Temple University Press, Philadelphia.
Klasa, K., Greer, S.L. and van Ginneken, E. 2018, 'Strategic purchasing in practice: Comparing ten European countries', *Health Policy*, 155(5), pp. 457–72.
Klein, R. 2010, 'The eternal triangle: Sixty years of the centre-periphery relationship in the national health service', *Social Policy and Administration*, 44(3), pp. 285–304.
Kutzin, J., Yip, W. and Cashin, C. 2016, 'Alternative financing strategies for Universal Health Coverage', *World Scientific Series in Global Health Economics and Public Policy*, 3, pp. 267–309.

Levy, J.D. 1999, 'Vice into virtue? Progressive politics and welfare reform in continental Europe', *Politics and Society*, 27(2), pp. 239–73.

Löblová, O. 2016, 'Three worlds of health technology assessment: Explaining patterns of diffusion of HTA agencies in Europe', *Health Economics, Policy and Law*, 11(3), pp. 253–73.

Lynch, J. 2020, *Regimes of Inequality: The Political Economy of Health and Wealth*, Cambridge University Press, Cambridge.

Mätzke, M. 2011, 'Political competition and unequal social rights', *Journal of Public Policy*, 31(1), pp. 1–24.

Mätzke, M. 2012, 'The institutional resources for communicable disease control in Europe: Diversity across time and place', *Journal of Health Politics, Policy, and Law*, 36(1), pp. 967–76.

Mätzke, M. 2013, 'Federalism and decentralization in German health and social care policy', in Costa i Font, J. and Greer, S.L. (eds), *Federalism and Decentralization in European Health and Social Care*, Palgrave Macmillan, Basingstoke, pp. 190–207.

Mätzke, M. and Stöger, H. 2015, 'Austria', in Fierlbeck, K. and Palley, H.A. (eds), *Comparative Health Care Federalism*, Ashgate, Farnham, pp. 15–29.

Mayntz, R. 1990, 'Politische Steuerbarkeit und Reformblockaden: Überlegungen am Beispiel des Gesundheitswesens', *Staatswissenschaften und Staatspraxis*, 1(3), pp. 283–307.

Moran, M. 2003, *The British Regulatory State*, Oxford University Press, Oxford.

Offer, A. and Söderberg, G. 2016, *The Nobel Factor: The Prize in Economics, Social Democracy, and the Market Turn*, Princeton University Press, Princeton.

Palier, B (ed.) 2010, *A long Goodbye to Bismarck?: The Politics of Welfare Reform in Continental Europe*, Amsterdam University Press, Amsterdam.

Pamphilis, N.M., Singh, S., Jeffery, C. and Slowik, M. 2019, 'Germany: The rise of territorial politics?' in Greer, S.L. and Elliott, H. (eds), *Federalism and Social Policy: Patterns of Redistribution in 11 Democracies*, Unviersity of Michigan Press, Ann Arbor, pp. 147–74.

Pierson, P. 2001, *The New Politics of the Welfare State*, Oxford University Press, Oxford.

Powell, M.A. 1997, *Evaluating the National Health Service*, Open University Press, Maidenhead.

Robinson, R. and Le Grand, J. 1993, *Evaluating the NHS Reforms*, King's Fund Institute, London.

Sagan, A., Webb, E., Azzopardi-Muscat, N., de la Mata, I., McKee, M. and Figueras, J. 2021, *Health Systems Resilience During COVID-19: Lessons For Building Back Better*, European Observatory on Health Systems and Policies, Health Policy Series 56, accessed 21 December 2022, <https://eurohealthobservatory.who.int/publications/i/health-systems-resilience-during-covid-19-lessons-for-building-back-better>.

Schmid, A., Cacace, M., Götze, R. and Rothgang, H. 2010, 'Explaining health care system change: Problem pressure and the emergence of "hybrid" health care systems', *Journal of Health Politics, Policy and Law*, 35(4), pp. 455–86.

Schroeder, W. and Paquet, R. 2009, *Gesundheitsreform 2007: Nach der Reform ist vor der Reform*, VS Verlag für Sozialwissenschaften, Wiesbaden.

Scott, J.C. 1998, *Seeing Like A State: How Certain Schemes to Improve the Human Condition Have Failed*, Yale University Press, New Haven.

Scott, J.C. 2009, *The Art of Not Being Governed*, Yale University Press, New Haven.

Streeck, W. and Schäfer, A. (eds). 2013, *Politics in the Age of Austerity*, Polity Press, Cambridge.

Timmermans, S. and Berg, M. 2003, *The Gold Standard: The Challenge of Evidence-based Medicine and Standardization in Health Care*, Temple University Press, Philadelphia.

Van Middelaar, L. 2013, *The Passage to Europe: How a Continent Became a Union*, Yale University Press, New Haven.

Wendt, C., Grimmeisen, S., Helmert, U., Rothgang, H., Cacace, M. 2004, 'Convergence of divergence of OECD health care systems', TranState Working Papers, No. 9, Universität Bremen, Collaborative Research Center 597 -Transformations of the State, Bremen.

White, J. 2013, 'The 2010 US health care reform: Approaching and avoiding how other countries finance health care', *Health Economics, Policy and Law*, 8(3), pp. 289–315.

Williams, G.A., Rajan, S. and Cylus, J.D. 2021, 'COVID-19 in the United Kingdom: How austerity and a loss of state capacity undermined the crisis response', in Greer, S.L., King, E.J., Massard da Fonseca, E. and Peralta-Santos, A. (eds), *Coronavirus Politics: The Comparative Politics and Policy of COVID-19*, University of Michigan Press, Ann Arbor, pp. 215–34.

Williams, I. 2013, 'Institutions, cost-effectiveness analysis and healthcare rationing: The example of healthcare coverage in the English National Health Service', *Policy and Politics*, 41(2), pp. 223–39.

PART V

Alternative paths toward health and healthcare

34

SOCIAL WELFARE AND ALTERNATIVE FORMS OF HEALTH PROVISION

The UK experience and radical new frontiers

Chris Thomas[1]

The 2007/8 Global Financial Crash engendered a crisis in orthodox economic thinking. Neoclassical economics – defined by Dequech (2008) according to its emphasis on rationality, utility maximization, and equilibrium, but neglect of uncertainty – was demonstrated to be both a poor theoretical explanation of how real economic processes work, and an inadequate source of solutions in the face of a severe crisis. Standing in contrast was a community of economic theories, broadly understood as 'heterodox economics': a conceptual corpus bound by a focus on political economy, examining the 'historical process of social provisioning within the context of a capitalist economy' (Lee 2009: 8–9).

Over a decade after the Financial Crisis (after which many countries pursued austerity policies), three years of the global COVID-19 pandemic, and with inflation and energy prices creating a cost-of-living crisis in many countries, orthodox health economics faces a similar (albeit more nascent) crisis – especially in high-income countries. These orthodox approaches and their codification in neoliberal policy – based on efficient resource allocation of healthcare as a commodity – are failing to meet people's health needs. While gains in life expectancy had not stopped in high-income countries before the pandemic began, they had already slowed markedly (OECD 2021). Some countries were experiencing a reverse rather than stagnation – including the UK and the USA (CDC 2022; King's Fund 2022) – with the OECD (2022) warning the consequences of COVID-19 could mean they are joined by Belgium, Sweden, Italy, Spain, and France. This is indicative of a widespread stalling of gains in both longevity and good health, and a decline in individual and national health security.

In reaction to these increasingly clear limitations in orthodox health economics, a body of research has looked to connect health and healthcare with a clearer understanding of political economy (see also: Thomas 2022a). This literature posits that health is defined by the social, political, and economic structures in which people live. In turn, it has brought into scope the 'social determinants of health' – and implicated our access to public services, the distribution of income and wealth, the nature and availability of work, and the performance of national economies in defining our health (WHO 2022). That is, it accounts for the material conditions in which we live, and how these are defined by society, material conditions, politics, and (intersectional) identity.

DOI: 10.4324/9781003017110-39

This theory of health has had notable successes, including broad adoption by the World Health Organization (WHO).[2] What is missing, however, is a common conception of how this evidence can support a reconceptualization of the role of the state in health creation. To redress this lacuna, the present chapter explores how the state can be reoriented to reflect the political economy of health, with a focus on the welfare state. It focuses on health in England as a case-study – a country with a notably binary view of the role of the state in health creation. On healthcare, the role of the state is broadly understood and rigorously defended. Yet, the mainstream view on the social determinants of health remains defined by belief in a neoliberal conception of individual responsibility. The chapter explores how this divide has emerged; the mechanisms by which the state is kept out of health creation (beyond healthcare); and articulates broader models of the welfare state that could yet offer the means to secure progressive health outcomes.

The evolution of the state's role in healthcare delivery

The notion that the state should be involved in the (universal, free) delivery of healthcare is a relatively recent invention (Gaffney 2018). In the specific case of the UK, its evolution can be traced from the Nineteenth Century.

During the 1800s, public health provision was largely administered by the New Poor Law (the *Poor Law Amendment Act 1834*). This governance mechanism offered only very limited, and often reluctant, provision to the poor, and was often subject to abuse (Brown 2017). The role of the state in delivering healthcare rapidly accelerated during the Twentieth Century, marked by two key moments: first, Prime Minister David Lloyd George's *Ministry of Health Act* (1919) and, second, the creation of the National Health Service (NHS) under Prime Minister Clement Atlee (1948). It is, perhaps, no coincidence that both quickly followed the conclusion of the two World Wars, during which time the socio-economic consequences of poor health had become clear as the state struggled to recruit healthy, fighting men, and was forced to deliver more healthcare services directly – both in the field and at home.

The Ministry of Health – the country's first national department for health – was formed as a direct consequence of the experience and challenges of providing healthcare during World War One. Having struggled with coordination and consistency of healthcare services, Lord Rhondda initially proposed a state Ministry of Health in 1917 – a recommendation eventually accepted and implemented in 1919. It formally brought New Poor Law healthcare provision, national insurance schemes, midwifery, public health, and school health programs into the function of national government (see: Parliament 1917).

Of course, it is the NHS that represents the more famous and extensive formalization of the role of the state in healthcare provision. It transitioned the role of the state from constituting a partial funder and overseer of healthcare, to providing direct and universal care. Under a broader expansion of welfare during the first Atlee Ministry (1945–50), Nye Bevan's system was founded on a commitment to the state providing a healthcare regime that is (i) free at the point of delivery, (ii) based on need, (iii) funded by general taxation, and (iv) publicly owned. Accordingly, Bevan's concept was a healthcare service where the state would provide a permanently preferable option to the market, through a commitment to 'universalizing the best'. That is, unlike many other components of the UK welfare state – including social security – the NHS would not compromise on quality or means-test people. Instead, it would provide the best possible interventions to all who need them.

A narrow and broad definition of health

While not formalized as part of the UK welfare state's 'health offer', both the Lloyd George and Atlee governments recognized health as broader than healthcare. That is, their definition of health encompassed the fact our material circumstances define our health, even before diagnosis. Lloyd George's Ministry for Health (1919) was accorded not only power over hospitals, but also significant powers over local government, housing, air quality, and social security. Similarly, Bevan was jointly Minister for Health and Housing, and envisioned an NHS-style system for social housing as a public service.

However, in both cases, the welfare state was never given formal means to intervene in the social determinants of health, based on the *value of health as a good in its own right*. That is, by restricting their capacity to reshape the broader material conditions shaping health, both initiatives remained limited at state levels to promote greater health outcomes. In turn, these measures have continued to constrain the capacity of the state, in its present form, to act on the 'social determinants of health' or the 'commercial determinants of health'. The former are defined by the WHO (2022) as including:

- Income and social protection
- Education
- Unemployment and job insecurity
- Working life conditions
- Food insecurity
- Housing, basic amenities, and the environment
- Early childhood development
- Social inclusion and non-discrimination
- Structural conflict
- Access to affordable health services of decent quality.

The latter are defined most succinctly by West and Marteau (2013: 686) as 'factors that influence health which stem from the profit motive'. The two categories are non-exclusive – poverty pay and low income, for example, straddle both categories. However, they are equally important in demonstrating the inadequacies of an approach to health creation that only includes a role for the state in *healthcare provision*. Or, to put it another way, we can see the evolution of the role of healthcare in England as embodying only a narrow view of health.

Research within the social sciences has also established a clearer differentiation between narrow and broad definitions of health (*e.g.* Rothstein 2002). As summarized in Table 34.1, the former views good health in medicalized terms as 'the absence of any disease or impairment' (Sartorius 2006: 662). Sickness must be evidenced by the presence of a particular illness. The latter, in contrast, views health as a spectrum of wellbeing – as 'an equilibrium that an individual has established within himself and his social and physical environment'. It defines poor health around the capability and means to live a healthy life, even before a symptom occurs. This distinction provides an alternative means to understand the approach to health by the UK welfare state. It has embodied a narrow comprehension of health, in which the state swings into action through care only once illness or disease has been identified. That is, as expansive as the English NHS might be – and as much as it is often championed as a source of significant pride and progress – it is also innately limited as an approach to meeting health needs. In turn, the third category in

Table 34.1 Conceptualizing state involvement in health creation

Extent of role	*Description*
Narrow	Little state intervention in either health or healthcare – leaving both, to the extent practically possible, to individuals and the market
Broad	More extensive state intervention in healthcare, but less scope for state intervention to meet wider health needs
Broader	More extensive state intervention in healthcare, usually as a provider – combined with extensive means to meet a range of health needs linked to the social and commercial determinants of health

Table 34.1 – constituting a 'broader' role still – will be outlined shortly as an alternative to both the narrow and broad definitions.

Nevertheless, the narrow-broad distinction is a relatively blunt categorization and requires some subjective interpretation. For instance, there are a few areas where the state plays a public health role beyond healthcare delivery – water sanitation, for example. Equally, while health is not core to their *raison d'*être, or even a key component of how they are evaluated, other components of the UK welfare state afford the government capacity to act on the social determinants of health, as outlined below. Judgment on the extent to which the government adopts a narrow or a broad approach, therefore, needs to be determined by how effectively population health needs are met *outside of healthcare*.

Overall, the capacity of the UK state to address the wider health needs of its populace is very poor. Consider, for example, the state's approach to *housing* policy. The *English Housing Survey* (Department for Levelling Up, Housing and Communities 2022) reveals that 10 percent of the UK's housing stock has a 'category 1 hazard', the highest level of public health threat. Over 800,000 households in England are overcrowded. Despite this, the social housing stock is decreasing. In 2021, 29,000 social homes were sold or demolished, but less than 7,000 were built (Shelter 2022). Analogously, the state has failed to address persistent problems of *poverty* in the country. At the time of writing, the Joseph Rowntree Foundation (2022) estimates that more than one in five people in the UK live in poverty. Other research has shown that one in six working households are in poverty – indicating that work does not effectively safeguard people from poverty (McNeil *et al.* 2021). Finally, the state continues to fail to provide sufficient, quality *education* to the populace. Education and the school setting are important predictors of our health through the life course. The *Deaton Review* (Institute of Fiscal Studies 2022) of inequalities points out that education inequalities translate, reliably, to income inequalities – a further determinant of health. The same review finds unequal access to, and success in, the education system:

> [D]espite decades of policy attention, there has been virtually no change in the 'disadvantage gap' in GCSE attainment over the past 20 years […] 16-year-olds who are eligible for free school meals are still around 27 percentage points less likely to earn good GCSEs than less disadvantaged peers.
>
> (Institute for Fiscal Studies 2022: 2)

England is equally poor at acting on the corporate determinants of health. While there has been some painstaking success in limiting the harms of tobacco – with the UK government pledging a tobacco-free future by 2030 – it has struggled in other policy areas. Indicatively, a review in England by Theis and White (2021: 126) found that:

> Obesity policies have been largely proposed in a way that does not readily lead to implementation: that government rarely commission evaluations of previous government strategies or learn from policy failures; that governments have tended to adopt less interventionist policy approaches; and that policies largely make high demands on individual agency.

In other words, there is a paucity of policies to restrict the corporate determinants of health, and the policy that does exist is created in a way that makes real implementation difficult or unlikely.

What limits a more systematic state role in health creation?

The question this begs is: what prevents the state from taking a more active role in health creation in England? The answer to this question cannot be attributed to a lack of levers – there are, equally, institutions, instruments, and discourses that actively guard against an expansion of the state. Put differently, the architecture of government and public commonsense ties us to the small state logic of neoliberalism, even as the health orthodoxy struggles to provide better health or greater health security. At least three factors are particularly important in limiting the role of the state, in this regard.

Personal responsibility

Personal responsibility discourse has a particularly powerful role in culturally delegitimizing the potential for state intervention in health beyond healthcare. Studies repeatedly show that responsibility for health is ultimately perceived to reside with the individual, rather than the state. A 2018 study by the Frameworks Institute showed the responsibility for obesity was intuitively and predominantly assigned to individuals by people interviewed in Southwark and Lambeth (L'Hôte *et al.* 2018). Analysis by the *British Attitudes Survey* from the Health Foundation (2022) showed that 61 percent of individuals thought individuals had a greater responsibility for their own health than the government, with only 9 percent believing that government had a greater responsibility than individuals. This, in turn, reflects a curious dichotomy in the UK. Alongside this emphasis on personal responsibility, an overwhelming majority of the UK public continue to hold that the NHS should be comprehensive and be exclusively delivered by the state. In effect, where the welfare state failed to formalize its role in health creation, a highly neoliberal concept of personal responsibility has emerged – wrapped in a rationalist understanding of human behavior, in a limited role of the state, and in free governance of the self.

What we measure

Gross Domestic Product (GDP) is one of the core instruments of neoliberal economics. While many of its critics still recognize the measurement of output production as useful (see: Coyle 2014), it is the absolute dominance of GDP that is problematic. It suggests that the sole purpose of the economy – and, thus, how it is measured – is defined in terms of ever-increasing production.

GDP supports a welfare model based on a narrow definition of health in two direct ways. First, it takes into account only health activity that formally contributes to GDP. The UK's particular approach to measuring GDP comparatively stresses non-market healthcare activities such as healthcare appointments and prescriptions. This means, at least in the short-term, healthcare activity is good for GDP, but preventative action counter-intuitively reduces the healthcare sector's contribution to this indicator. Second, and worse, GDP also incorporates business activities that harm human health. Even industries with little social value and high health harms – tobacco and gambling, for example – make a strong contribution to GDP. This is regularly cited by lobbyists in making the case that government should avoid regulation and other kinds of intervention in these industries. Combined, these two factors work to strongly disincentivize the role of the state in both providing more preventative intervention on the social determinants of health, and strongly regulating harmful business sectors and activities.

What we value

Another safeguard against a broader role for the state in health creation is the definition of 'value' in public sector and welfare institutions. As Mazzucato and Kattel (2019) (among others) have posited, mainstream economic theory locates value in business – with the role of government, at best, seen as fixing market failures. This logic has extended into our approach to health: the government has a largely reactive role in providing a service handled poorly by the market (healthcare), but not as an active agent in seeking and creating good health as a primary objective. Accordingly, a more capacious state role in health is unlikely until we '[understand] public value [...] as a way of measuring progress towards the achievement of broad and widely accepted societal goals that are agreed on by participatory processes', and which 'can only be achieved through collaboration between both private and public sectors' (Mazzucato and Kattel 2019: 3).

Defining an alternative approach

So far, this chapter has established that the UK welfare state's definition of health is narrow and that this is a choice embedded as mainstream by a combination of discourse and institutions, rather than constituting an inevitable outcome. However, this conclusion not only acts as a critical reflection on the political-economic status quo, but also offers a foundation from which we can begin to imagine a radically different alternative. This imagining constitutes the remainder of this chapter. It does not limit itself to rethinking how the traditional 1940s model of the welfare state can directly provide good health, as important as this is. Building on new political-economic research on the commercial determinants of health (see: Mialon 2020), it also offers reflections on the role of business in securing positive health outcomes. That is, both the welfare state itself and a potentially positive complementary role for business are encompassed in my vision for a more expansive role of the state in health. These two factors will be considered in turn.

The state as a provider (social determinants)

Despite its universal healthcare orientation, the UK has a small public health system. Its scope and funding are both very limited. Between national and local government, the funding for public health services – covering measures such as smoking addiction clinics, childhood health programs, sexual health providers, and mental health at work support – is just £3.417 billion per year, or the equivalent of around 2 percent of the NHS's budget (DHSC 2022). In real terms, this budget is decreasing, with research indicating that cuts are most severe in the especially deprived parts of the country (Thomas 2019, 2020). Despite this small budget, public health interventions are highly successful. Return on investment is particularly strong, with King's Fund (2014) analysis showing that for every £1 invested in sexual health services, there is a return worth £11, while for each £1 spent preventing children from taking up smoking, there is a return worth £15. Another study showed that public health investment is three-to-four times more productive than the same money spent in the NHS (Martin *et al.* 2020).

On delivery, the COVID-19 pandemic showed the comparative quality of this country's public health services – and provided a direct contrast to private sector service delivery. Initially, the UK outsourced its COVID-19 Test and Trace program, with poor results. Later in the process, Test and Trace was more regularly given to public health teams within local government. The success rates were much higher, with contact rates of 90 percent, compared to 60 percent for one outsourced company (Robertson 2020).

Increasingly, there are calls to build on the success of this kind of preventative public health service. Among the most extensive policy calls is for a Universal Public Health Service, run locally and designed to universalize preventative interventions on the social determinants of health. In my book, *The Five Health Frontiers* (Thomas 2022a), I put forward an idea for just such a service, formed around five core activity areas. The first would be *education* – with prescriptions ranging from more money for schools, ring-fenced for specific pupils, to funding for vocational activities and hobbies. The second would be *free, nutritional food* for all who need it – based on a strong, but overlooked, evidence base on the impact of food subsidies in securing positive health outcomes. The third would be *healthy housing*, targeting the extant UK social housing deficit and concomitant overcrowding. The fourth would be financial support for *utilities* – a recommendation proposed before the current, international energy crisis, and which has now been embedded in many high-income countries (albeit not on health grounds, nor to the extent that health optimization would demand). The fifth would be *financial support* for those experiencing deep poverty.

These are all areas where the state could play a significant role in delivering better health outcomes as a direct service provider. The definition of universality would remain the same as in the NHS: free at the point of delivery, based on need, funded through general taxation. As such, the *modus operandi* of interventions would center on need, rather than the means-testing that defines much of the current UK social security system.

The cost of the universal public health service would be around £42 billion per year initially. Around £13 billion of this cost would be increased workforce to rollout, administer, and deliver services. The model for public health staffing could resemble general practice, providing a single and expert front door for all who have health (but not healthcare) needs. Yet, the service could equally be adapted to work with the kind of relational state models and staffing developed by Cottam (2018) and others.

As either an addition or alternative to a Universal Public Health Service, we might also look at budgetary mechanisms to reorient existing welfare state services toward the goal of health creation. The purpose of the welfare state is not fixed. At certain points in the last 70 years, the purpose of the welfare state has centered on reducing poverty, inequality, and destitution. At others, particularly since the late-1990s, the social security system has been conceptualized as a means to get people into work – often, by strengthening conditionality and regimes of sanctions. Conversely, a Universal Public Health Budget would aim to reconfigure the welfare state toward health creation, rather than leaving this exclusively to the NHS. A functioning public health budget has been imagined by the Institute for Public Policy Research as follows (Thomas 2022b):

- First, the measures we prioritize should be expanded beyond GDP. A dashboard of measures could supplement GDP with indicators of resource depletion, wealth and income distribution, and health. In this vein, the Office for National Statistics (ONS) has recently developed the

Health Index: a stock and flow measure of health, which changes year on year. That is, it works in a similar way to GDP, and could be used to identify and evaluate health policy priorities.
- Second, the public health budget would need some money to spend. A 2022 IPPR report recommended that the public health budget be allocated 5 percent of total government expenditure, worth around £35 billion per year in the UK (Thomas 2022c)
- Third, the public health budget would need to be tied to political capital. As much as it is an important fiscal event, the salience of the UK's annual budget and three-yearly Comprehensive Spending Review is supported by its status as a political event. There are weeks of build-up; the chancellor is photographed with his distinctive red box; and there is a full-attendance speech in parliament, with a formal response. Announcing the public health budget each year, through its own fiscal event, could help replicate some of this political capital.

The ONS' health index and other UK data even allow for measurement of where the greatest possible marginal health gains may be sourced. Analysis from 2021 by actuarial firm Lane, Clark, and Peacock showed that the following would have the biggest impact on population health:

- Action on income inequality
- Action on rough sleeping, homelessness, and poor quality, crowded housing
- Better social security, and action on poverty
- Progress on childhood obesity
- Higher levels of education and better jobs (see: Thomas 2022b).

Notably, the results did not indicate that the NHS could achieve significant marginal gains, echoing research that suggests gains possible through better healthcare are smaller than those possible through greater social and economic equality (*e.g.* Marmot *et al.* 2010). These domains can then be used to develop policy. Using the Lane, Clark, and Peacock findings, the IPPR has suggested one possible policy package, based on expanding good jobs, rolling-out housing-first policies across the UK, increasing universal credit social security payments, and introducing a new (cash) benefit to support healthier diets (Thomas 2022b).

As with any instrument or measure, this tool is not above politics and ideology. Debates will continue over the best way to secure change. That is to say, it is not a technocratic solution that, in-and-of-itself, guarantees better health. Rather, it is a tool to reorient the welfare state toward health creation, and to legitimize a more capacious scope for the state to meet the health needs of the populace.

The state as a protector (commercial determinants)

There are some industries that have a particularly clear capacity to harm health, particularly among communities already enduring impoverishment and marginalization. Big tobacco – a business that, despite perceptions, continues to toast record-breaking profits annually – sells a product that kills, and is a pioneer of aggressive lobbying to avoid regulation. Increasingly, big food pushes a high-profit model of low-nutrition, low-sustainability ultra-processed food. Gambling and alcohol industries also fit typically into a business model built on aggressive marketing and regulatory avoidance.

These actors attract the vast majority of social movement, political, media, and public interest, yet they are not the only businesses that profit at the expense of poor health. All businesses that contribute to income inequality, gender or racial injustice, chronic stress, occupational health hazards, or rates of poverty pay contribute to poor health outcomes. For some, these harms will be offset by the health benefits of secure and well-paid jobs, or the health benefits of their products. For a great many others, however, the impact will be net negative. Accordingly, critical reflection should not fall on individual businesses and sectors alone, but must consider how the dynamics of capitalism structures the relationship between human health and output production/profit. In the current context, the former is too easily subordinated to, and exploited by, capital in pursuit of the latter.

Many policy studies have explored how this dynamic might change. Most effectively, such reflections have considered how the state might look to protect human health by borrowing from some of the mechanisms through which it has looked to protect planetary health in light of the climate emergency. One recommendation has been the use of a target similar to net-zero (Thomas 2022a). In this context, '*public health net-zero*' would describe a state in which the capacity to profit from health was eliminated. That is, commercial organizations would be unable to profit at the expense of health (Thomas 2022a)

One of the purest embodiments of public health net-zero, in this respect, would comprise shifting the cost of the health consequences of commercial activity from individuals to capital. This makes health externalities analogous to a form of pollution and embeds the principle of 'polluter pays'. This kind of policy has proved effective in the limited instances in which it has been implemented. Consider, for instance, the 2016 Soft Drinks Industry Levy (SDIL), which added a charge based on sugar content per 100ml to the price of drinks. However, while some revenue was generated, this was not the central aim of the policy. Instead, the core hope was that sugary drink manufacturers, in a highly competitive and saturated market, would modify their drinks to avoid the tax. This is exactly what transpired. Between 2015 and 2018, the total volume of sugars sold from soft drinks decreased 29 percent – driven by a reduction in the sugar content in products included in the SDIL (Bandy *et al.* 2020). The reaction to the Levy by affected businesses was highly negative, but the pecuniary impact on business has been lower than initially predicted. An analysis of stock market returns from affected companies demonstrated that, over the long-term, they have actually experienced growth as a result of the policy (Law *et al.* 2020). It has forced them to innovate more quickly than anticipated, but in a way that reduced their social burden and, with it, increased their company values.

Beyond the UK, more extensive fiscal policies have been implemented in a similar manner. In Mexico and Hungary, for example, a non-essential food tax has targeted most pre-packaged food high in fat, salt, and/or sugar. An evaluation of the policy in Hungary found that 73 percent of people had reduced consumption of the relevant products following its introduction (Martos 2015). Similarly positive results have been observed in Mexico (Smith *et al.* 2018). Accordingly, there is great scope to proceed further with these taxes in the UK. They could be extended to other unhealthy product categories, or they could be expanded to other commercial behaviors that are detrimental to health. Today, UK companies over a certain size are compelled to report on their gender pay-gap – an intervention that has done little to reduce it. A far more effective policy might be to levy their gender pay-gap on the basis of, and in a manner proportionate to, the health consequences of income inequality.

A second lever available in the pursuit of public health net-zero is the use of a creative ownership model, particularly where there is demonstrable proof that commercial actors cannot safely be left as responsible for an unhealthy product, market, or sector. Direct state control of distribution, for example, has been useful in reducing harm in the instances and nations where it has been used. State ownership of alcohol offers a prudent case-study. The Swedish Alcohol Retailing Monopoly is one example. Its stated purpose is 'to minimize alcohol related problems by selling alcohol in a responsible way, without a profit motive' (GoS 2022). That is, its objective is not to sell less alcohol, or move toward abolition of alcohol. Rather, it aims to ensure that alcohol is not sold in an actively harmful way, while the proceeds of sales can be reinvested in services and the public good. In turn, evaluation of the scheme has been excellent. Research has found that without the alcohol monopoly, consumption would be 31 percent higher. This would, in turn, have engendered 42 percent more alcohol-related deaths (Stockwell *et al.* 2018). Popularity is also high, with polling showing 78 percent favor the policy (Olsen 2019).

These two categories – shifting the cost of the health consequences of commercial activity from individuals to capital and creative ownership models – are not exhaustive of the methods through which public health net-zero could be pursued. Equally, as suggested above, our understanding of these levers must not be subject to a single industry focus. The public health movement in England has been criticized recently for committing a 'bad egg fallacy' and focusing on a few, particularly bad industries (Thomas 2022a). This is to the exclusion of a more fundamental critique of how capitalist economies work to exploit health in the interest of growth, output production, and profit. Accordingly, the levers must be used broadly to reduce the broad capacity of a capitalist economy to harm human health, not to constrain one or two sectors.

Indeed, this goes some way to explaining why a public health net-zero is fundamentally useful as an instrument. As a target, it forces the public health movement to look above single-issue campaigns – against big tobacco, gambling, food, or alcohol. Instead, emphasis is placed on bigger-picture issues concerning how prevailing models of ownership, regulation, tax, and broader state functions across the whole economy continue to subordinate human health to profit. Acknowledging and subverting this extant orientation is how we can ensure contemporary state measures are not limited to humanizing the worst practices of capitalism, but instead focus on fundamentally reconfiguring extant discourses and hierarchies of power as the means to secure more positive health outcomes.

Standing at a crossroads

This chapter has outlined some of the dynamics shaping the relationship between the UK welfare state and health promotion. Underpinning it is a normative assumption that meeting health needs should be desirable. Yet, morality alone has not proved a sufficient argument to bring about a more capacious, active role for the state in pursuing this objective. The detrimental political-economic and broader health effects likely to accrue from continuing along present lines, in turn, provide an equally compelling justification for moving toward a broader conception of health.

Both the UK and the world face great health uncertainty in the coming decades, as exemplified by the COVID-19 pandemic. Evidence suggests that the threat of such emerging infectious diseases (EIDs) is rising, with one study putting the annual risk of a COVID-19 scale breakout at 2 percent (Mirani *et al.* 2021). Yet, EIDs are not the only source of health risk. Antimicrobial resistance threatens our ability to rely on antibiotics. Moreover, climate change has its own health consequences – from extreme heat, cold, drought, floods, and pollution. More gradual health threats, like the rise in chronic conditions due to an aging population, or the rise in obesity driven by capitalist food systems, are further threats.

As well as the sheer human cost of these threats, their impact on the global economy – and on prosperity, more broadly – would be severe. Indeed, COVID-19 provides a natural experiment from which we can discern the relationship between health and economy. Indicatively, analysis has shown that the rise in long-term illness linked to the pandemic forced 200,000 people out the UK labor market (IPPR 2022). In the UK, the pandemic also led to the biggest drop in GDP in over 300 years (UK Parliament 2021).

Ultimately, perhaps, we stand where the climate movement did just decades ago: ahead of huge, existential disruptions, which threaten the foundations of human life, while armed with mainstream economic analyses and neoliberal prescriptions that fail to provide much analytical or policy succor. Human flourishing depends on our capacity to meet novel and complex health needs in the face of such unprecedented challenges and uncertainty. As with the ongoing climate emergency, addressing these concerns in a progressive and efficacious manner necessitates radically rethinking the ideas with which we understand human health, the material conditions shaping health outcomes, and the institutions structuring the trajectory of political-economic processes affecting health. As this chapter has demonstrated in the specific case of the UK, while its efforts will inexorably be contested, the state should play a pivotal role in securing such transformations – through reconsidering both the complexity of 'health' as a political-economic phenomenon and the scope of policy means necessary to secure it.

Notes

1 The views expressed in this chapter were written in the author's personal capacity, and do not necessarily reflect those of the Institute for Public Policy Research at which he is employed.

2 For an example of ambitious World Health Organisation work embodying the idea that inequality drives poor health, see the recent formation of the WHO Council on the Economics of Health for All.

References

Bandy, L.K., Scarborough, P., Harrington, R.A, Rayner, M. and Jebb, S.A. 2020, 'Reductions in sugar sales from soft drinks in the UK from 2015 to 2018', *BMC Medicine*, 18(20).

Brown, D. 2017, 'Workers, workhouses and the sick poor: Health and institutional healthcare in the long Nineteenth Century', *Journal of Urban History*, 43(1), pp. 180–8

CDC. 2022, 'Provisional life expectancy estimates for 2022', *NVSS Vital Statistics Rapid Release*, accessed 11 September 2022, <https://www.cdc.gov/nchs/data/vsrr/vsrr023.pdf>.

Cottam, H. 2018, *Radical Help: How We Can Remake the Relationships Between Us and Revolutionise the Welfare State*, Virago, London.

Coyle, D. 2014, *GDP: A Brief But Affectionate History*, Princeton University Press, New Jersey.

Department for Health and Social Care [DHSC]. 2022, *Public Health Ringfenced Grant 2022 to 2023: Local Authority Circular*, accessed 21 November 2022, <https://www.gov.uk/government/publications/public-health-grants-to-local-authorities-2022-to-2023/public-health-ringfenced-grant-2022-to-2023-local-authority-circular>.

Department for Levelling Up, Housing and Communities and Ministry of Housing, Communities and Local Government. 2022, *English Housing Survey*, accessed 11 September 2022, <https://www.gov.uk/government/collections/english-housing-survey>.

Dequech, D. 2008, 'Neoclassical, mainstream, orthodox, and heterodox economics', *Journal of Post Keynesian Economics*, 30(2), pp. 279–302.

Gaffney, A. 2018, *To Heal Humankind: The Right to Health in History*, Routledge, London.

Global Health Security Index. 2019, *Building Collective Action and Accountability*, accessed 11 September 2022, <https://www.ghsindex.org/wp-content/uploads/2019/10/2019-Global-Health-Security-Index.pdf>.

Government of Sweden [GoS]. 2022, *Swedish Alcohol Retailing Monopoly*, accessed 21 November 2022, <https://www.government.se/government-agencies/swedish-alcohol-retailing-monopoly--systembolaget-aktiebolag/>.

Health Foundation. 2019, 'Public opinion on the determinants of and responsibility for health', accessed 11 September 2022, <https://www.health.org.uk/blogs/public-opinion-on-the-determinants-of-and-responsibility-for-health>.

Institute for Fiscal Studies. 2022, *IFS Deaton Review of Inequalities*, accessed 11 September 2022, <https://ifs.org.uk/inequality/>.

Institute for Public Policy Research. 2022, *Introducing the Commission on Health and Prosperity*, <https://www.ippr.org/research/publications/health-and-prosperity>.

Joseph Rowntree Foundation. 2022, *Overall UK Poverty Rates*, accessed 11 September 2022, <https://www.jrf.org.uk/data/overall-uk-poverty-rates>.

King's Fund. 2014, *Making the Case for Public Health Interventions*, accessed 11 September 2022, <https://www.kingsfund.org.uk/audio-video/public-health-spending-roi>.

King's Fund. 2022, *What Is Happening to Life Expectancy in England*? accessed 11 September 2022, <https://www.kingsfund.org.uk/publications/whats-happening-life-expectancy-england>.

Law, C., Cornelsen, L., Adams, J., Penney, T., Rutter, H., White, M. and Smith, R. 2020, 'An analysis of the stock market reaction to the announcements of the UK soft drinks industry levy', *Economics and Human Biology*, 18(1), p. 100834.

Lee, F. 2009, *A History of Heterodox Economics: Challenging the Mainstream in the Twentieth Century*, Routledge, London.

L'Hôte, E., Volmert, A. and Fond, M. 2018, *Communicating About Obesity*, Frameworks Institute, accessed 11 September 2022, <https://www.frameworksinstitute.org/publication/communicating-about-obesity/>.

London School of Economics. 2021, *Partnership for Health Sustainability and Resilience: Interim Report of the Pilot Phase*, accessed 11 September 2022, <https://www3.weforum.org/docs/WEF_PHSSR_Interim_Report_of_the_Pilot_Phase.pdf>.

Marmot, M., Allen, J., Goldblatt, P., Boyce, T., McNeish, D., Grady, M. and Geddes, I. 2010, *Fair Society, Healthy Lives*, Institute for Health Equity, accessed 11 September 2022, <https://www.instituteofhealthequity.org/resources-reports/fair-society-healthy-lives-the-marmot-review>.

Martin, S., Lomas, J. and Claxon, K. 2020, 'Is an ounce of prevention worth a pound of cure? A cross-sectional study of the impact of English public health grant on mortality and morbidity', *BMJ Open* 10.

Martos, E. 2015, *Assessment of the Impact of a Public Health Product Tax*, World Health Organization, accessed 11 September 2022, <https://www.euro.who.int/__data/assets/pdf_file/0008/332882/assessment-impact-PH-tax-report.pdf>.

Mazzucato, M. and Kattel, R. 2019, 'Getting serious about value', *Institute for Innovation and Public Purpose*, accessed 11 September 2022, <https://www.ucl.ac.uk/bartlett/public-purpose/sites/public-purpose/files/iipp_policybrief_07_getting_serious_about_value.pdf>.

McNeil, C., Parkes, H., Garthwaite, K. and Patrick, R. 2021, *No Longer 'Managing': The Rise of Working Poverty and Fixing Britain's Broken Social Settlement*, IPPR, accessed 11 September 2022, <https://www.ippr.org/files/2021-05/no-longer-managing-may21.pdf>.

Mialon, M. 2020, 'An overview of the commercial determinants of health', *Globalization and Health*, 16, Article 74.

Ministry of Housing, Communities and Local Government. 2020, *English Housing Survey 2019 to 2020: Headline Report*, accessed 11 September 2022, <https://www.gov.uk/government/statistics/english-housing-survey-2019-to-2020-headline-report>.

Mirani, M., Katul, G.G., Pan, W.K. and Parolari, A.J. 2021, 'Intensity and frequency of extreme novel epidemics', *PNAS*, 118(35), p. e2105482118.

OECD. 2021, 'Trends in life expectancy', accessed 11 September 2022, <https://www.oecd-ilibrary.org/sites/da5bba97-en/index.html?itemId=/content/component/da5bba97-en>.

OECD. 2022, 'Health spending', accessed 11 September 2022, <https://data.oecd.org/healthres/health-spending.htm>.

Office for National Statistics. 2015, 'How has life expectancy changed over time?' accessed 11 September 2022, <https://www.ons.gov.uk/peoplepopulationandcommunity/birthsdeathsandmarriages/lifeexpectancies/articles/howhaslifeexpectancychangedovertime/2015-09-09>.

Olsen, T. 2019, 'Explaining the strong support for the Swedish alcohol retail monopoly', *Institute for Alcohol Studies*, accessed 11 September 2022, <https://www.ias.org.uk/2019/05/24/explaining-the-strong-support-for-the-swedish-alcohol-retail-monopoly/>.

Parliament. 1917, *Pamphlet On the Need for a Ministry of Health*, Archives, accessed 11 September 2022, <https://www.parliament.uk/about/living-heritage/transformingsociety/livinglearning/coll-9-health1/health-09/>.

Public Health England. 2014, 'Diptheria cases and deaths, England and Wales, 1914–2013', <https://webarchive.nationalarchives.gov.uk/ukgwa/20140714111350/http:/www.hpa.org.uk/Topics/InfectiousDiseases/InfectionsAZ/Diphtheria/EpidemiologicalData/dip005DataCasesDeaths/>.

Robertson, M. 2020, 'Don't repeat the mistakes of Test and Trace by outsourcing the COVID-19 vaccine programme', *Trade Unions Congress*, accessed 11 September 2022, <https://www.tuc.org.uk/blogs/dont-repeat-mistakes-test-and-trace-outsourcing-covid-19-vaccine-programme>.

Rothstein, M.A. 2002, 'Rethinking the meaning of public health', Journal of Law, Medicine and Ethics, 30(2), pp. 144–9.

Sartorius, N. 2006, 'The meanings of health and its promotion', *Croatian Medical Journal*, 47(4), pp. 662–4.

Shelter. 2022, *The Social Housing Deficit*, <https://england.shelter.org.uk/professional_resources/policy_and_research/policy_library/briefing_the_social_housing_deficit>.

Smith, E., Scarborough, P., Rayner, M. and Briggs, A. 2018, 'Should we tax unhealthy food and drink', *Proceedings of the Nutrition Society*, 77(3), pp. 314–20.

Stockwell, T., Stockwell, T., Sherk, A., Norström, T., Angus, C., Ramstedt, M., Andréasson, S., Chikritzhs, T., Gripenberg, J., Holder, H., Holmes, J. and Mäkelä, P. 2018, 'Estimating the public health impact of disbanding a government alcohol monopoly: Application of new methods to the case of Sweden', *BMC Public Health*, 18(1), pp. 1–16.

Sustain. 2021, *What Is Food Poverty?* accessed 11 September 2022, <https://www.sustainweb.org/foodpoverty/whatisfoodpoverty>.

Theis, D. and White, M. 2021, 'Is obesity policy in England fit for purpose? Analysis of government strategies and policies, 1992–2020', *Milbank Quarterly*, 99(1), pp. 126–70.

Thomas, C. 2019, *Hitting the Poorest Worst?* IPPR, accessed 11 September 2022, <https://www.ippr.org/blog/public-health-cuts>.

Thomas, C. 2020, *Resilient Health and Care*, IPPR, accessed 11 September 2022, <https://www.ippr.org/research/publications/resilient-health-and-care>.

Thomas, C. 2022a, *The Five Health Frontiers*, Pluto Press, London.

Thomas, C. 2022b, *Disease of Disparity*, IPPR, accessed 11 September 2022, <https://www.ippr.org/research/publications/disease-of-disparity>.

Thomas, C. 2022c. *The State of Health and Care 2022.* IPPR, accessed 11 September 2022, <https://www.ippr.org/research/publications/state-of-health-and-care-2022>

UK Parliament. 2021, *Coronavirus: Economic Impact*, Research briefing, accessed 11 September 2022, <https://commonslibrary.parliament.uk/research-briefings/cbp-8866/>.

West, R. and Marteau, T. 2013, 'Commentary on Casswell (2013): The commercial determinants of health', *Addiction*, 108(4), pp. 686–7.

World Health Organization. 2022, 'Social determinants of health', accessed 11 September 2022, <https://www.who.int/health-topics/social-determinants-of-health#tab=tab_1>.

35
THE NEED FOR COMPREHENSIVE PRIMARY HEALTHCARE

Toby Freeman and Fran Baum

Primary healthcare (PHC) is a fundamental element of health systems. PHC refers to that sector of the health system that serves as the first point of contact, and provides holistic treatment, prevention, and promotion services to the population. It includes primary medical care in the community, maternal and child healthcare, and public health strategies (Keleher 2001). PHC has been shown to be a key driver of population health (Starfield *et al.* 2005). The history and practice of primary healthcare is a contest of approaches to health and ideas about how healthcare should be structured and governed, what disciplines it should include, and what activities it ought to undertake. Underpinning these competing approaches are economic models, power relationships, and vested interests that are critical to unpack through a political economy analysis.

This chapter outlines comprehensive and selective visions of primary healthcare, and uses political economy to understand why the selective vision has dominated, the discordance between comprehensive approaches to PHC and neoliberalism, and what is needed to pursue a comprehensive vision that can place equity and health promotion – including action on the social determinants of health – at the heart of our health system.

Primary healthcare: competing visions

In 1978, an international conference organized by the World Health Organization (WHO) under the direction of then-Director General, Halfdan Mahler, produced the *Alma Ata Declaration* (WHO 1978), which set down the principles of PHC as a novel approach to healthcare and health promotion. The *Declaration* articulated a *comprehensive* formulation of PHC, stressing the imperative for action by national and international institutions to protect and promote the health of all. Specifically, it articulated a vision of health as a fundamental human right, oriented around principles of equity and community participation. Realizing this objective, in turn, necessitated an understanding of healthcare that extended beyond the activities of doctors and hospitals alone, instead prioritizing a more holistic, multi-actor approach to address the social determinants of health, and which centered on principles of social justice.

In this respect, the *Declaration* was informed and inspired by emerging models of healthcare that emphasized accessibility, community health workers, and disease prevention and health promotion, as well as treatment of existing ill-health. Examples included the 'barefoot doctor'

DOI: 10.4324/9781003017110-40

community health workers in China, rural Indian healthcare models, and the work of the Christian Medical Commission (Cueto 2004). Many of these models emerged from struggles and social movements, presenting a grassroots vision of what communities wanted health services to look like, and placed community health workers at their center (Cueto 2004).

The Alma Ata conference was a product of international cooperation that occurred amidst the backdrop of decolonizing African nations, and easing of Cold War tensions. Government representatives from over 130 countries and 67 international organizations attended (Cueto 2004). The membership of the WHO was shifting: while less than half of member-states were developing countries when the institution was established in 1948, this figure ballooned to over two-thirds by the 1970s (Williams 1988). This allowed the Alma Ata vision to be informed by growing criticism of health and healthcare inequalities between nations at different levels of economic development (Williams 1988), and of the hegemony of the developed West in emphasizing vertical disease-based approaches to health and the role of medicine and technology in treating ill-health (Cueto 2004).

In May 1979, the World Health Assembly unanimously endorsed the *Alma Ata Declaration*, committing member-states to implementing the vision of PHC (Williams 1988). The goal of PHC, as envisioned in the *Declaration*, was to achieve 'Health for All by the Year 2000'. Yet, over 20 years beyond the objective of Health for All by 2000, global health equity remains as elusive as ever. There is a 32-year life expectancy gap between the least healthy countries (Sierra Leone and the Central African Republic) and the most healthy (Japan and Hong Kong) (World Bank 2019), and health inequities within countries, by socioeconomic status, ethnicity, gender, and other factors, are rife and increasing.

Following Alma Ata, a call for an alternative, '*selective* PHC' approach was published just one year later (Walsh and Warren 1980). Walsh and Warren (1980: 145), two US authors, described the Alma Ata vision as 'unattainable', and presented an 'interim' plan targeting the most cost-effective treatment and prevention of the most critical health issues prevalent in the developing world, such as diarrheal diseases, measles, and malaria. Thus, the 'selective' PHC approach articulated exactly the kind of vertical disease-based approach the Alma Ata vision sought to redress. The authors justified the selective approach due to scarcity of resources to provide a more comprehensive PHC strategy. The editors of *Social Science and Medicine* noted that:

> By the mid 1980s it was apparent that several donor agencies had accepted the line of argument put forward by Walsh and Warren. As a result resources were increasingly being directed into vertical programs that sought quick technical solutions to health programs.
>
> (Editorial 1988: 877)

The two different approaches to PHC outlined above – 'comprehensive' and 'selective' – are underpinned by very different political economy assumptions. These differences are summarized in Table 35.1.

There have been sustained calls for comprehensive PHC since 1978. The WHO entitled their 2008 *World Health Report*, 'Primary health care now more than ever' (WHO 2008). Similarly, the Commission on the Social Determinants of Health (2008), which reports on how our living circumstances – including education, employment, working conditions, and housing – affect our health, has argued for the importance of comprehensive PHC. The Commission (2008: 8) notes that healthcare systems secure better health outcomes when oriented around a PHC model 'that emphasizes locally appropriate action across the range of social determinants, where prevention and promotion are in balance with investment in curative interventions'. More recently, assessment

Table 35.1 Contrasts between selective and comprehensive PHC

Characteristics	*Selective*	*Comprehensive*
Main aim	Reduction of specific disease – technical focus	Improvement in overall health of the community and individuals – and Health for All as overall social and political goal
Sectors involved	Strong focus on health sector – very limited involvement from other sectors	Involvement of other sectors central
Strategies	Focus on curative care, with some attention to prevention and promotion	Comprehensive strategy with curative, rehabilitative, preventive, and health promotion that seeks to remove root causes of ill-health
Planning and strategy development	External, often 'global', programs with little tailoring to local circumstances	Local and reflecting community priorities professional 'on tap not on top'
Participation	Limited engagement, based on terms of outside experts and tending to be sporadic	Engaged participation that starts with community strengths and the community's assessment of health issues, is ongoing, and aims for community control
Engagement with politics	Professional and claims to be apolitical	Acknowledges that PHC is inevitably political and engages with local political structures
Forms of evidence	Limited to assessment of disease prevention strategy based on traditional epidemiological methods, usually conducted out of context and extrapolated to situation	Complex and varied research methods including epidemiology, and qualitative and participatory methods

Source: Baum (2007).

of the impact of the COVID-19 pandemic has highlighted the ways in which social determinants of health have made certain populations more vulnerable to infection and less responsive to treatment. These include being in informal or casual work without provision for sick leave, being a migrant or refugee who does not speak the local language, living in over-crowded housing, and not having access to welfare payments (Paremoer *et al.* 2021).

Why has comprehensive PHC never been fully achieved?

Implementation of comprehensive PHC has never been fully achieved, and political economy concerns have been central to this. Even in the best examples of PHC (from countries like Sri Lanka, Thailand, Ethiopia, and China, along with sectors such as Aboriginal Community Controlled Health Services in Australia), the implementation of the original vision has been incomplete. A global stock-take of comprehensive PHC in 2017 found that it was consistently sidelined, and failed to be institutionalized as the dominant health system (Labonté *et al.* 2017). We examined why this was the case in high-income countries, and concluded that the comprehensive PHC vision was constrained by two factors. First, neoliberal approaches to healthcare, emphasizing individual responsibility for health and the role of the private sector and market forces in shaping healthcare, have engendered unsupportive policy environments. Second, the power of biomedicine and the medical workforce has created barriers to less hierarchical, multidisciplinary teamwork in PHC, and to the promotion of a social view of health that understands and addresses social determinant of health (Baum and Freeman 2022).

The new international economic order

The *Alma Ata Declaration* indicates that the conference participants behind it recognized such political-economic barriers to their vision for PHC, arguing that realization of comprehensive PHC necessitated a radically New International Economic Order. Building on a series of negotiations through conferences and other forums in the early-1970s, the New International Economic Order movement sought global equity, including trade terms that favor low- and middle-income countries, and rights to regulate multinational corporations. It sought to rebalance the unequal power relationships that benefited the developed world at the expense of the developing world. Nevertheless, it failed to address the manner in which these power relationships were entwined in the history of, and perpetuated, imperialism (Cox 1979), and remained essentially pro-market and pro-liberalism in orientation (Nicholls 2019).

A group of 77 countries presented the New International Economic Order strategy in the UN General Assembly in 1974 (Nicholls 2019). This led to a period of initial promise; however, after several years, the movement floundered, unable to enact the strategies or bring the proposal to debate. The New International Economic Order ultimately failed to gain traction because it was not supported by Western elites, the US in particular, under the new neoliberal Reagan government (Nicholls 2019). The developed nations favored trade settings and regulations that ensured they would continue to enjoy the status quo of their hegemony in the international economy (Cox 1979). This failure did not bode well for comprehensive PHC.

As well as calling for this New International Economic Order, the *Alma Ata Declaration* argued that PHC could be resourced through redirecting government spending. It posited that:

> An acceptable level of health for all people of the world by the year 2000 can be attained through a fuller and better use of the world's resources, a considerable part of which is now spent on armaments and military conflicts.

While global military expenditure dropped from 3.6 percent of global GDP in 1978 to 2.2 percent of GDP in 2019 (World Bank 2021), this still leaves over $1.9 trillion in military spending in 2019, an increase of 7.2 percent since 2010 in real terms (SIPRI 2020). Reflecting the importance of war and conflict, one of the key themes of the People's Health Movement is 'War and Conflict, Occupation and Forced Migration and Health' (People's Health Movement 2021).

Neoliberalism and comprehensive PHC

A major ideological adversary of the New Economic Order was neoliberalism, which has influenced government practice in many countries since the late-1970s. Critical of the viability of comprehensive PHC, international agencies including the International Monetary Fund (IMF), World Bank, and Word Trade Organization (WTO) have embraced a neoliberal approach to global governance and, through their policy activities, consequently sought to restructure myriad countries around a market-oriented political-economic rationality.

The rise of neoliberalism shortly after the *Alma Ata Declaration* saw the vision for comprehensive PHC wane. We outline three key reasons for this: (1) neoliberalism's fundamental conflicts with the principles of comprehensive PHC; (2) the structural adjustment and austerity policies that have undermined the potential for comprehensive PHC in many countries; and (3) the neoliberal approach of international donor agencies and the practices of philanthrocapitalism.

The conflicts between neoliberalism and comprehensive PHC

Neoliberalism manifests in policy emphases on cost-efficiencies in health systems, privatization and corporatization of public health services, and subjecting these services to a competitive economic rationality. Healthcare is conceived as a commodity for purchase, reliant on the capacity of the citizen to purchase it from the market, rather than approaching health and healthcare as a right (Sakellariou and Rotarou 2017). This logic underpins capitalism more generally. However, while somewhat comprehensive PHC services have existed in capitalist societies, the introduction of neoliberalism has heavily emphasized this market approach to healthcare and essentially expunged most comprehensive PHC from health systems. The starting point of healthcare as a commodity has ramifications for services' capacity to pursue accessibility strategies, such as transport services, community engagement activities, and outreach to reach those most in need (Baum *et al.* 2016). To a neoliberalized health service, the non-user is invisible and irrelevant. By being community-driven and whole-of-population focused, the comprehensive PHC service takes responsibility for the health of the whole community it serves in a way a neoliberalized health service never will.

Neoliberalism, as with the broader liberal tradition on which it builds, has a strong emphasis on the rights and responsibilities of individuals. In health, this translates into a focus on individual responsibility for health. This view aligns strongly with the dominant biomedical approach to health, which focuses on curing diseases in individuals, backed by medical power that helps shape health systems to suit the views of doctors (Baum *et al.* 2020; Illich 1975; Perera 2021). Together, individualist and biomedical perspectives of health have reigned over health systems in many countries, and this has constrained the potential for comprehensive PHC. The power and privilege of doctors has been cited as one of the barriers to the implementation of comprehensive PHC, resisting the role of community health workers and the political nature of comprehensive PHC (Cueto 2004). This individualist approach also tends to prohibit any consideration of inequities, as individualism leaves no room to identify and act on disparities or gradients in the population, and adopts a victim-blaming approach.

Furthermore, neoliberalism has seen the mimicking of private sector managerialism in public services that have not been privatized. This managerialism emphasizes narrow, short-term key performance indicators, which forces services to focus on immediate, measurable outcomes rather than the more transformative, long-term strategies outlined in the *Alma Ata Declaration* (Baum and Dwyer 2014; Baum *et al.* 2016). It is a direct threat to the principle of community control and community participation, reorienting services away from being responsive to the community, to compelling adherence to the dictates of imposed managerial performance indicators aimed at cost reduction (Baum *et al.* 2016).

Comprehensive PHC includes in its scope challenging social and economic drivers of ill-health and health inequities. This element of comprehensive PHC presents a fundamental challenge to the basic precepts of neoliberalism, which looks to markets to solve healthcare, and to reduce government intervention and expenditure. Neoliberal governments relentlessly use the provision of government funding to silence advocacy in NGOs or public services, demanding a sole focus on direct service provision (Glasius and Ishkanian 2015; Ishkanian 2014).

Structural adjustment and austerity policies

As neoliberalism was ascending in developed countries in the 1980s and 1990s, foreign debt was increasing in developing countries. The World Bank and IMF were powerful international institutions that set the terms of the loans provided to the latter, and certified whether they were deemed to have responsible economic and social policies (Werner *et al.* 1997). The structural adjustment policies adopted a neoliberal approach to healthcare that developing countries viewed as 'imposed by economists from North America and Europe' (Hall and Taylor 2003). This approach moved heavily away from the human rights approach to health and multi-sectoral strategy of the *Alma Ata Declaration*, instead emphasizing the role of the private sector in healthcare provision, private health insurance, and user payments, while cutting public spending on health (Hall and Taylor 2003; Werner *et al.* 1997). The result was increased child mortality and greater health inequities (Werner *et al.* 1997). Bassett and colleagues (1997) tracked the impact of a structural adjustment program in Zimbabwe in the 1990s, and showed how a health system that started as free for 90 percent of the population changed as user fees were enforced. This led to reduced attendance at health services, underpayment of nurses, worsening drug shortages, and declining quality of care. Oppong (2018) reported similar outcomes for Ghana.

The World Bank's 1993 *Investing in Health* report was a key document in global population health, signaling the dominance of a market-based approach to healthcare (Baum and Sanders 1995). Werner (1995a: 150) labeled the report 'the last nail in the coffin of the *Alma Ata Declaration*'. The report ignored the social determinants of health, and advocated for increased user fees for health services, limiting government spending to selective health measures that were deemed cost-effective, and a private, for-profit health system that encouraged competition (Baum and Sanders 1995; Labonte *et al.* 2008; Werner 1995a). The World Bank calculated cost-effective health interventions according to the 'Disability Adjusted Life Years' (DALY) purchased for each dollar invested. One example of the absurdity of the World Bank's evaluations of health interventions based on cost-effectiveness relates to water supply and sanitation, where the report argues:

> People want safe water and good sanitation and are willing to pay for these services [...] If households pay the total cost of water and sanitation services because of the productivity and amenity benefits, substantial health gains are an added bonus achieved at no cost per DALY [...] gained. When willingness to pay is much less than costs, it is usually a mistake to justify subsidies on the basis of health benefits alone [...] if publicly financed investments in these services are being considered for health reasons, it should be noted that such investments generally cost more per DALY gained than other health interventions recommended in this Report.
>
> (World Bank 1993: 93)

This example exemplifies the broader problems associated with adopting a narrow approach to evaluating PHC, where broad community development activity and action on social determinants of health are reduced to simplistic cost-benefit measures. Moreover, it is problematic to ascertain attribution or causality when taking upstream action in a complex social system that affects the health of the community (Labonte *et al.* 2008). The overwhelming dominance of such reductive cost-effectiveness evaluation methods since the World Bank report has been a further impediment to political acceptability of comprehensive PHC.

After the 2008 Global Financial Crisis, the IMF, European Central Bank, and European Commission argued that implementation of austerity measures was necessary to secure recovery (Labonté 2012). These were introduced in high-income countries, as well as low- and middle-income countries historically targeted by structural adjustment policies, even in countries that did not experience severe recessions (Labonté and Stuckler 2016). Such austerity measures included cuts to healthcare budgets, along with cuts that affected many social determinants of health, driving profuse ill-health (Labonté and Stuckler 2016).

Greece was the first country to undertake this new wave of austerity measures (Labonté 2012). When Greece received a bailout with austerity stipulations from the European Union and IMF, the nation instituted PHC reforms aimed at improving the PHC system. In fact, the austerity measures meant that accessibility and funding for PHC and public health reduced (Economou *et al.* 2015). The Greek experience highlights the fundamental contradiction between cuts to prevention and healthcare funding (which led to increased user fees and a reduction in clinic locations) with the establishment of a comprehensive PHC system (Economou *et al.* 2015). This demonstrates the short-term absurdity of such austerity cuts – as comprehensive PHC will, in the long-term, reduce expenditure through preventing ill-health requiring more costly healthcare. The severe shortcomings of the PHC system in Greece led to a grassroots movement establishing over 100 'solidarity clinics' funded by voluntary contributions, and staffed by volunteer and salaried staff to provide free PHC and engage in anti-austerity advocacy (Evlampidou and Kogevinas 2019).

International donor agencies and philanthrocapitalism

'Philanthrocapitalism' – that is, the increasing reconfiguration of philanthropic activities to better resemble the for-profit orientation of corporate processes – has profoundly shaped global health efforts (Baru and Mohan 2018), rising from 19 percent of financial global health assistance in 1998 to over 26 percent in 2007 (Rushton and Williams 2011). The selective vision of PHC was co-authored by Kenneth Warren of the Rockefeller Foundation – a US philanthrocapitalist foundation established by the Rockefeller family of banking and petroleum magnates, which has engaged in global health debates and efforts for many decades. Their selective vision was taken up by UNICEF and other donor agencies, to whom the promise of apolitical, rapid technological solutions appealed (Editorial 1988; Werner 1995b). Wealthy individuals and corporations are using private wealth to fund and direct global health efforts (Baru and Mohan 2018). This is supported by neoliberalism's concentration of wealth, producing 2153 ultra-wealthy billionaires in 2020 that own more wealth than the poorest 4.6 billion people (Coffey *et al.* 2020), and its undermining of the role of democratic governments in providing well-resourced healthcare for their citizens.

Donor global health programs have been critiqued for focusing on vertical solutions to specific diseases, rather than strengthening health systems (*e.g.* by supporting comprehensive PHC) (Balabanova *et al.* 2010; Koivusalo and MacKintosh 2011), for their links with transnational corporations that are contributing to ill-health (Ruckert *et al.* 2016), for lacking accountability and scrutiny (Bruen *et al.* 2014), and for representing the will of private actors rather than democratically elected governments (Rushton and Williams 2011). Baru and Mohan (2018: 5) argue that philanthrocapitalist global health foundations have 'shared a belief in narrow technology-centered biomedical approaches and tended to overlook the social, political and economic determinants of health', in direct opposition to the *Alma Ata* vision of PHC. The rise of private donor agencies has also undermined the role and authority of the WHO (Baru and Mohan 2018; Bruen *et al.* 2014), weakening its position to promote comprehensive PHC, while enabling these organizations to themselves exert considerable political influence on health policy (Global Health Watch 2014).

Recent debates: Universal Health Coverage

Universal Health Coverage (UHC) is one of the targets underpinning Sustainable Development Goal 3: 'Good Health and Well-Being'. UHC was defined as 'access to key promotive, preventive, curative and rehabilitative health interventions for all at an affordable cost' (WHO 2005). At first glance, this definition seems well aligned with comprehensive PHC. However, the goal hides a multitude of problems.

The language of UHC often reflects an economistic worldview centered on markets. Its focus is on financial systems, rather than on ensuring health systems promote health and prevent disease, or act on the social determinants of health. It is a far less radical goal than the *Alma Ata Declaration's* vision of Health for All. The affordability element on which UHC focuses is only one barrier to equity in access to healthcare (O'Connell *et al.* 2014). There is no mention of PHC in the Sustainable Development Goals to complement the focus on UHC (Hone *et al.* 2018).

The choice of UHC as a goal has focused attention largely on insurance-based models, opening up the potential for an increased role by private health insurance and the private sector in healthcare provision (Sanders *et al.* 2019). Much discourse around UHC has emphasized 'essential' curative medical care (Schmidt *et al.* 2015). In this way, UHC has acted to promote expensive medical care and technology at the expense of health promotion and disease prevention – contrary to the *Alma Ata* vision (Schmidt *et al.* 2015).

In 2018, the 40-year anniversary of the *Alma Ata Declaration*, the WHO released the *Astana Declaration*. This argues that PHC is critical to achieving UHC. However, the call for PHC in the *Astana Declaration* is a weak shadow of the vision laid out in the original *Alma Ata Declaration*.

Necessary political-economic conditions

Comprehensive PHC is needed more than ever at a time when health inequities – between and within countries – are increasing. Selective PHC is poorly suited to health promotion, disease prevention, management of health challenges such as COVID-19-like pandemics, and management and prevention of chronic non-communicable diseases. Critically, selective PHC is unable to change the living conditions that are driving ill-health and health inequities.

So how can the *Alma Ata* vision of PHC be revived? This has been the subject of a number of articles (Baum 2007; Bhatia and Rifkin 2010; Labonté *et al.* 2014; Lawn *et al.* 2008). Here, we discuss the necessary political-economic conditions for comprehensive PHC to flourish.

We have argued that neoliberal approaches in many countries have undermined capacity for comprehensive PHC. Others have argued that inequalities are inherent in capitalism, such that comprehensive PHC – by seeking to redress social and economic inequities – presents a more systemic challenge to capitalism. For instance, David Sanders (1985: 174–5) argues that comprehensive PHC is not compatible with a capitalist approach to healthcare:

> To change the nature of the medical contribution means creating a situation in which health care is no longer a commodity owned and purveyed by doctors and other health workers. This can only be by establishing an economic system that differs from the capitalist one, which is based on the generalized production and exchange of commodities for private profit. Indeed it is only in those countries where the capitalist system has been overthrown

> and the economic system is oriented to social need rather than private profit, that the medical contribution has changed fundamentally.

This is supported by comprehensive PHC achievements in non-capitalist countries, such as Cuba and China. While Cuba's PHC system can be criticized for being too biomedical, it nevertheless demonstrates an instance of the successful national implementation of PHC in the form of community-based polyclinics that adhere closely to the *Alma Ata Declaration* (González and Choonara 2019; Reed 2008), and has been effective in meeting the challenges of COVID-19 in the country (Reed 2020; Yaffe 2020). However, some level of comprehensive PHC has also prospered under social democratic capitalist governments. Even in strongly neoliberal countries such as Australia, the Aboriginal Community Controlled Health Organization sector, for instance, has maintained a very strong commitment to, and operationalization of, comprehensive PHC (Freeman *et al.* 2016).

In one of the largest recent research programs on comprehensive PHC, a global study led by Labonté *et al.* (2014) concluded that such measures are 'more likely in countries that include political commitments to equity, a legal or constitutional right to health guaranteed by the state, and commitments to universally funded health and social programs'. Certainly, a political commitment to equity, and health as a human right, is essential to allow comprehensive PHC. In Australia, there is political will to address Aboriginal and Torres Strait Islander health inequities, albeit in a way that does not challenge historic and ongoing colonization. There is much less political interest in redressing any socioeconomic inequities, including socioeconomic inequities in health.

A strong civil society sector is also critical to the success of comprehensive PHC. There are many examples of comprehensive PHC reliant on strong civil society globally, including India, Bangladesh, Nepal, and Ethiopia. The People's Health Movement[1] is a global civil society movement that was established in response to the failure to meet the *Alma Ata Declaration's* objective of Health for All by 2000. The Movement advocates for community-driven comprehensive PHC in all countries as a response to health inequalities.

Labonté also notes that political commitment to universal healthcare is necessary for comprehensive PHC. However, as the previous section on UHC shows, this commitment is far from a sufficient condition. The emphasis of comprehensive PHC on inter-sectoral action to address the social determinants of health necessitates governmental openness to considering health in all sectors, and for governments to see their role as governing for health *and* economic performance (Baum 2018). The importance of these broader conceptions of the role of PHC has been highlighted during the COVID-19 pandemic. About half of all COVID-19 deaths recorded globally have occurred in patients with diabetes and hypertension. These diseases are caused by the increased supply of high fat and sugar products – goods that are increasingly sold in sub-Saharan Africa, Latin America, and India, thereby creating new threats to health (Bump *et al.* 2021). Comprehensive PHC includes a role in advocating against the marketing practices of transnational food and beverage corporations and opposing new outlets.

Lastly, it is clear that global action and strategy are required, as well as nations working toward comprehensive PHC (Baum and Sanders 1995, 2011). The world is more globalized than when the *Alma Ata Declaration* was written. The influence of transnational corporations on health and healthcare systems, the approaches of international organizations such as the World Bank, and philanthropist foundations, all shape the possibilities for securing comprehensive PHC. Trade structures and other financial system elements that maintain wealth inequities between low- and middle-income countries and high-income countries also need to be addressed to ensure all countries have the resources to pursue comprehensive PHC. The COVID-19 pandemic has been a stark reminder of the interconnectedness of countries' health, as well as of inequities between countries.

Conclusion

Comprehensive PHC was a bold vision outlined in the late-1970s that has since failed to be fully implemented. A key barrier to its widespread adoption has been the dominance of neoliberal approaches to public policy in many countries and within the global finance system, which are incompatible with comprehensive PHC. Conversely, the latter has flourished to a greater extent in more social democratic and non-capitalist countries that have prioritized governing for health rather than for economic performance and elite interests alone.

As global income, wealth, and health inequalities continue to grow, and have been augmented still further by the COVID-19 pandemic, calls have amplified for restructuring governance configurations and policy environments, as well as the global political economy more broadly, to create healthier and fairer societies, as manifest in the movement for a Green New Deal. Comprehensive PHC sits well within this reform agenda, and will be critical to addressing health inequities into the future.

Note

1 See: <https://phmovement.org/>.

References

Balabanova, D., McKee, M., Mills, A., Walt, G. and Haines, A. 2010, 'What can global health institutions do to help strengthen health systems in low income countries?' *Health Research Policy and Systems*, 8(1), pp. 8–22.

Baru, R.V. and Mohan, M. 2018, 'Globalisation and neoliberalism as structural drivers of health inequities', *Health Research Policy and Systems*, 16(1), article 91.

Bassett, M.T., Bijlmakers, L. and Sanders, D.M. (1997), 'Professionalism, patient satisfaction and quality of healthcare: Experience during Zimbabwe's structural adjustment programme', *Social Science and Medicine,* 45(12), pp. 1845–52.

Baum, F. 2007, 'Health for all now! reviving the spirit of Alma Ata in the twenty-first century: An introduction to the Alma Ata declaration', *Social Medicine*, 2(1), pp. 34–41.

Baum, F. 2018, *Governing for Health*, Oxford University Press, New York.

Baum, F. and Dwyer, J. 2014, 'The accidental logic of health policy in Australia', in Miller, C. and Orchard, L. (eds), *Australian Public Policy: Progressive Ideas in the Neoliberal Ascendency*, Policy Press, Bristol, pp. 187–208.

Baum, F., Freeman, T., Sanders, D., Labonté, R., Lawless, A. and Javanparast, S. 2016, 'Comprehensive primary health care under neo-liberalism in Australia', *Social Science and Medicine*, 168, pp. 43–52.

Baum, F. and Freeman, T. 2022, 'Why community health systems have not flourished in high income countries: What the Australian experience tells us', *International Journal of Health Policy and Management*, 11, pp. 49–58.

Baum, F. and Sanders, D. 1995, 'Can health promotion and primary health care achieve health for all without a return to their more radical agenda?', *Health Promotion International*, 10(2), pp. 149–60.

Baum, F. and Sanders, D.M. 2011, 'Ottawa 25 years on: A more radical agenda for health equity is still required', *Health Promotion International*, 26(suppl 2), pp. ii253–7.

Baum, F., Ziersch, A., Freeman, T., Javanparast, S., Henderson, J. and Mackean, T. 2020, 'Strife of interests: Constraints on integrated and co-ordinated comprehensive PHC in Australia', *Social Science and Medicine*, 248, p. 112824.

Bhatia, M. and Rifkin, S. 2010, 'A renewed focus on primary health care: Revitalize or reframe?' *Globalization and Health*, 6(1), article 13.

Bruen, C., Brugha, R., Kageni, A. and Wafula, F. 2014, 'A concept in flux: Questioning accountability in the context of global health cooperation', *Globalization and Health*, 10(1), article 73.

Bump, J.B., Baum, F., Sakornsin, M., Yates, R. and Hofman, K. 2021, 'Political economy of COVID-19: Extractive, regressive, competitive', *British Medical Journal*, 372(73).

Coffey, C., Espinoza Revollo, P., Harvey, R., Lawson, M., Parvez Butt, A., Piaget, K., Sarosi, D. and Thekkudan, J. 2020, *Time to Care: Unpaid and Underpaid Care Work and the Global Inequality Crisis*, Oxfam, Oxford.

Commission on Social Determinants of Health. 2008, *Closing the Gap in a Generation: Health Equity Through Action on the Social Determinants of Health*, World Health Organisation, Geneva.

Cox, R.W. 1979, 'Ideologies and the new international economic order: reflections on some recent literature', *International Organization*, 33(2), pp. 257–302.

Cueto, M. 2004, 'The origins of primary health care and selective primary health care', *American Journal of Public Health*, 94, pp. 1864–74.

Economou, C., Kaitelidou, D., Kentikelenis, A., Maresso, A. and Sissouras, A. 2015, 'The impact of the crisis on the health system and health in Greece', in Maresso, A., Mladovsky, P, Thomson, S., Sagan, A., Karanikolos, M., Richardson, E., Cylus, J., Evetovits, T., Jowett, M., Figueras, J. and Kluge, H. (eds), *Economic Crisis, Health Systems and Health in Europe: Country Experience*, European Observatory on Health Systems and Policies, Copenhagen, pp. 103–42.

Editorial. 1988, 'The debate on selective or comprehensive primary health care', *Social Science and Medicine*, 26(9), pp. 877–8.

Evlampidou, I. and Kogevinas, M. 2019, 'Solidarity outpatient clinics in Greece: A survey of a massive social movement', *Gaceta Sanitaria*, 33, pp. 263–7.

Freeman, T., Baum, F., Lawless, A., Labonte, R., Sanders, D., Boffa, J., Edwards, T. and Javanparast, S. 2016, 'Case study of an aboriginal community-controlled health service in Australia: Universal, rights-based, publicly funded comprehensive primary health care in action', *Health and Human Rights: An International Journal*, 18(2), pp. 93–108.

Glasius, M. and Ishkanian, A. 2015, 'Surreptitious symbiosis: Engagement between activists and NGOs', *VOLUNTAS: International Journal of Voluntary and Nonprofit Organizations*, 26(6), pp. 2620–44.

Global Health Watch. 2014, *Global Health Watch 4*, Zed Books, London.

González, M.C. and Choonara, I. 2019, 'Cuba's success in child health: What can one learn?' *British Medical Journal Paediatrics Open*, 3(1), p. e000573.

Hall, J. and Taylor, R. 2003, 'Health for all beyond 2000: The demise of the Alma-Ata Declaration and primary health care in developing countries', *Medical Journal of Australia*, 178(1), pp. 17–20.

Hone, T., Macinko, J. and Millett, C. 2018, 'Revisiting Alma-Ata: What is the role of primary health care in achieving the sustainable development goals?', *The Lancet*, 392(10156), pp. 1461–72.

Illich, I. 1975, *Medical Nemesis*, Caldar and Boyars, London.

Ishkanian, A. 2014, 'Neoliberalism and violence: The big society and the changing politics of domestic violence in England', *Critical Social Policy*, 34(3), pp. 333–53.

Keleher, H. 2001, 'Why primary health care offers a more comprehensive approach to tackling health inequities than primary care', *Australian Journal of Primary Health*, 7(2), pp. 57–61.

Koivusalo, M. and MacKintosh, M. 2011, 'Commercial influence and global nongovernmental public action in health and pharmaceutical policies', *International Journal of Health Services*, 41(3), pp. 539–63.

Labonté, R. 2012, 'The austerity agenda: How did we get here and where do we go next?' *Critical Public Health*, 22(3), pp. 257–65.

Labonté, R., Sanders, D., Baum, F., Schaay, N., Packer, C., Laplante, D., Vega-Romero, R. Viswanatha, V., Barten, F., Hurley, C., Ali, H.T., Manolakos, H., Acosta-Ramirez, N., Pollard, J., Narayan, T., Mohamed, S., Peperkamp, L., Johns, J., Ouldzeidoune, N., Sinclair, R. and Pooyak, S. 2008, 'Implementation, effectiveness and political context of comprehensive primary health care: preliminary findings of a global literature review', *Australian Journal of Primary Health*, 14(3), pp. 58–67.

Labonté, R., Sanders, D., Packer, C. and Schaay, N. 2014, 'Is the Alma Ata vision of comprehensive primary health care viable? Findings from an international project', *Global Health Action*, 7, p. 24997

Labonté, R., Sanders, D., Packer, C. and Schaay, N. 2017, *Revitalizing Health For All: Case Studies of the Struggle for Comprehensive Primary Health Care*, University of Toronto Press, Toronto.

Labonté, R. and Stuckler, D. 2016, 'The rise of neoliberalism: How bad economics imperils health and what to do about it', *Journal of Epidemiology and Community Health*, 70(3), pp. 312–8.

Lawn, J.E., Rohde, J., Rifkin, S., Were, M., Paul, V.K. and Chopra, M. 2008, 'Alma-Ata 30 years on: Revolutionary, relevant, and time to revitalise', *The Lancet*, 372(9642), pp. 917–27.

Nicholls, S.T. 2019, *A Moment of Possibility: The Rise and Fall of the New International Economic Order*, unpublished PhD dissertation, University of Adelaide.

O'Connell, T., Rasanathan, K. and Chopra, M. 2014, 'What does universal health coverage mean?' *The Lancet*, 383(9913), pp. 277–9.

Oppong, J. 2018, 'Structural adjustment and the healthcare system: Ghana's experience, 1983–1999', in K. Konadu-Agyemang (ed), *IMF and World Bank Sponsored Structural Adjustment Programs in Africa*, Routledge, London, pp. 357–70.

Paremoer, L., Nandi, S., Serag, H. and Baum, F. 2021, 'COVID-19 pandemic and the social determinants of health', *British Medical Journal*, 372(129).

People's Health Movement. 2021, 'War and conflict, occupation and forced migration and health', accessed 14 July 2021, <https://phmovement.org/health-for-all-campaign/war-and-conflict-occupation-and-forced-migration-and-health/>.

Perera, I.M. 2021, 'What doctors want: A comment on the financial preferences of organized medicine', *Journal of Health Politics, Policy and Law*, 46(4), pp. 731–45.

Reed, G. 2008, 'Cuba's primary health care revolution: 30 years on', *World Health Organization Bulletin of the World Health Organization*, 86(5), pp. 327–9.

Reed, G. 2020, 'Mobilizing primary health care: Cuba's powerful weapon against COVID-19', *MEDICC Review*, 22(2), pp. 53–7.

Ruckert, A., Labonté, R., Lencucha, R., Runnels, V. and Gagnon, M. 2016, 'Global health diplomacy: A critical review of the literature', *Social Science and Medicine*, 155, pp. 61–72.

Rushton, S. and Williams, O. (eds) 2011, *Partnerships and Foundations in Global Health Governance*, Palgrave Macmillian, Hampshire.

Sakellariou, D. and Rotarou, E.S. 2017, 'The effects of neoliberal policies on access to healthcare for people with disabilities', *International Journal for Equity in Health*, 16(1), article 199.

Sanders, D. 1985, *The Struggle For Health: Medicine and the Politics of Underdevelopment*, Macmillan, London.

Sanders, D., Nandi, S., Labonté, R., Vance, C. and Van Damme, W. 2019, 'From primary health care to universal health coverage: One step forward and two steps back', *The Lancet*, 394(10199), pp. 619–21.

Schmidt, H., Gostin, L.O. and Emanuel, E.J. 2015, 'Public health, universal health coverage, and sustainable development goals: Can they coexist?', *The Lancet*, 386(9996), pp. 928–30.

SIPRI. 2020, *Trends in World Military Expenditure, 2019*, SIPRI, Solna.

Starfield, B., Shi, L. and Macinko, J. 2005, 'Contribution of primary care to health systems and health', *The Milbank Quarterly*, 83(3), pp. 457–502.

Walsh, J.A. and Warren, K.S. 1980, 'Selective primary health care: An interim strategy for disease control in developing countries', *Social Science and Medicine, Part C: Medical Economics*, 14(2), pp. 145–63.

Werner, D. 1995a, 'Turning health into an investment: Assaults on third world healthcare', *Economic and Political Weekly*, 30(3), pp. 147–51.

Werner, D. 1995b, 'Who killed primary health care?' *New Internationalist*, accessed 19 September 2021, <https://newint.org/features/1995/10/05/who>.

Werner, D., Sanders, D., Weston, J., Babb, S. and Rodriguez, B. 1997, *Questioning the Solution: The Politics of Primary Health Care and Child Survival; With an In-Depth Critique of Oral Rehydration Therapy*, Health Wrights, Palo Alto.

WHO. 1978, *Declaration of Alma-Ata, International Conference on Primary Health Care, USSR, 6–12 September*, WHO, Geneva.

WHO. 2005, 'WHA58, Resolution 33. Sustainable health financing, universal coverage and social health insurance', paper presented at the Fifty Eighth World Health Assembly, accessed 7 April 2021, <http://www.who.int/health_financing/HF%20Resolution%20en.pdf>.

WHO. 2008, *World Health Report: Primary Health Care Now More Than Ever*, WHO, Geneva.

Williams, G. 1988, 'WHO: Reaching out to all', *World Health Forum*, 9, pp. 185–99.

World Bank. 1993, *World Development Report 1993: Investing in Health*, World Bank, Washington, DC.

World Bank. 2019, 'Life expectancy at birht, total (years)', accessed 19 September 2021, <https://data.worldbank.org/indicator/SP.DYN.LE00.IN≥.

World Bank. 2021, 'Military expenditure (% of GDP)', accessed 19 September 2021, <https://data.worldbank.org/indicator/MS.MIL.XPND.GD.ZS>.

Yaffe, H. 2020, 'Leading by example: Cuba in the Covid-19 pandemic', *CounterPunch*, accessed 19 September 2021, <https://www.counterpunch.org/2020/06/04/leading-by-example-cuba-in-the-covid-19-pandemic/>.

36

THE POLITICAL ECONOMY OF HEALTHCARE AS COMMONS

Exploring the commons health system and Indigenous peoples

Young Soon Wong

In debating the relative strengths and weaknesses of public versus private healthcare systems, the underlying basis from which they originate – property arrangements – is rarely interrogated. Property rights, as one of the sacred tenets of economic theory, has long pivoted between private property regimes or state property regimes, depending on which branch of political-economic thought was ascendant. With the dominance of neoliberal policy in most countries today, market-led solutions have become the favored option for organizing healthcare systems. Not unexpectedly, then, issues of inequality of access that are characteristic of other private property regimes have also surfaced in the healthcare sector.

In the midst of ideological contestations between the duopoly of private and public systems, it is often overlooked that there are more than two ways to organize property arrangements. A third way concerns common property regimes, or what is commonly known as 'the commons'. The idea of the commons may seem like a relic from a romanticized past, but in reality, common property regimes form the basis of many contemporary localized or traditional natural resource management systems. From fisheries to forest (Arnold 1993; McKean and Ostrom 1995; Holland and Ginter 2001; Pomeroy *et al.* 2001; Chaudhary *et al.* 2015), from watersheds to pasturelands (Kerr 2007; Eychenne and Lazaro 2014; Watanabe and Shirasaka 2018), many local communities organize communally held systems to equitably and sustainably utilize resources within their locations.

Such property arrangements are particularly common among indigenous peoples where communally held resources are a natural extension of their societal structures. While the majority of common property regimes apply to natural resources, does the same arrangement extend to healthcare? In this chapter, we explore healthcare as commons: proposing a conceptual framework of a commons health system and using the traditional healthcare practice of the Orang Asli, Malaysia's indigenous peoples group, to demonstrate its broader applicability as a model from which other health systems may learn.

Healthcare as a common-pool resource

To conceptualize a health system as commons, we must first determine whether health fits the criteria of a common-pool resource. Three criteria are normally understood as comprising this:

DOI: 10.4324/9781003017110-41

(1) it is an economic good or resource; (2) it is finite and diminishes with (over)use; and (3) it is available to be consumed by all and to which access can be limited but only at high cost (Ostrom and Hess 2008). Put differently, a common-pool resource is a hybrid of private and public goods. It shares characteristics with private goods, in that its use by one person subtracts from what is available for others due to its finite quantity, or what is known as the 'subtractability' factor. Conversely, it has characteristics of public goods in that it is difficult to exclude people from using it, also known as the 'excludability' factor (Ostrom and Ostrom 1977; Ostrom *et al.* 1994).

While the World Health Organization (2000) defines a healthcare system as all the activities whose primary purpose is to promote, restore, or maintain health, we also know that health is intricately tied to social and economic factors that are often not under the purview of a country's healthcare systems. The social determinants of health approach (WHO 2008; Marmot 2013) highlight the linkages between ill-health and poor infrastructure, lack of livelihoods, low education, and degraded ecology. Conversely, investments in health bring economic returns or, as the WHO (Sachs 2001) puts it: good health is good for the economy. The rationale is that a labor force and population that is healthy will be able to engage fully in economic production and activities.

In its economic function, a common-pool resource consists of a resource system that comprises a stock facility and a flow of benefits, or what is termed as resource units from the resource system (Ostrom 2000). For a modern healthcare system, this may be categorized into the stock facility of hospital buildings and its attendant infrastructure, medical and supporting equipment, medicines, personnel and their skills, and medical and health knowledge – all of which are tangible or intangible resources. The flow of benefits or resource units from a healthcare system are the various healthcare services that are offered to the target population, such as accident and emergency services, maternal and child health, public health, and others.

Healthcare exhibits both subtractibility and excludability characteristics. Subtractibility here means that finite resources available for health budgets, trained personnel, and availability of facilities place limits on how many people can be served at any given time. This characteristic was exemplified during the COVID-19 pandemic amidst resource scarcity. Health systems across the world were severely stretched in attending to both COVID-19 cases and the typical caseloads of any given year, thereby giving rise to complex debates about priorities and ethics in triage and ICU admission criteria (Joebges and Biller-Andorno 2020; Leclerc *et al.* 2020; Swiss Academy Of Medical Sciences 2020; White and Lo 2021).

The most widespread excludability approach in contemporary healthcare systems is via pricing, where access is controlled by an individual's ability to pay for services. Despite its prominence as a key feature in private health systems, excludability is constantly challenged because access to healthcare is considered a fundamental human right under Article 25 of the Universal Declaration of Human Rights (United Nations 1948). A key feature in public health systems, signatory states are obligated to ensure that the right to health is respected, protected, and provisioned, thereby making it morally indefensible to exclude or discriminate against individuals or segments of a population from health services. However, although prevalent, excludability is not as easy to apply as it would seem, because the moral dimension places a high social, if not financial, cost if perceived as excessive.

Political economy of the commons

However, defining a common-pool resource solely by its economic attributes would diminish its overall value, since a resource has social and cultural value that may or may not include the economic. Which attribute has greater or less weightage is often expressed in the type of institutional property arrangement under which a resource is governed.

Four types of property regimes are widely recognized as operative in managing a resource system. First, there are open access property regimes, which describe resources that are not the legal property of any party, nor are there any arrangements for it to be managed by any entity. Access to it is unrestricted, often resulting in uncontrolled and unsustainable use of the resources (Berkes *et al.* 1989; Ostrom and Hess 2008).

Second, state property regimes describe the state's ownership of, and control over, decision-making as to usufruct rights of the resources. The state can either directly manage the property, or grant usufruct rights to individuals or groups to manage it (Bromley 1989; Bromley and Cernea 1989). Third, private property regimes describe an individual or corporation that has ownership and exclusive usufruct rights to resources, insofar as it is within legal and socially accepted perimeters of usage (Bromley 1989; Bromley and Cernea 1989; Ostrom and Hess 2008).

Fourth, common property regimes constitute a group or community sharing usufruct rights alongside duties over the use and management of a common-pool resource (Ostrom 1990; Bromley 1992). These rights are recognized either formally in specific legislation, or informally through tradition or customs. The community has relatively free but monitored access to use the resource within agreed limits to ensure its sustainability, and has built-in mechanisms by which they can exclude outsiders from utilizing the resource.

Of these institutional arrangements, two have become dominant since the Industrial Revolution. With private goods and services, the market is seen as the optimal institution for organizing the flow of benefits, while for public goods and services, the state is considered the optimal institution, as it can impose rules and regulations on self-interested parties. The hegemony enjoyed by private and state property regimes has meant that common property arrangements – emphasizing cooperative efforts by multiple groups to solve human social dilemmas – were bypassed for market or state solutions, as they were seen as chaotic and overly complex.

The recent renewal of interest in common property arrangements has arisen, first, because of numerous examples of the failure of state or markets to sustainably and equitably manage common-pool resources. This is best exemplified by the crisis of climate change (Andrew 2008; Bhuyan 2010) and the enormous wealth gap between rich and poor (Oxfam 2022). Second, the intellectual and theoretical boundaries of complex cooperative arrangements have expanded significantly, most notably in the work of Elinor and Vincent Ostrom on polycentric governance, or polycentricity, to foster better understanding and management of complex governance systems.

The concept of 'polycentricity' is credited to Michael Polanyi (Aligica and Tarko 2012) in his writings seeking to understand the social conditions that best preserved freedom of expression and the rule of law. Expanded by Ostrom's work into the field of public administration, and common-pool resource and public goods governance, polycentricity is defined as a complex, cooperative, competitive form of governance with multiple centers of decision-making – each of which operates with some degree of autonomy, but is capable of resolving inter-group conflict (Ostrom *et al.* 1961; Marshall 2005; Ostrom 2010). This contrasts with monocentric governance systems, comprising a single center of decision-making – whether a state or private entity. These monocentric systems are often considered simpler and more efficient than polycentric systems.

However, some advantages associated with polycentric governance systems are as follows: (1) they have better adaptive capacity toward dynamic social and environmental conditions; (2) their institutional design has greater congruence with complex natural resource systems; and (3) they have redundant features that help mitigate risk (Carlisle and Gruby 2019). On the flip side, some potential disadvantages are as follows: (1) their complexity increases transaction costs, as coordination between multiple stakeholders can be quite high (Huitema *et al.* 2009; Wyborn 2014); and (2) dispersion of responsibilities may result in poorer accountability (Huitema *et al.* 2009; Lieberman 2011).

Perhaps the most important attribute about polycentric systems concerns the issue of power. Unlike monocentric governance systems, where power is centralized, the exercise of power and its attendant coercive capability in a polycentric system is not monopolized by a single decision structure, but constrained and shared under a rule of law system (Aligica and Tarko 2012). This attribute enables poorer communities to maintain control and ownership over their resources.

Limitations of the current duopoly in healthcare provision

In tracing the historical threads of structured health systems, state formation was the precursor for the birth of both public and private health variants. Initially intended for the ruling and elite classes of society (Garrison 1914; Robinson 1994), health services provided via these systems were gradually extended to the rest of society as notions of statehood evolved and expanded (Rosen 1958; Porter 2005). Prior to the formation of modern states, commons-based health systems constituted the earliest form of health organization in non-state societies, and continue to prevail in many indigenous societies today (Service 1975). Despite existing over millennia, the near-ubiquity of such systems has almost disappeared with the rise of states and entrenchment of private property rights.

Contemporary healthcare systems are primarily governed under two forms of property regime: state and private. The structural attributes of each regime engender its own set of advantages and limitations to the governance of such a common-pool resource. In the case of health provision, one of the main limitations of for-profit private healthcare services is that of access for those who cannot afford to pay, such that it serves a limited and exclusive market. For example, in Malaysia, for-profit private healthcare providers are situated in cities and major towns where populations, infrastructure, and wealth are concentrated (Abdullah and Ng 2009), making their price and location largely inaccessible to poorer, often rural populations. Private healthcare is also not structured, nor motivated, to provide universal health coverage, despite sharing obligations with the state to guarantee the right to health for all (Gruskin *et al.* 2007).

Conversely, the purview of public health services typically encompasses the direct provisioning of services, public health policy, and regulation of services for a country's population. The role of the state is to safeguard and ensure the equitable allocation of resources through managing resources between competing demands, while public trust in the state is critical to whether it is perceived as having upheld this objective (Chanley *et al.* 2000; Marien and Hooghe 2011; Sae-chang *et al.* 2021). During the COVID-19 pandemic, three factors that influenced public trust in this institution were as follows: (1) the type of political regime; (2) the socio-economic policies implemented before the crisis; and (3) the capacity of state institutions to deliver services (Greer *et al.* 2020). Indigenous peoples' historical experience with state or private entities – marked by pervasive exploitation, marginalization, and genocide – has not inspired such trust (Burger 1987; Hinton 2002). These monocentric governance systems centralized power to varying degrees and, ultimately, implemented policies based on their own political philosophies and material interests.

For example, colonial Britain and its post-independence successor in Malaya used health services to draw the Orang Asli away from communist influence during the Malayan Emergency (Nicholas and Baer 2007; Bedford 2009). Apartheid South Africa used health policies as part of its effort to maintain the dominance of its white population (McIntyre and Gilson 2002), while Mexico used health services in its counter-insurgency effort to suppress the Zapatista rebellion in Chiapas (Farmer and Gastineau 2002). Within the contemporary neoliberal market system, biopiracy of indigenous medicinal plants (Bhattacharya 2014; Mgbeoji 2014; Imran *et al.* 2021) and patenting of indigenous knowledge (Ratuva 2009; Harry 2011) are arenas of contestations over natural resources and intellectual property.

Undoubtedly, the progress of extant modern health systems, with their technological advances in medicine and public health, has vastly improved the overall health of populations. Yet, the systemic limitations within their monocentric structural attributes appear to have capped their ability to address the huge diversity, complexity, and motivational structures of contemporary societies, particularly impoverished and marginalized populations. By adopting a more polycentric approach with the inclusion of community institutional arrangements, the health of populations can be improved – particularly among communities experiencing difficulty fitting into existing 'one-size-fits-all' governance configurations.

Conceptualizing commons-based health systems

Institutional property arrangements are social constructs endowed with legal rights, which function to facilitate economic growth and provide social security. Drèze and Sen (1991) view social security as the social means to prevent deprivation and vulnerability in populations. Economic growth alone is inadequate for preventing severe deprivation and poor health. State policy is essential for improving living standards and maintaining basic needs. Private property regimes do this indirectly through wealth accumulation, allowing individuals to raise their living standards and secure access to insurance markets and essential services such as healthcare, education, and housing. Conversely, state property regimes provide social services at varying intensities depending on the priorities of the state and the impact of political interests in shaping these.

Common property regimes, on the contrary, provide directly for social security needs through guaranteed access to vital resources and through risk pooling (Swallow 1997). Common property regimes guarantee access for everyone in a community to extract the resources they need to meet livelihood and health needs by recognizing the rights of members to vital resources. In risk pooling, common property regimes moderate the effects of disasters from affecting every productive resource through the practice of scattering and spatial diversification. It also allows the risk of failure to be pooled among the group instead of individuals, where reciprocity and mutual insurance help individuals tide over periods of ill-health, and severe or unexpected deprivation. Risk pooling and access to vital resources are particularly important for poorer groups, as Jodha (1990) found in studying Indian rural communities, which derived larger proportions of their subsistence needs from common property resources compared to the wealthy.

Social security systems in common property regimes are largely based on social relationships such as kinship, loyalty, or patronage relations within a village society (Platteau 1991). Such networks yield many social benefits, such as minimizing risk, fulfilling social obligations, credit favors, and enhancing personal prestige (White and Runge 1994), which may not be readily quantifiable, though require enormous amounts of personal effort, time, and material investment to build. Considerable transaction costs are, thus, involved in establishing such social networks, and any induced shift toward a new or different system would potentially cause considerable social and economic disruption.

The emphasis on securing the social security needs of everyone in the community demonstrates the underlying values of inclusivity and equity of common property regimes. This suggests congruence between a common property regime's primary function and the organization of a healthcare system that is inclusive and equitable.

According to Ostrom (1990), eight key design principles contribute toward the long-term sustainability and integrity of a common property regime. Seven of these are evident in the case-study below:

1 Clearly defined boundaries
2 Rules in use are well matched to local needs and conditions
3 Individuals affected by operational rules can participate in modifying these
4 A system for self-monitoring members' behavior
5 A graduated system of sanctions
6 Community members have access to low-cost conflict-resolution mechanisms
7 The right of community members to devise their own rules is respected by external authorities

As a tangible representation of some of the earliest forms of human organization, indigenous peoples' healthcare is the most relevant source of information to determine the presence of these design principles in practice. The following study of the traditional healthcare practices of Malaysia's Orang Asli indigenous people will seek to uncover the workings of their health system, and determine whether it matches the conceptual framework of a commons health system (Wong *et al.* 2014; Wong *et al.* 2016).

The Orang Asli: a brief history

The Orang Asli are the indigenous peoples of Peninsula Malaysia and the oldest population group recorded to inhabit the Peninsula (Zainuddin 2012), with pre-histories dating back from 10,000 to 2,000 years (Dentan *et al.* 1997). The state has officially classified them into three main groups and further sub-divided them into 18 ethnic sub-groups, with an approximate population of 217,000[1] or 0.7 percent of Malaysia's total population of 32.7 million (Government of Malaysia 2021a). Disaggregated official government statistics on the Orang Asli are undisclosed, making it difficult to determine the exact population of the group or the crucial indicators of socio-economic disparities (Horton 2006; United Nations 2008).

Traditionally, the Orang Asli mostly lived in the forested upland interiors, isolated from the reach of state politics. Some shared features among the different ethnic groups included the following:

- Small- to medium-sized bands of kinship-related households (Dentan *et al.* 1997), which enabled them to exploit ecological resources in a sustainable fashion, provided protection from state control, and facilitated mobility when there was a perceived threat (Scott 2010).
- Egalitarian social structures, particularly within the Negrito and Senoi groups (Dentan *et al.* 1997; Lye 2002), less so with the Aboriginal Malay groups (Nicholas 2000). These structures supported the sharing of knowledge and skills among group members to ensure survival.
- Most of their livelihood and daily needs were derived from their natural environment: the sea for coastal groups and the forests for those in the hinterland (Nicholas 2000). The forest was a source for nourishment, medicine, leisure, and household, building and trading materials (Barbara *et al.* 2008; Dounias and Colfer 2008).
- Land and natural resources were held communally to allow every community member access to vital resources (Barbara *et al.* 2008).
- Communities maintained some interaction with the state, but remained largely outside its control (Benjamin and Chou 2002). This particular feature relates to the history of slavery (Endicott 1983).

The organization and social structures in indigenous communities guaranteed availability and accessibility to basic resources for nourishment, shelter, and social and health needs which, coupled with limited wants, played a key role in enabling bands to both survive and thrive in difficult ecological conditions (Sahlins 1972; Mies and Bennholdt-Thomsen 1999).

The arrival of the modern developmental state – first with Western colonial government, followed and accelerated by the nation-state of Malaysia – meant that many of the features described above changed significantly. Almost all Orang Asli now live in one of the 853 officially recognized settlements in Malaysia (Government of Malaysia 2018). Where land and forests are still intact, the Orang Asli are able to maintain key traditional practices, such as swidden cultivation, hunting, and gathering. Even then, most are tied to the cash economy in varying degrees – either as farmer producers, traders of forest products, or wage laborers. Egalitarian leadership structures have been supplanted by state-appointed male-only headmen, and village development and security committees and the state have assumed control over almost every aspect of Orang Asli life. Land and natural resources remain held communally but, in many places, are increasingly threatened by encroachment and appropriation from state or commercial interests, and the influence of capitalism.

Modernity, however, has not brought the promise of development to the Orang Asli when compared to the national population. Socio-economic indicators demonstrate that the Orang Asli have the highest poverty rates (Idrus 2013; Government of Malaysia 2021b) and low education rates (Wong and Abdillah 2017; Government of Malaysia 2021b), and bear a higher burden of disease (Baer 1999; Nicholas and Baer 2007; Saibul *et al.* 2009; Wong *et al.* 2015). Such marginalization is a common theme for indigenous people across the globe, including in healthcare provision, suggesting that current modes of development are not working for a community like the Orang Asli (Wong *et al.* 2019).

Orang Asli healthcare as a commons health system

Beyond the herbal medicines and healing ceremonies that comprise popular images of traditional indigenous healthcare, there lies a framework that is theoretically and practically more multi-dimensional than mainstream health systems. Specifically, the concept of health therein inextricably links individual and communal health to social, cultural, spiritual, and environmental factors (Nicholas and Baer 2007). Compartmentalization of such elements in mainstream health systems is slowly being bridged through initiatives such as the social determinants of health approach, Millennium Development Goals, and Sustainable Development Goals. Nevertheless, the medicalization of health remains a prominent feature in public and private healthcare, driven by technological developments in the medical field and a changing social context (Rose 2007; van Dijk *et al.* 2016; Busfield 2017).

There are three features nested in the Orang Asli traditional healthcare system that conforms to the design principles, outlined above, of a resource system held and managed under a common property regime.

Natural resource base

For forest-dwelling communities like the Orang Asli, the land and tropical rainforest constitute their primary resource base: providing their sustenance, medicinal plants, and functioning as their spiritual and cultural foci. In itself, forest systems are recognized as a common-pool resource, with various examples of successful management under common property regimes (Ostrom 1990; Arnold 1993; Pagdee *et al.* 2006).

Orang Asli view forest resources and the land on which the forest grows as communally held. Land is regarded as a living entity, and features in the landscape and its wildlife are endowed with spiritual qualities. A band exercises rights to regulate and use these resources, yet no individual has permanent ownership, so much as usufruct rights. Resources from the natural forests are accessible to anyone from that band. However, crops planted by individuals belong to the specific individual and their household (Lim 1997; Nicholas *et al.* 2003). This perspective of ownership introduces an ethic of guardianship or stewardship over the land and forest resources, which helps to ensure these are used sustainably for the benefit of the entire band in perpetuity.

Items key to Orang Asli health that are obtained from the tropical rainforest, such as medicinal plants, are accessible to all members of the band in their territory. Food sources such as meat and vegetables come from both cultivated and natural sources – the former is harvestable only by the owners or with their consent, while the latter is accessible again to members from that band. A study by Samuel *et al.* (2010) identified 62 species of plants used for medicinal purposes by one Orang Asli community, while an earlier study by Dunn (1975) identified 104 fruit species that are harvested in another community from forest and forest swiddens.

During the onset of the COVID-19 pandemic in Malaysia, many Orang Asli communities retaining access to communal forest areas retreated into these to isolate from outside infection (Idrus *et al.* 2021), and were able to sustain themselves for the short-term. The natural resource base is the foundation on which the Orang Asli's traditional healthcare system rests, and enables them to thrive and survive during such crises.

Knowledge base

The ability to use and manage a natural resource base for medicinal, nutritional, shelter, spiritual, or cultural purposes comes from a community's knowledge repository accumulated over generations. This constitutes the second feature of a commons-based health system, where communally held indigenous knowledge underpins the workings of the system. Indigenous knowledge is central to the maintenance of the people's identity (Posey *et al.* 1996). It is an identity that is visibly community-oriented, communal, and with roles, reciprocities, and obligations of the individual to the band and vice versa.

Many indigenous communities, like the Orang Asli, hold their indigenous knowledge in common (Joranson 2008), thereby enabling it to be open and accessible to anyone in a band interested to learn the skills needed to survive in specific environmental niches. Indigenous knowledge is a resource that equips the band to obtain food, water, shelter, medicinal products, work, and tend the land, maintain social ties and health of the band, and negotiate spiritual and cultural rules. The accumulated knowledge and skills are then passed from generation to generation.

The egalitarian social structure of small bands, surviving in such an environment, requires a communal effort, and so the knowledge required to do that is shared and managed jointly. The more members who share the necessary information and skills for survival, the more the band are able to thrive. Accordingly, knowledge is non-subtractive in that one person's ability to use it does not compromise that of another.

This common access to knowledge, however, does not mean that every member will put into practice all available knowledge, as different genders, age groups, or lineages utilize different sets of knowledge to fulfill their different roles in the social setup of a band, though it remains accessible to interested band members. An individual's knowledge of health and health treatment is, accordingly, determined more by personal attentiveness than factors such as gender, while children gain this knowledge through observation and instruction by following adults in a band.

Not only is knowledge held in-common, but is also generated and used in-common through the participation of every band member in learning and decision-making. It is self-organized through collective-action and self-governance by a band. Communal decision-making is the norm in Orang Asli communities, with members collectively deciphering and providing information and knowledge to inform decisions affect the band. Some examples of this include decisions about opening up rice swiddens (Nicholas *et al.* 2003), moving the village to another location, marriage, death, and issues dealing with external or state authorities.

An approach to ownership and access to knowledge analogous to that of indigenous peoples that is increasingly being adopted by mainstream scholars is the concept of a 'knowledge commons' (Stiglitz 1999; Hess and Ostrom 2007; Kranich 2007; Joranson 2008). In such setups, knowledge is communally owned, jointly used, and managed by a group; cumulatively builds on past knowledge; is accessible to all in a group and at times beyond; is self-organized; and is non-subtractive, unlike other common-pool resources (Hess and Ostrom, 2007).

Social protection base

The third feature in the Orang Asli traditional healthcare system that makes it a commons health system is its social protection function. Broadly defined by the United Nations (2000) as 'a set of public and private policies and programs undertaken by societies in response to various contingencies to offset the absence or substantial reduction of income from work' and also 'to provide assistance to families with children as well as provide people with basic health care and housing', forms of social protection vary depending on traditions, cultures, and organizational and political structures.

In the subsistence context from which traditional Orang Asli society originated, livelihoods were not income-based, and so income and employment security were not relevant. Instead, livelihoods centered on obtaining food, water, and other materials for subsistence needs. Traditional social protection, then, consists in guaranteed sustenance, care, and health treatment for kin who are ill, incapacitated, disabled, and too young or old to meet their own livelihood needs (Baer 1999; Colfer 2008). This is achieved through risk pooling, when band members who are healthy or appropriately skilled provide those services embedded within social customs of reciprocity, kinship obligation, and cultural sanctions.

These customs are transmitted orally and through practice, and are a shared resource – utilized and owned jointly as a common property regime for the benefit of the band. Through habitual usage, they become an uncodified form of rules and precedents similar to common law (Thompson 1991) practiced by band members. The communal nature of these social customs helps to ensure a band's survival through mutual guarantee of basic health and survival needs within the capacity of a band, and a common understanding of what constitutes the rights of band members.

Summary of the health commons system

Functioning in an interrelated and interdependent way, the three features described in the preceding section provide the full range of essential services that ensure the health and well-being of an indigenous community. A communally managed natural resource base ensures that the Orang Asli have equitable and guaranteed access to shelter, water, nutrition, livelihood, and medicines. In addition, it provides the cultural backdrop of identity (Durie 1997; Kent and Bhui 2003) and recreational space for the population, which is essential for mental health (Litwiller *et al.* 2016).

Sustainably managing a large natural resource base, such as forests, is a complex planning, logistical, and monitoring undertaking. The Orang Asli draw upon their indigenous knowledge base from generations of accumulated knowledge, skill, and experience to utilize and manage it so that the objectives of providing basic health services and livelihood needs are achieved. Lastly, the social protection base practiced traditionally in the Orang Asli community provides the functionality of social health insurance, patient care, and after-care services, as well as social welfare services. Often underdeveloped in mainstream health systems, social protection is usually left for families to shoulder. In the commons-based health system, these support services are built-in as part of the social customs of the people, thereby guaranteeing care. This not only provides care for the ill and weak, but also ensures that those temporarily incapacitated are restored to productive roles and cushioned from the risk of falling into destitution.

Notwithstanding the limitations of the medical technology available among indigenous people groups, the commons-based health system has key attributes of equity, multi-dimensionality, and sustainability that present an immense challenge for the current duopoly of contemporary health systems. Yet, its continuation in today's political-economic environment is its biggest challenge. As with the Orang Asli, indigenous populations around the world find their freedom to exercise their customary rules increasingly constricted and compromised. The loss of customary land and forest to development, lack of political and legal recognition of indigenous rights, the erosion of traditional practices due to socio-economic changes, and the supplanting of indigenous knowledge with mainstream education have caused a steady decline, and may engender the eventual loss of commons-based health systems.

Conclusion

In conceptualizing and detailing the workings of commons health systems, this chapter does not suggest that it is inherently superior to public or private health systems, nor that it should supplant the current duopoly. Depending on the setting, one system may perform better than another. Nevertheless, the gaps in extant monocentric systems, particularly concerning the health of indigenous peoples, can be addressed with alternative polycentric commons systems that undergird indigenous health systems.

Accordingly, this chapter advocates not a standalone commons-based system isolated from public and private health systems, but one operating in conjunction with them to provide universal healthcare and to secure the surrounding social and economic determinants that are essential to the health and well-being of communities. More broadly, it posits that there is more diversity in the governance of health systems than is often understood, and that fostering more holistic, diverse approaches in current health provisioning will lead to better health outcomes. Examples of such innovations include the incorporation of indigenous health practices into extant health services, such as the Inuulitsivik Midwifery services in Nunavik, Canada (Van Wagner *et al.* 2012), and deployment of Aboriginal community-controlled health services in Australia (Panaretto *et al.* 2014). These are promising steps at the level of direct service provision, but greater possibilities exist – particularly at the governance level where policies are made. By placing priority on health, state policies recognizing and supporting indigenous communal ownership over its natural resources, intellectual property, and social protection practices may help to foster a secure environment for its continuation. Additionally, collaboration from public and private health sectors with indigenous owners to adapt and apply technology, management systems, and research capacity into active communal health regimes may help address a sizable bottleneck that has capped the effectiveness of commons health systems.

Public policy-making is a profoundly political process. This is especially so with health given its moral claim on human rights, identity, and personal and societal well-being (Carpenter 2012). As such, regardless of which governance regime is operating, healthcare provisioning and policies necessarily involve contested political interests and ideological considerations. Rather than adopting a more dogmatic approach, inclusivity makes room for the diversity through which human societies have organized to meet their health needs for millennia. Polycentric systems, such as the commons, empower communities to organize according to local conditions and needs. Moreover, its institutional design provides a tested framework for cooperative or competitive arrangements across multiple actors and levels, while retaining the capability to resolve conflicts. In the challenging conditions confronting human and planetary health, health system resilience will be increasingly tested, thereby requiring greater embrace of diverse and holistic approaches, and construction of cooperative arrangements such as the polycentric system of the commons explored in this chapter.

Note

1 Personal communication with Armani Williams-Hunt, an Orang Asli activist lawyer.

References

Abdullah, N.R.W. and Ng, D.K.E. 2009, 'Private health insurance in Malaysia: Policy options for a public-private partnership', *Institutions and Economies*, 1(2), pp. 234–52.

Aligica, P.D. and Tarko, V. 2012, 'Polycentricity: From Polanyi to Ostrom, and beyond', *Governance*, 25(2), pp. 237–62.

Andrew, B. 2008, 'Market failure, government failure and externalities in climate change mitigation: The case for a carbon tax', *Public Administration and Development*, 28(5), pp. 393–401.

Arnold, J.E.M. 1993, 'Management of forest resources as common property', *The Commonwealth Forestry Review*, 72(3), pp. 157–61.

Baer, A. 1999, *Health, Disease, and Survival: A Biomedical and Genetic Analysis of the Orang Asli of Malaysia*, Center for Orang Asli Concerns, Selangor.

Barbara, V., Eyzaguirre, P. and Johns, T. 2008, 'The nutritional role of forest plant foods for rural communities', in C.J.P. Colfer (ed), *Human Health and Forests: A Global Overview of Issues, Practice and Policy*, Routledge, New York, pp. 63–96.

Bedford, K. 2009, 'Gombak hospital, the Orang Asli hospital', *Indonesia and The Malay World*, 37, pp. 23–44.

Benjamin, G. and Chou, C. 2002, *Tribal Communities in the Malay World: Historical, Cultural, and Social Perspectives*, Institute of Southeast Asian Studies, Singapore.

Berkes, F., Feeny, D., McCay, B.J. and Acheson, J.M. 1989, 'The benefits of the commons', *Nature*, 340(6229), pp. 91–3.

Bhattacharya, S. 2014, 'Bioprospecting, biopiracy and food security in India: The emerging sides of neoliberalism', *International Letters of Social and Humanistic Sciences*, 12, pp. 49–56.

Bhuyan, D. 2010, 'The failure of states and international bodies to combat global warming: Disintegration of a vital global issue', *World Affairs: The Journal of International Issues*, 14(1), pp. 12–24.

Bromley, D.W. 1989, 'Property relations and economic development: The other land reform', *World Development*, 17(6), pp. 867–77.

Bromley, D.W. 1992, 'The commons, common property, and environmental policy', *Environmental and Resource Economics*, 2(1), pp. 1–17.

Bromley, D.W. and Cernea, M.M. 1989, *The Management of Common Property Natural Resources: Some Conceptual and Operational Fallacies*, World Bank, New York.

Burger, J. 1987, *Report from the Frontier: The State of the World's Indigenous Peoples*, Zed Books, Cambridge.

Busfield, J. 2017, 'The concept of medicalisation reassessed', *Sociology of Health and Illness*, 39(5), pp. 759–74.

Carlisle, K. and Gruby, R.L. 2019, 'Polycentric systems of governance: A theoretical model for the commons', *Policy Studies Journal*, 47(4), pp. 927–52.

Carpenter, D. 2012, 'Is health politics different?' *Annual Review of Political Science*, 15(1), pp. 287–311.

Chanley, V.A., Rudolph, T.J. and Rahn, W.M. 2000, 'The origins and consequences of public trust in government: A time series analysis', *The Public Opinion Quarterly*, 64(3), pp. 239–56.

Chaudhary, P., Chhetri, N.B., Dorman, B., Gegg, T., Rana, R.B., Shrestha, M., Thapa, K., Lamsal, K. and Thapa, S. 2015, 'Turning conflict into collaboration in managing commons: A case of Rupa Lake Watershed, Nepal', *International Journal of the Commons*, 9(2), pp. 744–71.

Colfer, C.J.P. (ed), 2008, *Human Health and Forests: A Global Overview of Issues, Practice and Policy*, Routledge, New York.

Dentan, R.K., Endicott, K., Hooker, M.B. and Gomes, A.G. 1997, *Malaysia and the 'Original People': A Case Study of the Impact of Development on Indigenous Peoples*, Allyn and Bacon, Boston.

Dounias, E. and Colfer, C.J.P. 2008, 'Sociocultural dimensions of diet and health in forest-dwellers' systems', in C.J.P. Colfer (ed), *Human Health and Forests: A Global Overview of Issues, Practice and Policy*, Routledge, New York, pp. 275–92.

Drèze, J. and Sen, A. 1991, *Political Economy of Hunger, Volume 1: Entitlement and Well-Being*, Clarendon Press, Oxford.

Dunn, F.L. 1975, *Rainforest Collectors and Traders: A Study of Resource Utilization in Modern and Ancient Malaya*, MBRAS, Kuala Lumpur.

Durie, M.H. 1997, 'Maori cultural identity and its implications for mental health services', *International Journal of Mental Health*, 26(3), pp. 23–5.

Endicott, K. 1983, *The Effects of Slave Raiding on the Aborigines of the Malay Peninsula*, in Reid, A. and Brewster, J. (eds), *Slavery, Bondage and Dependency in Southeast Asia*, University of Queensland Press, St. Lucia, pp. 216–45.

Eychenne, C. and Lazaro, L. 2014, 'Summer pastures: Between "commons" and "public goods"', *Journal of Alpine Research*, 102(2), pp. 65–93.

Farmer, P. and Gastineau, N. 2002, 'Rethinking health and human rights: Time for a paradigm shift', *The Journal of Law, Medicine and Ethics: A Journal of the American Society of Law, Medicine and Ethics*, 30, pp. 655–66.

Garrison, F.H. 1914, *An Introduction to the History of Medicine*, W.B. Saunders Company, Philadelphia.

Government of Malaysia. 2018, *Senarai Kampung Orang Asli di Seluruh Malaysia Beserta Kepadatan Penduduk*, MAMPU, accessed 20 May 2021, <https://www.data.gov.my/data/ms_MY/dataset/senarai-kampung-orang-asli-di-seluruh-malaysia-beserta-kepadatan-penduduk/resource/16c3ccc9-edeb-4946-8650-0b5e3f6d18b1>.

Government of Malaysia. 2021a, *Population of Malaysia 2021*, Department of Statistics Malaysia Official Portal, accessed 19 September 2021, <https://www.dosm.gov.my/v1/index.php?r=column/cthemeByCatandcat=155andbul_id=ZjJOSnpJR21sQWVUcUp6ODRudm5JZz09andmenu_id=L0pheU43NWJwRWVSZklWdzQ4TlhUUT09>.

Government of Malaysia. 2021b, *Twelfth Malaysia Plan, 2021–2025*, Economic Planning Unit, 19 September 2021, <https://rmke12.epu.gov.my/en>.

Greer, S.L., King, E.J., da Fonseca, E.M. and Peralta-Santos, A. 2020, 'The comparative politics of COVID-19: The need to understand government responses', *Global Public Health*, 15(9), pp. 1413–6.

Gruskin, S., Mills, E. and Tarantola, D. 2007, 'History, principles, and practice of health and human rights', *Lancet*, 370, pp. 449–55.

Harry, D. 2011, 'Biocolonialism and Indigenous Knowledge in United Nations Discourse', *Griffith Law Review*, 20(3), pp. 702–28.

Hess, C. and Ostrom, E. 2007, *Understanding Knowledge as a Commons*, MIT Press, Cambridge.

Hinton, A.L. 2002, *Annihilating Difference: The Anthropology of Genocide*, University of California Press, Berkley.

Holland, D.S. and Ginter, J.J.C. 2001, 'Common property institutions in the Alaskan groundfish fisheries', *Marine Policy*, 25(1), pp. 33–42.

Horton, R. 2006, 'Indigenous peoples: Time to act now for equity and health', *The Lancet*, 367(9524), pp. 1705–7.

Huitema, D., Mostert, E., Egas, W., Moellenkamp, S., Pahl-Wostl, C. and Yalcin, R. 2009, 'Adaptive water governance: Assessing the institutional prescriptions of adaptive (co-) management from a governance perspective and defining a research agenda', *Ecology and Society*, 14(1), article 26.

Idrus, R. 2013, 'Left behind: The Orang Asli under the New Economic Policy', in Gomez, E.T. and Saravanamuttu, J. (eds), *The New Economic Policy in Malaysia: Affirmative Action, Ethnic Inequalities, and Social Justice*, NUS Press, Singapore, pp. 265–92.

Idrus, R., Man, Z., Williams-Hunt, A. and Chopil, T.Y. 2021, 'Indigenous resilience and the COVID-19 response: A situation report on the Orang Asli in Peninsular Malaysia', *AlterNative: An International Journal of Indigenous Peoples*, 17(3), pp. 439–43.

Imran, Y., Wijekoon, N., Gonawala, L., Chiang, Y.-C. and De Silva, K.R.D. 2021, 'Biopiracy: Abolish Corporate Hijacking of indigenous medicinal entities', *The Scientific World Journal* 2021, e8898842.

Jodha, N.S. 1990, 'Rural common property resources: Contributions and crisis', *Economic and Political Weekly*, 25(26), pp. A65–78.

Joebges, S. and Biller-Andorno, N. 2020, 'Ethics guidelines on COVID-19 triage: An emerging international consensus', *Critical Care*, 24(1), p. 201.

Joranson, K. 2008, 'Indigenous knowledge and the knowledge commons', *International Information and Library Review*, 40(1), pp. 64–72.

Kent, P. and Bhui, K. 2003, 'Editorial: Cultural identity and mental health', *International Journal of Social Psychiatry*, 49(4), pp. 243–6.

Kerr, J. 2007, 'Watershed management: Lessons from common property theory', *International Journal of the Commons*, 1(1), pp. 89–109.

Kranich, N. 2007, 'Countering enclosure: Reclaiming the knowledge commons', in Hess, C. and Ostrom, E. (eds), *Understanding Knowledge as a Commons*, MIT Press, Camridge, pp. 85–122.

Leclerc, T., Donat, N., Donat, A., Pasquier, P., Libert, N., Schaeffer, E., D'Aranda, E., Cotte, J., Fontaine, B., Perrigault, P.-F., Michel, F., Muller, L., Meaudre, E. and Veber, B. 2020, 'Prioritisation of ICU treatments for critically ill patients in a COVID-19 pandemic with scarce resources', *Anaesthesia, Critical Care and Pain Medicine*, 39(3), pp. 333–9.

Lieberman, E.S. 2011, 'The perils of polycentric governance of infectious disease in South Africa', *Social Science and Medicine*, 73(5), pp. 676–84.

Lim, H.F. 1997, *Orang Asli, Forest, and Development*, Forest Research Institute Malaysia, Kuala Lumpur.

Litwiller, F., White, C., Gallant, K., Hutchinson, S. and Hamilton-Hinch, B. 2016, 'Recreation for mental health recovery' *Leisure/Loisir*, 40(3), pp. 345–65.

Lye, T.-P. 2002, Forest peoples, conservation boundaries, and the problem of "modernity" in Malaysia', in Chou, C. and Benjamin, G. (eds), *Tribal Communities in the Malay World: Historical, Cultural and Social Perspectives*, Institute of Southeast Asian Studies, Leiden, pp. 160–84.

Marien, S. and Hooghe, M. 2011, 'Does political trust matter? An empirical investigation into the relation between political trust and support for law compliance, *European Journal of Political Research*, 50(2), pp. 267–91.

Marmot, M. 2013, 'Universal health coverage and social determinants of health', *The Lancet*, 382(9900), pp. 1227–28.

Marshall, G. 2005, *Economics for Collaborative Environmental Management: Renegotiating the Commons*, Routledge, New York.

McIntyre, D. and Gilson, L. 2002, 'Putting equity in health back onto the social policy agenda: Experience from South Africa', *Social Science and Medicine*, 54(11), pp. 1637–56.

McKean, M.A. and Ostrom, E. 1995, *Common Property Regimes in the Forest: Just a Relic from the Past?* Duke University Press, Durham.

Mgbeoji, I. 2014, *Global Biopiracy: Patents, Plants, and Indigenous Knowledge*, UBC Press, Vancouver.

Mies, M. and Bennholdt-Thomsen, V. 1999, *The Subsistence Perspective: Beyond the Globalised Economy*, Zed Books, Cambridge.

Nicholas, C. 2000, *The Orang Asli and the Contest for Resources: Indigenous Politics, Development and Identity in Peninsular Malaysia*, IWGIA, Kuala Lumpur.

Nicholas, C. and Baer, A. 2007, 'Health care for the Orang Asli: Consequences of paternalism and non-recognition', in Chee, H.L. and Barraclough, S. (eds), *Health Care in Malaysia: The Dynamics of Provision, Financing and Access*, Routledge, New York, pp. 119–36.

Nicholas, C., Chopil, T.Y. and Sabak, T. 2003, *Orang Asli Women and the Forest: The Impact of Resource Depletion on Gender Relations Among the Semai*, Center for Orang Asli Concerns, Kuala Lumpur.

Ostrom, E. 1990, *Governing the Commons: The Evolution of Institutions for Collective Action*, Cambridge University Press, Cambridge.

Ostrom, E. 2000, 'Reformulating the commons', *Swiss Political Science Review*, 6(1), pp. 29–52.

Ostrom, E. 2010, 'Beyond markets and states: Polycentric governance of complex economic systems', *American Economic Review*, 100(3), pp. 641–72.
Ostrom, E., Gardner, R., Walker, J., Walker, J.M. and Walker, J. 1994, *Rules, Games, and Common-pool Resources*, University of Michigan Press, Ann Arbor.
Ostrom, E., and Hess, C. 2008, 'Private and common property rights', in Bouckaert, B. and De Geest, G. (eds), *Encyclopaedia of Law and Economics, Volume 2*, Edward Elgar, Northampton.
Ostrom, V. and Ostrom, E. 1977, 'Public goods and public choices', in Savas, E.S. (ed), *Alternatives for Delivering Public Services*, Routledge, New York, pp. 7–49.
Ostrom, V., Tiebout, C.M. and Warren, R. 1961, 'The organization of government in metropolitan areas: A theoretical inquiry', *The American Political Science Review*, 55(4), pp. 831–42.
Oxfam. 2022, *Inequality Kills: The Unparalleled Action Needed to Combat Unprecedented Inequality in the Wake of COVID-19*, Oxfam Policy and Practice, January 17, accessed 1 March 2022, <https://policy-practice.oxfam.org/resources/inequality-kills-the-unparalleled-action-needed-to-combat-unprecedented-inequal-621341/>.
Pagdee, A., Kim, Y. and Daugherty, P.J. 2006, 'What makes community forest management successful: A meta-study from community forests throughout the world', *Society and Natural Resources*, 19(1), pp. 33–52.
Panaretto, K.S., Wenitong, M., Button, S. and Ring, I.T. 2014, 'Aboriginal community controlled health services: Leading the way in primary care', *Medical Journal of Australia*, 200(11), pp. 649–52.
Platteau, J.P. 1991, *Traditional Systems of Social Security and Hunger Insurance: Past Achievements and Modern Challenges*. Clarendon Press, Oxford.
Pomeroy, R., Katon, B. and Harkes, I. 2001, 'Conditions affecting the success of fisheries co-management: Lessons from Asia', *Marine Policy*, 25, pp. 197–208.
Porter, D. 2005, *Health, Civilization and the State: A History of Public Health from Ancient to Modern Times*, Routledge, New York.
Posey, D.A. and Dutfield, G. 1996, *Beyond Intellectual Property: Toward Traditional Resource Rights for Indigenous Peoples and Local Communities*, IDRC, Ottawa.
Ratuva, S. 2009, 'Commodifying cultural knowledge: Corporatised western science and Pacific indigenous knowledge', *International Social Science Journal*, 60(195), pp. 153–63.
Robinson, O.F. 1994, *Ancient Rome: City Planning and Administration*, Routledge, New York.
Rose, N. 2007, 'Beyond medicalisation', *The Lancet*, 369(9562), pp. 700–2.
Rosen, G. 1958, *A History of Public Health*, MD Publications, Missouri.
Sachs, J. 2001, *Macroeconomics and Health: Investing in Health for Economic Development*, World Health Organization, Geneva.
Saechang, O., Yu, J. and Li, Y. 2021, 'Public trust and policy compliance during the COVID-19 pandemic: The role of professional trust', *Healthcare*, 9(2), p. 151.
Sahlins, M. 1972, *Stone Age Economics*, Routledge, New York.
Saibul, N., Shariff, Z.M., Lin, K.G., Kandiah, M., Ghani, N.A. and Rahman, H.A. 2009, 'Food variety score is associated with dual burden of malnutrition in Orang Asli (Malaysian indigenous peoples) households: Implications for health promotion', *Asia Pacific Journal of Clinical Nutrition*, 18(3), pp. 412–22.
Samuel, A.J.S.J., Kalusalingam, A., Chellappan, D.K., Gopinath, R., Radhamani, S., Husain, H.A., Muruganandham, V. and Promwichit, P. 2010, 'Ethnomedical survey of plants used by the Orang Asli in Kampung Bawong, Perak, West Malaysia', *Journal of Ethnobiology and Ethnomedicine*, 6(1), p. 5.
Scott, J.C. 2010, *The Art of Not Being Governed: An Anarchist History of Upland Southeast Asia*, Yale University Press, New Haven.
Service, E.R. 1975, *Origins of the State and Civilization: The Process of Cultural Evolution*. Norton, New York.
Stiglitz, J.E. 1999, 'Knowledge as a Global Public Good', in Kaul, I., Grunberg, I. and Stern, M. (eds), *Global Public Goods*, Oxford University Press, Oxford, pp. 308–25.
Swallow, B.M. 1997, *The Multiple Products, Functions and Users of Natural Resource Systems*, IFPRI, Washington.
Swiss Academy of Medical Sciences. 2020, 'COVID-19 pandemic: Triage for intensive-care treatment under resource scarcity', *Swiss Medical Weekly*, 150, p. w20229.
Thompson, E.P. 1991, *Customs in Common*, Merlin Press, London.
United Nations. 1948, *Universal Declaration of Human Rights*, United Nations, Paris.
United Nations. 2000, *Enhancing Social Protection and Reducing Vulnerability in a Globalizing World*, United Nations, New York.

United Nations. 2008, *State of the World's Indigenous Peoples*, United Nations, New York.

van Dijk, W., Faber, M.J., Tanke, M.A.C., Jeurissen, P.P.T. and Westert, G.P. 2016, 'Medicalisation and overdiagnosis: What society does to medicine', *International Journal of Health Policy and Management*, 5(11), pp. 619–22.

Van Wagner, V., Osepchook, C., Harney, E., Crosbie, C. and Tulugak, M. 2012, 'Remote midwifery in Nunavik, Québec, Canada: Outcomes of perinatal care for the Inuulitsivik health centre, 2000–2007', *Birth*, 39(3), pp. 230–7.

Watanabe, T. and Shirasaka, S. 2018, 'Pastoral practices and common use of pastureland: The case of Karakul, North-Eastern Tajik Pamirs', *International Journal of Environmental Research and Public Health*, 15(12), p. 2725.

White, D.B. and Lo, B. 2021, 'Mitigating inequities and saving lives with ICU triage during the COVID-19 pandemic', *American Journal of Respiratory and Critical Care Medicine*, 203(3), pp. 287–95.

White, T.A. and Runge, C.F. 1994, 'Common property and collective action: Lessons from cooperative watershed management in Haiti', *Economic Development and Cultural Change*, 43(1), pp. 1–41.

WHO. 2000, *The World Health Report 2000: Health Systems - Improving Performance*, World Health Organization, Geneva.

WHO. 2008, *Closing the Gap in a Generation: Health Equity Through Action on the Social Determinants of Health*, Commission on Social Determinants of Health Final Report, World Health Organization, Geneva.

Wong, B. and Abdillah, K. 2017, 'Poverty and primary education of the Orang Asli children', in Joseph, C. (ed), *Policies and Politics in Malaysian Education: Education Reforms, Nationalism and Neoliberalism*, Routledge, New York, pp. 54–71.

Wong, C.Y., Zalilah, M.S., Chua, E.Y., Norhasmah, S., Chin, Y.S. and Siti Nur'Asyura, A. 2015, 'Double-burden of malnutrition among the indigenous peoples (Orang Asli) of Peninsular Malaysia', *BMC Public Health*, 15(680).

Wong, Y., Allotey, P. and Reidpath, D. 2014, 'Health care as commons: An indigenous approach to universal health coverage', *The International Indigenous Policy Journal*, 5(3), pp. 1–14.

Wong, Y.S., Allotey, P. and Reidpath, D.D. 2016, 'Sustainable development goals, universal health coverage and equity in health systems: The Orang Asli commons approach', *Global Health, Epidemiology and Genomics*, 1, e12, pp. 1–10.

Wong, Y.S., Allotey, P. and Reidpath, D.D. 2019, 'Why we run when the doctor comes: Orang Asli responses to health systems in transition in Malaysia', *Critical Public Health*, 29(2), pp. 192–204.

Wyborn, C. 2014, 'Cross-scale linkages in connectivity conservation: Adaptive governance challenges in spatially distributed networks', *Environmental Policy and Governance*, 25(1), pp. 1–15.

Zainuddin, Z. 2012, *Genetic and Dental Profiles of Orang Asli of Peninsular Malaysia*, Universiti Sains Malaysia, Penerbit.

37

DIVERSE ECONOMIES OF CARE-FULL HEALTHCARE

Banking and sharing human milk

Lindsay Naylor

Contemporary systems of healthcare and other industries are largely defined by their neoliberal, capitalist character. However, this parochial approach to understanding the political economy of healthcare misses the myriad activities that make up the 'care' in healthcare. Receiving care is not isolated to capitalist exchanges, nor is it unquestionably tied to the neoliberal marketplace. There exist diverse economies of care within, outside, and alongside neoliberal capitalist ones. Moreover, multiple means by which we may examine care are often overlooked. In many cases, healthcare that cannot be counted does not count, as it relates to capitalist exchange. In this chapter, using the example of the banking and sharing of human milk, I demonstrate that other economies of care are happening, and stress that they should be valued in their own right, not solely in relation to capitalism.

Milk *banking* relies on diverse forms of labor by humans – volunteer and paid – and non-humans, while also involving monetary exchange. Conversely, milk *sharing* encompasses barter and trade systems, gift exchange, and the distribution of surplus. Human milk is universally recognized as the best first food for infants. Accordingly, these two forms of accessing human milk make possible the provision of care to infants for parents who are not able to provide milk themselves. Simultaneously, the banking and sharing of human milk raises political-economic questions about access and who benefits from these diverse forms of care. Here, I argue that the banking and sharing of milk represents economic diversity, yet there are structural limitations related to who can participate in these exchanges. Reading through this lens makes a twofold contribution: it demonstrates healthcare that sits within, alongside, and outside capitalism, while also revealing how it destabilizes the neoliberal (or individual responsibility) character of healthcare, by showing that care is not an autonomous act, but is made multiple and possible by a number of actors. This has the effect of breaking down the idea that there is no alternative to capitalism, which can be world-making – put differently, it exposes the existence of capitalism's others and supports their continuous becoming.

While human milk is an important part of health(care) for lactating parents and infants, when disembodied as donor human milk, it takes on a multiplicity that, when read through a diverse economies lens, demonstrates a complexity to that care. To better understand human milk exchanges as care-full, I first draw out the theoretical foundations for this chapter in a discussion of diverse and community economies. With specific attention to labor/work and exchange/transactions,

DOI: 10.4324/9781003017110-42

I then discuss how we might read care through a diverse economies lens, and what this perspective allows for. Finally, I turn to the case-study, drawing out the collective work and interdependent exchanges occurring in the banking and sharing of human milk.

Diverse and community economies

Here, I use a diverse economies framing to shape the conversation about the already existing care-full healthcare that takes place all around us. The diverse economies framework suggests that scholars should read economic activity for difference (Gibson-Graham and Dombroski 2020). To illustrate the implications of this approach, I focus on the US for two reasons: first, due to the neoliberal character of its healthcare system, and second, because there are very low rates of feeding human milk to infants in the country. These characteristics make the US an ideal place to examine alter- and non-capitalisms of human milk. In the US, healthcare is deeply steeped in the capitalist marketplace, and access to medical care is grounded in neoliberal understandings of individual ability to pay (amounts vary based on employment and personal wealth). The sharp increase in the use of crowdfunding services such as GoFundMe to provide for healthcare in recent years is clear evidence that the provision of commodified healthcare under capitalism is failing society (see: Berliner and Kenworthy 2019). Simultaneously, other forms of care exist alongside capitalist-style paid medical care. A diverse economies approach to thinking about care helps to identify and name these diverse sites of care, and also examine and analyze their entanglements.

To maintain a myopic view of the US healthcare system, where we view healthcare and its supporting industries through a neoliberal capitalist lens, falls into Gibson-Graham's critique of 'capitalocentrism' (2006a [1996]), where economic activities are at all times considered capitalist, or compared as capitalism's Other. By looking to economic activities that are not located at the tip of the iceberg (see: Figure 37.1) – wage work, profit, ownership over the means of production – as 'alternative' to capitalism, we maintain capitalism's hegemony. In turn, we accord less value to those activities that are not captured by capitalism – those activities under the water line.

Capitalocentric approaches mean that we only value and acknowledge as 'economic' those things that can be quantified, such as monetary exchanges that contribute to GDP, or wages that can be taxed. This practice has the effect of rendering many activities and exchanges invisible. Gibson-Graham (2006b), instead, urged scholars to look below the water line and read enterprise, labor, transactions, property, and finance for difference. To conduct such investigations is to make visible the myriad activities that exist within, alongside, and outside of their capitalist counterparts. To reframe the way we think about economy(ies) is to also recognize that we are interdependent, human, and non-human, and that we are in the process of collectively building and practicing community economies (Gibson-Graham and Dombroski 2020). Moreover, the normative implication of this work centers on demanding a system that is just and refocuses our attention on ethical action; when we see, name, and practice these community economies, we are doing the work of transformation (Gibson-Graham *et al.* 2013; Gibson-Graham and Dombroski 2020). A diverse economies approach is significant because it does not just *see* difference; it *enacts* difference.

Diverse economic thinking reads economies for difference, with attention to how we are sustained through interdependence (Miller 2019). As I have noted elsewhere, 'community economies are spaces of collective action where, in striving to create livable worlds, groups are actively reshaping their economic practices, identities, and exchanges […] and [they] are sites of care, interdependence, and being in common' (Naylor 2019: 29). Thus, community economies are sites of ethical decision-making and spaces where we can see care-full social relations around exchange. There are a number of different ways to apply this to healthcare. We can read healthcare through

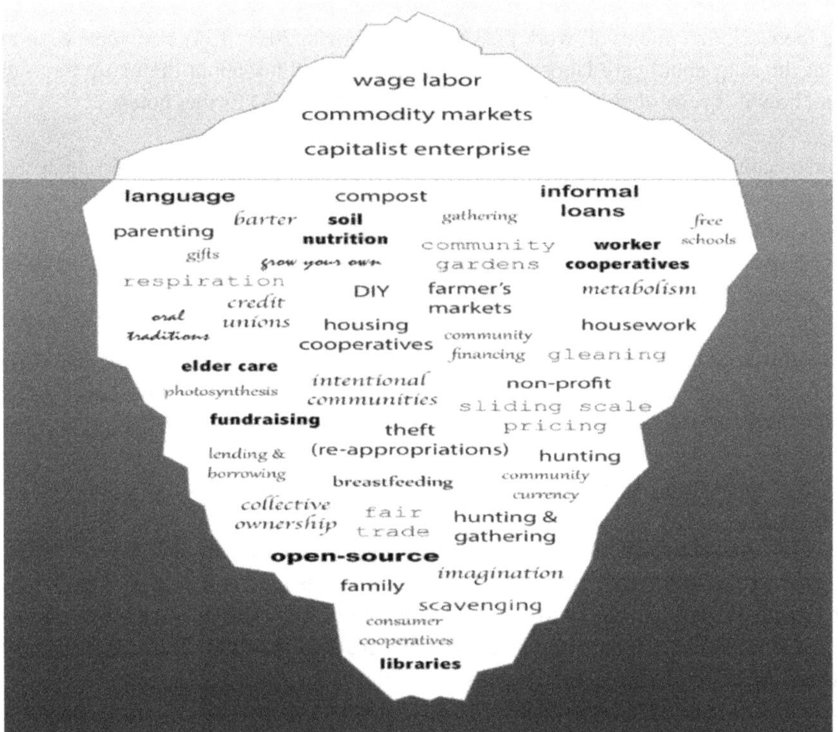

Figure 37.1 Diverse economies iceberg.

Source: Community Economies Collective (n.d.), as licensed under a Creative Commons Attribution-ShareAlike 4.0 International License.[1]

enterprise, labor, transactions, property, *and* finance.[2] For the purposes of this chapter, I focus on economies of care labor and transactions in the exchange of human milk in the US. Specifically, I argue that the banking and sharing of human milk represents another site of economic diversity. Reading the labor and transactions around human milk for difference is important because it both challenges and exposes the efforts of capitalism to capture it. Here, I consider 'livelihood and wellbeing,' as well as 'ethically responsible encounters,' as they relate to the banking and sharing of human milk (Gibson-Graham and Dombroski 2020: 19).

Dombroski *et al.* (2019) suggest that to rethink economies, we should start with care: who does care work, what constitutes care work, and how it can be expanded. Starting with care signals recognition that it is foundational and fundamental to economies. There is a gendered and power dynamic to care work as well, and feminist thinkers often point to the disproportionate labor burdens on people who identify as women in care work. However, in taking a diverse economies approach, scholars expand on the 'who' of care (including our non-human Others, which may include machinery, animals, bacteria – in this case, for example, pumping technologies, refrigerators, pasteurization processes; see also: de la Bellacasa 2017) and recognize that a diverse economy of healthcare is not and cannot be individual (or neoliberal). Dombroski *et al.* (2019) point to the multiple and joined effort of care that encompasses many beings and non-living things as a collective of care.

Care

'Care is the work that makes all work possible' (Dombroski 2020: 154). A diverse economies approach to thinking about care labor provides an avenue to think about the many forms that care takes and how it is rewarded (or not). As Dombroski (2020: 155) further notes:

> Diverse economies scholars include consideration of care labour as part of a more general consideration of diverse forms of labour including labour compensated for by wages and salary (paid labour), labour only partially compensated by wages and salary (alternative paid labour), and labour that is compensated completely outside of a system of payments or not at all (unpaid labour).

However, this approach is simultaneously expansive and limiting when thinking about care labor as a site of interdependence. It is expansive in that we are able to examine how care labor is valued. Yet, it is limiting, as a compensation lens does not easily allow for incorporation of the non-human others that are enrolled in care work. As a result, focusing less on the compensation component and privileging the formations of collective care is an important corollary exercise in reading care for difference.

Care work is also a form of exchange, a transaction, which may or may not involve money. A diverse economies approach extends to thinking about engagement within exchanges and multiplies the range of transactions (Diprose 2020). Ethical questions around care are a central component of reading transactions for difference, as exchanges are not neutral. Encounters involving care can take multiple forms and, again, demonstrate collectivity.

The care work that undergirds all labor matters. Often referred to by feminist scholars (largely from the global core) as 'social reproduction,' care work is many times undervalued and subject to patriarchal and white supremacist power dynamics. Indeed, whether caring labor is a choice in many cases remains an open question. Despite care work being essential to our lives, it remains overlooked and marginalized (Lawson 2009). It is work that is often taken up by, or imposed upon, people who are women or female-identifying (*cf.* Federici 2020 [2012]). Additionally, historically and contemporarily, white women are more often able to redistribute the work of social reproduction to Black, Indigenous, and women of color. By reading care for difference, we can see the formation of diverse and community economies, as well as the dynamics of who gets to participate and how care is valued.

Human milk and its exchange

Human milk is widely considered the best first food for infants (Updegrove 2013a, b; Smith *et al.* 2017). It is a biological process and practice of care across the globe (albeit unevenly), with scientifically agreed-upon benefits, including: protection against many health issues (*e.g.* asthma and cardiovascular disease) (Mosca and Gianni 2017), the provision of immunoprotective properties (Bode *et al.* 2014; Lorenzetti *et al.* 2021), increased health of the parent (Bode *et al.* 2014; Mosca and Gianni 2017), and improved cognition (Feldman and Eidelman 2003). The composition of milk changes during the period of feeding or pumping, and as the infant ages. It is made at the site of the body and defies the logics of capital. However, a diverse economies read for difference demonstrates how human milk, and the multiple actors involved in the labor and transactions surrounding it both defy and accommodate neoliberal capitalist logics. Simultaneously, as illustrated by Figure 37.2, milk is multiple: taking on additional properties besides that of being infant food

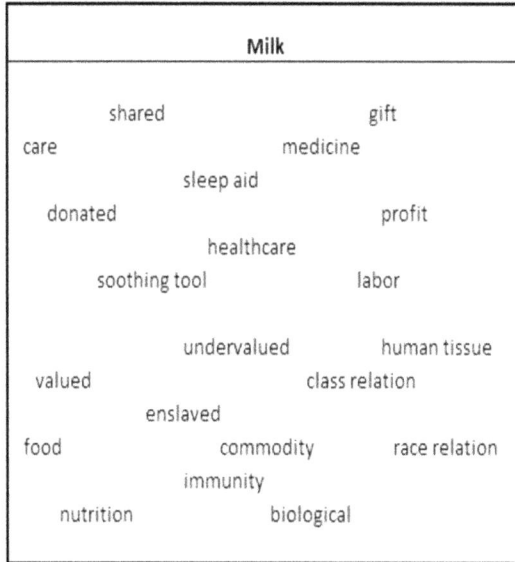

Figure 37.2 Diverse and community economies of human milk.

(Brown 2016; Naylor *et al.* 2020). Human milk is also contested and controversial, especially in the case of places such as the US or UK, when infants are fed at the site of the body in public settings (*cf.* Boyer 2011; Dillard 2015; Matthews 2018; Bartlett 2019; Naylor 2022). However, not all parents can make milk: some birth parents may not be able to produce any or enough milk, some may choose not to provide milk, or some may be adoptive parents, for example.[3] In these cases, if the preference is to supplement formula with human milk, or provide human milk exclusively, some parents and hospitals may turn to formal sites for donor human milk and/or additional channels for milk sharing.

Historically, utilizing another person's milk to feed an infant is fraught with inequity (Swanson 2009, 2014). It has entailed, for instance, the hiring of wet nurses, reciprocal breastfeeding, and the mandate of enslaved peoples breastfeeding through the violently enforced practice of rendering people as property by differential othering categories such as race, class, religion, and caste. These histories are well documented and are important as they relate to foundational thinking on whether or not to provide human milk to infants, as well as personal choices in breastfeeding or accessing other sources of human milk.[4] While infant feeding remains commoditized and rife with class and race-based inequities in the US, it simultaneously has a more recent history of being a gift, a donation, bereavement site, and/or product of over-supply (*cf.* Swanson 2014; Falls 2017).

Although there is a broader context for milk sharing that displays difference across the globe, here I focus on the US, where rates of breastfeeding remain low (CDC 2020). While channels to access human milk existed prior to formalization, including sharing and 'kitchen milk banks' (Swanson 2014), the first institutionalized milk bank was established in 1910 (Falls 2017: 52). There were also milk stations and bureaus that proliferated across the country in major cities through the early-1900s. These were places where people would donate, or sometimes be paid for their milk, and where parents could be given, or pay a fee for, the milk (Swanson 2014: 161–2). The numbers of these sites varied over time in the US. The formal milk bank arena today consists of 29 not-for-profit member milk banks that are affiliated with the Human Milk Banking

Association of North America (HMBANA) and, at the time of writing, two for-profit milk banking corporations (Prolacta Bioscience and Medolac). The cost of donor milk varies across state, institution, and health insurance coverage, but is generally estimated to be $3–5 per ounce in this marketplace. It is important to note, however, that Prolacta Bioscience and Medolac have higher price points and that medical institutions are their main market – particularly Neonatal Intensive Care Units, where pre-term and critically ill infants are medically treated. The for-profit milk banks reconstitute donor milk into proprietary fortified products aimed at treating very low-weight infants.

My interview data, and that from other scholars (*cf.* Caroll 2014; Falls 2017), confirm the lengthy and rigorous screening process that is undertaken to become a milk donor in formalized sites of exchange, such as milk banks. When donating to a HMBANA site, donors are first screened by staff through a phone interview. If eligible, they are then given a screening packet that queries health history and asks for additional information about the parent, their infant, and the status of feedings if they are taking place. There is also a medical consent process to be completed. Finally, a blood test is administered that screens for HIV/AIDS, hepatitis B and C, HTLV-1 and HTLV-2, and syphilis. In the case of Prolacta Bioscience, there are additional screening measures, which include a drug test and obtaining verification from their physician that they are able to provide milk without it being detrimental to their own child. As an interviewee from the company explained: 'we guarantee that the milk came from the donor and that it is excess milk.' In part, this measure is due to the paid character of the exchange by the for-profit company. In the same interview, it was suggested that paid donors have a 'better medical profile' than volunteer donors.

While these formalized contexts exist, in many cases they remain unaffordable or otherwise inaccessible to many (Swanson 2014; Carter and Reyes-Foster 2016). In those cases, some turn to milk sharing. There are now multiple groups across the US that use online resources to establish connections for peer-to-peer sharing of milk. Websites that advocate for sharing, at the time of writing, include the following: Eats on Feets, Milk Share, and Human Milk 4 Human Babies. In these cases, parents seeking milk determine the level of screening necessary and the lengths at which to go to procure milk from their peers. The buying, selling, and sharing of milk are unregulated, and milk is generally treated as a 'food/beverage' in terms of legal status.[5] However, many professionals strongly caution against peer-to-peer sharing of milk, citing safety concerns, such as the transfer of harmful substances and viruses and bacteria (AAP 2017).

Since 2017, I have been conducting research on access to human milk in a non-breastfeeding context. Put differently, I am asking questions about corporeally disassociated flesh (see: Dixon 2015): human milk outside of the context of the body, and what barriers and inequities exist to provisioning it as infants' first food. To date, I have interviewed mothers, NICU staff, breastfeeding coalition members, milk bank staff, and milk banking organizations, as well as surveyed mothers, about breastfeeding and donor human milk (n=81 interviews; n=113 survey respondents; n=9 milk bank staff).[6] Here, I draw on interviews I conducted with milk bank staff, recipients and donors of human milk, and both primary and secondary data on human milk sharing and donating.[7] Interviews were conducted by phone, virtually, and in-person at milk banks, and were entirely focused on experiences relating to donor human milk. For mothers (in this case, all of the non-milk bank interviewees identified as women and birth mothers), I focused on the experiences of breastfeeding (or not), considerations of human milk, donations of milk, and sharing of milk. For milk bank staff, I focused on processes and practices, production and distribution, cost and access, and perceived benefits and drawbacks of human milk banking.

These forms of accessing human milk demonstrate a collective of care, which includes many actors and non-human others (see: Figure 37.3).

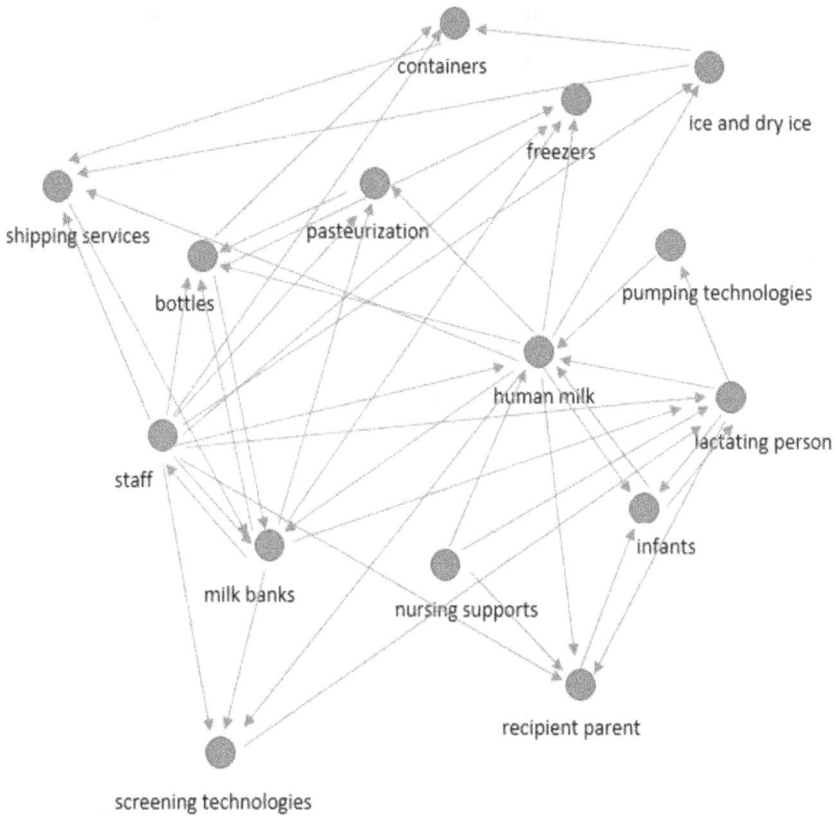

Figure 37.3 Assemblage of the collective of care.

When disembodied, the care work/labor of providing human milk is undertaken by a number of beings and made possible by non-human others (see: Table 37.1). Medical technologies, refrigeration and pasteurization technologies, transportation, lab, and service labor all make it possible for people to receive human milk.

Ways of accessing human milk further demonstrate such forms of care as related to the health of infants as a diverse economic relation. It is both embodied and disembodied. Mann (2017: 19–20) notes that:

> Embodied care is an *ethic* that understands individual and social morality as deeply bound up with the caring relationships and communities in which human beings are embedded. Care is also a set of practices where individuals take up the work of caring for the bodies of others predominantly with and through their own bodies.
>
> (emphasis in original)

Donors are providing care through their bodies and, in some cases, are receiving care or practicing a form of self-care (see also: Caroll 2015) as they share their milk with a real or imagined community. Donors in this study fall into three main groups. The first group includes those who are sharing excess milk due to overproduction (generally many donations over time) or frozen surplus after weaning their own child (generally a one-time donation). Mothers talked about keeping their

Table 37.1 Labor relations in contemporary exchanges of human milk

Labor	*Encounter*
Non-remunerated	Non-monetary or none
Earth others	Non-monetary or none
Social reproduction	Non-monetary or none
Volunteer	Non-monetary or none
Care	
Waged	Payment for services
Contract	
Other compensation	In-kind labor
Reciprocal	In-kind exchange
Barter	

Source: Adapted from Dombrowski and Gibson-Graham (2020: 13).

freezers well-stocked and then, when they were full or after a certain period of time, donating any excess. As one interviewee put it: 'and then I filled my freezer up again.' The second group includes those who are producing and donating, or otherwise sharing, their milk after the loss of an infant. These donors may donate to a milk bank or through other means. However, on average, the milk bank staff I spoke with reported having hundreds of donors, with one reporting approximately 800 donors in 2018, of which 10 percent constituted bereaved mothers who donate as part of processing the trauma of losing their infant. For HMBANA milk banks, in the case of bereavement, screening is minimal and all milk is accepted. Any milk that does not meet the standard for processing is used for research.

The third donor group consists of mothers who had previously had an infant in the NICU and were using donation as a form of reciprocity. Their infant had received donor human milk in the first few days of their life – generally prior to their birth mother's ability to produce their own milk. This form of reciprocity is often framed by milk banks and in the literature on donation as a form of gift-giving, or altruism. However, as I learned from the parents with whom I spoke, it was characterized in a number of different ways: donors largely emphasized its labor intensity and as a form of care work, while recipients focused on its qualities as a form of barter or contract (see: Table 37.1). One mother explained, 'breastfeeding and providing milk is hard work, many do not recognize the effort.' Others framed it is care: 'it's not like this is just about nutrition for the baby; it's also psychological care for the mother, so you're taking care of the mother and the baby.' The hard work and care came through in most interviews, and many mothers I spoke with balked at the idea of exchanging their milk through a commodity relation. Indeed, one mother laughed, saying: 'I could have bought or sold milk on EBay because a friend of mine told me about that, and boy would I have made a ton of money but that wasn't my scene so much.' At least among this group of interviewees, the labor relations of providing milk are, thus, more often considered as non-remunerated.

Donor human milk is not covered by health insurance in the US, except in some cases of medical care, such as when it is reframed as medicine and prescribed to treat very low birthweight and premature infants in the NICU (Naylor *et al.* 2020). This demonstrates the need to rethink and reframe milk differently in the US healthcare system. Specifically, what if it was considered multiple? As a commodity and market-based relation when secured in the formal setting of the milk bank, it can be cost-prohibitive for many parents. Accordingly, while donor milk is a form of care and care labor, distribution of access to this care is based in long-standing class relations and healthcare inequities. At some milk banks, there are charitable funds that are used to offset costs for parents who cannot afford the high cost of screened and processed donor human milk. However, the majority (80–100 percent) of donor human milk that enters this channel (both in the non-profit and in for-profit arenas) is sold to hospitals for use in the NICU (payment by consumer) and, in some cases, protected (insurance claims). When asked about human milk as a medically necessary intervention, an interviewee who had previously had an infant in the NICU replied:

> It's a commodity yeah, and it becomes a commodity [...] And the thing is too, and I don't mean to be cynical, but somebody's making money off this milk production, at the end of the day, and milk sharing is free, so somebody's making money off of, is monetizing the medical fragility of children and the production value of women, you know what I mean?

By distancing from capitalist exchanges, we can see other viewpoints that signal that the donation and sharing of milk is a care-full practice and not one that is limited to capitalist dictates and/or social reproduction. Specifically, beyond market-based forms of access and exchange, there are other exchanges that take place beyond the market (see: Table 37.2). The exchange of human milk can take place within a household, can be a gift, and is bound up in rituals of maintenance (*e.g.* the cleaning and sanitizing of pumping equipment). One of the recipients I spoke with who received donor human milk both as a part of medical treatment for her infant in the NICU, and then later as a gift exchange described this sharing of milk as a social experience via a communal freezer:

> it's informal, it's a drop-off, and so we have essentially on our mom board or whatever, and it's definitely a little more like hippie and I would describe myself that way, I would definitely describe myself that way as a parent, but people ask, the freezer's empty can somebody come drop off, so there's definitely a sense on this board that people know that milk is available to them, and they totally take advantage of it.

When I asked further about screening, she replied:

> No this is like, this is, you see on Facebook that this person's friends with the person you went to high school with and you're like oh I'm getting milk from my blah blah blah blah [...]

Table 37.2 Transactions in contemporary exchanges of human milk

Transaction	*Encounter*
Outside of market	
Household	Household negotiation
Gifting	Cultural norms
Earth other exchanges	Personal maintenance
Market-based	
Sale	Payment by consumer
Protected	Insurance claim payment
Earth other exchanges	Paid maintenance
Other exchange	
Local trade	Producer-consumer negotiation
Underground	Producer-consumer negotiation
Barter	Trade negotiation

Source: Adapted from Dombrowski and Gibson-Graham (2020: 14).

so some moms, I mean the screening process is like a mom that says I need no-restriction milk or caffeine-free milk or whatever it is.

She further explained that there was no money involved in these exchanges, noting: 'absolutely not, no, and people are honest with us, people are like, "look I'm on Zoloft but you're welcome to my milk" […] so it's just all completely open.' Other parents formed long-term relationships, such as the ones that Falls (2017) describes in their account of milk sharing. For example, in one case that was related to me, a mother shared: 'a friend of mine […] was an overproducer and she ended up developing a relationship with a mom locally who had adopted a child and they just had a relationship where they just met up all the time.' These forms of gifting and local trade show a community of care that is made possible by negotiation and trust, as well as the maintenance and care of non-human others. Receiving milk from a milk bank is a monetary exchange, but largely a non-monetary form of care made possible by a donor and a bevy of technologies. The transactions taking place are bound to a diversity of transactions that show a basis within, outside, and alongside capitalism.

These forms of labor and transactions in contemporary exchanges exemplify milk in its multiplicity and diversity. However, of the parents with whom I have been able to speak, all are able to be donors and recipients due to access that is tied to their race (white), class (middle-to-upper), and status within well-resourced communities. Thus, while it is important to recognize human milk exchanges through decentering capitalism, it is additionally crucial to see where imbalances in access to these forms of exchange exist, along with the white supremacist and patriarchal systems that perpetuate exclusion.

Concluding thoughts

As noted earlier, human milk is an important part of the health(care) of lactating parents and infants. It enters the formal healthcare arena in postnatal and NICU settings and, in the case of donor human milk, through non- and for-profit milk banks. However, the contemporary exchange of human milk is not centered on capitalist relations alone. Indeed, the banking and sharing of human milk is a care-full practice that takes multiple forms. That milk and care in this case are multiple, and that in its exchange, donors and recipients enter an assemblage of caregiving beings and non-human others, show a diversity of exchange and the caring forms they take. What this suggests is that when we examine healthcare, it is important to think about the 'care' therein and decenter it as an activity based in solely capitalism, where remunerated laborers provide medical care at a cost. Reading for difference using human milk as an example demonstrates how even as capitalism attempts to commodify and create an industry around it, opportunities still exist for it to function as a diverse and multiple form of care. That is, it can never be fully captured or replaced through market exchanges. Moreover, we must consider who can participate in this care, and what barriers and inequities exist to it operating effectively to nurture the reproduction of human life.

Notes

1 See: <https://www.communityeconomies.org/resources/diverse-economies-iceberg>.
2 See, for example: Williams and Onoschenko (2013); Dombroski *et al.* (2016); Dombroski (2020); and McKinnon (2020).
3 Please note that it is not my intention to wade into the debates over infant feeding.
4 These histories are beyond the scope of this chapter. However, see: Golden (2001); Swanson (2014); Falls (2017); and Mieso *et al.* (2021).

5 Prolacta Bioscience is currently advocating to the FDA that the classification of milk as a 'food' be amended.
6 Interviews in a NICU, and an online survey conducted between 2017 and 2018, were completed as part of a research team working on understanding barriers to breastfeeding and the practice of kangaroo care in the NICU. These data influence, but are not part of, the dataset drawn on in this chapter. Initial findings from this ongoing work are published as: Clarke-Sather *et al.* (2018); Clarke-Sather and Naylor (2019); Naylor and Clarke-Sather (2020); Naylor *et al.* (2020); and Weber *et al.* (2021).
7 A forthcoming component of this larger project is recruiting HMBANA donors to discuss their experiences in interviews. This fieldwork was due to start in early 2020, but was interrupted by the COVID-19 pandemic.

References

American Academy of Peadiatrics. 2017, 'Donor human milk for the high-risk infant: Preparation, safety, and usage options in the United States', *Pediatrics*, 139(1).

Berliner, L.S. and Kenworthy, N.J. 2017, 'Producing a worthy illness: Personal crowdfunding amidst financial crisis', *Social Science and Medicine*, 187(August), pp. 233–42.

Bode, L., McGuire, M. Rodriguez, J.M., Geddes, D.T., Hassiotou, F., Hartmann, P.E. and McGuire, M.K. 2014, 'It's alive: Microbes and cells in human milk and their potential benefits to mother and infant', *Advances in Nutrition*, 5(5), pp. 571–3.

Boyer, K. 2011, '"The way to break the taboo is to do the taboo thing": Breastfeeding in public and citizen-activism in the UK', *Health & Place*, 17(2), pp. 430–7.

Carroll, K. 2015, 'Breastmilk donation as care work', in Cassidy, T. and El Tom, A. (eds), *Ethnographies of Breastfeeding: Cultural Contexts and Confrontations*, Bloomsbury Publishing, London, pp. 173–86.

Carroll, K. 2017, 'Practicing the multiplicity of donor milk in neonatal intensive care', in Smith, P.H., Labbok, M. and Chambers, B.D. (eds), *Breastfeeding, Social Justice, and Equity*, Praeclarus Press, Amarillo, Texas, pp. 249–56.

Carter, S.K. and Reyes-Foster, B.M. 2016, 'Pure gold for broken bodies: Discursive techniques constructing milk banking and peer milk sharing in US news', *Symbolic Interaction*, 39(3), pp. 353–73.

Clarke-Sather, A.R., Cobb, K., Maloney, C. and Young, H. 2018, 'Contextual design theory applied to wearables that facilitate kangaroo care by interviewing mothers of hospitalized infants', in *2018 Design of Medical Devices Conference*, American Society of Mechanical Engineers, Minneapolis, Minnesota.

Clarke-Sather, A. and Naylor, L. 2019, 'Survey as a contextual design method applied to breastfeeding wearables for mothers caring for infants in NICUS', in *Proceedings of the 2019 Design of Medical Devices Conference*, American Society of Mechanical Engineers, Minneapolis, Minnesota.

Dillard, D.M. 2015, 'Nurse-ins, #notcoveringup: Positive deviance, breastfeeding, and public attitudes', *International Journal of Childbirth Education*, 30(2), pp. 72–6.

Diprose, G. 2020, 'Framing essay: The diversity of transactions', in Gibson-Graham, J.K. and Dombroski, K. (eds), *The Handbook of Diverse Economies*, Edward Elgar, Cheltenham, pp. 195–205.

Dixon, D.P. 2015, *Feminist Geopolitics: Material States*, Ashgate, Burlington, Vermont.

Dombroski, K. 2020, 'Caring labour: Redistributing care work', in Gibson-Graham, J.K. and Dombroski, K. (eds), *The Handbook of Diverse Economies*, Edward Elgar, Cheltenham, pp. 154–62.

Dombroski, K., Healy, S. and McKinnon, K. 2019, 'Care-full community economies', in Bauhardt, C. and Harcourt, W. (eds), *Feminist Political Ecology and the Economics of Care: In Search of Economic Alternatives*, Routledge, New York, pp. 99–115.

Dombroski, K., Mckinnon, K. and Healy, S. 2016, 'Beyond the birth wars: Diverse assemblages of care', *New Zealand Geographer*, 72(3), pp. 230–9.

Falls, S. 2017, *White Gold: Stories of Breast Milk Sharing*, University of Nebraska Press, Lincoln.

Federici, S. 2020, *Revolution at Point Zero: Housework, Reproduction, and Feminist Struggle*, PM Press, Oakland.

Feldman, R. and Eidelman, A.I. 2003, 'Direct and indirect effects of breast milk on the neurobehavioral and cognitive development of premature infants', *Developmental Psychobiology*, 43(2), pp. 109–19.

Gibson-Graham, J.K. 2006a, *A Postcapitalist Politics*, University of Minnesota Press, Minneapolis.

Gibson-Graham, J.K. 2006b, *The End Of Capitalism (As We Knew It): A Feminist Critique of Political Economy*, University of Minnesota Press, Minneapolis.

Gibson-Graham, J.K., Cameron, J. and Healy, S. 2013, *Take Back the Economy: An Ethical Guide for Transforming Our Communities*, University of Minnesota Press, Minneapolis.

Gibson-Graham, J.K. and Dombroski, K. 2020, *The Handbook of Diverse Economies*, Edward Elgar, Cheltenham.

Golden, J. 2001, *A Social History of Wet Nursing in America: From Breast to Bottle*, Ohio State University Press, Ohio.

La Bellacasa, M.P. de. 2017, *Matters of Care: Speculative Ethics in More than Human Worlds*, University of Minnesota Press, Minneapolis.

Lawson, V. 2009, 'Instead of radical geography, how about caring geography?' *Antipode* 41(1), pp. 210–3.

Lorenzetti, S., Plösch, T. and Teller, I.C. 2021, 'Antioxidative molecules in human milk and environmental contaminants', *Antioxidants*, 10(4), p. 550.

Mann, H.S. 2017, 'Breastfeeding as embodied care: On its goodness, awfullness, and irreducible pleasure', in Smith, P.H., Labbok, M. and Chambers, B.D. (eds), *Breastfeeding, Social Justice, and Equity*, Praeclarus Press, Amarillo, Texas, pp. 19–25.

McKinnon, K. 2020, *Birthing Work: The Collective Labour of Childbirth*, Springer, Singapore.

Mieso, B.R., Burrow, H. and Lam, S.K. 2021, 'Beyond statistics: Uncovering the roots of racial disparities in breastfeeding', *Pediatrics*, 147(5).

Miller, E. 2019, *Reimagining Livelihoods: Life Beyond Economy, Society, and Environment*, University of Minnesota Press, Minneapolis.

Mosca, F. and Giannì, M.L. 2017, 'Human milk: Composition and health benefits', *La Pediatria Medica e Chirurgica: Medical and Surgical Pediatrics*, 39(2), p. 155.

Naylor, L. 2019, *Fair Trade Rebels: Coffee Production and Struggles for Autonomy in Chiapas*, University of Minnesota Press, Minneapolis.

Naylor, L. 2022. 'The body as a site of care: Food and lactating bodies in the U.S.' *Gender, Place and Culture*, 29(3), pp. 440–9.

Naylor, L. and Clarke-Sather, L. 2020, 'Factors impacting breastfeeding and milk expression in the neonatal intensive care unit', *International Journal of Caring Sciences*, 13(2), pp. 970–81.

Naylor, L., Clarke-Sather, A. and Weber, M. 2020, 'Troubling care in the Neonatal Intensive Care Unit', *Geoforum*, 114(August), pp. 107–16.

Swanson, K.W. 2009, 'Human milk as technology and technologies of human milk: Medical imaginings in the early Twentieth-Century United States,' *WSQ: Women's Studies Quarterly*, 37(1), pp. 20–37.

Swanson, K.W. 2014, *Banking on the Body*, Harvard University Press, Harvard.

Updegrove, K. 2013, 'Nonprofit human milk banking in the United States,' *Journal of Midwifery and Women's Health*, 58(5), pp. 502–8.

Updegrove, K.H. 2013, 'Donor human milk banking: Growth, challenges, and the role of HMBANA,' *Breastfeeding Medicine* 8(5), pp. 435–7.

Weber, M.J., Clarke-Sather, A., Cobb, K. and Naylor, L. 2021, 'Proof of concept simple conductive thread stitch sensor to measure the duration of kangaroo care', *Journal of Textile Engineering and Fashion Technology*, 7(1), pp. 16–22.

Williams, C. and Onoschenko, O. 2013, 'The diverse livelihoods of healthcare workers in Ukraine: The Case of Sasha and Natasha', in Morris, J. and Polese, A. (eds), *The Informal Post-Socialist Economy: Embedded Practices and Livelihoods*, Routledge, New York, pp. 21–34.

38

THE POLITICAL ECONOMY OF HEALTH AND DEGROWTH

Jean-Louis Aillon and Mauro Bonaiuti

This chapter argues that it is not possible to promote and protect global health population within the current neoliberal and capitalist system. Neither would this task be achievable within other socio-economic configurations (such as socialism, communism, or sustainable development) that remain dependent on economic growth (Latouche 2009). A socio-economic model primarily oriented toward economic growth, after a certain threshold, becomes counter-productive: over time, its advantages decrease exponentially (diminishing marginal returns) until its negative effects outweigh its positive ones (Illich 1976; Bonaiuti 2014). Health is not immune from this process. In fact, growth is based on the indiscriminate exploitation of natural and human capital: undermining the principal determinants of health via producing increasing damage to the environment, greater inequalities, and unhealthy consumeristic cultures and lifestyles (INHS 2014).

Conversely, the chapter contends that degrowth represents a radical alternative to the current political-economic system and its hegemonic orientation toward growth (Latouche 2009). Instead, degrowth favors democratically led redistributive initiatives that engender production and consumption downscaling in industrialized countries to secure objectives of environmental sustainability, social justice, and welfare. In making this case, central tenets of degrowth theory will be explicated, focusing on how the socio-economic and cultural changes promoted by degrowth would have substantial positive repercussions for planetary health, and represent the prerequisites to implement several progressive health policies that remain largely proscribed in existing neoliberal and capitalist systems (Borowy and Aillon 2017). In turn, an alternative model of medicine and health systems will be presented by applying degrowth principles to the health field (Aillon and D'Alisa 2020), and through outlining some examples of its concrete application in other contexts (De Vogli and Owusu 2015; Borowy 2017). Finally, we explore the practical challenges of implementing a degrowth model in the health field, and the necessary conditions for achieving such a societal and medical revolution.

Health and its determinants

'Health' is not an objective and fixed category, but rather a peculiar social and cultural construction (Kleinman 1978), which differs among cultures, places, and time. However, it is important to fix at least some coordinates that can orient the following discussion. We will refer to health, within a

DOI: 10.4324/9781003017110-43

Western scientific biomedical framework, as constituting 'not merely the absence of disease or infirmity', or as physical health, but as a state of 'physical, mental and social well-being' (WHO 1946).

Similarly, several researchers in public health show that health does not depend mostly on healthcare services. Rather, it stems from broader socio-economic, cultural, and environmental conditions (structural factors, including macroeconomic policies) that influence more proximal determinants of health (agricultural and food production, air quality, education, working conditions, housing, water and sanitation, social and community networks, and individual lifestyles) (Dahlgren and Whitehead 1993). With the exception of unmodifiable factors (genetics), healthcare accounts for 10 percent to 25 percent of people's overall health status (Kuznetsova 2012; 11; McGinnis 2002), while health is mainly related to socio-economic (50 percent) and physical environment (10 percent) (Canadian Institute of Advanced Research 2012).

The unsustainability of a socio-economic system based on growth

The current socio-economic system can be described in several ways: capitalism, neoliberalism, globalization, consumer society, and so forth. Each reflects some distinctive features of the current society. As a means of critical reflection, however, degrowth focuses on the fact that the present socio-economic configuration is principally oriented around promoting economic growth within a system that can function properly only through significant and continuous economic growth. Some economic systems can be based on growth even without being capitalist and neoliberal, such as the Twentieth Century Soviet economies. In this context, degrowth scholars argue that at the current level of development within neoliberal-capitalist systems, economic growth is not sustainable from an environmental, social, and psychological perspective. In fact, to continue growing, such economies must continue progressively exploiting the environment and human beings (natural and human capital), thereby cultivating mounting environmental damages (in particular, climate change and pollution), inequalities, and stressful and unhealthy lifestyles (Latouche 2009; Demaria *et al.* 2013; D'Alisa *et al.* 2014).

In the past century, there has been a clear correlation between GDP growth and health (within and between countries), a phenomenon known as the 'Preston effect' (1975). However, this process is subject to a diminishing marginal returns effect. After a certain threshold of income increase, the rise in life expectancy has decreased exponentially until plateauing (Figure 38.1), while decreasing after a certain threshold (nearly US$40,000 dollars per capita), according to a more recent analysis (Gordon and Biciunaite 2014).

Furthermore, according to Preston, income explained only 10 to 25 percent of increases in life expectancy. The remainder likely stemmed from other hexogen factors, and depends on how wealth is redistributed to the poorest part of the society to reduce inequalities. If it is used to improve public expenditures in health, social, and cultural services, it produces positive health outcomes. If the contrary happens – in particular, after a certain threshold of economic development – GDP growth produces negative health outcomes related to the effects of rising inequalities, disruption of social networks and cohesion, overconsumption, and unhealthy lifestyles (such as tobacco and alcohol consumption, less healthy diets, and cultural habits) (Anand and Ravallion 1993; Gordon and Biciunaite 2014; Borowy 2017). In fact, Szreter (2005) shows that during some periods of strong economic growth and rising wages in Britain (as between 1820 and 1870), population mortality has actually augmented. That led him to affirm that 'economic growth should be understood as setting in train a socially and politically dangerous, destabilizing, and health-threatening set of forces' (Szreter 2005: 204).

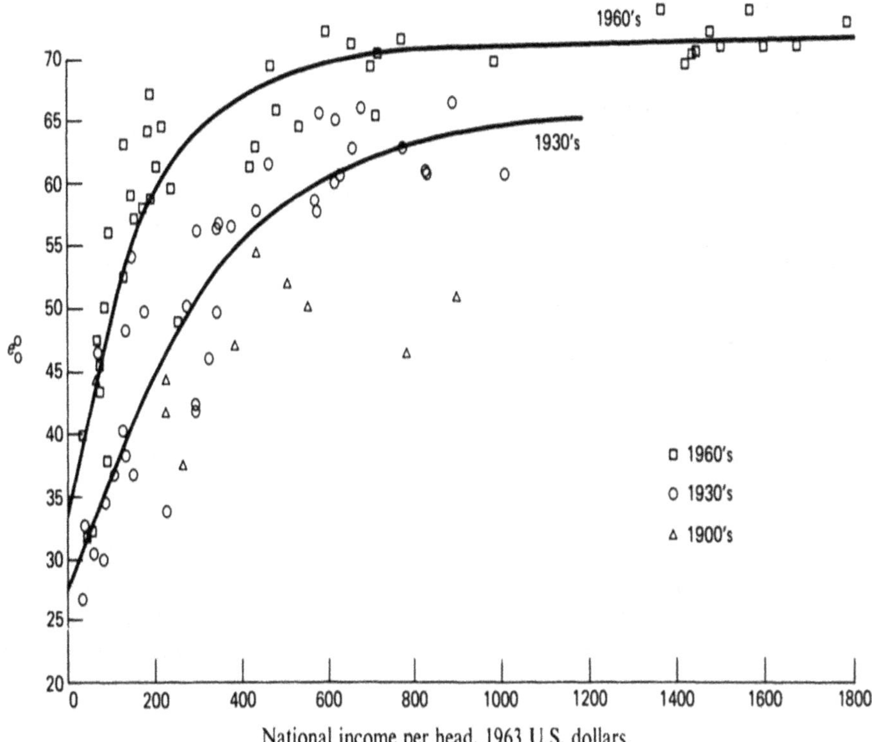

Figure 38.1 Preston curve.

Source: Preston (1975). With permission from Taylor and Francis.

Growth and healthcare

Sustained economic growth within Western capitalism – significantly based on colonialism, the slave trade, and exploitation of the Global South – has enabled rich countries to invest a great amount of resources into healthcare and sustain complex health systems that have strongly improved life expectancy relative to other countries. Indeed, over the past 300 years, life expectancy and body weight in OECD countries' populations have augmented over 50 percent (Fogel 2012). However, even if there is a general positive correlation between healthcare expenditure and life expectancy – similar to the growth of GDP – after a certain threshold (approximately US$4,000 PPP), growth in healthcare expenditure produces minimal gains in life expectancy (OECD 2016). After this threshold, it also engenders increasing costs in terms of iatrogenesis and overconsumption. Accordingly, '[i]ndividualization in modern health systems is […] reaping diminishing returns while incurring rising costs at the level of society and ecology' (Zywert and Quilley 2018: 202).

An excellent example of this complex relation is provided by healthcare expenditure in the US. In 2006, despite the country's total healthcare expenditure tallying nearly double that of

Cuba (15.3 percent v. 7.7 percent of the gross domestic product), and its total per-capita health expenditure extending to over 19 times that of Cuba (US$6719 v. $US362), the two countries had a comparable average life expectancy at birth (78 years old) (WHO 2009). Similarly, Tainter (2006) demonstrates how the US healthcare system has been subject to diminishing returns since the late-1950s. While expenditure on the health system (as a percentage of GDP) has increased, life expectancy has not comparably increased.

As the complexity of an organization (or a process) increases, the marginal benefits increase according to an S-shaped trend (illustrated in Figure 38.2). After an initial phase of growth in benefits, once the first mutation threshold (C1) is exceeded, there are decreasing returns, and finally, negative benefits are generated after the second threshold (C2).

Within healthcare, this phenomenon was illustrated over 40 years ago by Ivan Illich, one of the most important pioneers of degrowth. In a few seminal books such as *Tools for Conviviality* (Illich 1973) and *Medical Nemesis* (Illich 1976), he illustrates his idea that more medicine does not necessarily mean better health. In other words, he shows how different services/institutions (schools, medicine, cars), after a certain threshold of growth, become *counter-productive*. Thus, '[w]hen an enterprise grows beyond a certain point [...], it first frustrates the end for which it was originally designed, and then rapidly becomes a threat to society itself', while 'during the last fifteen years, professional medicine became a major threat to health' (Illich 1973: 8, 14). For Illich, the counter-productivity of the medical system can be understood not only as a clinical phenomenon, but also as a social and cultural form of iatrogenesis. Social iatrogenesis consists in 'health policies that reinforce an industrial organization that generates ill health', while '[c]ultural iatrogenesis consist in the fact that medically sponsored behaviour and delusions restrict the vital autonomy of people' and 'cripples personal responses to pain, disability, impairment, anguish and death' (Illich 1976: 270–1). The last two are difficult to quantify and, rather than life expectancy or mortality,

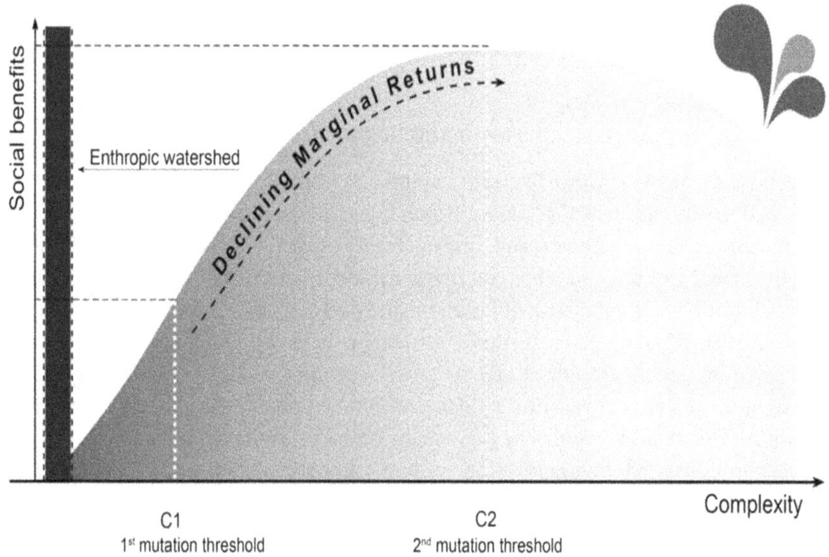

Figure 38.2 Diminishing marginal returns curve.

Source: Bonaiuti (2014). With permission from Taylor and Francis.

underline the loss of individual 'autonomy' in front of the medical institution as a critical aspect of modern healthcare.

Even if the time thresholds proposed by Illich were not supported by an adequate empirical foundation, his basic intuition – namely, that there is 'too much medicine', that more healthcare does not necessarily engender better health (Moynihan and Smith 2002; Saini *et al.* 2017), and that 'doing more does not mean doing better within the medical field' (Vernero *et al.* 2014) – remains relevant today. Since 2017, life expectancy in the US has dropped by three years (Murphy *et al.* 2018), with the proximate cause of this phenomenon identified as the opioid epidemic (Gomes *et al.* 2018) that caused the loss of 1,681,359 years of life in 2016 alone. That crisis is a result of a clinical, social, and cultural iatrogenic process: it commenced with the overconsumption of prescription pharmaceuticals, which were legally produced and marketed by pharmaceutical corporations, and legally prescribed by medical practitioners (Hadland *et al.* 2019; Hensher 2020b).

More broadly, healthcare expenses (public and private) comprise 6.6 percent of world GDP and, in the US, reached 17.1 percent compared to 8 percent in the EU (WHO 2019). As with other sectors of the economy, the efficiency and efficacy of healthcare has been affected by the imperative of the economy to continuously grow under neoliberalism. Accordingly, even in healthcare, 'there is strong evidence of the existence of supplier-induced demand, and of the impact of various forms of financial incentives on clinical practice' (Hensher 2017: 77). That has led to the growing medicalization of normal life events (disease mongering), overdiagnosis, overtreatment, overuse, and 'low value care' (Aillon and D'Alisa 2020; Hensher 2020a; Hensher *et al.* 2020).

Meanwhile, estimates of 'waste' in healthcare systems (not just overuse) comprise perhaps 20 percent of OECD health expenditure (OECD 2017), while the overall cost of waste in the US healthcare system tallies between 21 and 47 percent of total health spending (Berwick and Hackbarth 2012). Such waste in healthcare represents potential harm to patients and inefficiency for health systems, as well as a form of ecologically damaging overconsumption (Hensher *et al.* 2017; Hensher *et al.* 2020). In fact, 'in terms of emissions of greenhouse gases and air pollutants, the healthcare sector causes a large share of the total footprint (4.4% of greenhouse gases)' (Lenzen *et al.* 2020: e274) – especially in the US, where the country's health system produces nearly 10 percent of national greenhouse gases (Eckelman and Sherman 2016). Finally, clinical iatrogenesis is not a fringe phenomenon. It is highly harmful and costly: emerging as the fourteenth largest contributor to the global disease burden, with a cost that comprises 15 percent of total healthcare expenses in high-income countries (Slawomirski *et al.* 2017). Starfield (2000) estimated that, in the US, total annual deaths from iatrogenic causes average around 225,000, constituting the third largest cause of death after heart disease and cancer.

Growth will not be sustainable and healthy in the future

Recent studies highlight that 'there is no empirical evidence that absolute decoupling from resource use can be achieved on a global scale against a background of continued economic growth (Hickel and Kallis 2019: 469; Parrique *et al.* 2019). Thus, in the long-term, the choice will not be between sustainable development or green growth (both arguing in favor of economic growth) and degrowth, but rather between voluntary degrowth' or 'involuntary degrowth' (Bonaiuti 2014, 2018; Hensher and Zywert 2020). Continuous global growth, even if green, will not be sustainable into the future and, in its current capitalist and neoliberal configurations, will produce an increasingly unfair, environmental damaged and neurotic/alienated world (Fromm 1955; Latouche 2009). Diminishing marginal returns, if ignored, will lead to overlapping crises[1] and, after the second mutation threshold, may lead to scenarios such as authoritarian/technocratic involutions, or even global collapse (Bonaiuti 2014, 2018).

Health is determined mostly by social (inequalities), environmental (climate change, pollution, loss of biodiversity, change in land use), and cultural factors (overconsumption, stress, alienation). At the current level of development, such determinants will be increasingly detrimentally affected by economic growth. Together with the counter-productivity of the healthcare systems after a certain threshold (growth of economic and ecologically costs, diminishing marginal returns of care and iatrogenesis), this has led several researchers to argue that 'the present prevailing paradigm based on unlimited growth [...] is not sustainable from an economic, social and environmental point of view'. Equally, 'it is unable to safeguard the health of present and future generations', such that securing socio-ecological health into the future necessitates an alternative political-economic configuration transcending the extant orientation around growth (Italian Network for Sustainability and Health, 2014: 1; Borowy and Aillon 2017; Aillon and D'Alisa 2020; Hensher 2020a).

In turn, the most pertinent question for consideration should not be how to continue to foster indefinite growth, which that would likely lead to an 'involuntary degrowth' path: a significant diminution of complexity that could destroy modern society and healthcare. Rather, focus should be placed on investigating how to promote a planned and deliberate contraction of the economy ('voluntary degrowth') that could allow humanity to respect planetary boundaries and live in a fairer, more serene, and sustainable world. Concomitantly, we should plan how to adapt healthcare 'to a world of tightening ecological constraints' and diminished social complexity (Hensher and Zywert 2020). Degrowth offers a coherent framework for such systemic change.

What is degrowth?

From a macroeconomic perspective, contrasting with other post-growth scenarios (*e.g.* steady state), degrowth 'calls for a democratically led redistributive downscaling of production and consumption in industrialized countries as a means to achieve environmental sustainability, social justice and well-being' (Demaria *et al.* 2013: 209). Degrowth highlights that for high-income countries, a voluntary, democratic, and planned reduction in material and energy consumption – and, thus, in economic activity (GDP) – will be necessary to secure long-term social and ecological sustainability, while still allowing (different forms of) growth in low-income countries. Degrowth thereby breaks not only with capitalism and neoliberalism, but also with other models aimed at promoting economic growth (green growth, sustainable development, or conventional communist approaches). From an economic standpoint, the aim of degrowth is not the diminution of GDP alone. Indeed, this constitutes a transitory means to achieve real, long-term sustainability. After having reached a certain threshold, which allows for ecological boundaries to be respected, degrowth of GDP does not need to necessarily continue. In turn, a 'steady-state economy' could be maintained, focusing on promoting human flourishment while maintaining a stable societal metabolism (flow of energy and materials) (Daly 1992; Kerschner 2010). In this respect, such 'voluntary' degrowth is a planned and deliberate process to be promoted alongside a paradigm shift in economic, social, and cultural perspectives. As mentioned above, it differs from the diminishment of GDP within existing socio-economic systems, which can be defined as 'involuntary degrowth' or recession (Bonaiuti 2014, 2018).

Degrowth is, however, not only an economic concept. It simultaneously implies deep cultural critical reflection on the colonization of growth on Western imaginaries and bodies, and is a practical political project for a new kind of society transcending the tyranny of growth. Hence, Latouche

(2009) describes degrowth not as a theory, but as a 'political slogan with theoretical implications' aimed at strongly underlining the need to abandon the dogmatic goal of exponential growth. In turn, rather than constituting a fixed paradigm, degrowth represents 'a frame constituted by a large array of concerns, goals, strategies and actions [...] a confluence point where streams of critical ideas and political action converge'. It 'is not the alternative, but a matrix of alternatives which reopens a space for creativity by raising the heavy blanket of economic totalitarianism' (Latouche 2010: 520). Sources of degrowth are different and multidisciplinary, ranging from advocates of bio-economy and deep ecology, and critics of development, to proponents of democracy and socio-ecological justice, reflections on the meaning of life and wellbeing, and exponents of non-violence, ecofeminism, and no-borders (Demaria *et al.* 2013: 193–4). Degrowth is also a framework for a growing social movement, and a motivator for systemic change that will commence at the grassroots level, but that simultaneously involves joint efforts by multifarious actors and strategies (researchers, oppositional activists, practitioners, reformists in existing institutions, artists). For example, degrowth is inspired by Marxist and anarchist visions, especially in their critical reflections on the links between growth and capitalism, as well as their advocacy of a grassroots construction of the desired new world (Chertkovskaya *et al.* 2019).

In order to promote a concrete degrowth transition, Latouche (2009) proposes a path composed of eight interdependent changes:

1 Re-evaluate our worldview through the decolonization of the imaginary from growth ideology;
2 Reconceptualize the world with a new vision, culture, and values aimed at sufficiency, sobriety, commoning and cooperation, social and ecological justice, 'autonomy', and authenticity;
3 Restructure coherently to the new vision of the socio-economic system;
4 Redistribute the land, money, and work between and within countries, and across the Global North and South;
5 Relocalize the economy, society, and politics on a local basis ('open localism');
6 Reduce overconsumption, waste, work time, displacements, and mass tourism;
7 Reuse;
8 Recycle.

Building on these principles, within a degrowth framework, people will consume less and better (reduction of waste and overconsumption), and need to work less and have more time to dedicate to creative, meaningful, and nourishing activities (Pallante 2011). Markets will still exist but, instead of being totalizing, will function as a means for human flourishment. Their political-economic weight will, thus, be reduced and supplanted by other forms of exchange, by commoning, or by the gift economy. Economic wealth will be reduced, as will taxes and the welfare economy. This vision will, of course, engender great challenges to implement. However, from a long-term perspective, social and ecological justice will dramatically reduce societal problems compared to maintaining business-as-usual. Simultaneously, the building of local, convivial, and autonomous communities will allow economic processes to meet – within a non-market sphere and in a participative manner – the basic needs of communities (Latouche 2009).

Rethinking health and healthcare in a degrowth frame

Based on the broad contours outlined above, degrowth would promote a society with greater equity and environmental sustainability – shifting the main driver of human activity from economic growth to the health and wellbeing of humans, non-humans, and their environment. This principle is concisely embodied in the recent concept of 'planetary health' (Whitmee *et al.* 2015). As such, degrowth could be seen as a prerequisite for ensuring the efficacy of several health policies that have been largely undermined under extant neoliberal processes (*e.g.* sobriety and healthy lifestyles v. overconsumption). Moreover, several degrowth political proposals would have significant positive repercussions on the social determinants of health. In addition to the above-mentioned principles outlined by Latouche, some examples could include the following:

- Maximum and basic income, job guarantee, work sharing (fewer working hours);
- Empowering autonomous, local and convivial communities;
- Strengthening social networks, community care and welfare;
- Decommodification and self-sufficiency v. overconsumption;
- Community currencies, co-operatives, and commons;
- Carbon and green taxes;
- Agro-ecology, eco-communities, and urban gardening (Latouche 2009; D'Alisa *et al.* 2015; Borowy and Aillon 2017).

More specifically, adapting the model of Latouche from above, Aillon and D'Alisa (2020) have developed a theoretical framework around four principles to rethink health and healthcare within a degrowth frame. This four-step archetype will be used to articulate how health and healthcare systems could be reshaped within a voluntary degrowth transition, while also incorporating reflections by other scholars on the topic.

Re-evaluation and reconceptualization of the ideas of health, illness, and care

To re-evaluate the concept of health within a degrowth framework, it is first necessary to 'decolonize its imaginary' (Latouche 2009) from extant growth colonization processes. That is, it is imperative to question the ordinary values and epistemological principles that underpin mainstream scientific medical culture and practice. From this perspective, it is necessary 'to go beyond a certain vision of science and progress (materialistic, mechanistic, reductionist) that considers the human being as an "object of study", splitting emotion from reason and neglecting different essential (non-material) dimensions' (Aillon and D'Alisa 2020: 310–1). Within this framework, care becomes a qualitative and systemic endeavor oriented around the patients themselves, where health workers attempt to understand their uniqueness and different dimensions (bio-psycho-social and spiritual). Health is, thus, understood not as a 'complete state of physical, social and psychological wellbeing' (WHO 1946) – a condition almost impossible to reach – but rather as 'a dynamic equilibrium resulting from several external (*e.g.* socio-economic, environmental, and cultural factors) and internal determinants (*e.g.* psychological factors such as "resilience" and "sense of coherence"' (Aillon and D'Alisa 2020: 311). Health is not a good to be purchased from health professionals, but something that people create themselves and with their surrounding socio-ecological context: the 'degree of lived freedom [...] the range of autonomy within which a person exercises control over his own biological states and over the conditions of his immediate environment' (Illich 1976: 91).

Moreover, in order to avoid repeating colonialist mistakes, it must be acknowledged that there is no one 'Health', but many 'healths' and health systems with their own standards of legitimacy and efficacy, even if they do not fit within the extant scientific biomedical epistemology and ontology prevalent within Western cultures (Kleinman 1978).

Restructuring health services following the new conceptualization of health, and adapting them to a post-growth scenario

Forthcoming changes in global ecological and economic systems will drastically alter the world in which healthcare operates. Accordingly, in the course of transitioning toward a sustainable society, healthcare processes must adapt to operate within a new social-ecological system defined by novel, complex challenges. These include the following: diminishing returns of the socio-economic system; reduced availability of material resources, such as money for public and private expenditure, and energy for ends such as medical procedures, pharmaceuticals, and infrastructure; declining complexity in social – and, thus, healthcare – systems; increasing risks related to climate change, environmental degradation and growing inequalities; relocalized living and production practices due to rising transport costs; and minimal opportunity for future healthcare expansion (Hensher and Zywert 2020).

Such developments pose multifarious structural and cultural uncertainties for healthcare. In order to address these matters, we tentatively propose four broad principles around which the transition in healthcare should occur.

Redistribute

Besides the cultural changes proposed above, it will be fundamental to redistribute the resources of health systems (from the Global North to Global South and within countries) in order to promote universalist public healthcare at the global level. This could fill the gap of declining budget reserves (related to diminishing returns), funded by progressive taxation of higher incomes (including big corporations and financial transactions) and carbon taxes. Public management of health will also promote more sobriety in resource use, compared to private healthcare businesses. Moreover, health should be seen as a basic human right and healthcare as commons-based (Aillon *et al.* 2019).

Relocalize

Healthcare should be relocalized and decentralized within communities, and based on primary healthcare and community medicine (WHO 2008), rather than on a reactive hospital-based approach. The existing growth orientation of capitalism and neoliberalism, in accordance with prevailing imperatives toward individualism and commodification, engenders a disembedding of individuals from their family and community bonds. Conversely, within a degrowth framework, emerging communities will enable the re-embedding of care within the family and community networks (Zywert and Quilley 2018). Thus, even with reduced monetary budgets for healthcare and welfare, the community will be able to guarantee basic needs and services with the reciprocity of its members.

Reduce

Medicalization and the consequent iatrogenesis should be drastically reduced. Specifically, doctors should become pioneers of demedicalization through a range of measures. These include the following: returning power to patients, fostering self-care and autonomy, pressing for a more equitable global distribution of simple effective healthcare, avoiding a medicalized classification of quotidian problems, promoting the deprofessionalization of primary care, and assisting policy decisions about which complex services should be available (Moynihan and Smith 2002).

Overdiagnosis, overtreatment, overuse, low care value, and waste should also be minimized or avoided. As detailed above, healthcare waste (unnecessary and non-beneficial care) substantially contributes to total healthcare costs across the OECD. Consequently, there could be a significant degrowth in Western healthcare without reducing population health quality. Furthermore, the money saved from such modifications could be redeployed to cover the minimal public taxes collected during the transition to a post-growth scenario.

Given healthcare has a major impact on environment, it will also be necessary to reduce the dependence of the sector on intensive use of energy and materials – both through avoiding waste and increasing efficiency of resource use (technical efficiency). This transition may be assisted, in part, by integrating myriad environmental effects into economic evaluations of healthcare systems (Hensher 2020c). These changes could contribute to a reduction in global healthcare costs.

Even with reduced healthcare expenses stemming from moderating avoidable harms, unnecessary and non-beneficial care, and promoting efficiency, a planned economic degrowth may require further reductions in healthcare expenses. Thus, while reducing less cost-effective interventions, it is necessary to retain those components of modern healthcare that produce the greatest population health returns, such as vaccination programs, health promotion initiatives, and dietary measures to counteract non-communicable diseases (Hensher and Zywert 2020). Health systems will, accordingly, need 'to reduce the scale and scope of services produced and provided through active prioritization and resource allocation decisions (allocative efficiency)', such that 'real scarcity will become the driver of prioritization decisions, not the marketing strategies of pharmaceutical firms' (Hensher 2020a: 115). This decision process would not be limited to health systems, but rather democratically determined by the whole society. Essentially, a limited pool of resources – compatible with intergenerational equity – should be allocated to health (choosing between healthcare and other sectors of society relevant to health).

In order to achieve the above-mentioned objectives, it will be fundamental to reduce the monopoly power and influence of big pharmaceutical corporations on healthcare processes, which have engendered conflicts of interest and corruption. Medical knowledge should be codified as commons-based and globalized: making knowledge freely available, using new approaches such as 'open-source drug research', and encouraging the public system to develop socially useful drugs or interventions (Todd 2019).

Reuse and recycle

Recycling and reuse of existing materials should be pursued to minimize the ecological footprint of healthcare, while also redesigning new products able to be more easily reused or recycled relative to disposable objects. Furthermore, other forms of medical knowledge (traditional and complementary medicine) should be reused, while self-care and the ability of individuals and communities to cope with affliction and death should be enhanced (WHO 2014; Aillon and D'Alisa 2020).

Health promotion acting on socio-economic, environmental, and cultural determinants of health

Transitioning to a post-growth economy would accord the possibility to promote health by acting on its social determinants. In particular, risk factors for non-communicable diseases that have been difficult to rectify within extant growth-based economies could, instead, be positioned as paramount to securing the reduction of deleterious and wasteful consumption activities. The latter include those relating to food, alcohol, addictive products, and physical inactivity, as well as the health impacts of pollution (Hensher and Zywert 2020).

Involvement of citizens in health management (autonomy)

For Illich (1976: 6), 'the recovery from society-wide iatrogenic disease is a political task, not a professional one', such that 'the layman and not the physician has the potential perspective and effective power to stop the current iatrogenic epidemic'. From this perspective, the task of revolutionizing health and healthcare within a degrowth transition should not be imposed from top-down (from medical experts or politicians), but rather be constructed from the bottom-up. Accordingly, the involvement and empowerment of citizens is crucial to securing a degrowth transition (WHO 1978), while achieving the desired transformation on a global scale requires that 'local action [...] be linked to global policies and governance for health' (Missoni 2015).

Conclusion

Realizing the four steps outlined above as the means to reconfigure health and healthcare systems within a voluntary degrowth transition will be a complex and challenging endeavor. Resistance to change will likely be encountered from those with a material interest in maintaining extant capitalist and neoliberal systems oriented around perpetual growth, as well as from everyday citizens due to pervasively entrenched cultural values favoring such growth. Nevertheless, as demonstrated in this chapter, securing a degrowth transition is imperative to beget a more sustainable and equal political-economic system, and desirable as a means to more equitably and efficaciously secure global human health and welfare. Thus, we hope that the provocations detailed above will help invigorate ongoing discussion – by scholars and social movements alike – on the potential for degrowth to inform a healthier, more socio-ecologically sustainable world.

Note

1 Global terrorism, economic crisis, global migrations, and the ongoing COVID-19 pandemic could be seen as a negative externality within a counter-productivity process of global economic growth (Aillon and Cardito 2020; Modonesi 2020).

References

Aillon, J.L., Bessone, M. and Bodini, C. 2019, *Un Nuovo mo (n) do per Fare Salute: Le Proposte della Rete Sostenibilità e Salute*, Celid, Torino.

Aillon, J.L. and Cardito, M. 2020, 'Health and degrowth in times of pandemic', *Visions for Sustainability*, 14, pp. 3–23.

Aillon, J.L. and D'Alisa, G. 2020, 'Our affluence is killing us: What degrowth offers health and wellbeing', in Zywert, K. and Quilley, S. (eds), *Health in the Anthropocene: Living Well on a Finite Planet*, University of Toronto Press, Toronto, pp. 306–22.

Anand, S. and Ravallion, M. 1993, 'Human Development in Poor Countries: On the Role of Private Incomes and Public Services', *The Journal of Economic Perspectives*, 7(1), pp. 133–150.

Berwick, D.M. and Hackbarth, A.D. 2012, 'Eliminating waste in US health care', *Journal of the American Medical Association*, 307, pp. 1513–16.

Bonaiuti, M. 2014, *The Great Transition*, Routledge, London.

Bonaiuti, M. 2018, 'Are we entering the age of involuntary degrowth? Promethean technologies and declining returns of innovation', *Journal of Cleaner Production*, 197, pp. 1800–9.

Borowy, I. 2017, 'Economic growth and health: Evidence, uncertainties, and connections over time and place', in Borowy, I. and Schmelzer, M. (eds), *History of the Future of Economic Growth: Historical Roots of Current Debates on Sustainable Degrowth*, Routledge, London, pp. 129–53.

Borowy, I. and Aillon, J.L. 2017, 'Sustainable health and degrowth: Health, health care and society beyond the growth paradigm', *Social Theory and Health,* 15(3), pp. 346–68.

Dahlgren, G. and Whitehead, M. 1993, 'Tackling inequalities in health: What can we learn from what has been tried?', working paper, King's Fund International Seminar on Tackling Inequalities in Health, Ditchley Park, Oxfordshire.

D'Alisa, G., Demaria, F. and Kallis, G. 2014, *Degrowth: A Vocabulary for a New Era*, Routledge, London.

D'Alisa, G., Forno, F. and Maurano, S. 2015, 'Grassroots (economic) activism in times of crisis: Mapping the redundancy of collective actions', *Partecipazione e Conflitto*, 2015(2), pp. 328–342.

Daly, H.E. 1992, *Steady-State Economics,* Earthscan, London.

Demaria, F., Schneider, F., Sekulova, F. and Martinez-Alier, J. 2013, 'What is degrowth? From an activist slogan to a social movement', *Environmental Values,* 22(2), pp. 191–215.

De Vogli, R. and Owusu, J.T. 2015, 'The causes and health effects of the Great Recession: from neoliberalism to 'healthy de-growth', *Critical Public Health*, 25(1), pp. 15–31.

Eckelman, M.J. and Sherman, J. 2016, 'Environmental impacts of the US health care system and effects on public health', *PLOS ONE*, 11(6), p. e0157014.

Fogel, R. 2012, *Explaining Long-Term Trends in Health and Longevity*, Cambridge University Press, Cambridge.

Fromm, E. 1955, *The Sane Society*, Harper and Row, New York.

Gomes, T., Tadrous, M., Mamdani, M.M., Paterson, J.M. and Juurlink, D.N. 2018, 'The burden of opioid-related mortality in the United States', *JAMA Network Open,* 1(2), p. e180217.

Gordon, L. and Biciunaite, A. 2014, 'Economic growth and life expectancy – Do wealthier countries live longer?' *Euromonitor International*, 14 March, accessed 20 January 2021, <https://blog.euromonitor.com/economic-growth-and-life-expectancy-do- wealthier-countries-live-longer/>.

Hadland, S.E., Rivera-Aguirre, A., Marshall, B.D.L., and Cerdá, M. 2019, 'Association of pharmaceutical industry marketing of opioid products with mortality from opioid-related overdoses', *JAMA Netw Open*, 2(1), e186007.

Hensher, M. 2020a, 'Anthropocene health economics: Preparing for the journey or the destination?', in Zywert, K. and Quilley, S. (eds), *Health in the Anthropocene: Living Well on a Finite Planet*, University of Toronto Press, Tonronto, pp. 107–39.

Hensher, M. 2020b, 'Human health and ecological economics', in Costanza, R., Erickson, J.D., Farley, J. and Kubiszewski, I. (eds), *Sustainable Wellbeing Futures: A Research and Action Agenda for Ecological Economics*, Edward Elgar Publishing, Cheltenham, pp. 188–208.

Hensher, M. 2020c, 'Incorporating environmental impacts into the economic evaluation of health care systems: Perspectives from ecological economics', *Resources, Conservation and Recycling*, 154, p. 104623.

Hensher, M., Canny, B., Zimitat, C., Campbell, J. and Palmer, A. 2020b, 'Health care, overconsumption and uneconomic growth: A conceptual framework', *Social Science and Medicine*, 266, p. 113420.

Hensher, M., Tisdell, J., Canny, B. and Zimitat, C. 2020a, 'Health care and the future of economic growth: Exploring alternative perspectives', *Health Economics, Policy and Law*, 15(4), pp. 419–39.

Hensher, M., Tisdell, J. and Zimitat, C. 2017, 'Too much medicine: Insights and explanations from economic theory and research', *Social Science and Medicine*, 176, pp. 77–84.

Hensher, M. and Zywert, K. 2020, 'Can healthcare adapt to a world of tightening ecological constraints? Challenges on the road to a post-growth future', *BMJ*, 371, p. m4168.

Hickel, J. and Kallis, G. 2019, 'Is green growth possible?' *New Political Economy*, 25(4), pp. 469–86.

Illich, I. 1973, *Tools for Conviviality*, Calder and Boyars, London.

Illich, I. 1976, *Medical Nemesis: The Expropriation of Health*, Pantheon Books, New York.

Italian Network for Sustainability and Health. 2014, 'The Bologna manifesto for sustainability and health', *Rete Sostenibilità e Salute*, 14 June, accessed 20 January 2021, <https://www.sostenibilitaesalute.org/the-bologna-manifesto-for-sustainability-and-health/>.

Kerschner, C. 2010, 'Economic de-growth vs. steady-state economy', *Journal of Cleaner Production,* 18(6), pp. 544–51.

Kleinman, A. 1978, 'Concepts and a model for the comparison of medical systems as cultural systems', *Social Science and Medicine, Part B: Medical Anthropology*, 12, pp. 85–93.Latouche, S. 2009, *Farewell to Growth*, Polity Press, Cambridge.

Latouche, S. 2010, 'Degrowth', *Journal of Cleaner Production*, 18(6), pp. 519–22.

Lenzen, M., Malik, A., Li, M., Fry, J., Weisz, H., Pichler, P.P., Chaves, L., Capon, A. and Pencheon, D. 2020, 'The environmental footprint of health care: A global assessment', *The Lancet Planetary Health*, 4(7), pp. e271–9.

McGinnis, J.M., Williams-Russo, P. and Knickman, J.R. 2002, 'The case for more active policy attention to health promotion', *Health Affairs*, 21(2), pp. 78–93.

Missoni, E. 2015, 'Degrowth and health: Local action should be linked to global policies and governance for health', *Sustainability Science*, 10(3), pp. 439–50.

Modonesi, C. 2020, 'The environmental roots of zoonotic diseases: From SARS-CoV-2 to cancer viruses – A review', *Visions for Sustainability*, 14, pp. 54–65.

Moynihan, R. and Smith, R. 2002, 'Too much medicine? Almost certainly', *BMJ*, 324, pp. 859–60.

Murphy, S. L., Xu, J., Kochanek, K.D. and Arias, E. 2018, *Mortality in the United States, 2017, NCHS Data Brief, No. 328*, National Center for Health Statistics, Hyattsville, MD.

OECD. 2016, *Society at a Glance 2016: OECD Social Indicators*, OECD Publishing, Paris.

OECD. 2017, *Tackling Wasteful Spending on Health*, OECD Publishing, Paris.

Pallante, M. 2011, *Meno e Meglio: Decrescere per Progredire*, Mondadori, Milano.

Parrique, T., Barth, J., Briens, F., Kerschner, C., Kraus-Polk, A., Kuokkanen, A. and Spangenberg, J.H. 2019, *Decoupling Debunked: Evidence and Arguments Against Green Growth as a Sole Strategy for Sustainability, European Environment Bureau*, 8 July, accessed 28 December 2021, <https://backend.dnr.de/sites/default/files/Publikationen/Themenhefte/Entkopplungsreport_EEB_07_2019.pdf>.

Preston, S. 1975, 'The changing relation between mortality and level of economic development', *Population Studies*, 29(2), pp. 231–48.

Saini, V., Brownlee, S., Elshaug, A.G., Glasziou, P. and Heath, I. 2017, 'Addressing overuse and underuse around the world', *The Lancet*, 390(10090), pp. 105–7.

Slawomirski, L., Auraaen, A. and Klazinga, N. 2017, *The Economics of Patient Safety: Strengthening a Value-Based Approach to Reducing Patient Harm at the National Level*, OECD, Paris.

Starfield, B. 2000, 'Is US health really the best in the world?' *Jama*, 284(4), pp. 483–5.

Szreter, S. 2005, *Health and Wealth*, Rochester University Press, Rochester.

Tainter, J.A. 2006, 'Social complexity and sustainability', *Ecological Complexity*, 3, pp. 91–103.

Todd, M.H. 2019, 'Six laws of open source drug discovery', *ChemMedChem*, 14(21), p. 1804.

Vernero, S., Domenighetti, G. and Bonaldi, A. 2014, 'Italy's "Doing more does not mean doing better" campaign', *BMJ*, 349, p. g4703.

Whitmee, S., Haines, A., Beyrer, C., Boltz, F., Capon, A.G., de Souza Dias, B.F., Ezeh, A., Frumkin, H., Gong, P., Head, P., Horton, R., Mace, G.M., Marten, R., Myers, S.S., Nishtar, S., Osofsky, S.A., Pattanayak, S.K., Pongsiri, M.J., Romanelli, C., Soucat, A., Vega, J. and Yach, D. 2015, 'Safeguarding human health in the Anthropocene epoch: Report of The rockefeller foundation-lancet commission on planetary health', *The Lancet*, 386(10007), pp. 1973–2028.

WHO. 1946, *Constitution of the World Health Organization*, accessed 20 January 2021, <https://www.who.int/about/who-we-are/constitution/>.

World Health Organization. 1978, *Declaration of Alma-Ata*, World Health Organization, Geneva.

World Health Organization. 2009, *World Health Statistics 2009*, World Health Organization, Geneva.

World Health Organization. 2014, *WHO Traditional Medicine Strategy: 2014–2023*, World Health Organization, Geneva.

World Health Organization. 2019, *Global Spending on Health: A World in Transition*, World Health Organization, Geneva.

Zywert, K. and Quilley, S. 2018, 'Health systems in an era of biophysical limits: The wicked dilemmas of modernity', *Social Theory and Health*, 16(2), pp. 188–207.

39

CUBAN MEDICAL INTERNATIONALISM

A radical alternative approach to medical 'aid'

John M. Kirk

Most people are unaware of Cuba's public healthcare system and its policy of exporting medical services abroad, mainly to developing countries. This lack of awareness changed somewhat in 2020–21 because of Cuba's involvement in sending medical brigades around the world in the struggle against COVID-19. Yet, even in that role, there remains astonishing ignorance in the Global North. The misinformation that exists about the medical role of Cuba is unfortunate because there is much to be learned from its experience.

In 2021, Cuba's Henry Reeve medical brigade was nominated by hundreds of people and organizations from around the world for the Nobel Peace Prize, largely due to the island's international response to COVID-19. In late-2019, when the planet became aware of the enormous impact of the COVID-19 pandemic, Cuba already had some 28,000 medical personnel working in 59 countries, including in 29 poverty-stricken countries in sub-Saharan Africa (Acosta Damas 2020). In other words, before anybody had heard of the pandemic, Cuba already had more medical personnel working abroad in the Global South than all the G-7 industrialized countries combined. During the COVID-19 crisis itself, while countries were struggling to stave off massive health challenges, Cuba responded to calls for help and sent brigades of specialists in pandemics and emergency healthcare to Asia, Europe, Latin America and the Caribbean, the Middle East, and Africa. In all, almost 5,000 Cuban medical personnel – in 57 medical brigades – travelled to 40 countries, mainly on three- to six-month contracts.[1] In late-February 2021, 25 Brigades remained abroad, with the support of 2,500 Cuban medics (MINSAP 2021a) – part of the 28,705 Cuban medical personnel working in six countries at that time (MINSAP 2021b).

As argued in the present chapter, this program of medical brigades is one of several key features of a broader, multifaceted approach to medical internationalism (MI) adopted by Cuba for decades. Since the 1960s, this internationalism has resulted in the service of over 420,000 Cuban medical personnel in internationalist missions in over 150 countries. According to data compiled by the Cuban Ministry of Public Health, they have performed over 14,500,000 surgeries, delivered 4,470,000 children, and saved 8,700,000 lives (Prensa Latina 2021). The values informing this internationalism have been inculcated in Cuba for decades and are now entrenched in its new Constitution, codified in February 2019. Article 72 of the latter states that 'Public health is a right of all people and it is the State's responsibility to guarantee access to quality medical attention, protection and recovery services, free of charge'. Similarly, its Preamble emphasizes

DOI: 10.4324/9781003017110-44

the significance of 'proletariat internationalism, fraternal friendship, the help, cooperation and solidarity of the people of the world, particularly those of Latin America and the Caribbean' (Constitute Project 2019).

How can a small country like Cuba adopt such an expansive, international approach to healthcare? What lessons can be gleaned from Cuba's MI and this alternative stance on human solidarity? This chapter provides a background to understand this medical collaboration, in existence for over six decades; offers a general panoramic overview of some of the specific alternative medical collaboration programs offered; and analyzes the components of the Cuban approach, which make it an alternative form of international medical collaboration to that prevailing in the Global North.

Setting the context

Cuban MI is based upon a model and philosophy of healthcare that offers a distinctive alternative approach to how medicine is practiced in the Global North. To appreciate its significance, it is first important to understand the origins and approach to public healthcare on the island. When the Cuban Revolution occurred in 1959, the country maintained some 6,000 physicians and a single faculty of medicine (at the University of Havana). By the end of 1961, approximately half of the doctors had left, and the faculty of medicine retained only a handful of professors. By 1975, however, the number of Cuban doctors had tripled to 9,328. By 2019, there were 13 medical universities and 29 faculties of medicine on the island, as well as 97,202 doctors (MINSAP 2019: 173, 120). Some comparable data with the US are worth noting. According to the CIA *World Fact Book* (2021), the infant mortality rate in Cuba is lower than in the US (4.19 per 1,000 live births, compared to 5.22), although life expectancy is slightly higher in the latter (80.43 against 79.41). Per capita, the Cuban Government spends about one-fourteenth of the US' expenditure on the cost of medical services, yet has similar health results.

Cuba has a national healthcare policy that ensures that it is accessible to all, regardless of income, social class, or location. According to the World Bank (2019), while the US had 2.6 physicians per 1,000 people, Cuba tripled this figure with 8.4-one of the best ratios in the world. In addition, all healthcare in Cuba is free and emphasizes a preventive rather than curative approach – an alternative strategy that is far more cost-effective, and employed in both domestic and international healthcare strategies. Cuba also produces about 60 percent of its own medicines, which are extremely inexpensive.[2] With 97,000 doctors, and three times the number of physicians per patient as found in the US, there is a surplus of medical talent. Therefore, about 20 percent of Cuba's doctors are working abroad at any given time – and payment for their services to the Cuban Government is its single largest source of hard currency. The funds generated by exportation of medical services are used to subsidize the Cuban public healthcare system.

Understanding medical internationalism *a la Cubana*: some examples

A series of interviews appearing in an article in the July 24, 2020, issue of the *Financial Times* provides a useful insight into the diverse international reactions to Cuba's role during the COVID-19 pandemic. The mayor of Turin, where a large Cuban delegation had worked for several months in 2020, praised 'the victory of the values represented by those who came from the other side of the ocean, of solidarity and generosity', while an unnamed Western diplomat termed Cuba's support 'a straight economic question – it's a cash cow' (Frank *et al.* 2020). While it might initially be assumed that Cuba is pursuing MI for financial reasons, the situation is more complex. Indeed, for decades before Cuba received payment for medical services, the island had been sending medical contingents to the Global South – the earliest being in 1960 (after an earthquake in Chile) and in 1963 (to develop the healthcare service in newly-independent Algeria).

In more recent times, three events illustrate the Cuban approach to providing medical support at a time of medical emergencies when financial benefit was not a feature. The 2010 earthquake in Haiti (killing 250,000 and injuring 300,000) is one of the more significant examples of Cuba's response to a major international health crisis (Kirk 2015: 189–214). When the earthquake struck, there were already 403 Cuban medical personnel working in Haiti – 6,094 Cuban medics had previously worked in the country – along with some 400 local physicians trained in Cuba. They were joined by 60 members of the Henry Reeve Brigade, and 138 fifth-year Haitian medical students and interns training in Cuba (Relief Web 2010). Similarly, consider the Cuban response to the Ebola crisis that devastated several West African countries between 2013 and 2016, when over 11,000 people died. Cuba was the first country to send doctors when the epidemic broke out, after the World Health Organization had appealed for help. In all, 256 medical personnel from Cuba participated in the campaign, although 15,000 had volunteered. A final pertinent example is Cuba's support following the meltdown at the Ukrainian nuclear reactor of Chernobyl in 1986, which affected six million people (Kirk 2015: 236–52). In this case, between 1990 and 2011, Cuba provided free medical treatment and accommodation on the island to 23,000 children affected by the accident, as well as for accompanying family members. Such support was offered at a desperate time in Cuba, following the implosion of the USSR which, in turn, took with it 85 percent of Cuba's foreign trade.

Also significant is Cuba's offer of support to the US in the immediate aftermath of Hurricane Katrina in 2005, which resulted in over 1,800 deaths, mainly in New Orleans. Cuba assembled some 1,200 specialists in emergency medicine, and had them waiting in Havana, ready to fly to New Orleans at a moment's notice, along with 32 tons of medicine. Sadly, the administration of George W. Bush rejected Cuba's offer of help. Fortunately, however, the preparations for Katrina led shortly afterward to the formation of the Henry Reeve Brigade, as discussed below.

The common denominator in these examples of medical collaboration is a clear humanitarian spirit, which informs its distinctive alternative to providing medical support to regions affected by natural disasters and medical emergencies. The revolutionary government reacted in the same way to the Ebola epidemic, the earthquake in Haiti, the Chernobyl nuclear meltdown, and Hurricane Katrina – offering support where it was needed. While they received some compensation for their role in the Ebola case from the WHO, their response to the Haitian earthquake and provision of medical treatment to families affected by Chernobyl involved no repayment from the countries affected. Cuba's response to these crises, and ongoing medical support to scores of countries in the Global South, reveals a radically different approach to international medical 'collaboration' compared to the self-interested 'aid' provided by industrialized nations, as discussed below. As Cuban officials often note, 'We don't offer what we have left over. We share what we have' (Trotta 2014).

In sum, internationalism is in the DNA of the Cuban revolutionary process. In the 1970s and 1980s, for example, the Cuban role in Africa grew rapidly – in both military cooperation, and provision of medical and educational services. Over 300,000 Cubans fought in Angola between 1975 and 1991, and 2,000 were killed. The civilian role was also important in Angola, and over 50,000 Cubans worked there. Indeed, by 1984, almost half of all Cubans working in Africa were providing medical support – mainly in sub-Saharan Africa at no charge – to over 30 countries. Nelson Mandela has summarized the Cuban role in Africa with clarity:

> Cubans came to our region as doctors, teachers, soldiers, agricultural workers, but never as colonizers. They have shared the same trenches as us in the struggle against colonialism,

> underdevelopment, and apartheid. Hundreds of Cubans have given their lives, literally, in a struggle that was first and foremost, not theirs but ours. As Southern Africans, we salute them. We vow never to forget this unparalleled example of selfless internationalism.
>
> (Edmonds 2013)

The remainder of this chapter analyzes the evolution of Cuba's medical collaboration since its origins in 1960. Specifically, it identifies three key areas where this approach has been critical, yet not restricted by geographical boundaries: medical education for developing countries; Operation Miracle (eye surgery provided at no cost to several million people in Latin America and the Caribbean); and the role of the Henry Reeve Brigade (formed to deal with epidemics and natural disasters). Each underscores a distinctive aspect of Cuba's commitment to MI, while collectively illustrating an extraordinarily multifaceted approach to providing international healthcare to the Global South. Moreover, when examined side-by-side, these examples also highlight the value of the Cuban model as an alternative rationale for medical internationalism to that informing the prevailing Western model of foreign aid. While the latter is largely based upon a concept of charity, often accompanied by an underlying superciliousness with regard to expertise and technology, the former is centered on a humanitarian belief that access to free, public healthcare for all is an alienable human right.

Medical education

All Cubans enjoy free education, including training to become a doctor. For foreign students, it is also largely free, and Cuba has trained thousands of doctors (almost all from developing countries), at no charge to the students. More recently, while medical education remains free for the vast majority of students from the Global South, a sliding scale has been introduced for others based upon their ability to pay. The Latin American School of Medicine (ELAM) was established in early-1999 after the government took over the country's Naval Academy and turned it into the world's largest medical school (Kirk 2015: 42–67). It was founded at the specific request of President Fidel Castro, following the destruction caused by Hurricane Mitch in Central America. Castro established ELAM for people of the affected countries, with the aim of training one doctor for every life lost and offered six-year medical scholarships to students from the region. Initially, almost all students at ELAM were from Central America, although the medical school gradually admitted students from other, mainly Latin American, countries.

However, unlike medical schools elsewhere, ELAM sought to train students from poor backgrounds who would possess the social *'conciencia'* (an amalgam of political awareness, empathy, and social commitment), and who would appreciate their educational opportunities. The concept was to ensure a 'brain gain' instead of a 'brain drain', so that graduates would be less attracted to financial siren calls from the Global North. Scholarship recipients should be bright students from poor families otherwise unable to pay the high medical school tuition to become a doctor. It was argued that they understood the health needs of the region, and since they would otherwise be unable to attend medical school, they were more likely to stay and help people in underserved communities.

ELAM has continued training doctors from Latin America, but now also accepts students from the Caribbean, Africa, and even the US. Recent figures show that some 29,000 students from 105 countries have graduated since its founding in 1999 – including 182 Americans, mostly from visible minorities (Cuba's Latin American School 2019). Speaking to faculty and staff of ELAM on October 27, 2009, Dr. Margaret Chan, then-Director General of the WHO, praised the nature of the pragmatic training received by students at the institution: 'You are being trained to be engaged members of the communities you serve, and not just doctors in white jackets waiting for the problems to show up, preferably by appointment, in your offices'. Students at ELAM, she noted, were receiving the skills needed to help the underprivileged enjoy good health as a basic human right (Kirk 2015: 66–7).

Cuba has also trained doctors (at no cost to students) in several other countries. This is especially true in Venezuela, where 25,000 have become Cuban-schooled medical doctors. Medical schools have also been established by Cuba in several developing countries, including Yemen, Gambia, Ethiopia, Uganda, Guyana, Equatorial Guinea, Guinea Bissau, and Ghana. However, perhaps the most interesting case of Cuba's medical training has been in Timor-Leste since 2004. After obtaining their independence from Indonesia in 2002, Timor experienced a mass exodus of professionals, leaving only a few dozen doctors in the country. Cuba responded by sending medical staff – almost 300 by 2008 – but then decided to extend the ELAM approach, inviting students from Timor to study medicine in Cuba (Walker and Kirk 2013). By 2019, almost 1,000 Timorese had graduated in medicine, with most of their studies being undertaken at ELAM, followed by internships back in Timor. Cuba also helped to establish a faculty of medicine at the national university in the country's capital, Dili. There, students from other small South Pacific Islands are also studying medicine under Cuban professors. As can be seen, Cuba's support for medical training – provided to developing countries at no charge, or significantly reduced rates – is quite different from the largely commodified form of education found elsewhere.

Operation miracle

For people in the Global North, having cataract surgery is easy and relatively inexpensive. Conversely, for those living in the developing world, the cost is often prohibitive, while the loss of sight regularly deprives people of their livelihood and the natural advantages accruing from normal vision. Starting in 2004, the Cuban and Venezuelan Governments developed 'Operation Miracle', a program that continues throughout the region. The goal, as drawn up by Presidents Fidel Castro and Hugo Chávez, was to restore sight to six million people in Latin America and the Caribbean – mainly the poor who could never afford such surgery. The program started almost by accident. Cuba had originally embarked on a regional literacy crusade ('Yo, sí puedo' or 'Yes I can') – another remarkable program that has taught basic literacy to over ten million people in 30 countries. It was discovered, however, that many were unable to read – not because of a lack of educational training, or academic ability, but rather due to severe vision problems. Cuba then decided to address the challenge in several ways. First, tens of thousands of patients from Latin America and the Caribbean were flown to Cuba for (free) eye surgery. When the patient numbers became so great that they could not all be treated on the island, Cuban ophthalmologists were sent to the countries with the greatest needs, and eye clinics were established. Simultaneously, Cuba opened its medical training facilities to Latin American doctors to become ophthalmologists, replacing the Cuban specialists in their home countries.

The program has been successful. Venezuela has so far benefited most, with almost three million patients receiving treatment in 20 clinics. Figures from July 2016 show that in Venezuela, almost 15,000 patients with eye problems were examined daily, and over 23 million medical consults had taken place since the program was implemented (Misión Milagro 2016). Recall that these services were freely provided to all patients. In all, over four million patients from some 30 countries (mainly in Latin America and the Caribbean) have benefited from the program, and clinics had been set up by Cuba in Bolivia, Argentina, Colombia, Costa Rica, Ecuador, El Salvador, Guatemala, the Dominican Republic, and Uruguay.

The Henry Reeve Brigade

A third major example of Cuban medical internationalism can be found in the work of the Henry Reeve Brigade, a large group of medical professionals trained to deal with epidemics and natural disasters. The Brigade is named after a Brooklyn native, who fought in the First War of Cuban Independence (1868–78), reaching the rank of Brigadier General, before dying while fighting against Spain. Since its formation in 2005, the Brigade has dealt with myriad disasters – from floods in Guatemala and Mexico to earthquakes in China and Sierra Leone, from hurricanes in Haiti to tsunamis in Sri Lanka. Its basic philosophy was expressed in a speech by Fidel Castro on September 15, 2005, announcing the formation of the Brigades:

> Not once throughout its generous revolutionary history has our people refused to offer medical solidarity whenever another country has been affected by a natural catastrophe and needed our help – regardless of ideological and political differences, or serious offences from the governments of those countries [...] Tens of thousands of Cuban doctors and health professionals scattered around the world are irrefutable proof of that. For them there will never be barriers based upon language, sacrifice, danger or other obstacles.
>
> (Garófalo and Gómez García 2011: 60)

Until the COVID-19 pandemic, the largest Cuban deployment was in Pakistan in 2005, when a large delegation of medical specialists (2,300) was sent to respond to a major earthquake in Kashmir. The impact of this medical assistance was significant. In addition to attending patients and performing surgeries (the most complicated cases were freely transported to Havana), Cuban medical staff developed a local educational program in preventive care alongside local medics. The Cubans stayed for seven months, during which time they treated 1,743,000 patients (73 percent of all medically assisted cases resulting from the earthquake). They performed 14,506 surgeries and treated some 166,000 people with rehabilitation and physiotherapy services (Kirk 2015: 129). In many ways, even more important was the legacy left by Cuba. When the Henry Reeve Contingent returned to Cuba, they donated the 32 field hospitals that they had brought and trained 450 Pakistani army doctors to operate them. They also provided 234 tons of medicine and supplies, and 275 tons of equipment to stock the hospitals. The most significant support, however, came in the form of medical scholarships for local students. As had been the case with students from Central America and Haiti (discussed above), Cuba offered students the chance to study medicine for free at ELAM. Ultimately, 1,000 Pakistani students accepted this offer, with the first cohort arriving in Havana in 2007.

Since the mission in Pakistan, the Henry Reeve contingent has participated in dozens of missions and broadened its mandate to include natural disasters and medical epidemics, epitomized by Ebola and COVID-19. It was formed with the support of 1,500 medical specialists with experience in these fields, and now has some 9,000 members. Prior to August 2020, it had not only provided medical support to 45 countries, including 22 states of Latin America and the Caribbean, but also sent specialists to countries in Asia and Oceania, Africa, the Middle East, and Europe. In 2017, at the 70th World Health Assembly in Geneva, the Henry Reeve Contingent was awarded the prestigious Lee Jong-wook Memorial Prize for its commitment to providing medical support to over 3.5 million people in 21 countries affected by disasters and epidemics. In presenting the prize, it was noted that an estimated 80,000 lives had been saved by the actions of Cuban medical personnel (Mitchell 2019).

The rationale for Cuba's medical internationalism program

So how has a small country like Cuba (with a population of only 11.2 million) maintained such a diverse program of medical cooperation for over six decades? Why does it do so? What is its value as an alternative form of MI? There are several explanations for Cuba's humanitarian commitment. All of them, however, depend upon a specifically Cuban interpretation of the significance of public health, based on ideas outlined and developed for decades by Fidel Castro:

> Although every person and every people have the right to a healthy life, and to enjoy the privilege of a long and useful life, the richest and most developed societies, ruled by the desire for profit and consumerism, have converted medical services into a vulgar form of merchandise, inaccessible to the poorest sectors of the population. In many countries of the Third World such services hardly exist.
>
> (Garófalo Fernández and Gómez García 2011: 60)

The Cuban approach to healthcare is the antithesis of this reasoning, rejecting it as a 'vulgar form of merchandise'. Instead, healthcare is perceived as the most basic human right. Cuban MI has, thus, developed on the fundamental principle of the need to provide healthcare to all, freely to the patient (not the 'client', Cuban doctors insist), and wherever needed.

On one level, there is a solid economic case for MI, since provision of medical services abroad is Cuba's largest source of hard currency. Carmelo Mesa-Lago has noted that the country that paid the most for these medical services was Venezuela, which in 2017 provided Cuba with $6 billion for professional services. To contextualize this, in pre-COVID times, Cuba received $3.5 million in remittances from family members living abroad, while the income generated by tourism was $3.3 billion (Diario de Cuba 2019). A sliding scale of payment is employed when contracting out medical services, with the key component being the recipient country's ability to pay. A recent study (Escobedo *et al.* 2021), for instance, showed that between 2011 and 2016, over 140,000 Cuban professionals worked in 67 countries. Payment was received in the following way: Cuba received payment for its assistance from over one-third of the countries (30), it fully funded just under one-third (20), and costs were shared in the remaining 17 countries.

One reason that Cuba has pursued MI stems from the opportunities for local medical staff to earn more income by working abroad, since their salaries are relatively low on the island. Following the demise of the Soviet Union, the Cuban economy failed badly. Between 1989 and 1994, GDP fell 35 percent, food was scarce (the average Cuban male lost 20 pounds in weight), and 85 percent of Cuba's trade with traditional allies disappeared within a year. The Government, in turn, decided to invest in tourism to generate hard currency, resulting in foreign investment flooding into Cuba. Castro warned that dependency on tourism would cause many societal problems, as professionals flocked to work as maids and waiters. An inverted employment pyramid resulted, with medical professionals earning significantly less than taxi drivers and hotel workers. There have since been significant salary increases for medical personnel – most recently in 2020 – but Cuban medical personnel remain underpaid.

Volunteering abroad as doctors helped to rectify this imbalance somewhat, since salaries were significantly greater during medical missions. For instance, until the Bolsonaro Government forced the closure of the 'Mais Médicos' program, over 8,000 Cuban physicians earned $1,200 monthly in Brazil – compared to the $80 they would have received in Cuba. The Cuban Government was aware of the salary imbalance resulting from the financial crisis of the 1990s, and saw exportation of medical services as a means to both secure hard currency for the national economy (since the recipient country paid Havana roughly three times the salary provided to each Cuban healthcare worker), and provide underpaid health personnel the opportunity to earn higher salaries. The monies generated from medical services abroad were used to support the domestic healthcare system.

Cuba is also often assumed to pursue MI for political or diplomatic relations – a form of 'soft power' or 'medical diplomacy', holding that a country is more successful in influencing or co-opting others through persuasion and aid, rather than by using coercive force. Analogously, by providing professional services (such as healthcare, education or construction), Havana is deemed better able to win support from other countries in international fora. It is instructive that, for many years, most developing countries in the United Nations General Assembly have supported the annual motion brought by the Cuban Government against the US embargo. In June 2021, for instance, 184 countries supported the Cuban position, with only two – the US and Israel – voting against. Some see this as clear evidence of Cuba's medical diplomacy in delivering votes at the United Nations.

This argument is problematic, however. As outlined above, Cuba was providing medical support to developing countries for decades before the embargo motion was first presented in 1992. Rather, the prime reason for Cuban medical collaboration was the development of a philosophy over decades that doing so was a moral obligation. In June 1965, Castro explained the essence of his philosophy:

> So never, looking ahead to the future decades, will we have too many doctors or dentists, teachers, engineers or technicians. We will need them all, and if we don't need them, other countries with greater needs than ours will. And so, we should prepare ourselves to meet our obligations to other peoples, since otherwise our concept of human solidarity will remain limited by our own needs and by our own borders.
>
> (Garófalo Fernández and Gómez García 2011: 10)

This Cuban approach to MI is very different from any form of 'aid' provided by industrialized nations. For Cuba, medical collaboration, particularly with countries of the Global South, is a moral duty. The need to provide solidarity and humanitarian support are values inculcated in Cubans from an early age, and there are few on the island without a relative or friend who has participated in 'internationalist missions'. Moreover, far from the idea promulgated by the former-Trump administration that members of these missions were forced to participate, Cuban medical personnel participate freely (Kirk 2015; Kirk and Erisman 2009).[3] These examples of cooperation provide a source of great pride for Cubans, who are also not blind to the practical benefits accruing to those participating in the missions. These medical experiences abroad are seen as a rite of passage that everybody goes through, and from which they benefit materially and spiritually.

An alternative model ahead of its time?

There are many criticisms of traditional medical aid, perhaps summarized best by the provocative title of an article by Welling *et al.* (2010), 'Seven sins of humanitarian medicine'. One major oversight is that foreign NGOs and government missions alike often arrive in developing nations to provide medical assistance without consulting the local government and, thus, implement their own agenda. Moreover, these organizations may well establish programs where the needs are not greatest. Often, local life can be disrupted when aid programs 'put their own needs before the needs of those whom they try to serve' (Sullivan 2019: 820). At times, there is a basic mismatch between local needs and imported technology, which is particularly felt when foreign experts leave. The lack of a follow-up strategy after their departure is also a common criticism. Often, the 'responders are poorly suited to help, with little or no experience in international relief, poor understanding of the local culture, and usually have no relationship with either local agencies or the affected population', with this influx phenomenon consequently described as 'disaster tourism' or 'parachuting' (Van Hoving *et al.* 2010: 202). Moreover, long-term reliance on relief aid – as opposed to collaborating with local medical staff – can often result in weakening local health systems.

Conversely, the Cuban experience of MI over six decades offers a pragmatic, successful alternative, suitable for implementation in the developing world. In this regard, as former-Secretary General of the UN, Ban Ki-moon (2014: n.p.) stated, '[The Cuban] doctors are with communities through thick and thin: before disasters strike, throughout crises and long after storms have passed [...] Cuba can teach the entire world about health care'.

Myriad elements have contributed to the success of this alternative. As discussed above, MI has significantly contributed to other nations obtaining (and maintaining) their political-economic freedom. Also important is the commitment of the leadership of the revolutionary government to maintain its broad policy of internationalism, particularly in the Global South. This is difficult to understand for anybody not accustomed to the socialization practiced in Cuba for six decades, or the sense of national unity resulting during these years of developing a national project and defending it from the self-declared enmity of the US. A series of humanitarian and moral values have been comprehensively drilled into Cubans, which are now profoundly rooted and have been honed with experience. Indeed, from their earliest education in preschool centers, Cubans are encouraged to think of their role in the collective and of the need to help others. Fidel Castro summarized this philosophy well in a 2005 speech about the essence of Cuban medical professionals:

> What is the secret of our philosophy? Basically, that human capital is far more important than money. Human capital implies not only knowledge but also – and especially – awareness and commitment, ethics, solidarity, truly human feelings, a spirit of sacrifice, heroism, and the capacity to do a lot with very little.
>
> (Garófalo Fernández and Gómez García 2011: 58–9)

Can MI be emulated in other countries? With difficulty, and then only with a major change in mindset, since it provides a stark contrast to the philosophy and practice characterizing existing models. Indeed, a long process of establishing political will was a key element in the success of the Cuban model of MI, manifest in a decades-long process in which Castro emphasized the need for collaboration, particularly in Latin America and the Caribbean. Venezuela under Chávez had made strides in this direction, but his death and the subsequent economic crisis (accompanied by political polarization) put paid to that experiment. It would likely require a radical government of the Global South to implement such a model. Even then, any such approach would almost certainly engender the hostility of medical associations, which – as demonstrated in several countries where Cuban medics have arrived – have criticized their (radically different) training.

However, this does not mean that the Cuban model should be discounted. There are invaluable lessons to be learned from MI as a clear, pragmatic alternative, particularly for developing countries. Most importantly, COVID-19 has revealed with enormous clarity that we are all interconnected in this rapidly deteriorating planet, and urgently need to collaborate on an international level to avoid future disasters – a point well made in a recent article on the transformation of post-pandemic global health and development (Igoe and Chadwick 2020). Therein lies a significant potential role for Cuba, which could provide a medical army of 9,000 specialists trained in emergency measures and epidemics on standby, ready to help wherever needed. This pragmatic alternative, perhaps rolled out as a UN program, deserves to be considered as a measure to be implemented on a broader scale, since we have seen how the methods used by wealthy nations have fallen short in dealing with COVID-19.

Before that can happen, however, some hard questions need to be raised. Will we, as members of the international community, be able to lay aside petty arguments and differences, realize that pandemics do not respect international borders and, in turn, work together to deal effectively with common medical threats? The nationalistic protectionism exhibited over controlling 'our' vaccines against COVID-19, the reluctance of governments to share resources in the Covax program of the WHO, the disinterest in ignoring patent limitations of drugs so that poor countries could vaccinate their populations, and the general 'Me first' mentality are all deeply ingrained. Despite some tentative steps toward ameliorating such entrenched attitudes during the pandemic through temporary reform to intellectual property rights laws in the World Trade Organization, it is unlikely that the global community will be prepared to permanently codify such changes. Cuban exceptionalism and its alternative approach to humanitarianism are, thus, ahead of their time.

By way of conclusion...

This chapter has sought to show how, for six decades, Cuba has pursued a policy of MI that is a clear alternative to the traditional concept of 'aid' promoted by the Global North. Solidarity, not charity, is the basic philosophy of the Cuban approach. In both its domestic public healthcare system and application of global outreach, Cuba offers a distinctive counterhegemonic model that is, in many ways, the antinomy of neoliberal approaches examined elsewhere in this volume. It attempts to ensure a more egalitarian approach to healthcare and geopolitical solidarity, particularly in relation to the Global South. Indeed, the essence of the strategy is its emphasis on South-South solidarity, as opposed to traditional North-to-South 'aid' and charity. The Cuban approach to public healthcare also debunks the long-held assumption that development of healthcare is necessarily related to national GDP, demonstrating that low-income countries can attain high health outcomes comparable to those in the Global North (Pineo 2019). Simultaneously, it proves the feasibility of training a new form of revolutionary physician, imbued with *conciencia*, and an alternative model of medical collaboration.

As discussed above, the Cuban approach to MI is different from any other type of medical aid practiced by the Global North, largely because it is based upon the same philosophical underpinnings as its domestic healthcare system. Cuban MI is primarily a moral obligation, inspired by deeply entrenched concepts of egalitarianism, human capital, and social justice, which has been honed over six decades of experience. In contrast to the dominant, short-term programs implemented by developed countries and NGOs, Cuba seeks to provide long-term solutions, exemplified by the medical education program at ELAM, now into its third decade of providing free medical training to thousands of students from the Global South. Similarly, the provision of family healthcare programs by Cuba in many developing countries – the Programa Integral de Salud (Comprehensive Health Program) – has seen collaboration between 19,818 medical personnel in 43 countries over a decade (Jiménez Expósito 2010).

The Cuban approach to MI evidently possesses a novel ideological and humanitarian foundation, and offers a distinctive alternative to the fragmented, often self-seeking, forms of medical aid provided by governments and NGOs in the Global North (Wenham *et al.* 2021). There is, in sum, much for the latter to learn from Cuba. Indeed, perhaps MI has been ignored by mainstream media in the industrialized world for so long because it offers a viable, yet radically different and potentially threatening approach to extant institutions and ideologies of healthcare.

Notes

1 Information on the Cuban role in dealing with COVID-19 in specific countries can be found at the website of the Cuban Ministry of Public Health: *https://salud.msp.gob.cu/category/cooperacion/*.

2 Indeed, at the time of writing, Cuba is the only country in Latin America to have developed and produced its own vaccines for COVID-19 and, in all, has manufactured five variants. By mid-2022, over 80 percent of the Cuban population has been vaccinated.

3 In Kirk (2015) and Kirk and Erisman (2009), I interviewed some 270 Cuban *internacionalistas* over a 15-year period. While almost all volunteered for medical missions as a means of earning a substantial deal of money, many also saw their experience as an excellent way of developing their medical education, since in the Global South, they saw diseases, which had long disappeared from Cuba, and which they had only seen in medical textbooks.

References

Acosta Damas, M. 2020, *57 Años de Internacionalismo Médico Cubano*, accessed 23 June 2021, <https://www.cubaenresumen.org/2020/05/57-anos-de-interncionalismo-medico>.

CIA. 2021, *World Factbook*, accessed 11 June 2021, <https:www.cia.gov/the-world-factbook>.

Constitute Project. 2019, *Cuba's Constitution of 2019*, accessed 17 May 2021, <constituteproject.org/constitution/Cuba_2019.pdf?lang=eng>.

Cubadebate. 2016, 'Misión Milagro cumple 123 años: el programa que cambió la vida de millones', *Cubadebate*, 8 July, accessed 10 March 2019, <http://www.cubadebate.cu/noticias/2016/07/08/mision-milagro-cumple-12-anos-el-programa-que-cambio-la-vida-de-millones/>.

Cubadebate. 2021, 'Médicos cubanos han llevado su solidaridad a casi un tercio de la población mundial', *Cubadebate*, 22 February, accessed 23 February 2021, <http://www.cubadebate.cu/noticias/2021/02/22/medicos-cubanos-han-llevado-su-solidaridad-a-casi-un-tercio-de-la-poblacion-mundial/>.

Diario de Cuba. 2019, 'Señor ministro de Economía, aquí algunas recomendaciones para usted si Maduro cae', *Diario de Cuba*, 11 March, accessed 13 March 2019, <americanuestra.com/señor-ministro-de-economia-de-cuba-aquí-algunas-recomendaciones-para-usted-si-maduro-cae/>.

Edmonds, K. 2013, 'Cuba's other internationalism: Angola 25 years later', *NACLA Report on the Americas*, 27 September, accessed 2 March 2019, <https://nacla.org/blog/2013/9/27/cubas-other-internationalism-angola-25-years-later>.

Escobedo, A., Auza-Santiváñez, C., Rumbaut, R., Bonati, M. and Choonora, I. 2021, 'Cuba: Solidarity, Ebola and COVID-19', *BMJ Paediatrics Open*, 5, p. e001089.

Frank, M., Stott, M. and Schipani, A. 2020, 'Pandemic deepens divide over Cuba's international medical squads', *Financial Times*, 24 July 2020, accessed 19 May 2021, <https://www.ft.com/content/06069a38-7066-4cc0-bbe3-285a1dcaa465>.

Garófalo Fernández, N. and Gómez García, A.M. 2011, *Pensamientos de Fidel Castro Sobre la Salud Pública*, Editorial Ciencias Médicas, Havana.

Igoe, M. and Chadwick, V. (2020), 'After the pandemic: How will COVID-19 transform global health and development?' *DEVEX*, 13 April, accessed 1 May 2020, <https://www.devex.com/news/after-the-pandemic-how-will-COVID-19-transform-global-health-and-development-96936>.

Jiménez Expósito, Y. 2010, 'El programa integral de salud de Cuba: Un modelo de cooperación Sur-Sur', *Revista Cubana de Salud Pública Internacional*, 1(1), <www.medigraphic.com/pdfs/revcubsalpubint/spi-2010/spi101g.pdf>.

Ki-moon, B. 2014, 'Secretary-general hails Cuba for training medical 'miracle workers', being on frontlines of global health', address to officials at the Escuela Latinoamericana de Medicina (ELAM) in Havana, 28 January, accessed 19 September 2022, < https://press.un.org/en/2014/sgsm15619.doc.htm>.

Kirk, J.M. 2015, *Healthcare Without Borders: Understanding Cuban Medical Internationalism*, University Press of Florida, Gainesville.

Kirk, J.M. and Erisman, H.M. 2009, *Cuban Medical Internationalism: Origins, Evolution and Goals*, Palgrave Macmillan, New York.

MEDICC. 2019, *Cuba's Latin American School of Medicine Graduates Hundreds of New Doctors*, 24 July, accessed 26 July 2019, <http://medicc.org/ns/cubas-latin-american-school-of-medicine-graduates-hundreds-of-new-doctors/>.

Ministry of Foreign Relations, Cuba. 2021, *Henry Reeve International Medical Brigade Specialized in Disaster Situations and Serious Epidemics*, Internal Report, Havana.

MINSAP [Ministry of Public Health, Cuba]. 2020, *Anuario Estadístico de Salud*, accessed 1 May 2021, <files.sld.cu/bvscuba/files/2020/05/Anuario-Electronico-2019-ed-2020.pdf>.

MINSAP. 2021a, *Brigadas Henry Reeve que han Colaborado en la Lucha Contra la COVID-19,* Facebook entry, 22 February, accessed 23 February 2021, <https://www.facebook.com/MINSAPCuba/photos/a.32168786470...>.

MINSAP. 2021b, 'La historia de Javier: Un médico profundamente humanista', 23 May, accessed 23 May 2021, <https://salud.msp.gob.cu/la-historia-de-javier-un-medico-profundamente-humanista/?doing_wp_cron=1621783305.2636060714721679687500>.

Mitchell, C. 2019, 'OPS/OMS, Brigada Médica Internacional Henry Reeve de Cuba recibe premio Lee Jong-wook de la OMS', accessed 3 February 2019, <https://www3.paho.org/hq/index.php?option=com_content&view=article&id=13375:cubas-henry-reeve-international-medical-brigade-receives-prestigious-award&Itemid=42353&lang=pt>.

Pineo, R. 2019, 'Cuban public healthcare: A model of success for developing nations', *Journal of Developing Societies*, 35(1), pp. 16–61.

Prensa Latina. 2021, *Cuba and 58 Years of Medicine Throughout the World*, 23 May, accessed 23 May 2021, <https://misiones.cubaminrex.cu/en/articulo/cuba-and-58-years-medicine-throughout-world>.

Relief Web. 2010, *Haiti: Cuban Aid to Earthquake Victims*, 19 January, accessed 20 February 2021, <https://reliefweb.int/report/haiti/haiti-cuban-aid-earthquake-victims>.

Sullivan, H.R. 2019, 'Voluntourism', *AMA Journal of Ethics*, 21(9), pp. 815–22.

Trotta, D. 2014, 'Cuban doctors proud to risk lives in mission to halt Ebola', *Reuters*, 21 October, accessed 15 November 2014, <reuters.com/article/uk-health-ebola-cuba-idAFKCN0IA27D20141021>.

Van Hoving, D.J., Wallis, L.A., Docrat, F. and De Vries, S. 2010, 'Haiti disaster tourism – A medical shame', *Prehospital and Disaster Medicine*, 25(3), pp. 201–2.

Walker, C. and Kirk, J. 2013, 'From cooperation to capacitation: Cuban medical internationalism in the South Pacific', *International Journal of Cuban Studies,* 5(1), pp. 10–25.

Welling, D.R., Ryan, J.M., Burris, D.G. and Rich, N.R. 2010, 'Seven sins of humanitarian medicine', *World Journal of Surgery*, 34(3), pp. 466–70.

Wenham, C., Kavanagh, M., Phelan, A., Rushton, S., Voss, M., Halabi, S., Eccleston-Turner, M. and Pillinger, M. 2021, 'Problems with traffic light approaches to public health emergencies of international concern', *The Lancet,* 297(10827), pp. 1856–8.

World Bank. 2019, 'Physicians (per 1,000 people)', accessed 1 May 2022, <https://data.worldbank.org/indicator/SH.MED.PHYS.ZS>.

40
THE TRANSITION TO POST-CAPITALIST HEALTH AND HEALTHCARE

Howard Waitzkin

How to change the political-economic conditions that cause illness, suffering, and early death, and how to construct a more humane version of healthcare are challenging questions. In particular, they lead to further questions about the compatibility between capitalism and the capacity to meet human needs. As argued in this chapter, securing favorable achievements in health and healthcare requires going beyond the contradictory socio-ecological dynamics of the existing capitalist system, in favor of different societal configurations that prioritize health and well-being over the accumulation of wealth.

In confronting such challenges and investigating the potential for systemic change, I first clarify the meaning of 'praxis' – the relationship between theory and practice. Praxis, here, refers to an activist practice aimed at changing the political-economic conditions that generate illness and impede humane healthcare, guided by theoretical analysis and understanding of those conditions. I then describe a post-capitalist alternative for health and healthcare. To do so, I consider how this transition can materialize through a 'rinky-dink revolution', and how this change may reshape the political economy of health and healthcare.

Praxis and the contradictions of reform

Praxis is the uniting of theory and practice, study, and action (Gramsci 1971: Part 3). Regarding health and healthcare, there is an obvious difference between *knowledge* about political-economic conditions and *changing* those conditions. Understanding the problems of health and healthcare is not enough. Knowledge alone will not solve the difficulties we face. Research and analysis must be linked to action that changes the conditions responsible for illness and early death, as well as those that impede humane healthcare. Moreover, meaningful improvements in health and healthcare require confronting the practicalities of activism.

Antonio Gramsci (1971) developed an understanding of praxis in his *Prison Notebooks*. Among his theoretical contributions, Gramsci analyzed 'hegemony', the dominant ideologies of a society. He argued that fascist governments could not obtain a population's acquiescence to domination by force alone. Instead, those who rule must communicate key ideas that justify their domination, and these ideas then become hegemonic in achieving a population's consent to otherwise unacceptable policies. A major part of the praxis that Gramsci advocated involved theoretical understanding

DOI: 10.4324/9781003017110-45

and then action to demystify those hegemonic ideas that helped preserve the wealth and power of society's ruling elite.

Healthcare workers and activists concerned about the relationship between social change and health face difficult challenges in their daily work. People's problems often have roots in social conditions. Consider, for instance, those who cannot find a job or adequate housing; the elderly or disabled who need periodic medical certification to obtain subsistence welfare benefits; prisoners who develop illnesses because of prison conditions; patients with cancer whose insurance does not cover treatment; and workers with high blood pressure or heart disease compelled to choose between buying medications, purchasing food, and paying rent. These problems are complex, and are usually 'patched' in a reactive, *ad hoc* manner rather than fixed at their source. At the individual level, patching allows patients to continue functioning in the same social system that often causes the problem. However, even health workers who are highly critical of these societal conditions devote most of their clinical time to patching the system's victims. Frequently, this work has the paradoxical effect of preserving the system's overall stability.

The contradictions of patching have no simple resolution. One implication is that health work in itself is not sufficient. Instead, health workers can try to link their clinical activities to efforts aimed directly at basic sociopolitical change. The goal is to encourage healthcare praxis that points to progressive change in the social order. If health workers do not address the social roots of medical problems, solutions will remain limited and unsatisfactory.

To achieve this goal, it is important to acknowledge the contradictions of reform, which can slide into reformism. That is, improved material circumstances may seem beneficial, but can actually reinforce the status quo by reducing the potential for social conflict. Then political praxis no longer seems needed, and reform morphs into reformism. In other words, people fight for reform when conditions grow more oppressive. Therefore, in the realm of health and welfare, a repetitive pattern takes place: reforms most often follow social protest, resulting in incremental improvements that do not change the overall patterns of oppression, and these limited improvements suffer cutbacks when protest recedes (Fox and Cloward 1971: 3–79). So, reform often proves unhelpful or temporary.

A distinction developed initially by French activist and journalist André Gorz (1973: 135–77) helps clarify this problem. 'Reformist reforms' provide small material improvements, while leaving current political and economic structures intact. These reforms may reduce discontent while helping to preserve the system in its present form. In contrast, 'non-reformist reforms' achieve lasting changes in the present system's structures of power and finance. They do not simply modify material conditions. Instead, they provide the potential for large-scale, transformative political action. Rather than obscuring sources of exploitation by small incremental improvements, non-reformist reforms expose and highlight structural inequities. Such reforms ultimately increase frustration and political tension in a society, and can contribute to revolutionary upheaval. According to Gorz, such reforms are dynamic phases in a progressive struggle, not ends in themselves.

In the context of contemporary public health initiatives, 'universal health coverage' (UHC) offers an important example of a reformist reform. UHC does not mean 'healthcare for all' (HFA) – a delivery system that provides equal services for the entire population regardless of an individual's or family's financial resources (Waitzkin 2015). Rather, it refers to the more limited policy objective of health insurance coverage (Frenk 2015; Waitzkin *et al.* 2021: 226–36). The UHC orientation has become 'hegemonic' in global health policy circles (Heredia 2015; Smithers and Waitzkin 2022). Yet, those limited studies that have analyzed UHC's outcomes in countries such as Colombia, Chile, and Mexico challenge its underlying assumptions concerning the benefits of managed care, competition in markets, economic efficiency, or securing substantial cost reductions without undermining quality. Under UHC, access barriers remain or worsen as costs and corporate profits expand (Stuckler *et al.* 2010; Waitzkin 2011: Chapter 9; Sengupta 2013; Laurell 2015). As explained elsewhere in this book, the *Affordable Care Act* ('Obamacare') in the US contains many features similar to these reformist health reforms in other countries implementing UHC proposals.

There are also multiple examples of countries that have not accepted such reformist health reforms, but instead have constructed health systems based on the goal of HFA. These countries have fought to achieve universal access to care, but without tiers of differing benefit packages for the rich and poor. Such a change comprises a non-reformist health reform. Canada, for instance, prohibits private insurance for services provided in its national health program. Wealthy people in Canada must participate in the publicly funded system, and the presence of the entire population in a unitary system assures a high-quality national program (Thever 2005). Analogously, countries trying to advance the HFA model in Latin America during recent years have included Bolivia, Brazil, Cuba, Ecuador, Uruguay, and Venezuela. The single-payer, 'Medicare for All' proposal in the US provides another example of a proposed non-reformist reform (Waitzkin *et al.* 2021: Chapter 10).

Moving beyond capitalism for our health

Praxis in health and healthcare requires asking another fundamental question: are humane social conditions that foster health and a humane healthcare system possible in a capitalist society (Waitzkin and Waterman 1974)? Previously, practitioners, activists, and scholars could point to some countries in Europe and elsewhere with mixed capitalist-socialist systems, such as the United Kingdom and Sweden, which created conditions fostering good health and access to needed services. However, all those countries have experienced attacks on their public sector national health programs (NHPs) under the proliferation of neoliberalism since the 1970s, and inequality and structural racism continue to cause ill-health and early death (Waitzkin *et al.* 2021: Chapter 4).

Non-reformist reforms aim to transform capitalist society and move beyond the contradictions of capitalism that weaken NHPs and create illness-generating social conditions. But how can that transition actually happen? How can we move beyond capitalism for our health? These questions have emerged as crucial, especially in our current period of history with its profound problems and opportunities for transformation (see: Waitzkin and the Working Group on Health Beyond Capitalism 2018).

'It is easier to imagine the end of the world than the end of our economic system'. This statement, attributed to Fredric Jameson (2003),[1] conveys how simple it is to visualize scenarios leading to the end of humanity and other life forms (global warming with rising oceans and hot, uninhabitable land masses, nuclear Armageddon, and so forth). The quotation also conveys a vacuum of creative thinking that continues to inhibit transcending global capitalism – a system that benefits an increasingly concentrated fragment of the world's population (now roughly 0.5 percent at the expense of the rest of us (Oxfam 2022). Yet, how to get from A to B, capitalism to post-capitalism, is the question that we need to answer during this critical period of history, when the destructive forces of this system threaten the survival of human beings and other species.

Most of us find that it is difficult to imagine a viable path from capitalism to post-capitalism (the 'TINA' perspective, that is, 'There Is No Alternative'). Because it is hard to imagine a viable path from capitalism to post-capitalism, most people addressing our world's challenges assume that capitalism will continue to exist. Therefore, we engage in peculiar ways of struggling to improve our most important problems without confronting capitalism, even though we recognize that capitalism generates these problems and continues to make them worse (Fisher 2009).

Regarding health, capitalism's structural characteristics and contradictions exert deleterious effects leading to illness and early death (Doyal and Pennell 1979; Bambra 2011). For instance, since its earliest years, the contradiction between safety and profit has led to dangerous conditions affecting workers and communities. Corporations' profits decrease when they invest in equipment and services to protect workers in illness-producing workplaces, and this disincentive contributes to chronic occupational illnesses and mortality. Likewise, environmental pollution generated by capitalist industries creates chronic and sometimes fatal health problems affecting communities in which these industries are located.

In one of the earliest studies in social epidemiology, Friedrich Engels (2009 [1887]) documented occupational diseases generated by capitalist workplace practices, such as lead poisoning, black lung, cotton-workers' lung diseases, and many other disorders generated by unsafe working conditions. He also demonstrated the effects of industrial pollution on the health of communities, including various environmental lung diseases, neurological disorders, and cancers. Because the owners and managers of capitalist industries understood these injurious processes, yet continued the processes to enhance profits, Engels argued that capitalists were guilty of premeditated 'social murder', a perspective that recently has become even more influential (Abbasi 2021; Waitzkin *et al.* 2021: Chapters 2–3; Medvedyuk *et al.* 2021).

In addition to health itself, capitalism stands in the way of achieving adequate healthcare. For instance, we struggle for single-payer systems, such as improved Medicare for All, without coming to grips with the continuing vulnerability of national health programs within capitalist states. Under the pretense of 'balancing the budget', we have seen this vulnerability manifest recently in the deleterious effects of resurgent austerity programs in undermining the scope of European NHPs (Gaffney and Muntaner 2018). Nevertheless, through devoting strategic political efforts solely to reforming healthcare institutions, our actions may reactively redress the harmful effects of capitalism without proactively confronting their root causes in the dynamics of the system.

It is time to change this attitude of acquiescence and consent. The moment has come for a shift in our approach so that we struggle to remedy our key political-economic problems by confronting and transcending capitalism itself through revolutionary transformation – even if this transformation involves everyday actions and inactions that appear not only unglamorous, easy, and even 'rinky-dink', but also safe and feasible in every person's life.[2] To this end, my co-workers and I propose a 'rinky-dink revolution' (see: Figure 40.1): one that clearly identifies the fundamental causes of illness and early death in global capitalism, and confronts these causes through transformations to create a post-capitalist political-economic system. This process entails simple and safe ('rinky-dink') actions that ordinary people can take to build a post-capitalist political economy based on social solidarity, rather than exploitation and the accumulation of capital. Among other favorable outcomes for humans and other beings, as well as the Earth, this new political economy fosters health rather than illness and early death, and facilitates accessible health and mental health services. The transformative process need not involve violent revolution, but rather strategies of 'creative constructions' that build the new political economy, as well as 'creative destructions' that slow down and stop the smooth functioning of capitalism.

Transitioning from capitalism to post-capitalism

The remainder of this chapter considers the transition from capitalism toward a post-capitalist order through such rinky-dink actions, with particular attention to transforming the political-economic determination of health and healthcare.

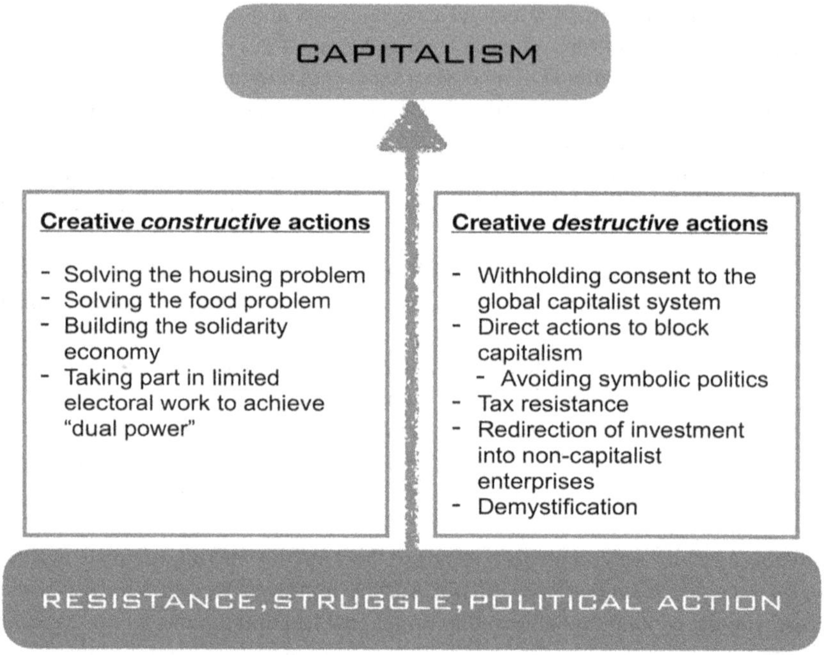

CAPITALISM

Creative *constructive* actions

- Solving the housing problem
- Solving the food problem
- Building the solidarity economy
- Taking part in limited electoral work to achieve "dual power"

Creative *destructive* actions

- Withholding consent to the global capitalist system
- Direct actions to block capitalism
  - Avoiding symbolic politics
- Tax resistance
- Redirection of investment into non-capitalist enterprises
- Demystification

RESISTANCE, STRUGGLE, POLITICAL ACTION

Figure 40.1 Rinky-dink revolution.
Source: Waitzkin (2020).

Elections, 'democracy', health, and healthcare

The question of how to achieve good health and accessible healthcare for populations often seems to revolve around who wins elections. Yet, elections only play a small role in the struggle to transform oppressive social conditions. Since the origins of modern democracy in the Greek Empire, elections have remained the tool of rich and powerful elites. Capitalism has only magnified the inherent social class characteristics of these electoral processes, such that a limited, 'bourgeois democracy' now prevails throughout the world, marked by a symbolic ritual of voting for representatives committed to the political-economic status quo (Hobsbawm 2000 [1975]). As social medicine nurse and anarchist, Emma Goldman (1910), pointed out long ago, voting in elections is mostly a symbolic action that never, in itself, delivers fundamental change.[3]

The problem, in large part, arises from the character of the state in which elected governments reside. In practice, this arrangement does not accord with the liberal vision of a neutral, beneficent state. Rather, the contemporary state – which assumes responsibility for protecting health and delivering healthcare, among other social services – remains a specifically *capitalist* state, functioning primarily as what Marx and Engels (2002 [1848]: Chapter 1) termed the 'executive committee of the bourgeoisie'. The capitalist state secures the conditions for perpetual capital accumulation. Accordingly, despite their seemingly benevolent impact, the welfare state's functions pertinent to health – provision of NHPs, as well as public education, housing, transportation, livable wages, and adequate food supplies – are inherently subject to several political-economic contradictions.

First, the welfare components of the capitalist state remain vulnerable to cutbacks and elimination during economic crises, as recently exemplified by the extension of austerity policies to the

NHPs of most European countries (Navarro and Muntaner 2014; Maresso *et al.* 2015; Reeves *et al.* 2015; Gaffney and Muntaner 2018). Important public programs of the welfare state predictably constrict or disappear as the capitalist state gears up to address the recurrent crises of capitalism. The state secures the conditions for ongoing accumulation, while displacing the costs of doing so elsewhere in the economy via budget cutbacks (Harvey 2014). These contradictory characteristics of the capitalist state also have manifested in the introduction of measures that undermine public health systems. As demonstrated during the COVID-19 pandemic, for instance, the ability of public health agencies to implement policies seeking to prevent spread of the infection was compromised by pressures from capital to reopen and resume economic activities that would increase community risk. Simultaneously, these public health agencies often could not overcome barriers to equitable provision of vaccines and medications due to the institutionalized monopoly power of pharmaceutical corporations that protected patent restrictions and profitability (Waitzkin *et al.* 2021).

Second, these welfare functions of the capitalist state contribute to false consciousness and hegemonic beliefs about the state's beneficent potential to ameliorate the excesses of the system. This ideological impact has been termed the state's 'legitimation function' (Offe 1996; Waitzkin 2000: Chapter 2, 2011: Chapter 3). By providing helpful services including healthcare through an NHP, the state legitimates the continuing inequalities and exploitation inherent in the capitalist system.[4] Many of us, especially if concerned about health and healthcare, respond to the suffering we encounter everywhere by advocating expansion, or at least maintenance, of the capitalist state's welfare components. We do this even though we understand that these welfare components remain perpetually vulnerable and legitimatize a system that inherently causes exploitation, inequality, hunger, ill-health, and early death. Moreover, we persist in advocating for the welfare state although we know that the global capitalist system has become weaker and more vulnerable due to deepening crises, loss of legitimacy, and its effects on the environment that threaten the survival of humanity and other life forms.

During the current period of world history, not only with all its dangers, but also with its deep potential for transformation, the time has come to move beyond our illusions that electoral politics and reforms to the capitalist state can achieve the revolutionary changes that are necessary for good health and accessible healthcare. So what is the praxis of that revolution, and what is the eventual aim? As detailed in Figure 40.1, this praxis entails two intertwined processes: 'creative constructions' and 'creative destructions'.

Creative constructions: a solidarity political economy

Many groups worldwide, including those that work in health and healthcare, are trying to achieve revolutionary change by creating a solidarity political economy beyond capitalism. This change entails production of goods and services within a political-economic system based on cooperation and mutual aid so that the economy is oriented not toward capital accumulation and growth, but rather sustaining the Earth and those who live here. Specifically, it aims to assure the comfortable survival of everyone, especially by solving the perpetual challenges of finding a place to live (the 'housing problem') and feeding oneself and others who depend on us (the 'food problem'). Within this political-economic configuration, energy comes from sources other than carbon, uranium, and plutonium; work involves more creative fun and fosters personal development, while technology reduces time devoted to work and expands leisure time (Waitzkin 2020). The transformation reconfigures the political-economic conditions that determine health – away from their primary goal of capital accumulation, and toward meeting socio-ecological needs.

In the US, over 200 organizations are currently collaborating to construct such a non-capitalist economy.[5] People in some of the poorest and most marginalized areas of the country (such as Jackson, Mississippi; the Rust Belt in the Midwest; and low-income neighborhoods of major cities) are pursuing this work, with some remarkable accomplishments. Similar organizations are growing in areas of the world most affected by imperialism and more recent austerity policies under neoliberalism, as in southern Europe and Latin America. These efforts often emphasize the health-centered goal of 'living well' (*sumak kawsay* in Quechua, *buen vivir* in Spanish). Activists in Latin American countries such as Bolivia, Ecuador, Venezuela, and Nicaragua have advanced this goal as a key component of proposed national health policies. Living well usually implies community-based solidarity and sustainability through 'mutual aid', moving away from the social conditions of capitalist society that worsen poverty, inequality, environmental pollution, and unacceptable health outcomes (Consejo Nacional de Planificación 2013; Hartmann 2019; Mamani 2018; Spiegel *et al.* 2019).

These efforts aim to free people from spending their lives as workers in precarious, proletarianized jobs (including jobs previously considered 'professional' employment), where we are unable to survive with healthy lives, let alone feel a sense of accomplishment in work and solidarity in community. To many people employed in this way, work also seems to accomplish little or nothing that feels meaningful, so positions of employment come to be understood as 'bullshit jobs' (Graeber 2018). In turn, the struggle for political-economic transformation reduces the need to work as 'wage slaves', without energy and time to create a new and different world. These conditions have led to growing stress, physical and mental health problems, and burnout among health and mental health professionals, with many of them leaving their professions (Waitzkin *et al.* 2018: Part 1). Such lived experiences of employment have contributed to the 'Great Resignation' during the COVID-19 pandemic, whereby millions of people left their jobs, creating a shortage of exploitable workers for capitalist corporations.

As suggested already, moving into a transformed, post-capitalist political economy means finding solutions to some perennial problems that are exacerbated by capitalism and fundamentally intertwined with health and healthcare. First, groups trying to achieve a solidarity political economy continue developing novel ways to solve the *housing problem*. For most people, paying for housing constitutes their biggest expense – thereby requiring continual laboring for wages in the capitalist economy – and is a major source of day-to-day insecurity. Accordingly, through finding ways to create cheap, small-scale, cooperative, pleasant, and comfortable housing units that require very little money, the solidarity political economy fosters collaborative solutions to avoid the exploitative social relations afflicting those who need housing within capitalism, such as extraction of rent, debt, burdensome taxes, and insurance. Housing co-ops, for instance, find inexpensive properties in cities or rural areas where housing can be rehabilitated or constructed with sophisticated technologies that reduce the costs of labor and improve the environmental sustainability of housing materials.[6] The objective is to maintain housing costs at around US$150 per person per month, which can be in federal currency, local currency of a city or town, or non-monetary time equivalents of donated work ('Mutual Exchange of Work' units, 'MEOWs').

Second, the path to a solidarity political economy includes solving the *food problem*, which of course is a key component of health and healthcare. The goal is sustainable, local food production and consumption with a low carbon footprint (meaning minimum petroleum products used for fertilizers, pesticides and, especially, transportation of food and its raw materials), and with a more favorable impact on the health of human beings, other living species, and the Earth. Community gardens and food cooperatives, for example, have figured as key components of achieving food sovereignty. In such cases, gardening focuses on cultivating plants that produce healthy nutrients, such as non-animal sources of proteins, with limited fats and carbohydrates. This approach helps redress the global epidemics of obesity and diabetes, which have arisen from a combination of food insecurity, 'food deserts' (where healthy foods are unavailable or too expensive for purchase in local areas), and promotion of sugar- and fat-rich foods by capitalist agricultural and food industries that produce and market processed food products (Albritton 2009). Animals for products like meat, fish, eggs, and milk are raised and slaughtered locally, and packaged for local consumption.

Broader objectives in addressing the food problem include independence from capitalist agriculture and sovereignty of local decision-making in the production and distribution of food. Food independence means giving up consumption of food that requires access to seasonal production in distant places delivered via carbon-based transportation, whose high financial costs and pollution contribute to climate change, depletion of fresh water supplies, and continuing exploitation of agricultural workers. Food sovereignty entails the formation of locally based cooperatives that assume control over food production and distribution. For families of average size, the aim again is restricting food costs to around US$150 per person per month, which can be paid through currency or time equivalents (such as MEOWs).[7]

While solving the housing and food problems are both crucial for health and 'good living', several other key elements of constructing the solidarity political economy are also important. For instance, we must replace economic activities that are ecologically unsustainable. In addition to its inherent need to exploit human beings and animals to produce commodified goods and services, capitalism also requires ongoing 'expropriation of nature' to fuel perennial economic growth and, thus, enable capital accumulation. Such expropriation engenders fundamental contradictions, because the natural resources consumed are actually limited or generate problems through their use that threaten the survival of humanity and other species (Foster and Clark 2018a, b). Among many examples, fossil fuels remain scarce, and their continued use undermines health and well-being by generating pollution and precipitating climate catastrophe.

Constructing the solidarity political economy requires not *less* growth, but *de-growth*. So, in addition to the above changes in economic production, simple changes in our patterns of economic consumption are essential. For instance, minimizing international travel, in the aggregate, can generate substantial socio-ecological transformations (Paulson *et al.* 2020).

Daily life in the solidarity political economy means engaging in cooperative economic activities to meet one's own needs and wants, as well as those of others in one's community. The underlying principle of such economic activities involves mutual aid (Kropotkin 1914: Chapters 7–8), by which people exchange goods and services without the exploitative structures and processes necessary for capital accumulation. Interestingly, one does not need money for many of these economic activities. Communities all over the world are discovering and implementing local economies that do not require much, if any, national currency, such as dollars. Instead, people are returning to simpler versions of economic exchange, where goods and services are produced and exchanged directly at the local level. For instance, through barter, people can directly exchange a good or service, thereby satisfying the needs or wants of each. Similarly, through time banking, a person can perform one hour of work anywhere in a specified community of participants. After doing so, they can request one hour of work from others through the time bank, which coordinates requests for services and keeps track of time worked. Health and mental health cooperatives within communities can operate through both these modes of simple exchange, with practitioners providing services in which they are trained and, in return, receiving goods and services that they need.

By participating in the solidarity political economy, community members thereby enhance local economic activities and reduce dependency on expensive and carbon-producing transportation of products and workers around the world. Within many communities, people are deciding to share their infrastructure, including tools, kitchens, libraries, workspaces, equipment, communications such as phone and internet, and buildings for housing, stores, clinics, hospitals, and other facilities that respond to common needs and wants. Such spaces become components of a 'commons', which is available for everyone to share but does not generate profits accrued by some at the expense of others.

Finally, the solidarity political economy involves limited forms of electoral 'democracy'. Communities worldwide that are attempting to construct economies beyond global capitalism have developed a profound skepticism about the capitalist state, including its welfare functions such as healthcare systems managed by the capitalist state. Rather than investing time, money, and energy in national electoral politics and politicians to advance goals like an NHP, activists have realized that non-capitalist NHPs cannot survive without social movements that transform the fundamental characteristics of capitalism itself.

As this understanding applies to elections, the focus moves from the national and state levels to the local level, usually within a county or municipality. Activists take part in limited electoral work to achieve 'dual power'. Implemented most clearly by Cooperation Jackson in Mississippi (Akuno and Nangwaya 2017), dual power involves two elements of power. First, activists build a network of strong community-based organizations that focus on different components of the solidarity political economy, such as housing, food, ecologically sustainable energy production and waste management, transportation, education, and health and mental health services. These organizations make decisions through direct participatory discussion and consensus within a 'communal' structure. Adapting their model from revolutionary struggles in other countries and theories of transition beyond the capitalist state, local communes eventually would assume the main responsibility for governance in a post-capitalist society and choose the regional and national leaders who implement policies shaped mostly from below.[8] Second, during a transitional period, activists achieve 'dual power' by winning local elections, especially for mayor and municipal or county councils, as occurred in Jackson. Local elections accomplish some narrow purposes, such as control of police departments and other wings of 'law enforcement' to prevent repression and brutality. Another key purpose involves access to funds and labor based in the public sector to help provide healthcare, housing, food, and other essential services.

Creative destructions

While efforts to build solidarity political economies will continue as a fundamental component of post-capitalist praxis, this innovative and often experimental work will not, in isolation, lead to a transformation of global capitalism and its pernicious effects on health and healthcare. Thus, in addition to the positive construction of a new world, praxis can also contribute to the peaceful, creative destruction of the current injurious system.

Of course, military routes to progressive revolutionary objectives – including the establishment of post-capitalist health and healthcare systems – are conceivable and sometimes necessary (Guevara 1960). However, the non-military wing of revolutionary action also opens up countless exciting possibilities for non-violent transformation. Research suggests that a small proportion of a country's population, estimated at 3.5–5 percent, can achieve revolutionary change through non-violent resistance, even in countries with brutal dictatorships (Chenoweth and Stephan 2012; Chenoweth 2017). Yet, such actions move far beyond electoral politics to include direct action, with the aim of slowing down and shutting down the capitalist system and the state that protects that system.

Mass protests in many countries often involve huge peaceful demonstrations, carried out with permits from the local police. Despite their importance, such actions do nothing to shut down the capitalist system. These important non-violent actions reverberate mostly in the realm of symbolic politics. Conversely, direct actions that disrupt the transport of fossil fuels, toxic chemicals, conventional and nuclear weapons, military equipment, precious metals, timber, and other items that keep the capitalist system afloat may enable activists to slow down or shut down the capitalist system. In the US, the heroic struggle by Indigenous communities at Standing Rock to stop the Dakota Access Pipeline was one such action. Here, the explicit purpose of the movement went beyond simply demonstrating against the socio-ecological devastation caused by constructing the pipeline. Instead, the struggle also aimed to block transport of oil to refineries and 'consumers' – thereby, slowing down and stopping one key component needed for the smooth functioning of the capitalist system (Estes 2019). Such activities sought to buttress the socio-ecological conditions necessary for health by protecting Indigenous lands from expropriation by capitalism, preserving accessibility of safe water supplies, and challenging the continued reliance on fossil fuels for economic growth.[9]

Besides direct action, activists trying to move beyond capitalism can change what we do with our money, especially in the realms of taxes, investments, and local economic activities. When large numbers of people participate, such efforts can disrupt, undermine, and create space for further actions to transform illness-generating conditions fostered by global capitalism. Consider tax resistance. For over a century, US pacifists have resisted taxes that pay for past and present wars, which currently comprises around half of the federal budget – roughly the same portion that pays for the combined total of health and mental health services, social security, public education, food and nutrition, housing and urban development, services for workers, children's services, and all other human resources (War Resisters League 2018–22). Thus, on a larger scale, tax resistance could obstruct the capitalist state's pursuit of perpetual war as a means of capital accumulation, with its associated destructive effects on health, well-being, and mortality. Similarly, shifting our investments away from corporate financial institutions can disrupt their often-pernicious investment activities, while moving these funds into solidarity political economies that protect our planet, support the health of communities, and nurture non-capitalist economic enterprises.

Praxis for post-capitalist political economies within capitalist countries

To conclude, I return to the situation occupied by most authors and probably most readers of this book, who live within global capitalism. Our societies arguably have become the most important spaces in which revolutionary transformation can occur. The purpose of this transformation is to create locally oriented, post-capitalist political economies as a means to improve the social conditions that determine ill-health and early death, and to construct systems that provide humane healthcare liberated from the destructive imperatives of capital accumulation.

To secure such transformational change, as outlined in this chapter, the praxis of 'rinky-dink revolution' involves actions and inactions that are easy, safe, mundane, unglamorous, and feasible for everyone. Adopting this praxis has become important especially for people concerned with health and healthcare, who spend much of their lives working within the very same political-economic system that causes most of the problems that we seek to correct. Accordingly, rinky-dink revolution includes withholding consent to processes that capitalism needs to maintain itself and grow, plus several creatively constructive and destructive efforts in which millions of people – albeit, still a minority of countries' existing populations – participate.

The transition to post-capitalism is already occurring throughout the world in the creative construction of communal organizations that govern themselves and that act to assure the survival and well-being of their participants. The resulting solidarity political economies, first, find ways to create cheap, small-scale, cooperative, pleasant, comfortable, and health-promoting housing units that require very little money, with collaborative solutions to exploitative rent, debt, taxes, and insurance. Second, communal organizations solve the food problem through local production and distribution of healthy food, achieving independence from capitalist agriculture, and local sovereignty in food production and distribution. The implementation of post-capitalist healthcare occurs mainly within locally organized solidarity political economies. Simultaneously, creative destructions do not take place by obtaining police permits for demonstrations, even large ones, but rather by direct actions that actually slow down or stop the smooth functioning of capitalism. Other creative destructions of capitalism involve diverting our investments and tax payments into post-capitalist solidarity political economies, with awareness of the predictably favorable impacts on health and healthcare. Through such actions, we can realize the joy of stopping our consent to, and unwitting support for, a system that we know damages our health, well-being, and happiness, and that stifles our ability to give and receive humane, high-quality, and accessible healthcare.

Notes

1 Jameson (2003: 76) actually said, ‘Someone once said that it is easier to imagine the end of the world than to imagine the end of capitalism. We can now revise that and witness the attempt to imagine capitalism by way of imagining the end of the world.’

2 This section is adapted from Waitzkin (2020).

3 As Tommy Douglas, the great left-wing Canadian politician and founder of the Canadian single-payer NHP, orated in his allegory of ‘Mouseland’ in 1944, mice vote for white cats or black cats, but never for mice. See: <https://youtu.be/SPOY3jDkuVw>. Analogously, the problem faced in contemporary capitalism is not just the presence of elected leaders who are neo-fascist, racist, sexist, and xenophobic, but rather a system that assures its elected leaders will remain representatives of the feline class. According to Vladimir Lenin (1935: Chapter 5), Marx described this process less metaphorically: ‘Every once in a while, the oppressed are allowed to decide which particular representatives of the oppressing class will represent them and oppress them.’

4 This legitimation function dates back to the initial traces of the welfare state in Nineteenth Century Germany, as Chancellor Bismarck initiated the world’s first national health program explicitly as a method to win support from the working-class and to prevent more fundamental revolutionary action. The ‘national socialism’ of Nazi Germany actually functioned as a version of the welfare state, as it implemented a strong public sector that provided unprecedented benefits for its Aryan population (the so-called *Volksgemeinschaft*), including affordable housing, accessible education, food security, and even health services. Similarly, in the midst of massive unrest and episodes of revolt in the US during the mid-1960s, Medicare and Medicaid became a tactic to prevent socialization of the entire healthcare system as part of a struggle to transform capitalism. See: Marmor (2000); and Piven and Cloward (1971).

5 The following websites provide overviews of efforts to create a solidarity political economy: <https://neweconomy.net/members>; <https://ussen.org>; <http://solidarityeconomy.us>; <www.solidarityeconomy.coop>; <www.solidaritystl.org>; and <https://cooperationjackson.org>.`

6 To illustrate, for information about Cooperation Jackson’s path-breaking efforts in Mississippi, see: Akuno and Nangwaya (2017).

7 Again, the efforts of Cooperation Jackson offer helpful perspectives on sustainable food production and distribution. See: Akuno and Nangwaya (2017).

8 For more on transition from the capitalist state to post-capitalist participatory governance, see: Mészáros (2010: esp. Chapters 13, 19, 20; 2022: Parts 1 and 2). Helpful discussions of the applications of Mészáros’s work on Venezuela’s Bolivarian Revolution, especially concerning its communal transition, appear in: Foster (2015: 1–17); Lebowitz (2015: Chapters 5–6); and Harnecker (2015: Chapters 7–9). A similar model of communal governance, but with more anarchist roots, has emerged in the autonomous region of Rojava in northern Syria, as part of the so-called Rojava Revolution. See: Knapp *et al.* (2016: Chapters 5–7, 11–13).

9 For reflections on similar direct actions against the Dakota Access Pipeline beyond that at Standing Rock, see: Democracy Now (2017). On the history of direct action, see: Kauffman (2017). Such actions targeting the infrastructure of corporate capitalism resemble the ‘roaming strikes’ that have become a component of

a resurgent US labor movement. The elite leadership of the largely debilitated labor unions in the country will not likely spearhead militant direct actions, such as a general strike. However, the militancy of non-unionized workers in struggles such as Fast Food Forward, OUR Walmart, Warehouse Workers United, Warehouse Workers for Justice, and Fight for 15 have achieved powerful effects by obstructing production through a roaming but escalating strategy (Early 2013).

References

Abbasi, K. 2021, 'COVID-19: Social murder, they wrote – elected, unaccountable, and unrepentant', *BMJ*, 372(314), pp. 1–3.

Akuno, K. and Nangwaya, A. 2017, *Jackson Rising*, Daraja Press, Montreal.

Albritton, R. 2009, *Let Them Eat Junk: How Capitalism Creates Hunger and Obesity*, Pluto Press, London.

Bambra, C. 2011, *Work, Worklessness, and the Political Economy of Health*, Oxford University Press, Oxford.

Chenoweth, E. 2017, 'It may only take 3.5% of the population to topple a dictator – with civil resistance', *The Guardian*, 1 February 1, accessed 21 December 2021, <www.theguardian.com/commentisfree/2017/feb/01/worried-american-democracy-study-activist-techniques>.

Chenoweth, E. and Stephan, M.J. 2012, *Why Civil Resistance Works: The Strategic Logic of Nonviolent Conflict*, Columbia University Press, New York.

Consejo Nacional de Planificación. 2013, *Buen Vivir: Plan Nacional, 2013–2017*, Government of Ecuador, Quito.

Democracy Now. 2017, 'Meet the two catholic workers who secretly sabotaged the Dakota Access Pipeline to halt construction', July 28, <www.democracynow.org/2017/7/28/meet_the_two_catholic_workers_who>.

Doyal, L. and Pennell, I. 1979, *The Political Economy of Health*, Pluto Press, London.

Early, S. 2013, *Save Our Unions: Dispatches from A Movement in Distress*, Monthly Review Press, New York.

Engels, F. 2009 [1887], *The Condition of the Working Class in England*, Oxford University Press, Oxford.

Estes, N. 2019, *Our History Is the Future*, Verso, New York.

Fisher, M. 2009, *Capitalist Realism: Is There No Alternative?* Zero Books, Hampshire.

Foster, J.B. 2015, 'Chávez and the communal state: On the transition to socialism in Venezuela', *Monthly Review*, 66(11), pp. 1–17.

Foster, J.B. and Clark, B. 2018a, 'The expropriation of nature', *Monthly Review*, 69(10), pp. 1–27.

Foster, J.B. and Clark, B. 2018b, 'The robbery of nature', *Monthly Review*, 70(3), pp. 1–20.

Frenk, J. 2015, 'Leading the way towards universal health coverage: A call to action', *Lancet*, 385(9975), pp. 1352–8.

Gaffney, A. and Muntaner, C. 2018, 'Austerity and health care', in Waitzkin, H. and Working Group on Health Beyond Capitalism (eds), *Health Care Under the Knife: Moving Beyond Capitalism for Our Health*, Monthly Review Press, New York, pp. 119–36.

Goldman, E. 1910, *Anarchism and Other Essays*, Mother Earth Publishing Association, New York.

Gorz, A. 1973, *Socialism and Revolution*, Anchor, New York.

Graeber, D. 2018, *Bullshit Jobs: A Theory*, Penguin, London.

Gramsci, A. 1971, *Selections from the Prison Notebooks*, International, New York.

Guevara, E.C. 1960, 'On revolutionary medicine', *Marxists Internet Archive*, August 19, accessed 2 November 2022, <www.marxists.org/archive/guevara/1960/08/19.htm>.

Harnecker, M. 2015, *A World To Build*, Monthly Review Press, New York.

Hartmann, C. 2019, '"Live beautiful, live well" ("Vivir Bonito, Vivir Bien") in Nicaragua: Environmental health citizenship in a post-neoliberal context', *Global Public Health*, 14(6–7), pp. 923–38.

Harvey, D. 2014, *Seventeen Contradictions and the End of Capitalism*, Oxford University Press, New York.

Heredia, N., Laurell, A.C., Feo, O., Noronha, J., González-Guzmán, R. and Torres-Tovar, M. 2015, 'The right to health: What model for Latin America?' *The Lancet*, 385(9975), pp. e34–7.

Hobsbawm, E. 2000 [1975], *The Age of Capital*, Abacus, London.

Jameson, F. 2003, 'Future city', *New Left Review*, 21 (May-June), pp. 65–79.

Kauffman, L.A. 2017, *Direct Action and the Reinvention of American Radicalism*, Verso, New York.

Kropotkin, P. 1914, *Mutual Aid*, Extending Horizon Books, Boston.

Knapp, M., Flach, A. and Ayboga, E. 2016, *Revolution in Rojava: Democratic Autonomy and Women's Liberation in Syrian Kurdistan*, Pluto Press, London.

Laurell, A.C. 2015, 'Three decades of neoliberalism in Mexico', *International Journal of Health Services*, 45(2), pp. 246–64.

Lebowitz, M. 2015, *The Socialist Imperative,* Monthly Review Press, New York.

Lenin, V.I. 1935 [1918], *The State and Revolution,* International Publishers, New York.

Mamani, F.H. 2018, 'BOLIVIA-Buen Vivir/Vivir Bien: Los 13 principios', accessed 2 November 2022, <https://caminantedelsur.com/2018/02/05/bolivia-buen-vivir-vivir-bien-los-13-principios-por-fernando-huanacuni-mamani/>.

Marmor, T. 2000, *The Politics of Medicare*, Transaction Publishers, Piscataway.

Marx, K. and Engels, F. 2002 [1848], *Manifesto of the Communist Party*, Penguin, London.

Medvedyuk, S., Govender, P. and Raphael, D. 2021, 'The reemergence of Engels' concept of social murder in response to growing social and health inequalities', *Social Science and Medicine*, 289, p. 114377.

Maresso, A., Mladovsky, P., Thomson, S., Sagan, A., Karanikolos, M., Richardson, E., Cylus, J., Evetovits, J., Jowett, M., Figueras, J. and Kluge, H. (eds) 2015, *Economic Crisis, Health Systems and Health in Europe: Country Experience*, WHO Regional Office for Europe/European Observatory on Health Systems and Policies, Brussels.

Mészáros, I. 2010, *Beyond Capital,* Monthly Review Press, New York.

Mészáros, I. 2022, *Beyond Leviathan,* Monthly Review Press, New York.

Navarro, V. and Muntaner, C. (eds), 2014, *The Financial and Economic Crises and Their Impact on Health and Social Well-Being*, Baywood Publishing, Amityville.

Offe, C. 1996, *Modernity and the State: East, West*, MIT Press, Cambridge.

Oxfam. 2022, 'Inequality kills: The unparalleled action needed to combat unprecedented inequality in the wake of COVID-19', January 17, accessed 2 November 2022, <https://www.oxfam.org/en/research/inequality-kills>.

Paulson, S., D'Alisa, G., Demaria, F. and Kallis, G. 2020, The Case for Degrowth, Polity Press, Cambridge.

Piven, F.F. and Cloward, R.A. 1971, Regulating the Poor, Vintage, New York.

Reeves, A., McKee, M. and Stuckler, D. 2015, 'The attack on universal health coverage in Europe: Recession, austerity and unmet needs', European Journal of Public Health, 25(3), pp. 364–5.

Sengupta, A. 2013, 'Universal health coverage: Beyond rhetoric', Municipal Services Project Occasional Paper No. 20, November, accessed 2 November 2022, <www.municipalservicesproject.org/sites/municipalservicesproject.org/files/publications/OccasionalPaper20_Sengupta_Universal_Health_Coverage_Beyond_Rhetoric_Nov2013_0.pdf>.

Smithers, D. and Waitzkin, H. 2022, 'Universal health coverage as hegemonic health policy in low- and middle-income countries: A mixed-methods analysis', Social Science and Medicine, 2022(302), p. 114961.

Spiegel, J. B., Ortiz Choukroun, B., Campaña, A., Boydell, K. M., Breilh, J. and Yassi, A. 2019, 'Social transformation, collective health and community-based arts: "Buen Vivir" and Ecuador's social circus programme', Global Public Health, 14(6–7), pp. 899–922.

Stuckler, D., Feigl, A.B., Basu, S. and McKee, M. 2010, 'The political economy of universal health coverage', Background paper for the Global Symposium on Health Systems Research, WHO, Montreux, November 16–19, accessed 2 November 2022, <www.pacifichealthsummit.org/downloads/UHC/the%20political%20economy%20of%20uhc.PDF>.

Thever, M.D. 2005, Health Care for All: Is Canada's System A Model for America? Xlibris, Philadelphia.

Waitzkin, H. 2000, The Second Sickness: Contradictions of Capitalist Health Care, Rowman and Littlefield, New York.

Waitzkin, H. 2011, Medicine and Public Health at the End of Empire, Routledge, New York.

Waitzkin, H. 2015, 'Universal health coverage: The strange romance of the Lancet, MEDICC, and Cuba,' Social Medicine/Medicina Social, 9(2), pp. 93–7.

Waitzkin, H. 2020, Rinky-Dink Revolution: Moving Beyond Capitalism by Withholding Consent, Creative Constructions, and Creative Destructions, Daraja Press, Ottawa, and Monthly Review Essays, New York.

Waitzkin, H., Pérez, A. and Anderson, M. 2021, Social Medicine and the Coming Transformation, Routledge, New York.

Waitzkin, H. and Waterman, B. 1974, The Exploitation of Illness in Capitalist Society, Bobbs-Merrill, Indianapolis.

Waitzkin, H. and the Working Group on Health Beyond Capitalism. 2018, Health Care Under the Knife: Moving Beyond Capitalism for Our Health, Monthly Review Press, New York.

War Resisters League. 2018–21, 'Where your income tax money really goes', War Resisters League, accessed January 2022, <https://www.warresisters.org/store/where-your-income-tax-money-really-goes-fy2021>.

INDEX

Note: **Bold** page numbers refer to tables; *italic* page numbers refer to figures and page numbers followed by "n" denote endnotes.

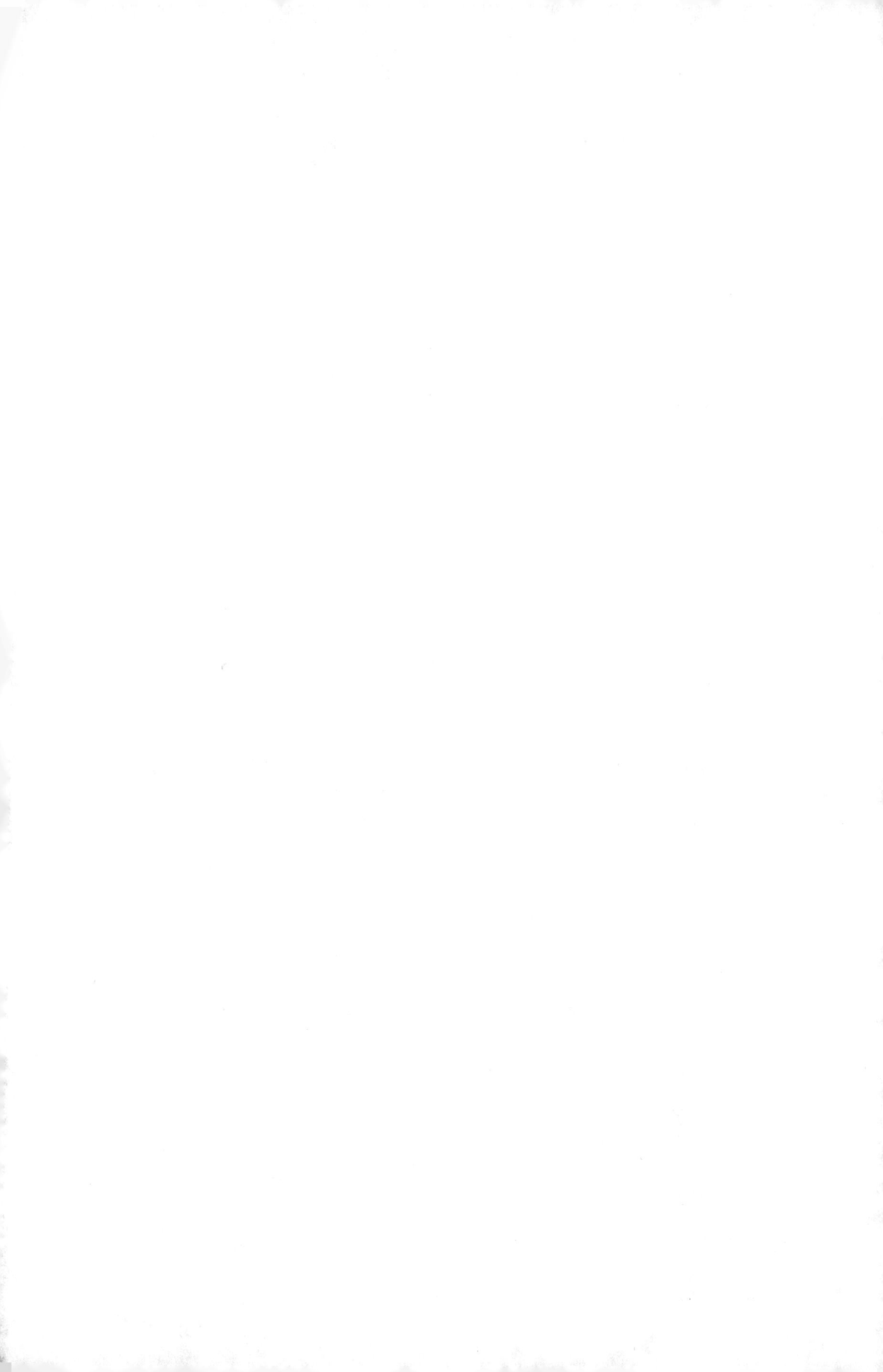

For Product Safety Concerns and Information please contact our EU representative GPSR@taylorandfrancis.com
Taylor & Francis Verlag GmbH, Kaufingerstraße 24, 80331 München, Germany

www.ingramcontent.com/pod-product-compliance
Lightning Source LLC
Chambersburg PA
CBHW072006230326
41598CB00082B/6809

* 9 7 8 1 0 3 2 6 5 0 6 7 8 *